Atlas of Pediatric Clinical Diagnosis

Binita R. Shah, M.D., F.A.A.P.

Professor of Clinical Pediatrics and Emergency Medicine
Departments of Emergency Medicine and Pediatrics
State University of New York
Health Science Center at Brooklyn
Brooklyn, New York

Director, Pediatric Emergency Medicine
Department of Emergency Medicine
Kings County Hospital Center
Brooklyn, New York

Teresita A. Laude, M.D., F.A.A.P., F.A.A.D.

Associate Professor of Pediatrics and Dermatology
Director, Division of Pediatric Dermatology
Departments of Dermatology and Pediatrics
State University of New York
Health Science Center at Brooklyn
Brooklyn, New York

W.B. SAUNDERS COMPANY

A Division of Harcourt Brace & Company

Philadelphia London Toronto Montreal Sydney Tokyo

W.B. SAUNDERS COMPANY
A Division of Harcourt Brace & Company

The Curtis Center
Independence Square West
Philadelphia, Pennsylvania 19106

Library of Congress Cataloging-in-Publication Data

Shah, Binita R.
Atlas of pediatric clinical diagnosis / Binita R. Shah, Teresita A. Laude.—1st ed.

p.   cm.

ISBN 0–7216–7639–1

1. Children—Medical Examination Atlases.   2. Children—Diseases—Diagnosis
   Atlases.   I. Laude, Teresita A.   II. Title. [DNLM: 1. Diagnosis—Infant
   Atlases.   2. Diagnosis—Child Atlases. WS 17 S525a 2000]

RJ50.S49 2000   618.92′0075—dc21

DNLM/DLC   99-19073

ATLAS OF PEDIATRIC CLINICAL DIAGNOSIS   ISBN 0–7216–7639–1

Printed in the United States of America.

Last digit is the print number: 9   8   7   6   5   4   3   2   1

To my father
Ratilal P. Patel, M.B., B.S.
From whom I inherited my love for medicine
and
To my premier teacher and mentor
Laurence Finberg, M.D.
Under whose influence I was "born" as a pediatrician
pursuing excellence for children

Binita R. Shah, M.D.

To my husband
Josef Q. Laude, M.D.
and
our granddaughter
Natalie

Teresita A. Laude, M.D.

Foreword

A budding clinician learns in a variety of ways: by memory of facts, by experiences with patients, and by accumulating visual images of conditions. This book by Drs. Binita Shah and Teresita Laude particularly assists with the last of these. From their own collection of photographs taken through many years of clinical experience in a very busy pediatric outpatient department they have provided the reader with a true visual journey through the observational side of pediatric practice. Even experienced pediatricians will find it useful to peruse this volume to refresh and to expand visual memory. Keeping the book at the workplace will facilitate both patient care and teaching.

The authors have particular qualifications for their work. Dr. Shah is one of the ablest clinicians I have known and she has been lauded for her teaching by generations of students and residents. Several years back she added certification in Pediatric Emergency Medicine to her credentials and has broadened her experience in that aspect of pediatric care.

Dr. Laude holds certification from the American Boards of Pediatrics and Dermatology. She too has diagnosed and treated patients while capably teaching students. Both authors are avid photographers who are now sharing with you, the reader, a facet of their clinical excellence through a teaching text and reference.

In addition, explanatory material accompanies each picture summarizing the entity with systematic discussion of etiology, epidemiology, pathophysiology (when appropriate), laboratory findings, differential diagnosis, and treatment. A good example of this feature may be seen in the chapter on bone disease where the various types of rickets and its mimickers are thoroughly characterized. The scope of the book is enormous, with hundreds of pictures, many in color. It belongs in the pediatric office, in urgent care clinics that have replaced the "walk in" sector of pediatric departments, and in emergency departments where children are seen. The 15 chapters separate the subject by anatomic site or by biologic system to help the reader find the place in the book of interest.

The authors have filled an important niche in the clinician's armamentarium for dealing with both common and rare entities that present with visual aspects.

Laurence Finberg, MD
Clinical Professor of Pediatrics, UCSF and Stanford
Professor and Chairman Emeritus
SUNY Health Science Center at Brooklyn

Preface

One wonders if, in this day and age of computed tomography and magnetic resonance imaging, anybody is interested in learning clinical diagnosis. Aside from being faster and more cost-effective than these technologies, a correct clinical diagnosis can be an extremely rewarding experience for those who make the diagnosis. A thorough history and physical examination still remain crucial in arriving at a correct diagnosis. Indeed, modern technology must be used when appropriate *only* to enhance the clinical assessment of the patient, not to replace it. In the new millennium, we believe there will be an increased demand for books in which important information is instantly accessible. One will have less time to read dense prose in traditional textbooks to learn about diseases. With these thoughts in mind, a clinical atlas in an outline format was conceived.

"Don't touch the patient . . . state first what you see; cultivate your powers of observation . . . " This quotation of Sir William Osler has always influenced our approach at the bedside while caring for patients. Among all the senses that help clinicians to arrive at a diagnosis, visual sense is by far the most helpful in detecting physical findings. *"A picture is worth a thousand words"* and *"I cannot define an elephant but I know one when I see one . . . "* These familiar old adages underscore the benefits of learning from photographs.

Over the years, we have acquired a huge collection of clinical photographs of pediatric patients that we have used for teaching purposes. We have attempted to link visual cues with the clinical diagnosis in this atlas. We believe that this is a great opportunity to share these materials with our colleagues caring for children.

This is a unique (and probably the first) pictorial clinical atlas in which diseases are presented in a consistent, easily retrievable format that includes (as appropriate): definition, etiology, epidemiology, pathogenesis, anatomy/pathology, inheritance, clinical features, laboratory, differential diagnosis, complications, treatment, prognosis, and prevention. Clinical material is also presented in tables and boxes for quick reference, and important facts are emphasized as key points.

This book emphasizes "must-know" clinical essentials that help one quickly diagnose and treat common diseases of children. The presentation of clinical photographs along with clinical facts will certainly help improve diagnostic skills of clinicians responsible for first-line diagnosis and management of pediatric diseases.

This atlas is primarily for educators and clinicians practicing pediatrics, family medicine, pediatric emergency medicine, or emergency medicine. Many residents are overworked, chronically sleep-deprived, and have "zero tolerance" for learning clinical facts from dense prose in a textbook. Residents in the training programs in any of the aforementioned fields and medical students during their pediatric clerkship will find this clinical atlas practical for quick and effective decision-making and immediate therapeutic intervention. "Physician extenders" such as nurse practitioners and physician assistants who care for children will also find this atlas valuable during their training and practice.

We hope that readers find this book as stimulating and enjoyable to study as we did in compiling it. There are a total of 638 illustrations (more than 300 in color) depicting 216 distinct entities. Nevertheless, we could not be as complete as we would have liked to be. There are deliberate omissions because it was impossible to include every pediatric condition. We think that Dr. Samuel Johnson put it best, upon completion of his *Dictionary* in 1755, when he wrote:

"In this work, when it shall be found that much is omitted, let it not be forgotten that much likewise is performed."

BINITA R. SHAH, M.D.
TERESITA A. LAUDE, M.D.

Acknowledgments

This book is a tribute to the children at Kings County Hospital Center and SUNY Health Science Center at Brooklyn. Each day we are reminded how precious children are and we acknowledge all those who devote time, energy, and love to the care of children.

We offer our deepest appreciation to our colleagues, residents, and medical students for referring patients to us; a pictorial book like this would not have been possible without their help.

We are indebted to Ms. Judith Fletcher at W.B. Saunders; her constant encouragement, sage advice, and enormous help in bringing this book to fruition will never be forgotten. We are also grateful to Saunders staff, including Donna Morrissey, Edna Dick, and Shelley Hampton, for their help in the final editing and printing of this book; their courteous service and patience are appreciated.

Finally, I wish to thank my husband Rajni P. Shah, M.D. and my children Ronak and Toral for their unconditional love, enthusiastic support, and long-suffering tolerance of my involvement in this challenging endeavor (BRS).

Binita R. Shah, M.D.
Teresita A. Laude, M.D.

Credits for Radiographs

Rona Orentlicher, M.D.
Assistant Professor of Clinical Radiology
Department of Radiology
State University of New York Health Science Center at Brooklyn, Brooklyn, New York

Director, Pediatric Radiology
Kings County Hospital Center, Brooklyn, New York

For writing legends for all the radiographs used in this book and contributing the following radiographs:

Figures 2–14 to 2–18, Child abuse

Figure 4–16, Bilateral retinoblastoma

Figure 5–11, Obstructive sleep apnea

Figures 7–11, 7–12, and 7–18, Sickle cell anemia

Figure 7–27, Metastatic neuroblastoma

Figures 7–28 and 7–29, Osteosarcoma

Figure 7–31, Bilateral ovarian teratoma

Figure 7–32, Hodgkin lymphoma

Figures 9–19 and 9–20, Intussusception

Figure 9–23, Hirschsprung disease

Figure 10–4, Chronic osteomyelitis

Figure 10–6, Septic arthritis

Figure 10–21, Blount disease

Figure 10–23, Osgood-Schlatter disease

Figure 10–26, Osteogenesis imperfecta

Figure 10–28, Slipped capital femoral epiphysis

Figure 11–6, Swallowed nails

Figure 12–26, Rheumatic carditis

Figure 13–8, Tuberous sclerosis

Figures 13–20 to 13–22, Craniosynostosis

Figure 13–23, Microcephaly

Figure 13–27, Hydrocephalus

Contents

1 Neonatology 1
Binita R. Shah, M.D. and Teresita A. Laude, M.D.

Transient Neonatal Pustular Melanosis
(TNPM) 1
Erythema Toxicum Neonatorum (ETN) 2
Subcutaneous Fat Necrosis 3
Neonatal Herpes Simplex Infection 4
Aplasia Cutis Congenita (ACC) 5
Mongolian Spot 7
Brachial Palsy 8
Cephalhematoma 9
Caput Succedaneum 11
Traumatic Facial Nerve Palsy 13
Asymmetric Crying Facies 15
Amniotic Constriction Bands 17
Neonatal Mastitis 19
Congenital Muscular Torticollis 20
Natal Teeth 22

2 Child Abuse and Sexual Abuse 24
Binita R. Shah, M.D.

Child Abuse 24
Shaken Impact Syndrome 30
Skeletal Injuries and Child Abuse 32
Sexual Abuse and Sexually Transmitted
Diseases (STDs) 36
Conditions Mistaken for Child Abuse and
Child Sexual Abuse 41

3 Infectious Diseases 50
Teresita A. Laude, M.D. and Binita R. Shah, M.D.

Varicella 50
Herpes Zoster 54
Herpes Simplex Infections 56
Measles 59
Rubella 62
Mumps 64
Infectious Mononucleosis (IM) 66
Gianotti-Crosti Syndrome 68
Roseola Infantum 69
Erythema Infectiosum 70

Hand-Foot-Mouth Disease 72
Herpangina 74
Molluscum Contagiosum 75
Warts 76
Human Immunodeficiency Virus (HIV)
Infection 78
Rocky Mountain Spotted Fever (RMSF) 81
Erysipelas 82
Scarlet Fever 84
Localized Streptococcal Skin Infections 86
Streptococcal Toxic Shock Syndrome 89
Necrotizing Fasciitis (NF) 91
Localized Staphylococcal Skin Infections 92
Staphylococcal Scalded Skin Syndrome
(SSSS) 94
Staphylococcal Toxic Shock Syndrome 96
Erythrasma 97
Ecthyma Gangrenosum 99
Pertussis 100
Buccal Cellulitis 101
Gonococcal Infections 102
Meningococcemia 104
Acquired Syphilis 106
Congenital Syphilis 107
Infant Botulism 109
Tinea Capitis 112
Tinea Corporis 115
Other Dermatophyte Infections 116
Tinea Versicolor 118
Candidiasis 120
Scabies 121
Pediculosis Capitis 124
Cutaneous Larva Migrans 125

4 Ophthalmology 127
Binita R. Shah, M.D.

Ophthalmia Neonatorum 127
Chlamydial Ophthalmia 129
Acute Conjunctivitis 131
Infantile Glaucoma 134
Hyphema 136
Hordeolum 139
Chalazion 140
Cataract 140
Retinoblastoma 143

Otolaryngology 147

Binita R. Shah, M.D.

Preseptal Cellulitis   147
Orbital Cellulitis   149
Acute Bacterial Sinusitis   153
Acute Mastoiditis   156
Facial Palsy with Acute Otitis Media   158
Obstructive Sleep Apnea   159

Dermatology 162

Teresita A. Laude, M.D.

Atopic Dermatitis (AD)   162
Postinflammatory Hyperpigmentation and
    Hypopigmentation   167
Allergic Contact Dermatitis   168
Diaper Dermatitis   170
Urticaria   171
Arthropod Bites   173
Popsicle Panniculitis   176
Exfoliative Dermatitis   176
Erythema Nodosum   177
Drug Eruptions   179
Stevens-Johnson Syndrome   181
Toxic Epidermal Necrolysis (TEN)   183
Pyogenic Granuloma   185
Henoch-Schönlein Purpura (HSP)   186
Seborrheic Dermatitis   189
Pityriasis Rosea   190
Lichen Striatus   191
Psoriasis   192
Acne   195
Infantile Acropustulosis   198
Granuloma Annulare   199
Perioral Granulomatous Dermatitis in
    Childhood   200
Granuloma Gluteale Infantum   201
Lichen Sclerosus et Atrophicus (LSA)   202
Linear IgA Disease of Childhood   203
Pemphigus   205
Dermatitis Herpetiformis   207
Bullous Pemphigoid   208
Vitiligo   209
Alopecia Areata   210
Hemangioma   212
Klippel-Trenaunay Syndrome   215
Congenital Pigmented Nevus (CPN)   216
Nevus of Ota, Nevus of Ito   217
Nevus Sebaceus of Jadassohn   219
Epidermal Nevus (EN)   221
Mastocytosis   222
Langerhans' Cell Histiocytosis   224
Ichthyosis   226
Netherton Syndrome   228
Epidermolysis Bullosa (EB)   230
Incontinentia Pigmenti   232
Hypomelanosis of Ito   233

Rothmund-Thomson Syndrome   235
Anhidrotic Ectodermal Dysplasia
    (AED)   236
Keloids   237
Acanthosis Nigricans   238
Phytophotodermatitis   239
Dermoid Cyst   240
Hidradenitis Suppurativa   241
Spider Bites   243

Hematology and Oncology 245

Binita R. Shah, M.D.

Iron Deficiency Anemia   245
Acute Hemolytic Anemia and Glucose-6-
    Phosphate Dehydrogenase (G6PD)
    Deficiency   248
Acute Immune Thrombocytopenic
    Purpura   250
Sickle Cell Anemia   253
Sickle Cell Anemia and Acute Sequestration
    Crisis   259
Sickle Cell Anemia and Transient Aplastic
    Crises (TAC)   260
Sickle Cell Anemia and Acute Chest
    Syndrome (ACS)   261
Sickle Cell Anemia and Stroke   263
Sickle Cell Anemia and Priapism   266
Hemophilia A   268
Acute Lymphoblastic Leukemia (ALL)   273
Neuroblastoma   276
Osteosarcoma   281
Mature Cystic Ovarian Teratoma   285
Hodgkin Lymphoma   288

Endocrinology 292

Binita R. Shah, M.D.

Adolescent Gynecomastia   292
Premature Thelarche   294
Juvenile Graves Disease   296
Autoimmune Thyroiditis   298
Addison Disease   301
Familial Glucocorticoid Deficiency
    (FGD)   304
Cushing Syndrome (CS)   307
Pheochromocytoma   311
McCune-Albright Syndrome   314
Ambiguous Genitalia   316

Urology and Surgery 320

Binita R. Shah, M.D.

Hydrometrocolpos with Imperforate
    Hymen   320
Labial Adhesions   321

Urethral Prolapse 323
Testicular Torsion 325
Torsion of the Appendix Testis 330
Epididymitis (Epididymo-orchitis) 332
Balanoposthitis 334
Paraphimosis 336
Intussusception 338
Hirschsprung Disease 342
Preauricular Sinus 345
Pilonidal Sinus and Abscess 346
Thyroglossal Duct Cyst 348

10 Bone Disorders and Orthopedics 350

Binita R. Shah, M.D.

Acute Hematogenous Osteomyelitis 350
Chronic Osteomyelitis 355
Septic Arthritis 357
Nutritional Vitamin D–Deficiency Rickets
    (NR) 360
Familial Hypophosphatemic Rickets
    (FHR) 366
Vitamin D–Dependent Rickets Type 1
    (VDDR, type 1) 369
Metaphyseal Dysplasia, Schmid Type 372
Blount Disease 374
Legg-Calvé-Perthes Disease (LCPD) 376
Osgood-Schlatter Disease 378
Osteogenesis Imperfecta Syndrome
    (OI) 381
Slipped Capital Femoral Epiphysis
    (SCFE) 384

11 Emergency Pediatrics 387

Binita R. Shah, M.D.

Anaphylaxis 387
Esophageal Foreign Body 389
Foreign Bodies in Stomach and Lower
    Gastrointestinal Tract 392
Ingestion of Cylindrical and Button (Disc)
    Batteries 395
Nursemaid's Elbow 399

12 Rheumatology 401

Teresita A. Laude, M.D. and Binita R. Shah, M.D.

Systemic Lupus Erythematosus (SLE) 401
Neonatal Lupus Erythematosus (NLE) 403
Juvenile Rheumatoid Arthritis (JRA) 405
Juvenile Dermatomyositis (JDM) 407
Lyme Disease 408

Kawasaki Disease 410
Serum Sickness 413
Sarcoidosis 415
Acute Rheumatic Fever (ARF) 416

13 Neurology 420

Binita R. Shah, M.D. and Teresita A. Laude, M.D.

Neurofibromatosis (NF) 420
Tuberous Sclerosis 423
Sturge-Weber Syndrome 425
Spinal Dysraphism 426
Bell's Palsy 428
Craniosynostosis 430
Neural Tube Defects 434
Anencephaly 437
Meningomyelocele 438
Meningocele 440
Encephalocele 441

14 Genetics 444

Binita R. Shah, M.D. and Teresita A. Laude, M.D.

Trisomy 21 Syndrome 444
Trisomy 21 and Atlantoaxial Instability 446
Turner Syndrome 448
Sotos Syndrome 451
TAR Syndrome 453
Albinism 456
Piebaldism 458
Waardenburg Syndrome 459

15 Miscellaneous 461

Binita R. Shah, M.D.

Oral Electrical Burns 461
Nursing-Bottle Caries 463
Ranula 464
Minimal Change Nephrotic Syndrome
    (MCNS) 465
Acute Poststreptococcal Glomerulonephritis
    (APSGN) 468
Lymphedema 471

Suggested Readings 475

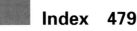

Index 479

1

Neonatology

Binita R. Shah, M.D. and Teresita A. Laude, M.D.

Transient Neonatal Pustular Melanosis (TNPM)

DEFINITION
TNPM is a benign eruption that is present at birth.

ETIOLOGY
Unknown

EPIDEMIOLOGY
1. Incidence
   a. Seen in 5% of African-American newborns
   b. Seen in 0.5% of white newborns
2. More commonly seen in full-term, otherwise healthy African-American newborns

LABORATORY
1. In rare cases, TNPM may have to be differentiated from other pustular conditions in the newborn. The following tests are helpful:
   a. KOH preparation (to rule out candidiasis)
   b. Gram stain (to rule out staphylococcal pustulosis)
   c. Tzanck smear and culture (to rule out HSV infection)
2. Skin biopsy, if done, shows a collection of neutrophils in the epidermis.

DIFFERENTIAL DIAGNOSIS (see Table 1-2)
Two conditions that are similarly benign, of unknown etiology, self-limiting, and that may be pustular should be considered:

1. Erythema toxicum neonatorum (ETN)
2. Infantile acropustulosis (IA)

TREATMENT
None

KEY POINTS

Transient Neonatal Pustular Melanosis

- Lesions are always present at birth.
- TNPM is seen in 5% of African-American newborns and 0.5% of white newborns.

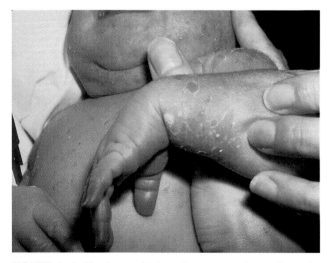

FIGURE 1-1. Newborn with transient neonatal pustular melanosis showing an intact pustule and a ruptured pustule with a collarette of scale.

TABLE 1-1

Clinical Features of Transient Neonatal Pustular Melanosis

Skin Lesions

Present at birth
Any of following three types of lesions may be present alone or in combination:
    Vesicopustules
    Ruptured vesicopustules with collarette of scales
    Pigmented macules
Most common distribution
    Trunk
    Extremities
Duration
    Vesicopustules last 48–72 hours
    Pigmented macules last 3 weeks to 3 months

TABLE 1–2
Differential Diagnosis

	TNPM	ETN	IA
Racial incidence	>African-Americans	= African-Americans and whites	>African-Americans
Onset of lesions	At birth	After 48 hours	Between 2 and 10 months
Maximum duration of lesions	3 months	3–4 weeks	3 years
Involvement of palms and soles	Variable	Spared	Involved

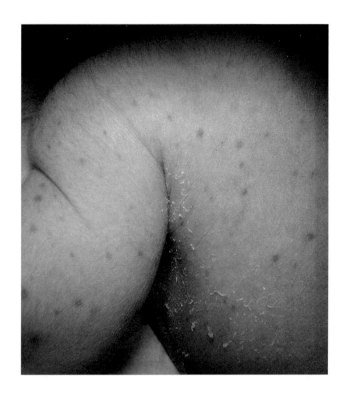

FIGURE 1–2. Pigmented macules of transient neonatal pustular melanosis.

Erythema Toxicum Neonatorum (ETN)

DEFINITION
ETN is a benign, transient, self-limiting eruption in the newborn.

ETIOLOGY
Some investigators think that ETN may be an allergic response to some unknown insult.

EPIDEMIOLOGY
1. The condition is seen in 40% of otherwise healthy full-term newborns.
2. It is not seen in premature newborns.

LABORATORY
1. Peripheral eosinophilia may be demonstrated.
2. A Tzanck smear shows eosinophils and neutrophils.
3. Skin biopsy, if done, shows follicular aggregates of neutrophils and eosinophils.

TREATMENT
None

KEY POINTS

Erythema Toxicum Neonatorum

- Lesions have the appearance of flea bites.
- They represent follicular aggregates of eosinophils and neutrophils.

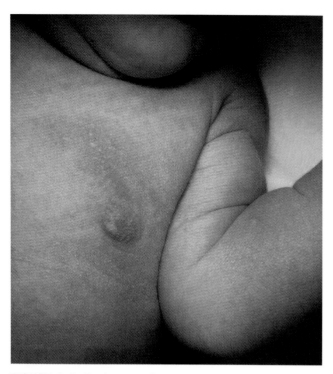

FIGURE 1–3. Erythema toxicum neonatorum lesions with appearance of flea bites.

TABLE 1–3
Clinical Features of Erythema Toxicum Neonatorum

Skin Lesions

Appear commonly as pale or ivory-colored papules surrounded by splotchy erythema
Flea bite appearance
Lesions may become confluent
Pustules may be seen (in 10% of cases)
Onset of eruption
   Between 2nd and 4th day of life
Distribution
   Chest
   Back
   Proximal extremities
   Head and neck
   Palms and soles *spared*
Duration
   Lesions may last 2 to 3 weeks

Subcutaneous Fat Necrosis

DEFINITION

A benign, self-limiting disorder of healthy newborns

ETIOLOGY/EPIDEMIOLOGY

1. The exact cause is unknown.
2. Theories about it include post-traumatic aftereffects of delivery, asphyxia, hypothermia, and calcium metabolic derangement.
3. The newborn is otherwise healthy.

LABORATORY

1. Serum calcium levels are high in a few infants with subcutaneous fat necrosis.
2. Skin biopsy, if done, demonstrates fat crystals in a sunburst arrangement in the subcutaneous tissue. Inflammatory cell infiltrates and Langhans giant cells are also present.

> **BOX 1–1**   *Differential Diagnosis of Subcutaneous Fat Necrosis*
>
> **SCLEREMA NEONATORUM**
> Seen in premature infants
> Seen in debilitated newborns with severe underlying diseases (e.g., sepsis, congestive heart failure, respiratory distress syndrome)
> Skin: diffusely hard, tight, and waxy
> Fatality rate: 50% to 75% of cases

COMPLICATIONS

There may be significant calcification of the lesion, which may later liquefy and drain onto the skin surface.

TREATMENT

1. No treatment is indicated in most instances.
2. Spontaneous resolution is the rule.

KEY POINTS

Subcutaneous Fat Necrosis

- Lesions are indurated subcutaneous plaques on the back, buttocks, and cheeks of otherwise healthy newborns.
- Hypercalcemia may be seen in 10% of infants with subcutaneous fat necrosis.

TABLE 1–4
Clinical Features of Subcutaneous Fat Necrosis

Skin Lesions

Well circumscribed
Indurated
Subcutaneous plaques
Surface may look uneven and lobulated
Overlying skin may be normal, erythematous, or dusky
Lesions are usually asymptomatic or mildly painful
Commonly seen in first few days of life
Most common location
  Back
  Buttocks
  Cheeks
  Occasionally extremities
Duration
  Lesions may last a few weeks to several months

Other Features

Hypercalcemia (about 10% of cases)

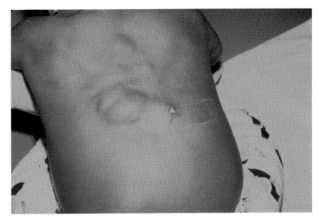

FIGURE 1–4. Subcutaneous fat necrosis in an 11-month-old infant that had been present from birth. The lesion had calcified.

Neonatal Herpes Simplex Infection

SYNONYM   Herpes Simplex Neonatorum

DEFINITION

A potentially serious infection with Herpes simplex virus (HSV) acquired by the newborn from the maternal birth canal

EPIDEMIOLOGY/PATHOGENESIS

1. Infection is usually acquired from maternal labial lesions.
2. Fifty percent of infants born to mothers with primary HSV-2 of the genitalia (herpes progenitalis) develop neonatal HSV infection.
3. Only 2% of infants born to mothers with recurrent HSV-2 infection develop the disease.
4. It can be transmitted to the neonate after delivery by cesarean section or when no rupture of the amniotic membranes has occurred.
5. A history of prior or current genital HSV infection is present in only 20% to 30% of mothers who give birth to an infected neonate.

BOX 1–2 *Etiology of Herpes Simplex Neonatorum*

Herpes simplex virus type 2: 80% to 90% of cases
Herpes simplex virus type 1: 10% to 20% of cases

LABORATORY

1. Tzanck smear for rapid diagnosis (see p. 56)
2. Viral culture
3. Lumbar puncture and examination of the cerebro-spinal fluid (CSF), liver enzymes, chest radiograph, complete blood count (CBC), and blood culture

TREATMENT

1. Hospitalization
2. Acyclovir 30 mg/kg/24 hours in three divided doses intravenously for minimum of 14 days
3. Ophthalmologic consultation

PROGNOSIS

1. Mortality from untreated neonatal infection: about 50%
2. Major sequelae in survivors
   a. Half of the survivors of those with central nervous system (CNS) involvement have neurologic sequelae
      (1) Microcephaly
      (2) Hydranencephaly
      (3) Seizure disorder
   b. Blindness

KEY POINTS

Neonatal Herpes Simplex Infection

- The infection is acquired at birth from a mother who usually has a primary HSV-2 infection of the genitalia.
- The central nervous system and the eyes may be involved. CSF examination and ophthalmologic consultation are indicated.

TABLE 1–5
Clinical Features of Herpes Simplex Neonatorum

Localized Skin, Mouth, or Eye Infection
Seen in one third of cases

Skin Infection
Grouped vesicles or pustules
Varying number
Sites: scalp, torso, extremities
Usually appear between the 3rd and 6th day of life
May be present at birth (ascending infection)
   With premature rupture of membranes
   With prolonged labor

Eye Infection
Keratitis
Chorioretinitis

TABLE 1–6
Clinical Features of Herpes Simplex Neonatorum

Disseminated Infection
Seen in one third of cases
Involves liver, lungs, adrenals, and brain
Presents as bacterial sepsis

Localized CNS Infection
Seen in one third of cases
Seen in 2nd or 3rd week of life
Often skin lesions are absent
Presents as encephalitis
   Seizures
   Irritability, lethargy
   Bulging fontanel

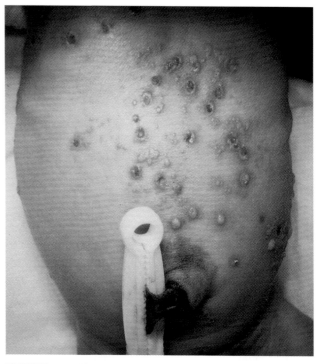

FIGURE 1–5. Herpes simplex neonatorum in a 3-day-old preterm infant; grouped vesicopustules are seen on the torso. She also had herpetic keratitis.

Aplasia Cutis Congenita (ACC)

DEFINITION
A congenital localized absence of skin

ETIOLOGY/EPIDEMIOLOGY (see Table 1–7)
Type 1 is the most common type; the child who has it is otherwise normal.

INHERITANCE
ACC may be inherited as an autosomal dominant trait.

LABORATORY
1. A complete history and physical examination must be done to determine the type of ACC.
2. An underlying skull defect and possible intracranial communication must be ruled out by proper studies.
   a. A plain film of the skull may be all that is necessary to diagnose type 1 ACC.
   b. MRI may be done depending on other findings.

> **BOX 1–3** *Differential Diagnosis of Aplasia Cutis Congenita*
>
> **SCALP LESION RESULTING FROM FETAL MONITORING**
> May be located on any part of the scalp
> Commonly appears as an eroded, crusted area
> May become infected occasionally
> Unlike ACC, lesion heals, and hair grows back

TREATMENT
Excision and simple repair or use of a tissue expander to correct the defect.

KEY POINTS

Aplasia Cutis Congenita

- Aplasia cutis congenita localized to the scalp is the most common clinical type.
- This must be differentiated from the lesion resulting from fetal scalp monitoring.

TABLE 1–7
Etiology/Epidemiology: Frieden's Classification of Aplasia Cutis Congenita

Type 1. Scalp ACC without multiple anomalies
Type 2. Scalp ACC with associated limb abnormalities
Type 3. Scalp ACC with associated epidermal and organoid nevi
Type 4. ACC overlying embryologic malformations
Type 5. ACC with associated fetus papyraceus or placental infarcts
Type 6. ACC associated with epidermolysis bullosa
Type 7. ACC localized to extremities
Type 8. ACC caused by specific teratogens
Type 9. ACC associated with malformation syndromes

TABLE 1–8
Clinical Features of Aplasia Cutis Congenita

Skin Lesion

Most commonly solitary
Well circumscribed
Varying size
May present as a healing ulcer, a scar, or a membrane
Lesion on scalp may be surrounded by a collarette of hair
Most common location: scalp near vertex
May be seen on any skin surface

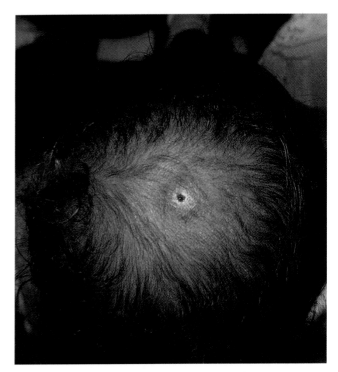

FIGURE 1–7. Crusted lesion resulting from fetal scalp monitoring.

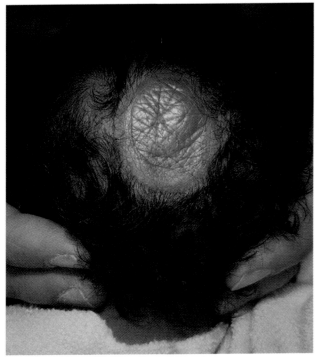

FIGURE 1–6. Cutis aplasia congenita presenting as a membrane in the vertex of the scalp.

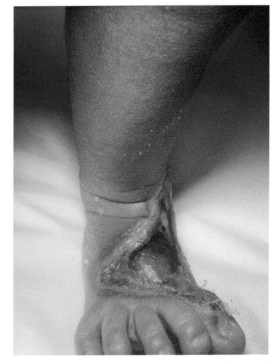

FIGURE 1–8. Cutis aplasia congenita presenting as absent skin on the dorsum of the right foot.

Mongolian Spot

DEFINITION

Mongolian spot is a benign transient birthmark.

ETIOLOGY/PATHOGENESIS

1. Mongolian spot is a form of dermal melanocytosis. During the embryonic period melanocytes move from the neural crest to the epidermis and may become arrested in the dermis, where they do not normally belong.
2. As a result, when light strikes the surface of the lesion, all colors of the spectrum are absorbed by the melanin in the dermis except blue, which is reflected back (Tyndall phenomenon).
3. As time goes on, these melanocytes lose their cell membranes and are processed by macrophages. Clinically this means that the lesion fades.

EPIDEMIOLOGY

It is seen in

1. 95% of African-American newborns
2. 70% of Asian and Hispanic newborns
3. 10% of white newborns

TABLE 1–9
Clinical Features of Mongolian Spot

Skin Lesion
A flat bluish-gray discoloration
Location
    Most common: sacrogluteal area (90% of cases)
    Outside sacrogluteal area (10% of cases)
Natural history
    Lesion generally fades gradually
    Disappears by 5–6 years of age

DIFFERENTIAL DIAGNOSIS

1. Accidental or inflicted injury
   a. In a white infant, Mongolian spot may be mistaken for ecchymosis resulting from accidental or inflicted injury.
   b. An ecchymosis, however, undergoes a color change and resolves within a few days, unlike Mongolian spot.
2. Other forms of dermal melanocytosis
   a. These are permanent lesions.
   b. Examples include blue nevus, nevus of Ota, nevus of Ito (see p. 217).

TREATMENT

None

PROGNOSIS

Resolves spontaneously and completely within 5 to 6 years in 98% of cases

KEY POINTS

Mongolian Spot

- Mongolian spots are benign lesions that eventually fade spontaneously.
- They are more common in African-American, Asian, and Hispanic infants.

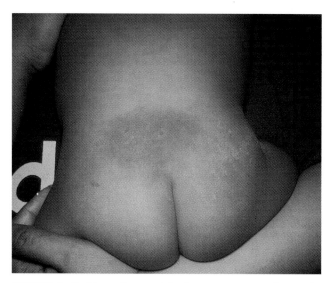

FIGURE 1–9. Mongolian spot in the sacrococcygeal area, its most common location.

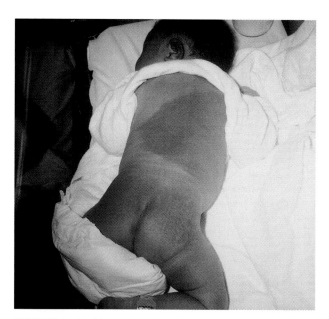

FIGURE 1–10. Mongolian spot on the posterior torso.

Brachial Palsy

DEFINITION

Traction, stretch, or avulsion injury to the brachial plexus (5th cervical through 1st thoracic spinal roots) during birth results in brachial palsy.

EPIDEMIOLOGY

1. Incidence: approximately 0.7 to 1 in 1000 live births.
2. The following three types are seen depending on the site of the injury:
   a. Erb-Duchenne palsy
      (1) Most common (70% to 80% of cases)
      (2) Upper arm paralysis results from injury to C5 and C6 roots.
   b. Paralysis of entire arm
      (1) Second most common (22% of cases)
      (2) Complete plexus is injured.
   c. Klumpke palsy
      (1) Extremely rare (8% of cases)
      (2) Lower arm paralysis results from injury to C8 to T1 roots.

BOX 1-4   *Clinical Features of Klumpke Palsy*

Injury to C8 to T1 roots
Paralysis of flexors and extensors of the forearm
Paralysis and wasting of intrinsic muscles of the hand resulting in a claw-like posture
Tendon reflexes usually intact with a poor or absent grasp response
Involvement of T1 root with sympathetic fibers results in Horner syndrome:
   Ipsilateral ptosis
   Miosis present at birth
   Heterochromia irides (later in life)

PREDISPOSING FACTORS

Most cases of brachial palsy are seen in large full-term newborns of primiparous mothers following a prolonged and difficult labor involving:

1. Lateral traction on the head and neck during delivery of the shoulder in the vertex presentation
2. Extension of arms over the head in the breech presentation
3. Excessive traction on the shoulder
4. Shoulder dystocia

ERB-DUCHENNE PALSY (ERB PALSY)

A. Clinical Features

1. For typical findings see Table 1–10.
2. Uncommon findings
   a. Ipsilateral phrenic nerve injury may be present (clinical signs include respiratory distress due to diaphragmatic paralysis).
   b. About 10% of newborns with brachial plexus injuries have fractures of the clavicle or humerus and facial nerve palsy.

B. Laboratory

1. Diagnosis is clinically apparent from the posture of the affected arm.
2. Radiographs of the clavicle, humerus, and shoulder (as indicated) to exclude fracture or dislocation or other injuries (pseudo Erb palsy)
3. Electromyography assesses severity of the injury and determines the prognosis in patients who show no improvement in 6 to 8 weeks.
4. Nerve root avulsion or rupture can be demonstrated by MRI.

C. Differential Diagnosis

1. Fracture of clavicle
2. Fracture, dislocation, or epiphyseal separation of humerus (pseudo Erb palsy)
3. Cerebral injury

D. Treatment/Prognosis

1. Pediatric neurology and rehabilitation consultations
2. Spontaneous recovery rates of 70% to 90% are reported, especially when paralysis is secondary to edema or hemorrhage surrounding the nerve fibers.
3. First signs of recovery appear within a couple of weeks in most patients, and full function usually returns within 3 months.
4. The earlier the beginning of recovery, the better the long-term prognosis.
5. Main goal of therapy is prevention of contractures by intermittent partial immobilization and appropriate positioning.
   a. Arm should be abducted 90 degrees with external rotation at the shoulder, full supination of the forearm, and slight extension at the wrist with the palm turned toward the face.
   b. This position can be maintained either by pinning a towel over the wrist and fixing it to the mattress or by using a brace or splint during the first 1 to 2 weeks.
6. Active physical therapy should be avoided in the immediate post-delivery period because of a painful traumatic neuritis. Gentle passive exercises should be started by 7 to 10 days of life.
7. With laceration of the nerve, damage is usually permanent, and surgical reconstruction of the plexus (e.g., nerve grafting, neuroplasty, and neurolysis) should be considered in infants who show no evidence of spontaneous recovery after 3 to 6 months.

KEY POINTS

Erb Palsy

- The brachial plexus is the most common site of injury to the peripheral nervous system during traumatic delivery.

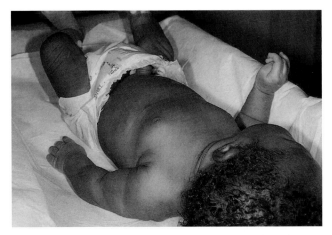

FIGURE 1–11. Asymmetric Moro reflex in a neonate with the typical posture of Erb palsy (left arm) noticed shortly after birth. This neonate had a birth weight of 4.5 kg and had breech presentation. Neonates with Erb palsy cannot abduct and rotate their arms externally from the shoulder, cannot supinate the forearm, and cannot extend the wrist because the shoulder abductors and external rotators, forearm flexors and supinators, and wrist extensors are paralyzed.

- The arm is limply adducted and internally rotated at the shoulder with extension and pronation at the elbow, so that partially flexed fingers face backward ("waiter's tip" posture).
- Presence of hand grasp is a favorable prognostic sign.

TABLE 1–10
Clinical Features of Erb Palsy

Unilateral involvement (90% of cases)
Right arm affected about twice as often as left
Bilateral (but not necessarily symmetric) involvement (10% of cases)
Characteristic posture of upper arm:
    Limply adducted and internally rotated at shoulder
    Elbow extended
    Forearm pronated
    Wrist flexed
Absent biceps and brachioradialis reflexes of affected arm
Absent triceps reflex (with C7 involvement) of affected arm
Absent Moro reflex and voluntary movements of affected arm
Intact grasp reflex
Sensory deficit on radial aspect of arm may be present

Cephalhematoma

DEFINITION

A traumatic subperiosteal hemorrhage overlying a cranial bone

ETIOLOGY

A cephalhematoma is caused by a rupture of the blood vessels that course from the skull to the periosteum, and is especially likely to occur during prolonged or difficult labor (see Figure 1–16).

BOX 1–5   *Sites of Cephalhematoma*

Most common: Parietal region
Rarely: Occipital region
Very rarely: Frontal bones

EPIDEMIOLOGY

1. Incidence ranges from 0.4% to 2.5% of live births.
2. Male-female ratio is 2:1.
3. Vaginal delivery is not necessarily a prerequisite for occurrence of this lesion, since it has been seen in infants born by cesarean section.
4. It occurs more commonly in infants born to primiparous mothers.

LABORATORY

1. A linear skull fracture is present in about 5% of newborns with unilateral cephalhematoma and in about 18% of newborns with bilateral cephalhematomas.
2. Radiographic findings vary with the age of the cephalhematoma.
   a. By end of the 2nd week, it may begin to calcify under the elevated pericranium at the margins of the hematoma, eventually forming a complete shell of bone overlaid on the entire lesion.
   b. Widening of the space between the new shell of the bone and the inner table may persist for years; the space originally occupied by the hematoma usually develops into normal diploic bone. However, cyst-like defects at that site may persist for months or years.

COMPLICATIONS

1. Presence of a skull fracture and associated intracranial hemorrhage (rare)

2. Cephalhematoma of a significant size may be associated with
   a. Anemia
   b. Hyperbilirubinemia (as a consequence of absorption of blood products)
3. Abscess formation within a cephalhematoma
   a. Metastatic seeding may occur in a septic newborn (e.g., associated with meningitis and septicemia).
   b. Secondary to contamination during an attempted needle aspiration
4. Focal infection within the cephalhematoma (during the course of a systemic infection) should be suspected from the following signs:
   a. Rapid enlargement of the mass
   b. Erythema of the overlying skin

DIFFERENTIAL DIAGNOSIS

1. Caput succedaneum (see Table 1–12)
2. Encephalocele (especially with midline occipital cephalhematoma)
3. Cranial meningocele characterized by
   a. Pulsations
   b. Increase in pressure during crying
   c. Radiographic evidence of a bony defect

TREATMENT

1. No treatment is required for cephalhematoma.
2. Rarely, blood transfusion may be required for massive blood loss.

3. No specific therapy is required for the underlying linear skull fracture. A radiograph may be taken at 4 to 6 weeks to ensure closure and to exclude formation of a leptomeningeal cyst.

PROGNOSIS

1. Most cephalhematomas are absorbed gradually by 2 to 12 weeks, depending on their size.
2. A pressure dressing *does not* hasten absorption of hematoma, and may contribute to skin breakdown and infection.
3. Rarely, a neonatal cephalhematoma may persist into adult life as a bony protuberance with no symptoms (cephalhematoma deformans of Schuller).

KEY POINTS

Cephalhematoma

- Cephalhematoma, unlike caput succedaneum, does not extend across the midline or across the suture lines of the affected bone.
- Needle aspiration or incision and drainage of cephalhematoma is contraindicated because of the risk of introducing infection.

TABLE 1–11
Clinical Features of Cephalhematoma

Swelling usually appears several hours or days after birth (subperiosteal bleeding being a slow process)
Usually unilateral
Swelling often larger on 2nd or 3rd day
Swelling limited to surface of one cranial bone
Swelling does not extend beyond suture lines of affected bone
Sharply demarcated boundaries are palpable
About 15% are bilateral; even if parietal, they are still palpably distinct from one another
Swelling does not transilluminate
Firm, fluctuant, and localized mass with a palpable rim that gives the impression of a shallow crater in the bone under the mass
No discoloration of overlying scalp

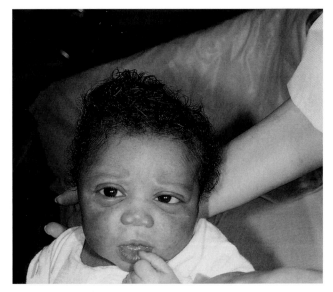

FIGURE 1–12. Newborn with a unilateral cephalhematoma over the parietal region.

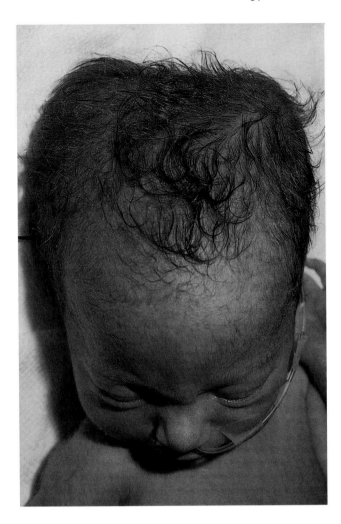

FIGURE 1-13. Newborn with bilateral cephalhematomas over the parietal region. Even bilateral cephalhematomas are still palpably distinct from one another. (Courtesy of Nathan Rudolph, M.D., State University of New York, Brooklyn, NY.)

Caput Succedaneum

DEFINITION

Edema or swelling of the soft tissues over the part of the body that was the presenting part during delivery (e.g., edema of the scalp during a vertex delivery)

ETIOLOGY/PATHOGENESIS

1. Normal transit of the fetal head through the birth canal induces marked molding of a very pliable fetal skull and scalp edema, especially with difficult labor.
2. Edema results from accumulation of serum or blood (or both) above the periosteum.
3. Soft tissue edema or injuries involving the external genitalia (scrotum or vulva) or buttocks may appear after a breech delivery.

CLINICAL FEATURES (see Table 1–12)

1. Head molding and overriding of the parietal bones occur commonly with caput and become more evident after the caput has resolved. These findings are transient.
2. An extensive caput may obscure various sutures and fontanels.
3. Diffuse swelling, discoloration, and distortion of the face are seen in infants born in a face presentation.

DIFFERENTIAL DIAGNOSIS (see Table 1–12)

1. Cephalhematoma (particularly with bilateral cephalhematomas)
2. Subgaleal hemorrhage (see Figure 1–16)
   a. A caput may be difficult to distinguish from the rare but serious subgaleal hemorrhage.
   b. Subgaleal hemorrhage is a collection of blood in the soft tissue space between the galea aponeurotica and the periosteum of the skull.
   c. Newborns with subgaleal hemorrhage show signs of central nervous system trauma (hypo-

tonia, seizures) and significant anemia (pallor, lethargy), and they deteriorate rapidly.

TREATMENT

1. No specific treatment is indicated, and it usually resolves within a few days.
2. Phototherapy may be indicated for hyperbilirubinemia as a result of extensive ecchymosis.
3. Rarely, a hemorrhagic caput may result in hypovolemic shock which requires blood transfusion or produces significant anemia.

PROGNOSIS

Caput succedaneum usually resolves within several days.

KEY POINTS

Caput Succedaneum

- A caput is present at birth.
- A caput, when present on the scalp, is external to the periosteum and unlike cephalhematoma, may extend across the sutures or midline of the skull.
- Spontaneous resolution within a few days is the rule.

TABLE 1–12
Differential Diagnosis: Caput Succedaneum versus Cephalhematoma

Caput Succedaneum	Cephalhematoma
Collection of serum/blood above the periosteum	Subperiosteal bleeding
Diffuse soft tissue swelling	Firm, localized, fluctuant mass
Vaguely demarcated	Sharply demarcated
Overlying skin: petechiae, purpura, ecchymosis	No discoloration of overlying scalp
Usually crosses suture lines	Does not cross suture lines
May extend across midline	Does not extend across midline
Present at delivery	Appears several hours after birth
Resolves in first few days	Gradually resolves in 2 to 12 weeks

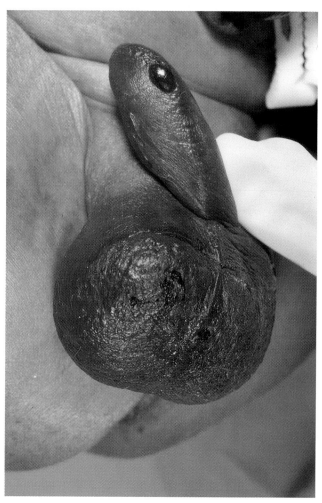

FIGURE 1–15. Scrotal edema/hematoma with ecchymosis and hemorrhagic blister on the penis in a neonate after breech presentation in a difficult delivery. Spontaneous resolution of such edema usually occurs in about 48 hours, and discoloration resolves within 4 to 5 days.

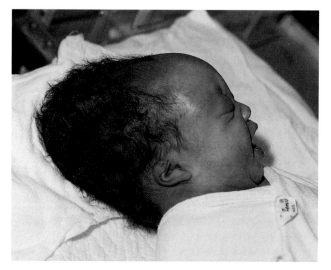

FIGURE 1–14. Newborn with a caput and associated normal head molding. (Courtesy of Nathan Rudolph, M.D., State University of New York, Brooklyn, NY.)

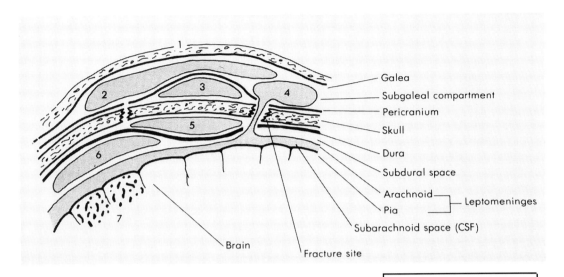

Galea
Subgaleal compartment
Pericranium
Skull
Dura
Subdural space
Arachnold ⎱
Pia ⎰ Leptomeninges
Subarachnoid space (CSF)

Brain
Fracture site

FIGURE 1–16. Traumatic head injuries. (From Barkin RM, Rosen P: Emergency Pediatrics, 3rd ed, St. Louis, Mosby-Year Book, 1990.)

1. Caput succedaneum
2. Subgaleal hematoma
3. Cephalhematoma
4. Porencephalic cyst or leptomeningeal cyst
5. Epidural hematoma
6. Subdural hematoma
7. Cerebral contusion

Traumatic Facial Nerve Palsy

DEFINITION

Facial nerve palsy following trauma (at birth or in utero)

ETIOLOGY/PATHOGENESIS

1. Facial palsy may be central or peripheral.
2. Peripheral facial palsy
   a. More common
   b. May be complete (involving the entire side of the face) *or*
   c. Partial (a small branch of the nerve is injured, and weakness is limited to the forehead, eyelid, or mouth)
   d. Usually due to hemorrhage and edema rather than avulsion
   e. During labor and delivery: The peripheral portion of the facial nerve may be compressed over the stylomastoid foramen (through which it emerges) or where the nerve traverses the ramus of the mandible.

(1) After forceps delivery—with prolonged application of forceps blade, especially when fetal head has been grasped obliquely
(2) After spontaneous delivery—with prolonged pressure exerted by maternal sacral promontory
   f. Injury sustained in utero (e.g., persistent position of fetal foot against the superior ramus of the mandible)
3. Central facial palsy
   a. Rare
   b. Intracranial injury (e.g., temporal bone fracture or intracranial hemorrhage or infarct) leading to facial palsy on the contralateral side

EPIDEMIOLOGY

Incidence varies from 0.05% to 1.8%.

CLINICAL FEATURES (see Boxes 1–6 and 1–7)

1. The clinical expression of palsy may be subtle and may not be apparent at birth.

2. Paralysis is usually apparent on the first or second day of life.

BOX 1-6 | *Clinical Features of Central Facial Palsy*

Involves only lower half or two thirds of the face
In a crying infant, the following signs are apparent:

    Flattening of nasolabial fold on contralateral side (of the lesion)

    Dropping of corner of the mouth on contralateral side (of the lesion)

    Unable to suck a nipple without dribbling milk on contralateral side (of the lesion)

    Sparing of muscles of forehead on both sides

    Sparing of muscles of eye on both sides

May be associated with other signs of intracranial injury (e.g., 6th cranial nerve palsy)

BOX 1-7 | *Clinical Features of Peripheral Facial Palsy*

Involves upper and lower face on the affected side
In a crying infant, the following signs are apparent:

    Flaccid paralysis of *all* facial muscles on the affected side

    Nasolabial fold remains flat on the affected side

    Unable to wrinkle forehead on the affected side

    Unable to close the eye on the affected side

    Drooping of corner of the mouth on the affected side

    Unable to suck a nipple without dribbling milk on the affected side

---

LABORATORY

1. Diagnosis is made clinically.
2. Electrodiagnostic testing
   a. Helps in predicting recovery
   b. Repeatedly normal nerve excitability indicates good prognosis.
   c. Decreased or absent excitability early in the course suggests a poor prognosis.

DIFFERENTIAL DIAGNOSIS

1. Mobius syndrome
   a. Bilateral facial palsies (secondary to agenesis of the facial nerve nucleus)
   b. Usually bilateral abducens palsy
   c. Involvement of several cranial nerves
   d. Other developmental defects
2. Asymmetric crying facies or congenital hypoplasia or aplasia of the depressor anguli oris muscle (see p. 15)

TREATMENT

1. No specific therapy is indicated for most facial palsies.
2. Protection of the cornea
   a. Methylcellulose drops (1%) to the affected eye several times a day
   b. Eye pad
3. Need for surgical intervention is rare unless the nerve has been lacerated at delivery.

PROGNOSIS

1. Excellent; high rate of spontaneous recovery
2. Resolution usually occurs within several days; total recovery may require several weeks or months.

KEY POINTS

Traumatic Facial Nerve Palsy

- Failure of eye closure on the affected side is usually the first noticeable sign of peripheral facial palsy.
- Facial asymmetry is diagnosed by observation of the crying newborn.
- Nasolabial folds are asymmetric with facial nerve palsy; nasolabial folds are symmetric with congenital hypoplasia of depressor anguli oris muscle.

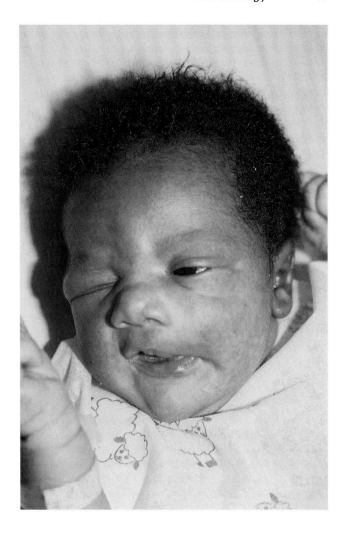

FIGURE 1–17. Traumatic peripheral facial nerve palsy in a 2-day-old neonate with birth by forceps extraction. Note involvement of whole left side of face, with failure of left eye to close (the normal right side, which appears to pull and distort the face, may be mistakenly thought to be paralyzed, and the paralyzed side may be thought to be normal.) (Courtesy of Nathan Rudolph, M.D., State University of New York, Brooklyn, NY.) (For asymmetric crying facies [absence of the depressor anguli oris muscle] see Figure 1–18.)

Asymmetric Crying Facies

SYNONYMS   Congenital Hypoplasia or Aplasia of Depressor Anguli Oris Muscle
Cardiofacial Syndrome
Cayler Syndrome (congenital heart disease with facial weakness)

DEFINITION
Congenital hypoplasia or aplasia of the depressor anguli oris muscle is a minor congenital anomaly that causes asymmetric crying facies.

EPIDEMIOLOGY
Prospective surveys of consecutive births yield an incidence of 0.5% to 1%.

PATHOGENESIS
1. No pathologic documentation is available.
2. Defect probably represents a hypoplasia or aplasia of the depressor anguli oris muscle.

INHERITANCE
1. Autosomal dominant with variable expression has been suggested in some families.
2. Complex multifactorial inheritance

CLINICAL FEATURES
1. For typical findings see Table 1–13.
2. Other associated congenital anomalies
   a. Cardiovascular anomalies (most common)
     (1) Often referred to as cardiofacial syndrome

| BOX 1–8 | *Differential Diagnosis of Asymmetric Crying Facies* |

TRAUMATIC FACIAL PALSY

Central facial palsy (rare, see page 14)
Peripheral facial palsy (more common; see also page 14)

PERIPHERAL FACIAL PALSY

Spontaneous recovery occurs within several days or weeks in majority of patients
With complete palsy
- Flaccid paralysis of *all* facial muscles on the affected side
- Nasolabial fold remains flat on the affected side
- *Unable* to wrinkle forehead on the affected side
- *Unable* to close the eye on the affected side
- Drooping of corner of the mouth on the affected side
With partial involvement
- Orbicularis oculi muscle most frequently *spared*

(congenital heart disease associated with facial weakness)
  (2) Heart defects may include ventricular septal defect, tetralogy of Fallot, patent ductus arteriosus, coarctation of the aorta, truncus arteriosus, single ventricle, tricuspid atresia, right ventricular hypoplasia, pulmonary stenosis
  b. Genitourinary
  c. Musculoskeletal (e.g., barrel thorax, high-set scapula)
  d. Cervicofacial (e.g., micrognathia, cleft palate, short neck)
  e. Respiratory (e.g., congenital lobar emphysema)
  f. Central nervous system

LABORATORY

1. Diagnosis is made by observation of the crying newborn.

2. Thorough examination and appropriate tests are needed to detect other associated anomalies (e.g., cardiac evaluation by electrocardiogram, chest radiograph, and echocardiogram).
3. Electromyographic studies
  a. Help in differentiating hypoplasia of the depressor anguli oris muscle from traumatic injury of the facial nerve
  b. In hypoplasia of the muscle:
    (1) Conduction velocity and latency of the facial nerve are normal.
    (2) Fibrillations are not present at the site of the depressor anguli oris muscle.
    (3) Motor unit potentials are absent or decreased in number at the site of the depressor anguli oris muscle.

TREATMENT

1. No treatment is needed for this entity.
2. Consultations are required for the associated anomalies.

PROGNOSIS

1. Absence of depressor anguli oris muscle in older children and adults is not noticed because it is not a significant component of facial expression.
2. As the child grows and increasingly uses the smiling muscles (risorius and zygomaticus), the facial asymmetry becomes less prominent.

KEY POINTS

Asymmetric Crying Facies

- Face of newborn appears symmetric at rest, but the mouth is pulled downward to one side when crying.
- Isolated unilateral weakness of the depressor anguli oris muscle is the most common cause of facial asymmetry at birth.
- Nasolabial folds are symmetric with hypoplasia of the depressor anguli oris muscle; nasolabial folds are asymmetric with unilateral facial nerve palsy.
- Asymmetric crying facies should be used as an index for a search for other congenital malformations.

TABLE 1–13
Clinical Features of Asymmetric Crying Facies

Typical Findings

Failure of one corner of mouth to move downward and outward with crying or grimacing
All other facial movements symmetric
Absence of muscle is palpable as a thinner lower lip on the paralyzed side
Not associated with feeding difficulties
Forehead wrinkling normal on both sides of face
Eye closure normal on both sides of face
Nasolabial folds normal on both sides of face
Seen as either an isolated anomaly or associated with other anomalies

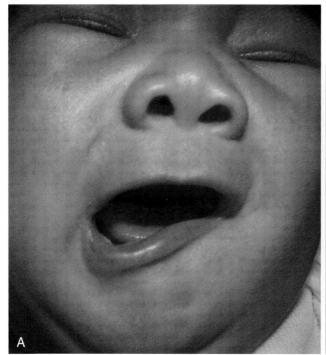

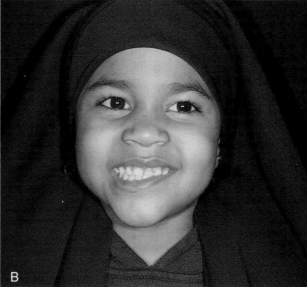

FIGURE 1–18. *A,* Asymmetric crying facies at birth. The left corner of the mouth fails to move downward and outward with crying. The nasolabial folds are symmetric, and the neonate is able to close both eyes (unlike the patient with facial palsy; see Traumatic facial nerve palsy, Figure 1–17.) *B,* Mild asymmetry of the angle of the mouth is still visible at 8 years of age. This patient's asymmetry was remarkable at birth and has improved greatly over the years. (Courtesy of Swati Mehta, M.D, State University of New York, Brooklyn, NY)

Amniotic Constriction Bands

SYNONYMS   Amniotic Rupture Sequence
Amniotic Band Disruption
  Sequence
Amniotic Bands

DEFINITION

Small strands of amnion as a result of amnion rupture lead to annular constrictions encircling the developing structures (usually extremities) and to various other anomalies.

ETIOLOGY

1. Amniotic membrane rupture sequence
   a. Idiopathic in most cases
   b. Amnion rupture occurs most likely before 12 weeks of gestation; however, disruptive defects resulting from amniotic bands may occur at any time during gestation.
   c. Disruptive defects: Constrictive tissue bands caused by primary amniotic rupture lead to subsequent entanglement of the fetal parts (e.g., limbs) in fibrotic amniotic bands.
   d. Deformational defects
      (1) Decreased fetal activity (e.g., secondary to tethering of a limb by an amniotic band)
      leads to other deformities (e.g., scoliosis, foot deformities).
      (2) Chronic leakage of amniotic fluid leads to oligohydramnios, which leads to hypoplasia of lung.
2. Vascular compromise with fibrous band formation
3. Other associated conditions with formation of constrictive tissue bands include:
   a. Abdominal trauma
   b. Amniocentesis
   c. Hereditary defects of collagen
      (1) Marfan syndrome
      (2) Ehlers-Danlos syndrome
      (3) Osteogenesis imperfecta

EPIDEMIOLOGY

1. Usually occurs as a sporadic event in an otherwise normal family
2. Incidence of partial or complete constriction bands that produce defects in extremities and digits: 1 in 10,000 to 1 in 45,000 live newborns (otherwise normal newborns)

CLINICAL FEATURES

1. As in all disruptive defects, no two affected fetuses have exactly the same defects.
2. There is no single feature that occurs consistently.

3. Deformities of limbs
   a. Intrauterine amputation
   b. Ring constriction
   c. Pseudosyndactyly
4. Cranial or facial deformities
   a. Cleft lip (from a strand interrupting fusion of the facial process)
   b. Deformities due to tearing apart of structures that have previously developed normally
5. Abdominal or thoracic wall defects
6. Skin defects
7. Umbilical cord constriction

LABORATORY

1. Examination of the placenta and membranes is diagnostic.
2. Multiple fibrous strands of amnion extend from the placental insertion of the umbilical cord to the surface of the amnion-denuded chorion or float freely within the chorionic sac.

TREATMENT

1. Plastic surgery consultation—for removal of partially constrictive bands (associated with vascular and lymphatic compromise) on the limbs.
2. Counseling and/or education of the family; recurrence risk for subsequent pregnancies is negligible.

KEY POINTS

Amniotic Constriction Bands

- As in all disruptive defects, no two affected fetuses have exactly the same defects, and there is no single feature that occurs consistently.
- Internal anomalies do not occur because amnion rupture results in external compression and/or disruption; thus, features evident on surface examination are usually the only abnormalities.

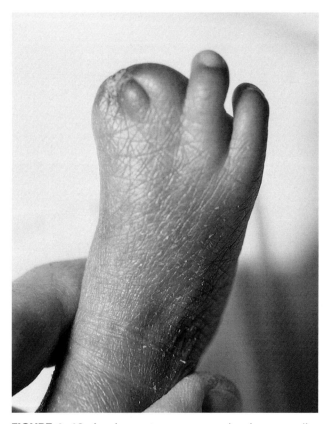

FIGURE 1–19. Amnion rupture sequence showing anomalies of the foot (this patient also had similar deformities of the hand). (Courtesy of Nathan Rudolph, M.D., State University of New York, Brooklyn, NY.)

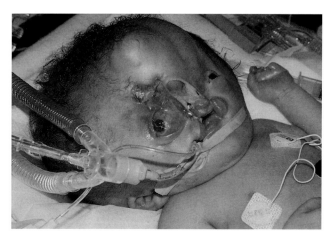

FIGURE 1–20. Craniofacial defects secondary to amnion rupture sequence. (Courtesy of Debra Day-Salvatore, M.D., St. Peter's University Hospital, New Brunswick, NJ)

Neonatal Mastitis

SYNONYMS Mastitis Neonatorum
Breast Abscess

DEFINITION

An infection of the breast tissue that affects full-term infants 1 to 5 weeks postnatally

EPIDEMIOLOGY

1. Incidence: low
2. Seen in full-term infants only
3. Not seen in premature infants (presumably due to underdevelopment of the mammary glands)
4. Female-male ratio 2:1

BOX 1-9 *Etiology of Neonatal Mastitis*

MOST COMMON PATHOGEN

- *Staphylococcus aureus* (85% to 95% of cases)

OTHER PATHOGENS

- Gram-negative bacteria: *Escherichia coli, Proteus,* group D streptococci, *Pseudomonas*
- Group B *Streptococcus*
- *Salmonella* species (in patients with gastroenteritis)
- Anaerobic bacteria (e.g., *Peptostreptococcus*)
- Mixed infection (e.g., *S. aureus* and *E. coli*)

PATHOGENESIS

1. Unilateral or bilateral breast engorgement may result from stimulation by maternal hormones that cross the placenta during gestation.
2. Breast engorgement occurs in both male and female term infants and usually subsides within several weeks.
3. Breast engorgement does *not* occur in premature infants.
4. Retrograde entry of bacteria present on the skin through the ducts into deeper hypertrophied glandular tissue leads to cellulitis or abscess formation.
5. Repeated manipulation of the engorged breast to express the milky discharge ("witch's milk") may be a contributory factor.

LABORATORY

1. Blood culture (usually negative)
2. Gram-stained smear of purulent material is obtained by either
   a. Gentle manipulation of the nipple *or*
   b. Needle aspiration or incision and drainage of the abscess
3. Culture of the purulent material for aerobic and anaerobic bacteria
4. Nose and throat culture may help to detect colonization with *Staphylococcus aureus*

COMPLICATIONS

1. Cellulitis with local spread
2. Bacteremia (rare)
3. Systemic spread or extramammary foci (rare)
4. Recurrence (rare)

DIFFERENTIAL DIAGNOSIS

Physiologic breast engorgement

TREATMENT

1. Hospitalization
2. Intravenous antibiotics based on Gram stain (pending culture result)
   a. For gram-positive cocci: Penicillinase-resistant penicillin (oxacillin or methicillin)
   b. For gram-negative bacteria: Cefotaxime or an aminoglycoside
   c. If no organism is seen: Oxacillin (or methicillin) *and* cefotaxime (or aminoglycoside)
3. Surgical consultation for incision and drainage, if fluctuance is present
4. Duration of therapy (depending on rate of response): usually 7 to 10 days

PROGNOSIS

1. Excellent for cure of the infection
2. Long-term: Some girls may have diminished breast tissue on the affected side.

KEY POINTS

Neonatal Mastitis

- Usually a unilateral, erythematous, and tender enlargement of breast in a full-term infant
- Physiologic enlargement of the breasts is bilateral with no signs of inflammation.

TABLE 1-14
Clinical Features of Neonatal Mastitis

Age at presentation
    Most common: 1–5 weeks of age
    Rare during first week of life
    Most frequently seen during 2nd and 3rd weeks of life
Involvement
    Unilateral: most common
    Bilateral: extremely rare
Localized signs of inflammation
    Warm, swollen, erythematous, tender, and firm
    More likely to be firm than fluctuant
    Discharge from nipple (if present): purulent
Systemic signs uncommon
    Low-grade fever (only 25% of cases)
    Leukocytosis

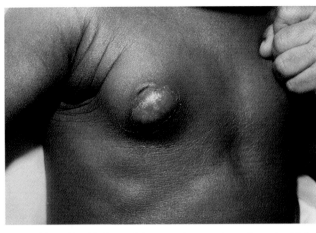

FIGURE 1-22. Unilateral breast abscess in a 3-week-old female neonate. Her mother admitted to repeated massaging of the engorged breast to express the milk.

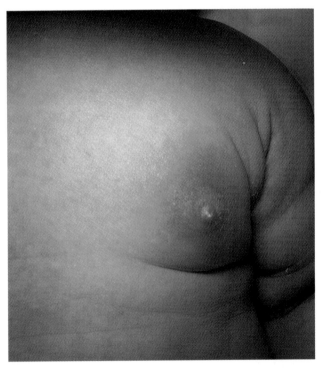

FIGURE 1-21. Neonatal mastitis presenting as an erythematous, indurated, unilateral swelling of the breast in a 2-week-old female infant.

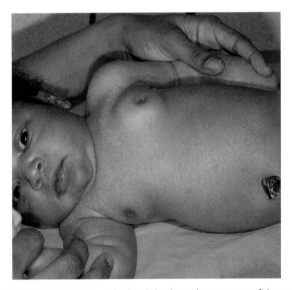

FIGURE 1-23. Bilateral physiologic enlargement of breasts with no signs of inflammation in a 2-week-old male infant.

Congenital Muscular Torticollis

DEFINITION

Torticollis means twisted or "wry neck." Birth injury to the sternocleidomastoid (SCM) muscle leading to torticollis is referred to as congenital muscular torticollis.

ETIOLOGY/PATHOGENESIS

1. Intrauterine or perinatal compartment syndrome
   a. Birth trauma
     (1) Difficult breech or vertex delivery of large infants involving hyperextension of the SCM muscle may result in tearing and bleeding within the muscle.
     (2) Since the SCM muscle is contained within a separate facial compartment, bleeding may result in compartment syndrome with subsequent ischemia, infarction, fibrosis, and contracture of the muscle.
   b. Abnormal pressure, position, or trauma to the muscle during intrauterine life
2. Hereditary defect in the development of the muscle

LABORATORY

1. Exclude underlying skeletal anomalies:
   a. Radiographs of the cervical spine and shoulders—anteroposterior and lateral views
   b. Computed tomography, if indicated
2. Ultrasonography—to define the quantity of normal muscle remnant surrounding the lesion

DIFFERENTIAL DIAGNOSIS

1. Klippel-Feil syndrome (fusion of two or more cervical vertebrae, short neck, low posterior hair line, and torticollis)
2. Congenital cervical vertebral anomalies
3. Sprengel's deformity

TREATMENT

1. Gentle stretching exercises to lengthen the contracted muscle (as early as possible)
   a. Tilt the head toward the opposite shoulder.
   b. Rotate the chin toward the affected side.
   c. Maintain the corrected position for 5 to 10 seconds at each attempt.
   d. A program of 10 to 15 attempts four times daily is usually sufficient in most patients.

TABLE 1–15
Clinical Features of Congenital Muscular Torticollis

Recognized at or shortly after birth
Common presenting complaint: tilting of head
Sternocleidomastoid mass ("pseudotumor" of infancy)
  Palpable mass in midportion of the muscle
  First noted usually 10–14 days after birth
  Occasionally mass may be felt at birth
  Mass well circumscribed, firm to hard, fusiform
  Usually 1–2 cm in diameter
  No signs of inflammation or skin discoloration
  Mass increases in size during first 2–4 weeks, then starts to regress gradually
  Mass usually disappears by 5–8 months of age
With subsequent fibrosis, torticollis develops soon after birth
Head tilts toward the affected side and the chin elevates and rotates to the opposite side
Passive rotation toward the side of torticollis is limited
Lateral side bending toward the side away from torticollis is limited
Flattening of head on involved side (may be present)
Slight facial asymmetry on involved side (may be present)
Other associated findings related to intrauterine malposition (may be present)
  Developmental hip dysplasia
  Metatarsus adductus

---

2. Stimulate the infant to turn the head spontaneously toward the affected side (e.g., by hanging a musical mobile on that side).
3. Conservative therapy is continued for at least 6 months.
4. Surgical intervention
   a. Options include muscle lengthening, release of contractures, and excision of the affected muscle and distal tenotomy.
   b. Surgery should be considered for patients who do not improve with stretching exercises.

PROGNOSIS

1. Most infants treated conservatively usually show complete recovery within 2 to 3 months.
2. If the deformity is not corrected, permanent contractures of the soft tissues on the side of the affected muscle with facial asymmetry will result.

KEY POINTS

Congenital Muscular Torticollis

- Normally an infant's head can be turned freely so that the chin can touch each shoulder and the ear can touch the ipsilateral shoulder.

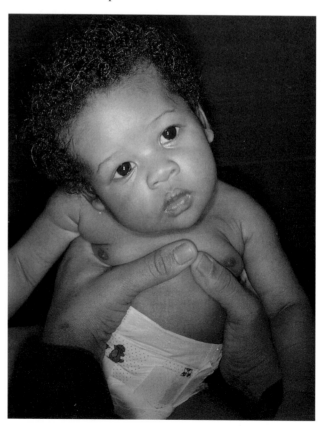

FIGURE 1–24. Congenital muscular torticollis. The head is held in the characteristic position of flexion, lateral bend, and contralateral rotation owing to fibrosis and shortening of the muscle (the head tilts toward the affected side while the chin rotates to the opposite side). A firm mass in the midportion of the sternocleidomastoid muscle was accidentally noted on the right side of the neck in this 4-week-old neonate by the grandmother during bathing.

Natal Teeth

DEFINITION

Teeth present at birth are called natal teeth. Teeth that erupt shortly after birth (within the 1st month of life) are called neonatal teeth.

ETIOLOGY/INHERITANCE

1. Unknown
2. Family history of natal teeth or premature eruption of teeth (15% to 20% of cases)
3. Natal teeth may be associated with
   a. Cleft lip and palate (secondary to disruption of the dental lamina, resulting in superficial placement of primary tooth buds)
   b. Syndromes: Pierre Robin, Ellis-van Creveld, or Hallermann-Streiff syndrome

EPIDEMIOLOGY

1. Incidence: approximately 1 in 1400 to 1 in 2000 live births
2. Natal teeth are more frequently seen than neonatal teeth.
3. Natal teeth
   a. In about 85% to 95% of cases: normal primary teeth (deciduous or milk teeth) that have erupted early
   b. In about 5% of cases: extranumerary or supernumerary teeth

---

BOX 1-10   *Clinical Features of Natal Teeth*

Most common location: mandibular central incisor area
Usual number: two
Common symptoms: pain and refusal to feed

PATHOLOGY

1. Natal teeth are usually poorly formed, have very little root formation or bony support, and have a thin hypoplastic enamel (as a result of premature eruption).
2. Attachment of natal teeth is superficial and is usually limited to the gingival margin.

3. Natal teeth may occur at the end of a stalk of granuloma-like uncalcified tissue that is extremely mobile and friable.

LABORATORY

Radiographs—to exclude the possibility of supernumerary teeth

DIFFERENTIAL DIAGNOSIS

Supernumerary teeth

TREATMENT

1. Consultation with oral surgeons
2. Treatment recommendations: either retention or extraction of the teeth
3. If possible, natal teeth should not be removed because they are primary teeth, and if removed they will not be replaced.
4. Many of these teeth exfoliate spontaneously because they have erupted superficially owing to inadequate root formation.
5. Temporarily covering the sharp incisal edges of the teeth with tooth-colored, acid-etched composite dental material may be indicated
   a. For symptomatic or significant ulceration of the tongue
   b. For alleviating discomfort or difficulties during breastfeeding
6. Indications for removal
   a. Risk of aspiration (detachment due to excessive mobility or looseness)
   b. Ulceration on the tongue
   c. Interference with mother's ability to breastfeed

PROGNOSIS

Removal of the natal teeth leaves a defect for several years until the permanent teeth appear. Removal may alter position of the permanent teeth and dental arch, requiring orthodontic treatment in later years.

KEY POINTS

Natal Teeth

- Natal teeth are present at birth, often in pairs.
- Most common location is in mandibular central incisor area.
- Most natal teeth represent primary teeth and not supernumerary teeth.

TABLE 1–16
Complications of Natal Tooth

Detachment and aspiration of the tooth
Interference with nursing due to abrasion or biting of the
    mother's nipple
Riga-Fede disease
    Ulceration or irritation of sublingual aspect of tongue due to
        contact with sharp teeth edges during sucking *or*
    Laceration of tongue *or*
    Rarely, amputation of tip of tongue during birth process
        (because tongue lies between the alveolar processes)

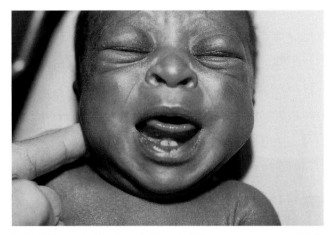

FIGURE 1–25. Natal teeth (in pairs) that were present at birth in the mandibular central incisor area in this neonate. (Courtesy of Nathan Rudolph, M.D., State University of New York, Brooklyn, NY.)

2 Child Abuse and Sexual Abuse

Binita R. Shah, M.D.

Child Abuse

DEFINITION

Child abuse is maltreatment of a child by parents, guardians, or caregivers. The maltreatment may be in the form of direct physical or sexual abuse or denial of nutrition or medical care or failure to provide a safe, nurturing environment.

EPIDEMIOLOGY

1. Annual reporting of child abuse in the United States is 2.4 million. Of these cases, 200,000 to 300,000 children are sexually abused.
2. Annual mortality is more than 4000 children as a result of abuse or neglect.
3. Abusive head trauma is the most common cause of death from child abuse.
4. Blunt abdominal trauma accounts for the second highest mortality among abusive injuries; mortality rate in abusive abdominal trauma is 40% to 50%.

PATHOGENESIS

Mechanisms of inflicted injury include direct impact (e.g., punching, slapping, hitting with an object), shaking, penetrating injuries, and asphyxiation.

RISK FACTORS FOR ABUSE

1. Characteristics of the abused child
   a. Premature birth
   b. Congenital defects
   c. Mental retardation
   d. Multiple births
2. Characteristics of an abusive family
   a. Single parent
   b. Very young mothers at first pregnancy
   c. Lack of education
   d. Interspousal violence

CLINICAL FEATURES

1. Presenting signs include asymptomatic swelling, bruising, seizures, mental status changes, skeletal fractures (up to 50% of patients), and death.
2. Abusive head trauma may present as any of the following:
   a. Shaken impact syndrome (see p. 30)
   b. Subgaleal hematoma

BOX 2-1 | *Suspect Child Abuse (with any of the following)*

Multiple injuries
Injuries (e.g., bruises) in different stages of healing
Delay in seeking medical care
Inconsistent history
Injuries inappropriate for child's stage of development
Alleged mechanism of injury is not consistent with either the clinical finding or the child's stage of development (e.g., a 3-month-old infant with a history of rolling off the bed and sustaining a subdural hematoma)
Frequent episodes of "accidental" poisoning

---

   c. Epidural hematoma
   d. Periorbital ecchymosis
   e. Traction alopecia
   f. Skull fracture
   g. Tin ear syndrome (a blow to side of the head causing the head to spin along the long axis of the neck)
      (1) Unilateral bruising of pinna of the ear
      (2) Ipsilateral cerebral edema
      (3) Ipsilateral subdural hemorrhage
      (4) Ipsilateral retinal hemorrhages
3. Skeletal injuries (see p. 32)
4. Abdominal trauma
   a. Suspect abusive abdominal trauma in any child with unexplained peritonitis or shock (especially in the presence of bilious vomiting and/or anemia).
   b. In order of decreasing frequency, inflicted abdominal injuries include
      (1) Ruptured liver or spleen
      (2) Intestinal perforation
      (3) Duodenal hematoma
      (4) Pancreatic injury
      (5) Kidney trauma
5. Bruises and contusions (see Table 2-1, and Box 2-2)

<table>
<tr><td>

BOX 2-2 *Bruises*

Presence of bruises on relatively protected skin sites suggests inflicted injuries. Examples:
- Cheeks
- Neck
- Trunk
- Genitalia
- Upper legs

Accidental bruises are seen on the skin over bony prominences. Examples:
- Anterior tibia—shins
- Knees
- Elbows
- Forehead
- Dorsum of hands

</td></tr>
</table>

a. A bruise results from application of a blunt force to the skin surface that produces disruption of capillaries (and larger blood vessels with a greater force).

b. For each contusion document the color, shape, pattern, location, and size.

6. Burns
   a. Inflicted burns are uniform in depth and include tap water scalds and flame burns.
   b. Inflicted tap water scalds
      (1) Most common type of nonaccidental burn injury
      (2) In children, 83% of inflicted burn injuries involve tap water–induced scalds (only 15% of accidental scald injuries involve tap water in the general pediatric population).
      (3) Immersion burns
         (a) Most common sites include perineum and/or extremities.
         (b) Inflicted immersion burns have a distinct line demarcating burned and unburned areas.
   c. Flame burns
      (1) Second most common type of inflicted burns
      (2) Well-circumscribed affected area
      (3) Outline of the hot object used is seen (e.g., an iron).

7. Poisoning
   a. Examples: Poisoning by table salt with water restriction (child presents with hypernatremia), over-the-counter and prescription drugs, laxatives, ipecac, pepper, carbon monoxide, illicit drugs
   b. Deliberate poisoning may continue while the child is in the hospital.

8. Munchausen syndrome by proxy is a serious disorder of parenting in which illness in a child is either produced or simulated by a parent.

LABORATORY

1. Complete blood count (screening for anemia, base line hemoglobin/hematocrit)
2. Liver function tests (elevation of transaminase levels in child with liver injury)
3. Radiographs
   a. Skeletal survey screening for occult fractures (see Box 2–3)
      (1) Mandatory for all patients less than 2 years of age with evidence of physical abuse
      (2) Indicated in infants less than 1 year of age with evidence of significant neglect and deprivation
      (3) The yield from skeletal survey decreases with increasing age as the frequency of occult fractures decreases in older children (between 2 and 5 years of age).
      (4) Instead of a skeletal survey, appropriate radiographs can be ordered based on complaints of pain and/or physical examination in older children.

<table>
<tr><td>

BOX 2-3 *Full Skeletal Survey*

Anteroposterior (AP) views of
   Chest/ribs
   Arms/shoulders
   Forearms
   Hands
   Pelvis
   Femurs
   Lower legs
   Feet

Skull: AP and lateral views including cervical spine

Spine: AP and lateral views of thoracolumbar spine including sternum and lower lumbar spine

KEY POINTS
- "Babygram" (a single complete body image) is *not* acceptable.
- All radiographs should be taken as separate exposures.
- Additional views (lateral and/or oblique) should be taken as indicated.
- At least two views of each fracture should be taken for complete delineation.

</td></tr>
</table>

   b. Skeletal survey is usually *not* indicated for
      (1) Children more than 5 years of age because acute occult fractures are rarely present in this age group
      (2) Siblings of an abused victim without clinical evidence of physical abuse
      (3) Victims of isolated sexual abuse

c. Dating of the fractures
 (1) Helps in estimating the age of injury
 (2) Helps in identifying multiple episodes of trauma, inflicted at different times
 (3) Is based on callus formation, appearance of periosteum, fracture line, and soft tissues as seen on radiographs
4. Radionuclide bone scan
 a. Bone scan can identify most fractures within the first 48 hours after an injury.
 b. Helpful in infants and young children with suspected abusive injuries in whom skeletal survey is negative
 c. Helpful in detecting fractures in locations that are difficult to see radiographically (e.g., hands, feet, or ribs)
 d. Helpful for detecting recent fractures (<7- to 10-day-old rib fractures or subtle diaphyseal fractures)
 e. Serves as a complementary test to radiographs, when additional evidence of abusive injuries is required to establish the diagnosis of child abuse
 f. Injuries cannot be dated on bone scans.
5. Computed tomography (CT) without contrast enhancement
6. Photographic documentation

DIFFERENTIAL DIAGNOSIS (see also Table 2–5)

1. Accidental trauma
2. Sudden infant death syndrome
3. Metabolic conditions associated with an increased tendency for fractures (e.g., osteogenesis imperfecta, rickets)

TREATMENT

1. Stabilization of vital signs (if indicated): "ABCDE" of primary survey approach (see p. 31)

2. Multidisciplinary team approach (as indicated): pediatrician, child abuse consultant, social worker, specialists in pediatric radiology, neurology, neurosurgery, and ophthalmology
3. Legal issues for physicians
 a. Reporting to child protective services, law enforcement agencies (e.g., investigation of death scene)
 b. Physicians in the United States are required under the laws of each state to report all suspected as well as known cases of child abuse or child sexual abuse to child protective services agencies.
 c. Reporting is mandatory; there are penalties for failure to report.
 d. Possibility of civil malpractice litigation against physicians for failure to recognize or diagnose child abuse or child sexual abuse
 e. For filing a "false report," statutes generally provide immunity as long as the report is done in "good faith."
4. Referral is made to mental health professionals for both victims and their nonoffending parents to help them cope with the emotional trauma.
5. Once a diagnosis of child abuse is made, all other siblings should be evaluated.

PROGNOSIS

Child abuse and neglect is associated with considerable physical morbidity and mortality.

KEY POINTS

Child Abuse

■ Prevention is the best management.

TABLE 2–1
Determination of Age of Bruise or Contusion

Day (approximate)	1, 2	3, 4, 5	6, 7	8, 9, 10	13, 21, 28
	Red-blue	Blue-purple	Green	Yellow-brown	Resolved

From Johnson CF: Inflicted injury versus accidental injury. Pediatr Clin North Am 37(4):791, 1990.

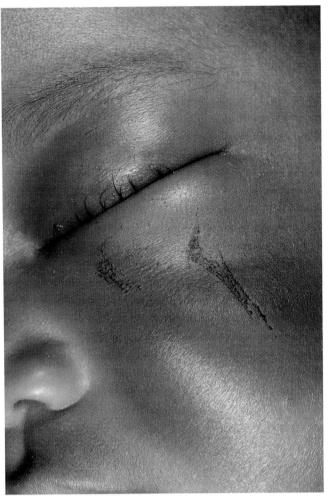

FIGURE 2–1. Acute "red" bruise (1 to 2 days old) with scratch marks inflicted on the eye and face of this 9-month-old infant who was left in the custody of a 12-year-old mentally retarded child. The infant also had a bite mark on the abdomen (see Figure 2–4).

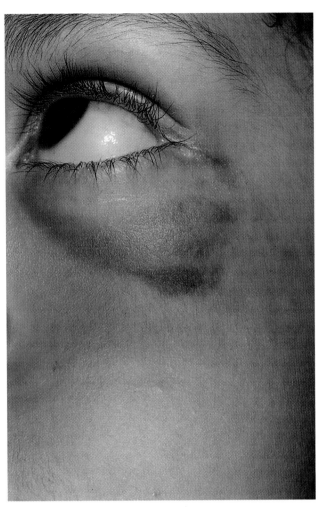

FIGURE 2–2. "Blue-purple" bruise (about 3 to 5 days old) in a 6-year-old child beaten by his stepfather.

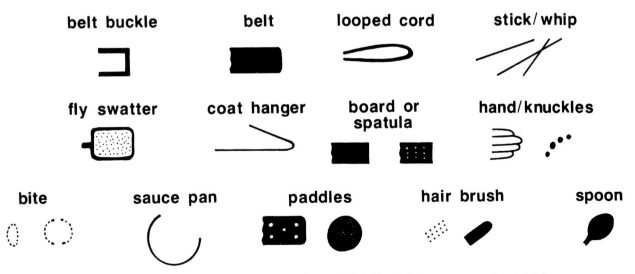

FIGURE 2–3. Marks from objects. (From Johnson CF: Inflicted injury versus accidental injury. Pediatr Clin North Am 37(4):803, 1990.)

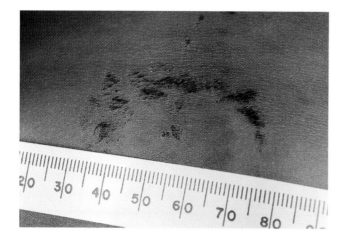

FIGURE 2–4. Bite marks. Bite marks should be suspected when ecchymosis, lacerations, or abrasions are found in an elliptical or oval form. Canine tooth marks in a bite are the most prominent (or deep) part of the bite. The normal distance between maxillary canine teeth in adult humans is 2.5 to 4.0 cm; in a child it is less than 3.0 cm. If the intercanine distance is less than 3 cm, the bite mark may have been inflicted by a child; if it is more than 3 cm, the bite was probably inflicted by an adult. As seen here, human bites compress the flesh, causing only contusions; bites made by dogs and other carnivorous animals tear the flesh.

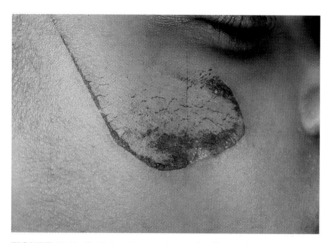

FIGURE 2–5. Belt buckle mark on the face of an 8-year-old girl who was beaten by her mother's boyfriend because of disciplinary problems and poor school performance. She had numerous other bruises as well.

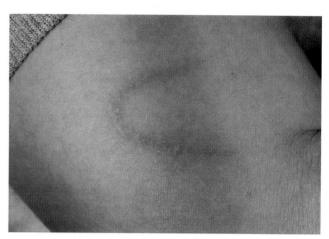

FIGURE 2–6. Looped cord mark on the arm of a 12-year-old girl beaten by her mother.

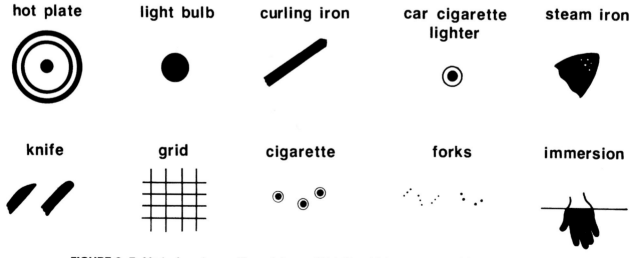

FIGURE 2–7. Marks from burns. (From Johnson CF: Inflicted injury versus accidental injury. Pediatr Clin North Am 37(4):807, 1990.)

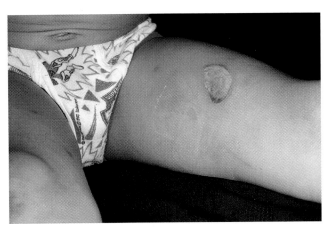

FIGURE 2–8. Burn inflicted by a hot spoon on the thigh of this child (and his sibling) by their uncle because they were "misbehaving."

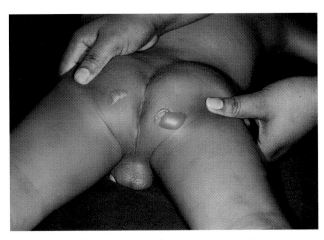

FIGURE 2–9. Second-degree burn on the buttocks (extending to scrotum) of a toddler showing a sharp demarcation between the burned and unburned areas.

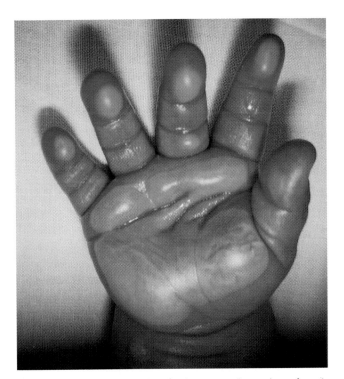

FIGURE 2–10. Second-degree burn on the palm of a 4-month-old infant. He had burns on both palms because his hands were forcibly applied to a hot radiator because he was "crying too much."

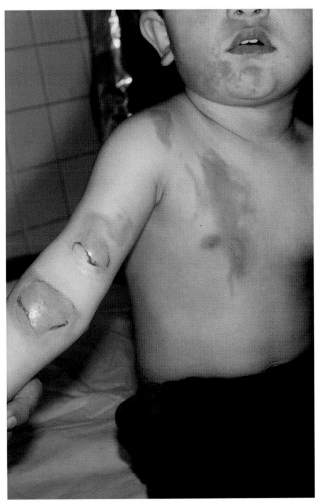

FIGURE 2–11. Accidental first- and second-degree burns on the lower face, shoulder, chest, and hand in a 3-year-old child. Hot tea was spilled on him when he reached up and pulled the mug filled with the tea from a table. In a typical spill burn, hot liquid usually falls onto the child's face and shoulder first. Usually the most severe burns are seen at these sites, but burns become less severe as the liquid runs down the body and cools.

Shaken Impact Syndrome

SYNONYMS   Shaken Baby Syndrome
Whiplash Shaken Baby Syndrome
Whiplash Shaken Infant Syndrome

INTRODUCTION

1. A clinicopathologic entity seen in infants with a constellation of intracranial injuries, retinal hemorrhages, and skeletal injuries
2. The mechanism of injury was initially postulated to be a violent back-and-forth shaking of the infant held by the chest. However, findings of skull fracture, subgaleal and subperiosteal hemorrhages, and focal cortical contusions suggest that the shaking episode is likely to be followed by some type of impact (e.g., roughly discarding the infant onto a sofa or into a crib).
3. Shaking may cause direct intracranial, cervical spine, and intraocular injuries or may act in combination with impact injuries (shaken impact syndrome). Brain injuries seen in this syndrome are diffuse and/or focal. Diffuse injuries are secondary to acceleration and deceleration caused by violent shaking; focal injuries are due to impact and contact.

EPIDEMIOLOGY

1. Abusive head trauma is the most common cause of death from child abuse.
2. About 95% of fatal or life-threatening head injuries in infants during the 1st year of life result from abuse.
3. Shaken impact syndrome is almost always seen in infants less than 2 years of age.
   a. Most common age: infants less than 1 year of age
   b. Most patients: infants less than 6 months of age

LABORATORY

1. Complete blood count with platelet count (mild to moderate anemia is a typical finding because of the intracranial blood loss)
2. Funduscopy after pupils are dilated (if required, by a pediatric ophthalmologist)
3. Coagulation profile (prothrombin time, partial thromboplastin time, fibrinogen, and bleeding time); bleeding diathesis may be seen (release of cerebral thromboplastin)
4. Liver chemistries (elevated transaminase levels indicate occult liver injury)
5. Urinalysis (to detect renal injuries)
6. Lumbar puncture
   a. Presence of blood is often mistaken for "bloody or traumatic" spinal tap.
   b. Centrifuged cerebrospinal fluid (CSF): xanthochromic supernatant suggests a past cerebral bleed (blood in CSF for at least 12 to 24 hours).
   c. Chronic subdural bleed: CSF is viscous and yellow.
7. Computed tomography (CT) without contrast enhancement

BOX 2–4	*Retinal Hemorrhage and Shaken Impact Syndrome*

HEMORRHAGE

Present in 75% to 90% of cases
Bilateral in 60% to 90% of cases
Unilateral in 10% to 30% of cases
Usually last 10–14 days; may persist for longer
Flame-shaped hemorrhages (superficial retinal nerve fiber layer)
Dot and blot hemorrhages (intraretinal)

MECHANISM

Retinal venous hypertension (resulting from significant accelerative or decelerative forces) leading to rupture of retinal veins

DIFFERENTIAL DIAGNOSIS

Birth trauma (mild; resolves within a few days to 3 weeks)
Severe accidental trauma (e.g., motor vehicle accidents, blunt eye trauma)
Nontraumatic (e.g., coagulopathy, carbon monoxide poisoning, sepsis, meningitis, severe hypertension)
Following cardiopulmonary resuscitation (*controversial*)

KEY POINT

Retinal hemorrhage in infants less than 2 years of age suggests shaken impact syndrome unless proven otherwise.

---

   a. Diagnostic study of choice for all suspected head injuries
   b. Demonstrates extra-axial and/or subarachnoid hemorrhage, mass effect, and bony pathology
   c. Identifies injuries that may need immediate intervention
   d. Dates injuries by documenting changes in chemical state of hemoglobin in the affected area
8. Skeletal survey (see Box 2–3)
   a. Mandatory for infants with shaken impact syndrome
   b. Skeletal survey may have to be repeated in 2 weeks to identify new fractures that may not have been apparent initially (healing is seen after 7 to 10 days).
9. Bone scan (see page 26) if skeletal survey is negative, and suspicion of abuse is very high
10. Magnetic resonance imaging (MRI)
    a. As adjunct to CT; complements CT findings
    b. Better characterization of extent of parenchymal injury; predicts clinical outcome

DIFFERENTIAL DIAGNOSIS

1. Sepsis or meningitis
2. Poisoning
3. Seizure disorder

4. Inborn error of metabolism
5. Hemorrhagic disease of the newborn (vitamin K deficiency)

TREATMENT

1. "ABCDE" assessment with simultaneous stabilization of vital signs and monitoring (cardiac, pulse oximetry)
   a. *Airway* (with C-spine stabilization)
   b. *Breathing;* 100% oxygen either by face mask/ reservoir for alert patients or by bag-valve-mask ventilation and intubation (if required) for patients with altered sensorium or apnea
   c. *Circulation* and hemorrhage control
   d. *Disability* (neurologic examination)
      (1) Pupils: size, symmetry (unequal pupil), response to light
      (2) Level of consciousness by *AVPU* system (*A,* alert; *V,* responds to verbal stimuli; *P,* responds to only painful stimuli; *U,* unresponsive)
      (3) Localizing signs (weakness or paralysis of an extremity)
   e. *Exposure/Environmental* (undress patient completely to see any occult injury; prevent hypothermia)
2. Hospitalization; neurosurgical and neurology consultations

3. Reporting to child protective agency (see p. 26)

PROGNOSIS

1. Death
2. Long-term neurologic morbidity may include any of the following:
   a. Mental retardation
   b. Chronic subdural effusions
   c. Hydrocephalus
   d. Spastic quadriplegia
   e. Seizures
   f. Cerebral atrophy
   g. Encephalomalacia
   h. Porencephalic cysts

KEY POINTS

Shaken Impact Syndrome

- One of the most common causes of intracranial injury in infants less than 1 year of age
- Suspect in any infant with a bulging fontanel, head circumference greater than 90th percentile, retinal hemorrhage, or altered sensorium.
- Suspect in any infant with an abnormal respiratory pattern despite normal pulmonary examination.
- Usually lack of external signs of trauma and minimal neurologic deficits

TABLE 2–2
Clinical Features of Shaken Impact Syndrome

Common Presenting Signs or Symptoms

Lethargy or irritability	Head circumference >90th
Coma	percentile
Poor feeding	Apnea
Seizures	Bradycardia
Vomiting	Usually minimal neurologic deficits
Bulging or tense fontanel	Typically absence of external bruising or visible injuries

TABLE 2–3
Common Findings of Shaken Impact Syndrome

Intracranial and spinal cord injuries
  Subdural hemorrhage
  Bilateral chronic subdural hematoma
  Intracerebral contusion/hemorrhage, interhemispheric hemorrhage
  Subarachnoid hemorrhage
  Cerebral edema
  Skull fracture
  Hematomas of the cervical spinal cord
  Injuries at the cervicomedullary junction of the spinal cord
Retinal hemorrhages (see Box 2–4)
Other eye findings
  Vitreous hemorrhages
  Retinal folds
  Traumatic retinoschisis
Skeletal injuries (strongly suggestive of shaken impact syndrome)
  Bilateral, multiple, posterior rib fractures
  Metaphyseal fractures of long bones

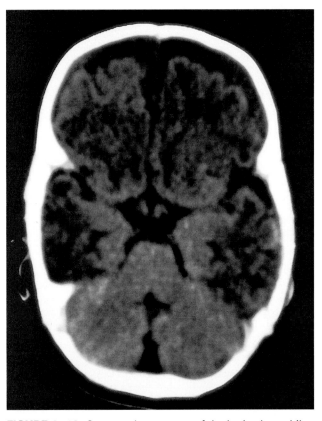

FIGURE 2–12. Computed tomogram of the brain shows bilateral chronic subdural hematomas. Multiple posterior rib fractures were also noted in this 3-month-old infant, who was admitted for seizures, a bulging anterior fontanel, and severe anemia (Hgb 7 g/dL).

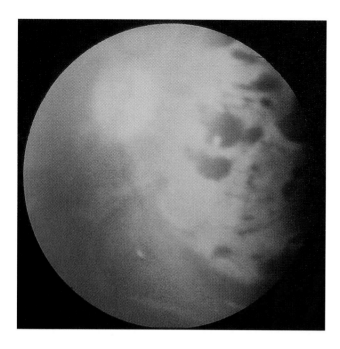

FIGURE 2-13. Retinal hemorrhage. (Courtesy of Alex Levin, M.D. From Giardino AP, Christian CW, Giardino ER (eds): A Practical Guide to the Evaluation of Child Physical Abuse and Neglect. Thousand Oaks, CA, Sage Publications, 1997.)

Skeletal Injuries and Child Abuse

INTRODUCTION

1. Recognition of a skeletal injury may be the first indication of child abuse.
2. Inflicted skeletal injuries may involve virtually any part of the axial and appendicular skeleton.
3. Presence of multiple fractures and/or fractures in different stages of healing suggests child abuse.

EPIDEMIOLOGY

1. The reported frequency of fractures associated with child abuse varies from 11% to 55%.
2. Intracranial and visceral injuries often coexist with abusive skeletal injuries.
3. Age is the single most important risk factor for abusive skeletal injuries.
   a. Seen more frequently in infants and young children than in older children.
   b. About 55% to 70% of all abusive skeletal injuries are seen in infants less than 1 year of age.
   c. About 80% of abuse fractures are seen in infants less than 18 months of age.
   d. Only 2% of accidental fractures are seen in infants less than 18 months of age.

CLINICAL FEATURES

1. Presentation of skeletal injuries in a young nonverbal infant:
   a. Pain manifested by inconsolable crying or irritability
   b. Crying with movement of the affected area or decreased use of a broken extremity
   c. Some skeletal injuries (e.g., rib or metaphyseal fractures) may not be apparent on physical ex-

---

BOX 2-5   *Rib Fractures and Child Abuse*

Most commonly seen in infants and toddlers

About 90% are seen in infants less than 2 years of age.

About 80% are located posteriorly near the costovertebral articulation.

Lateral and anterior fractures are uncommon.

Usually multiple ribs are involved.

Bilateral involvement may be seen.

Fractures are *not* apparent on the physical examination.

Fractures do *not* interfere with respiration in most patients.

Fractures are usually *not* associated with pulmonary or visceral injuries.

Detected by radiographs (healing fractures with callus formation)

May also be detected by bone scans (acute fractures less than 7 to 10 days old)

Usually occur with violent shaking involving anteroposterior thoracic compression in infants

Usually occur with direct blows to the chest in older children

KEY POINTS

Rib fractures should *not* be considered a complication of cardiopulmonary resuscitation in infants and young children.

Presence of rib fractures (in the absence of a severe vehicular accident or metabolic bone disease) should be considered *evidence of child abuse* unless and until proved otherwise.

amination and can be identified only by radiographs.

2. Most common injuries are fractures of the extremities.
   a. Most common types of fractures:
      (1) Diaphyseal fractures of long bones (humerus, ulna, radius, femur, tibia, fibula)
      (2) Fractures may be spiral, torus, transverse, oblique, or greenstick.
      (3) Local swelling and tenderness may be present.
      (4) External bruising may or may not be present over the fracture site.
      (5) Diaphyseal fractures are not specific of abusive injuries and can also result from accidental injuries.
3. Skull fractures
   a. Second most common form of abusive skeletal injuries.
   b. Plain radiographs are the method of choice for identifying fractures.
   c. Usually due to direct impact to the head with a solid object.
   d. Linear parietal skull fractures are the most common type of fractures (in abusive injuries as well as in accidental injuries).
   e. Soft tissue swelling overlying the fracture site may not be seen but may become apparent after a week, when the scalp hematoma liquefies.

f. No type of skull fracture is pathognomonic of abuse; however, skull fractures that are multiple or bilateral, or that cross suture lines are more likely to be nonaccidental.
   g. Absence of a skull fracture does not exclude the possibility of intracranial injury.

TREATMENT

1. Orthopedic consultation
2. Diaphyseal fractures
   a. Treatment depends on the type, location, and stage of the fracture and on the age of the patient.
   b. Usually immobilization is required.
   c. Limitation of weight bearing is necessary for lower limb fractures.
3. Metaphyseal fractures
   a. Most heal without specific treatment.
   b. Do not need immobilization.
4. Skull fractures
   a. Isolated skull fractures require no specific therapy in the majority of the cases.
   b. Observation for "growing skull fracture" or development of a leptomeningeal cyst
5. Rib fractures heal rapidly, and do not require any specific therapy.

BOX 2-6 *Pathognomonic or "Classic" Abuse Fractures*

METAPHYSEAL–EPIPHYSEAL FRACTURES

Examples: "bucket-handle" or "corner" fractures
Typically found in infants and young children
Associated with shaken impact syndrome (acceleration-deceleration forces associated with shaking)
Associated with traction and torsional forces applied to a long bone of an infant while being pulled or twisted by an extremity
Usually soft tissue swelling or external bruising is absent
Usually not identified by physical examination

KEY POINTS

Skeletal Injuries and Child Abuse

- The body mass of an infant less than 12 months old does not ordinarily generate sufficient force to fracture a normal bone in a simple fall from a crib, bed, or couch.
- Although diaphyseal fractures are the most common fractures seen in child abuse cases, they are not pathognomonic for abusive injuries.
- Metaphyseal or epiphyseal fractures require forces that are not produced by the usual accidental trauma of infancy, and their presence should raise a strong suspicion of child abuse.
- The hallmark finding in fractures caused by nonaccidental trauma is the lack of a plausible explanation.

TABLE 2–4
Fractures Strongly Suggestive of Child Abuse

Posterior rib fractures	Skull fractures (multiple, bilateral, or cross suture line)
Metaphyseal fractures of the long bones	Sternal fractures
Spiral fractures in an infant who is not yet walking	Scapular fractures
Clavicular fractures (not midshaft)	Avulsion fractures of the spinous process
Sternoclavicular	Compression fractures of vertebral body
Acromioclavicular	

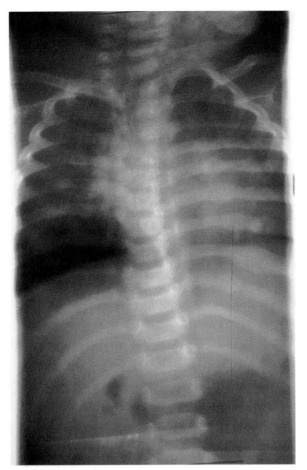

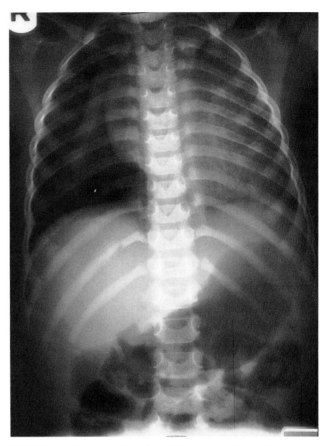

FIGURE 2–14. Multiple posterior rib fractures in a 14-month-old infant who was admitted because of multiple bruises found on the skin. A right pneumothorax was also noted.

FIGURE 2–15. Frontal view of the chest of a child who arrived dead at the emergency room showing a right tension pneumothorax. On closer examination, fractures of the right eighth, ninth, tenth, and eleventh ribs were seen posteriorly.

TABLE 2–5
Differential Diagnosis of Child Abuse Fractures

Accidental trauma
Disorders with an increased tendency toward fracture
  Osteogenesis imperfecta
  Rickets
  Scurvy
  Osteoporosis
  Hypervitaminosis A
  Infantile cortical hyperostosis
  Menke's kinky hair syndrome
  Congenital syphilis
  Leukemia

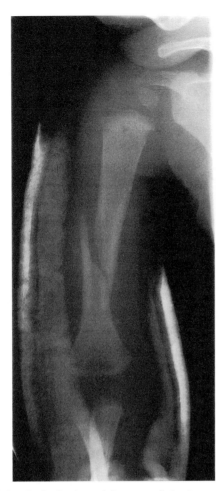

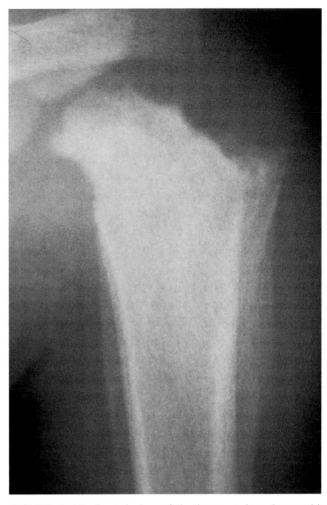

FIGURE 2–16. A diaphyseal fracture of the humerus in a 6-month-old infant. A humeral fracture in a child less than 3 years old is strongly suspicious of child abuse.

FIGURE 2–17. Frontal view of the humerus in a 2-year-old child. Note extensive periosteal reaction along the shaft with diffuse metaphyseal irregularity and a corner fracture seen laterally.

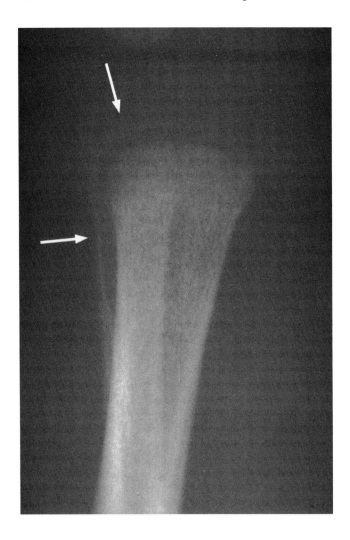

FIGURE 2-18. Frontal view of the distal tibia in a 4-month-old infant. Note the lifting off of a thin band of metaphysis, representing a bucket handle fracture.

Sexual Abuse and Sexually Transmitted Diseases (STDs)

DEFINITION

1. Sexual abuse is engagement of a child in sexual activity that involves any of the following:
   a. Sexual activities that the child cannot comprehend
   b. Sexual activities for which the child is not developmentally prepared and cannot give informed consent
   c. Sexual activities that violate the social and legal taboos of society
2. Sexual abuse includes a wide spectrum of activities ranging from nontouching abuses (e.g., exhibitionism) to activities involving direct genital, anal, or oral contact ranging from rape to gentle seduction.

EPIDEMIOLOGY/PATHOGENESIS

1. Statistics from the National Center for Child Abuse and Neglect 1993 study:
   a. Sexual abuse incidence: 3.2 in 1000 children
   b. About 1% of children experience some form of sexual abuse each year
2. About 80% to 90% of abused children are female; mean age 7 to 8 years old
3. Perpetrators are male in 75% to 90% of cases; they are adults or minors known to the child (usually a family member [father, stepfather, mother's boyfriend, or uncle or other relative]). Children are more frequently abused by males.
4. Abuse by family members or known acquaintances usually involves multiple episodes over periods of time ranging from weeks to years (as opposed to abuse by strangers or unknown assailants, which usually occurs in a single episode).
5. Vaginal or rectal penetration is more likely to lead to infection, whereas fondling is unlikely to lead to infection.
6. There are only five modes of transmission of STDs:
   a. Transplacental
   b. Perinatal
   c. Sexual abuse
   d. Consensual sexual intercourse
   e. Accidental (extremely unlikely)

ANATOMY

1. All girls are born with a hymen (in the absence of multiple congenital anomalies), and normal hymens have different configurations (e.g., fimbriated, crescentic, annular).
2. Hymenal diameter increases with age. Hymenal diameter is also dependent on position, degree of traction, and child's degree of relaxation during examination.
3. Hymenal notches between 9 o'clock and 3 o'clock positions, bumps, tags, and vestibular bands are normal findings.
4. Masturbation, tampons, or accidents are not likely to cause injury to the hymen or internal genital structures.

LABORATORY

1. Detailed records, drawings, or photographs must be kept because of the possibility of civil or criminal court involvement.
2. Use of dolls or line drawings is common in interviewing of children 3 to 6 years old.

BOX 2-7   *Clinical Findings* **Specific** *for Sexual Abuse*

Presence of sperm, semen, or acid phosphatase in the mouth, vagina, or anus
Pregnancy in early adolescence
Evidence of sexually transmitted diseases (not acquired perinatally) in prepubertal children

---

3. American Academy of Pediatrics, Committee on Child Abuse and Neglect recommendations (1994)
   a. Routine cultures and screening of all sexually abused children for gonorrhea, syphilis, human immunodeficiency virus (HIV), or other STDs are not recommended.
   b. The yield of positive cultures is very low in asymptomatic prepubertal children (especially those with a history of fondling only).
   c. Appropriate cultures and serologic tests are recommended "when epidemiologically indicated or when history and/or physical findings suggest the possibility of oral, genital or rectal contact."
4. Cultures for *Neisseria gonorrhoeae* on special culture media
   a. Girls: specimens collected from vagina, rectum, and pharynx; a cervical specimen is not recommended for prepubertal girls.
   b. Boys: specimens collected from rectum, pharynx, and urethra; urethral swab culture is performed if
      (1) Urethral discharge is present.
      (2) Dysuria is present.
      (3) Urine leukocyte esterase is positive.
      (4) Erythema is present.

5. Cultures for *Chlamydia trachomatis*
   a. Culture is still the preferred method of diagnosis.
   b. Nonculture antigen detection tests such as enzyme immunoassays (EIA) and direct fluorescent antibody (DFA) tests and DNA probes are not specific at rectogenital sites in children and are not approved for use in children.
   c. Girls: specimens collected from vagina and anus
   d. Boys: specimens collected from anus and urethra (if urethral discharge is present)
   e. Cultures for *C. trachomatis* are *not* recommended from the following sites:
      (1) Intraurethral specimen in the absence of urethral discharge in prepubertal boys (low yield, traumatic experience)
      (2) Pharyngeal specimen in either sex (low yield, persistence of perinatally acquired infection beyond infancy)
6. Rape kit protocol modified for child sexual abuse
   a. If alleged sexual abuse has occurred within 72 hours *and*
   b. Child provides a history of sexual abuse including ejaculation.
7. If more than 72 hours have elapsed since the alleged sexual abuse (and injuries needing immediate attention are absent), examination can be scheduled at the earliest convenient time for the child, investigative team, and physician.
8. Serologic tests for syphilis (VDRL)
9. Serologic tests for hepatitis B (hepatitis B surface antigen and antibody)
10. HIV serology (as indicated)
11. Culture and wet mount of a vaginal swab specimen for *Trichomonas*
12. Culture of lesions for herpes simplex virus

TREATMENT (see also p. 26 for legal reporting)

1. Attention to all acute injuries that may require immediate intervention
2. Multidisciplinary approach involving local or regional child abuse consultants and social workers
3. Once sexual abuse has been identified, all siblings of sexual abuse victims should be examined.
4. Treatment for STDs and reporting requirements (see Table 2–9)
   a. Presumptive treatment of children who have been sexually abused is usually not done.
      (1) Lower risk for ascending infection in girls than in adolescents
      (2) Close follow-up can be arranged.
   b. Treatment is given once a specific diagnosis has been confirmed.

FOLLOW-UP

1. A follow-up visit is scheduled about 2 weeks after the most recent sexual exposure.
   a. For collection of additional specimens (infecting pathogens may not be present in sufficient

quantity following a very recent exposure resulting in negative cultures initially)

b. For repeat physical examination

2. Follow-up is scheduled about 12 weeks after the most recent sexual exposure to collect sera for antibody (to allow sufficient time for antibody production).

KEY POINTS

Sexual Abuse and STDs

- A normal physical examination does *not* exclude child sexual abuse; diagnostic findings of sexual abuse are seen in only 3% to 16% of victims.
- Diagnosis of child sexual abuse is made on the basis of a child's history; the child's statement that he or she was sexually abused is often the most important evidence of molestation.
- Any STD in a child (nonperinatally acquired) strongly suggests sexual abuse unless and until proved otherwise.
- Gonorrhea is the most frequent STD found in abused children; infection in the pharynx and rectum is frequently asymptomatic.

TABLE 2–6
Signs and Symptoms Suggestive of Child Sexual Abuse

Behavioral Changes	Genitourinary/Anogenital Related
Appetite disturbances	Anal or genital pain
Withdrawal/depression	Genital or anal bleeding
Poor school performance	Painful urination
Precocious sexual behavior	Painful defecation
Sleep disturbances	Infections
Nightmares	Recurrent urinary tract
Enuresis	Recurrent vulvovaginitis
Encopresis	
Phobias	
Suicidal attempts or ideation	

TABLE 2–7
Clinical Findings "Suggestive" of Sexual Abuse

Hymenal injuries
  Most common sites of injury: between 3 o'clock and 9 o'clock positions
  Types of injuries: laceration, transection, disruption (strongly suggest abuse)
  Notches or midline scarring in lower portion of hymen
  Posterior or lateral concavities (indentations in hymenal tissues)
  Hymenal diameter > two standard deviations for age in presence of other findings
Anal injuries
  Fresh anal injuries (e.g., laceration) without adequate accidental history
  Anal dilatation >15 mm transverse with gentle buttock traction (in absence of stool in rectal vault this finding strongly suggests abuse)
Injuries in posterior fourchette (strongly suggest abuse)
Bruising of inner thighs or genitalia or bite marks
Unexplained erythema or petechiae of palate (especially at junction of hard and soft palate)

TABLE 2–8
Sexual Abuse and Sexually Transmitted Diseases (STDs)

STDs may be transmitted during sexual assault
In children, evidence of STD may be the first indication that abuse has occurred
STDs occur in 2% to 15% of sexually abused children
Prevalence of STDs in sexually abused children:
  Neisseria gonorrhoeae (most frequent [1% to 30% incidence reported in past; recent studies show <3%])
  Syphilis (infrequent; prevalence of positive serology 0 to 1.8%)
  Chlamydia trachomatis (infrequent; prevalence <5%)
  Human immunodeficiency virus (not acquired perinatally or blood borne; data unknown)
  Human papillomavirus (condylomata acuminata; prevalence 1% to 2%)
  Herpes simplex virus (data unknown)
  Trichomonas vaginalis (data limited)
  Gardnerella vaginalis (data limited)
  Ureaplasma urealyticum (data limited)

TABLE 2–9
Implications of Commonly Encountered STDs for the Diagnosis and Reporting of Sexual Abuse of Prepubertal Infants and Children

STD Confirmed	Sexual Abuse	Suggested Action
Gonorrhea*	Certain	Report
Syphilis*	Certain	Report
Chlamydia*	Probable	Report
Condylomata acuminata*	Probable	Report
Trichomonas vaginalis	Probable	Report
Herpes 1 (genital)	Possible	Report†
Herpes 2	Probable	Report
Bacterial vaginosis	Uncertain	Medical follow-up
Candida albicans	Unlikely	Medical follow-up

*If not perinatally acquired.
†Unless there is a clear history of autoinoculation.
From American Academy of Pediatrics. Committee on Child Abuse and Neglect: Guidelines for the Evaluation of Sexual Abuse of Children. Pediatrics 87 (2):254, 1991.

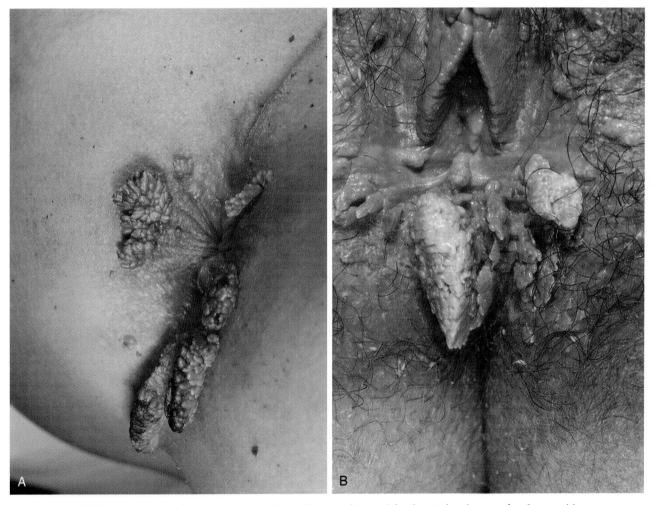

FIGURE 2–19. *A,* Condylomata acuminata (venereal warts) in the perianal area of a 3-year-old male who was abused by his maternal uncle. These are soft, flesh-colored, elongated lesions that occur around the mucocutaneous junctions and intertriginous areas (e.g., perianal area, mucosal surfaces of the female genitalia). Condylomata acuminata must be differentiated from condylomata lata because both occur in the same areas. *B,* Condylomata acuminata in a 13-year-old girl who was repeatedly abused by her stepfather.

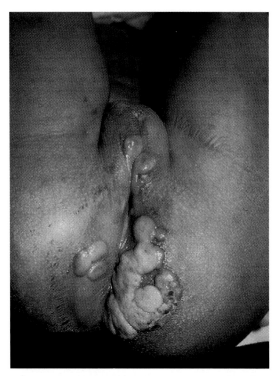

FIGURE 2–20. Condylomata lata in a 6-year-old girl. Her VDRL test was strongly positive. Lesions occur around the anus and genitalia as flat-topped, round to oval nodular lesions and plaques (formed by papules that coalesce) with a wide base. Unlike condylomata acuminata, these lesions are flat and are never covered by digitate vegetations.

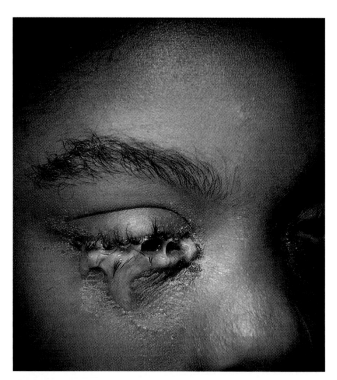

FIGURE 2–22. Gonococcal conjunctivitis in an 8-year-old girl who presented with profuse mucopurulent discharge. Pharyngeal and rectal cultures were also positive for *Neisseria gonorrhoeae*. Investigation among family members led to finding a 21-year-old uncle with gonococcal urethritis, and subsequently he confessed to abusing this girl.

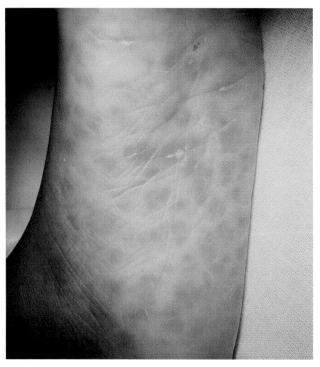

FIGURE 2–21. Acquired syphilis in a 6-year-old girl who had been in several foster homes since birth to a drug-addicted mother. Erythematous papulosquamous, nonpruritic lesions were present on her palms as well as feet. VDRL and fluorescent treponemal antibody absorption (FTA–ABS) tests were positive.

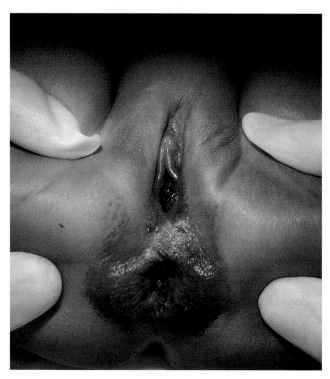

FIGURE 2–23. Fresh anal injuries and significant anal dilation with hematoma at the introitus in a 4-month-old infant brought to the emergency room dead. These injuries occurred when the infant was left by the mother in the custody of a boyfriend. This infant also had bruises on the abdomen and face, posterior rib fractures, and intra-abdominal injuries (splenic rupture, retroperitoneal hematoma).

Conditions Mistaken for Child Abuse and Child Sexual Abuse

MONGOLIAN SPOTS

1. Gray-blue pigmentation most commonly seen on lower back and buttocks
2. Can be seen anywhere on body
3. Most often seen in African-American infants (95%)
4. Uncommon in white infants (10%)
5. Present since birth
6. Number may vary from one lesion to several lesions extending up the back and shoulders
7. May be mistaken for bruises
8. Nontender, macular lesions
9. Usually resolve over a period of months

BOX 2-8   *Conditions Mimicking Child Abuse*

CONDITIONS MIMICKING ABUSIVE BRUISES

Accidental trauma (e.g., raccoon eyes from accidental trauma)

Birthmarks (e.g., mongolian spots, hemangioma [especially cavernous])

Coagulation defects (e.g., hemophilias [factor VIII, IX, or X deficiency])

Vasculitis (e.g., Henoch-Schönlein purpura)

Platelet dysfunction (e.g., acute or chronic immune thrombocytopenic purpura)

Traditional practices (e.g., coining, cupping, and moxibustion)

Dermatologic conditions (e.g., phytophotodermatitis [see pp. 239–240])

CONDITIONS MIMICKING INFLICTED BURN INJURIES

Accidental burns

Ecthyma (mimics cigarette burns; see pp. 87–88)

Blistering distal dactylitis (see pp. 87–88)

Epidermolysis bullosa (see pp. 230–231)

"CAO GIO" (COIN RUBBING)

1. This is a linear pattern of purpura produced when the skin is stroked by a coin after being smeared with oil in an attempt to get rid of an "ill wind."
2. It is commonly practiced by Southeast Asian mothers when a child is sick.
3. May be mistaken for child abuse

CUPPING ("VENTOSA")

1. Round identical purpuras are produced when the mouth of a jar full of lighted cotton soaked in alcohol is inverted onto the skin.
2. This is a cultural practice among some population groups (e.g., east Europeans); its purpose is to produce decongestion.
3. May be mistaken for child abuse

PURPURA FULMINANS

1. This is the presentation of disseminated intravascular coagulation (DIC) in the skin. It results in retiform necrotic areas corresponding to areas supplied by thrombosed dermal capillaries.
2. Meningococcal infection is the most common precipitating event.
3. Varicella with secondary group A beta-hemolytic streptococcal infection may also result in purpura fulminans.
4. An acquired state of protein C deficiency and the presence of lupus phospholipid antibody have been demonstrated in some cases.
5. Aggressive treatment of infection as well as heparin administration and platelet transfusion may be life-saving.

PROTEIN C DEFICIENCY

1. This is an autosomal recessive disorder characterized by absence of protein C as an anticoagulant.
2. It presents in the newborn as microvascular thrombosis and skin necrosis (neonatal purpura fulminans).
3. May also be an acquired disorder in some cases of fulminating sepsis.
4. Immediate administration of fresh frozen plasma may be critical.

BOX 2-9   *Conditions Mistaken for Child Sexual Abuse*

GENITOURINARY CONDITIONS

Labial agglutination (see pp. 321–323)

Urethral prolapse (see pp. 323–325)

Congenital vaginal anomalies

Accidental injuries (e.g., straddle injuries)

Lichen sclerosus et atrophicus (see p. 202)

Hemangioma

ANORECTAL CONDITIONS

Perianal streptococcal disease (see pp. 87–88)

Crohn disease

Chronic constipation, anal fissures

Rectal prolapse

Postmortem anal dilatation

Congenital anal anomalies

ACUTE IMMUNE THROMBOCYTOPENIC PURPURA

1. An *acquired* antibody-mediated platelet destruction
2. Most commonly seen in infants and young children between 1 and 4 years of age
3. Presents as pinpoint petechiae and ecchymoses
4. Ecchymosis is most commonly distributed *asymmetrically* over the lower extremities; however, it may be present anywhere on the body.
5. Mucous membrane bleeding, including bleeding from the gums and nose

HENOCH-SCHÖNLEIN PURPURA (HSP; see pp. 186–188)

1. Immune complex–mediated aseptic vasculitis of small blood vessels (arterioles, capillaries)
2. Most commonly seen in children between 2 and 8 years of age
3. Preceding viral infection or group A beta-hemolytic streptococcal infection
4. Palpable purpura; lesions may progress from hives to purpura
5. Lesions *symmetrically* distributed over buttocks, thighs, and extensor surfaces of arms and legs
6. Associated findings include abdominal pain, arthralgia or arthritis, and renal involvement (hematuria, proteinuria)
7. In young infants angioedema (scalp, trunk, hands, or feet) may be present with purpuric lesions

"RACCOON EYES" (PERIORBITAL ECCHYMOSIS) OR BLACK EYES (FROM ACCIDENTAL TRAUMA)

1. Bleeding into the subgaleal space leaks ventrally in an upright child along the facial soft tissues into the periorbital space.
2. Presents as darkening (secondary to degradation products of blood) of eyes and soft tissue swelling of the forehead few days after the trauma.
3. Bilateral periorbital ecchymosis results from a single blow to the forehead or to the basilar skull with resultant skull fracture.
4. This may be mistaken for direct trauma to the eyes (e.g., a punch); however, absence of other signs of eye trauma (e.g., abrasions, laceration, swelling of eyelids, tenderness, subconjunctival bleeding, hyphema) helps to differentiate the two.

HEMOPHILIA A (FACTOR VIII DEFICIENCY; see pp. 268–272)

1. Seen in males (sex-linked recessive transmission)
2. May present with extensive bruising, soft tissue bleeding, and hemarthrosis
3. Extent and severity of bleeding are more than would be expected with minimal trauma.
4. Family history and history of similar episodes are helpful in arriving at the diagnosis.

SCURVY

1. Deficiency of vitamin C (ascorbic acid)
2. Breast-fed infants receive adequate amounts of vitamin C (provided that the mother's diet contains adequate vitamin C). Infants fed evaporated milk formula must receive vitamin C supplements.
3. Majority of cases seen during infancy (age 6 to 24 months)
4. Generalized tenderness, especially pronounced in the legs
5. Edematous swelling along the shafts of the legs
6. Subperiosteal hemorrhage may be palpated at the end of the femur
7. Pseudoparalysis due to pain
8. Hemorrhagic manifestations
   a. Petechial hemorrhage in skin and mucous membranes
   b. Orbital hemorrhage
   c. Subdural hemorrhage
   d. Hematuria
   e. Melena

RICKETS (see also pp. 360–365)

1. Rickets is caused by undermineralization of the cartilaginous growth plate resulting in excessive accumulation of unmineralized matrix.
2. Rickets is seen only in growing children (growth plate exists only when skeleton is growing).
3. Conditions leading to development of rickets include inadequate exposure to sunlight, dietary vitamin D deficiency (e.g., food faddism, exclusively breast-fed infants who receive no vitamin D supplements), fat malabsorption, and metabolic bone diseases.
4. Failure to thrive, delayed growth development, rachitic deformities including bowlegs, and prominent "swelling" of wrists and ankles are some of the features.
5. Radiographic changes are best seen at the metaphyses and epiphyses (e.g., the knee or the most rapidly growing bones in infants) and can be mistaken for metaphyseal skeletal injuries characteristic of child abuse.
6. Pathologic fractures can occur in patients with rickets.

OSTEOGENESIS IMPERFECTA (OI; see also pp. 381–383)

1. Inherited disorder of connective tissue (defect in collagen biosynthesis) that primarily affects the musculoskeletal system
2. Four clinical types are seen with variable manifestations.
3. Blue sclera, increased bone fragility, susceptibility to fractures, and resultant deformities are some of the features.
4. Radiographic features include osteopenia, fractures, and angulation of healed fractures.
5. Patients with all forms of OI may show some degree of easy bruisability; clotting factors and platelet counts are normal.

URETHRAL PROLAPSE (see pp. 323–325)

1. Seen in prepubertal girls between 4 and 7 years of age

2. More common in African-American girls
3. Most common presenting complaint is painless vaginal bleeding
4. Other complaints may include urinary symptoms or presence of a vaginal mass.
5. A doughnut-shaped mass is seen at the introitus; the center of the doughnut is the urethral meatus.

PERIANAL STREPTOCOCCAL INFECTION
(see also pp. 87–88)

1. Group A beta-hemolytic streptococcal infection
2. Presenting complaints are rectal itching, pain, bleeding, or constipation.
3. Symptoms may be present for months before a correct diagnosis is made.
4. Findings are localized to the perineum; systemic signs or symptoms are absent.
5. Erythema and tenderness around anus
6. Anal fissures and bleeding may be seen.

LICHEN SCLEROSUS ET ATROPHICUS
(see also p. 202)

1. Involvement of the anogenital area

2. An area of hypopigmentation in the shape of an hourglass involving the anus and genitalia
3. Affected skin is atrophic and bleeds easily after minor trauma.
4. Hemorrhagic form with involvement of the labia and surrounding skin may mimic abuse.
5. One of the most common dermatitides mistaken for sexual abuse

BLISTERING DISTAL DACTYLITIS
(see pp. 87–88)

1. A tender, tense, cloudy, fluid-filled blister with surrounding erythema located over the volar fat pad on the distal portion of the finger or toe
2. May involve multiple fingertips or toes
3. Most common cause is group A beta-hemolytic streptococci; rarely caused by *Staphylococcus aureus*
4. Purulent exudate shows gram-positive cocci and polymorphonuclear leukocytes on Gram stain; can be confirmed by culture.

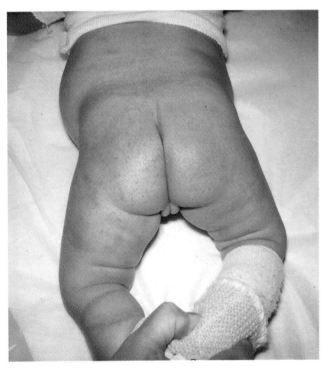

FIGURE 2–24. Mongolian spot on the buttocks of a white infant that was mistaken for abuse. The child was also in a cast for correction of his club foot; the findings of blue pigmentation and cast were the reasons for suspecting child abuse.

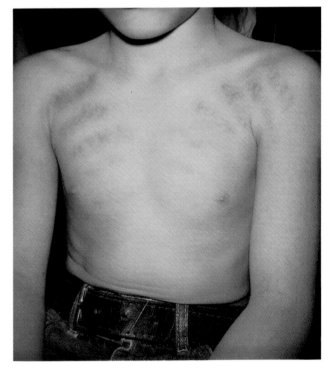

FIGURE 2–25. "Cao gio" (coin rubbing). This 6-year-old Cambodian boy was brought in by the school social worker because of suspected child abuse.

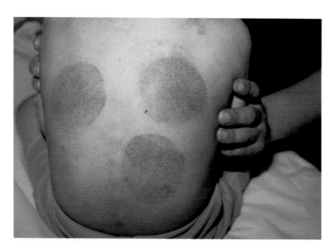

FIGURE 2-26. A Palestinian boy brought in for upper respiratory symptoms was found to have three identical round purpura on the back from cupping.

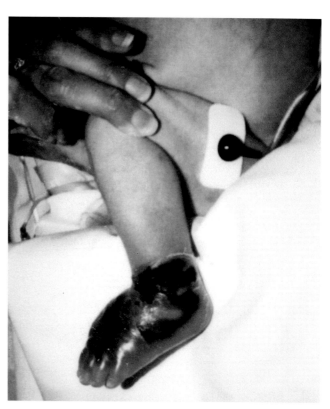

FIGURE 2-28. Newborn with protein C deficiency showing necrosis of the skin of the foot.

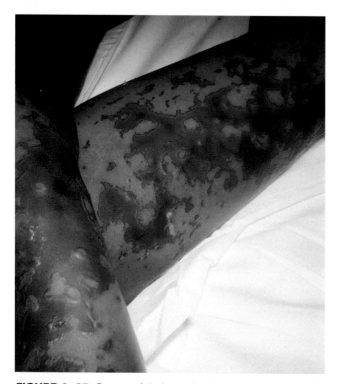

FIGURE 2-27. Purpura fulminans in a boy with meningococcemia.

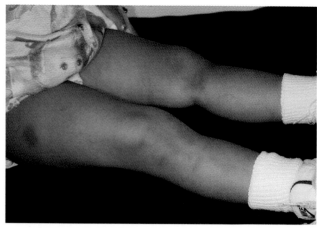

FIGURE 2-29. Acute immune thrombocytopenic purpura with *asymmetric* ecchymosis on the lower extremities in a 3-year-old girl. Physical examination and complete blood count were normal except for a platelet count of 15,000/mm³.

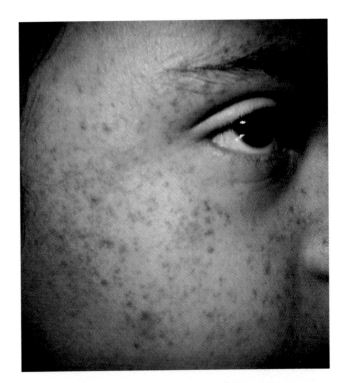

FIGURE 2–30. Petechiae on the face and upper thorax occur commonly in healthy children following intractable episodes of coughing, vomiting, or crying. This patient developed a petechial eruption localized to her face shortly after a tooth extraction.

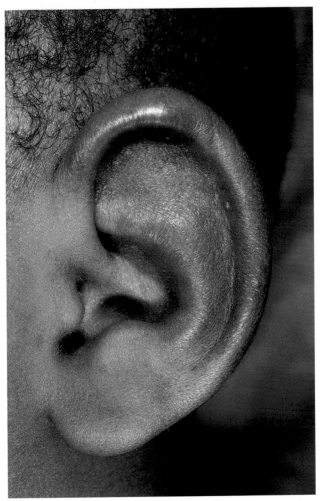

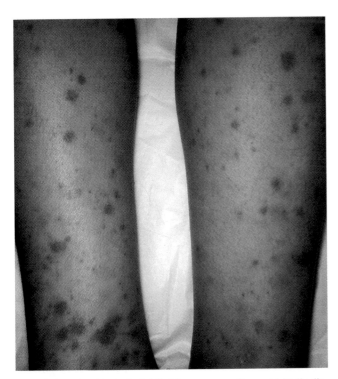

FIGURE 2–31. Henoch-Schönlein purpura. *Symmetrically* distributed purpuric lesions on both lower extremities in a 6-year-old girl whose throat culture was positive for group A beta-hemolytic streptococci.

FIGURE 2–32. Henoch-Schönlein purpura (HSP) with vasculitis involving the ear lobe. This is one of the characteristic findings of HSP and can be mistaken for abuse.

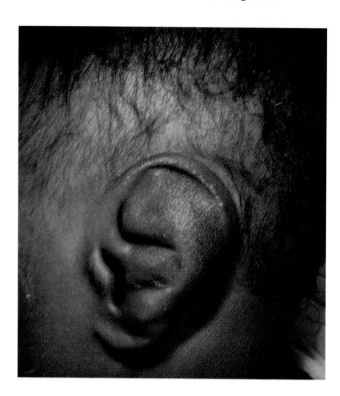

FIGURE 2–33. Bruising of the pinna secondary to child abuse in a 4-month-old infant. This patient had bruises on both ears that were mistaken for cellulitis and treated with antibiotics. Ears (and buttocks) are not frequently injured in childhood accidents, and bruises at these sites are strong indicators of abuse. Hematoma at this site may lead to formation of cauliflower ear or boxer's ear.

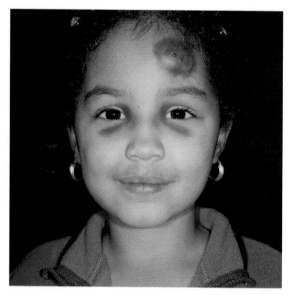

FIGURE 2–34. Periorbital ecchymosis occurred in this girl 3 days after she fell and hit her forehead against the bed railing while jumping in the bed.

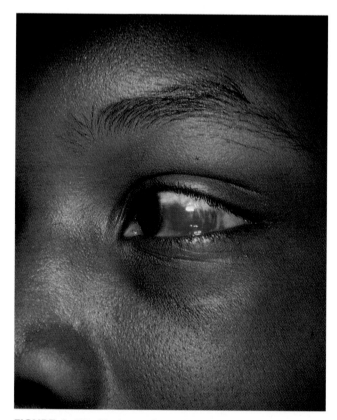

FIGURE 2–35. Black eye from direct trauma (the child was punched by her father). The presence of abrasion, subconjunctival bleeding, and eyelid swelling suggests direct trauma to the eye. This patient also had numerous bruises over her body.

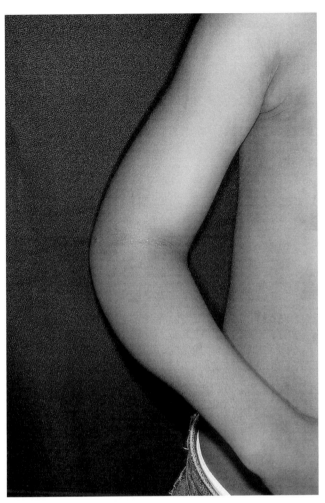

FIGURE 2-36. Hemophilia. Hemarthrosis of left elbow (swollen, warm, tender, limitation of movements) in an 8-year-old male child.

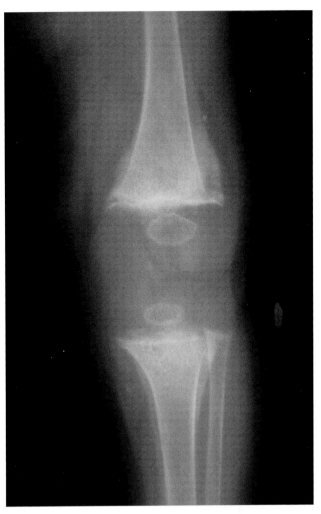

FIGURE 2-37. Scurvy. Frontal view of the knee in an infant. There is diffuse osteopenia and thickening of the provisional zones of calcification. In addition, there are multiple spurs at the ends of the femur and tibia with subperiosteal bone formation around the shafts. Wimberger ring is seen in the femoral and tibial epiphyses, and there is mild fibular cupping. (Courtesy of Laurence Finberg, M.D., University of California, San Francisco.)

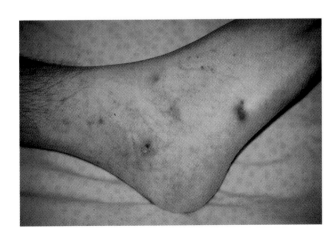

FIGURE 2-38. Petechial hemorrhages in the skin of a child with cystic fibrosis and scurvy. (Courtesy of R. Givsti, M.D., Long Island College Hospital, Brooklyn, NY.)

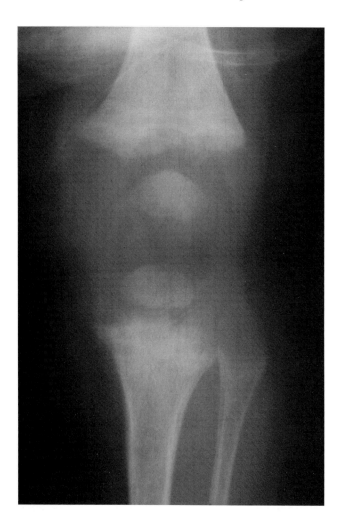

FIGURE 2-39. Rickets. Flaring and cupping of the distal femur and proximal tibia and fibula in a 2-year-old child with severe osteopenia and rickets secondary to nutritional vitamin D and calcium deficiencies. The family consumed a strict vegan diet devoid of any animal products including milk.

FIGURE 2-40. Osteogenesis imperfecta. Frontal view of chest and abdomen showing multiple fractures of long bones and ribs. Characteristic "ribbon" ribs and flattening of the vertebrae are seen. (Courtesy of Laurence Finberg, M.D., University of California, San Francisco.)

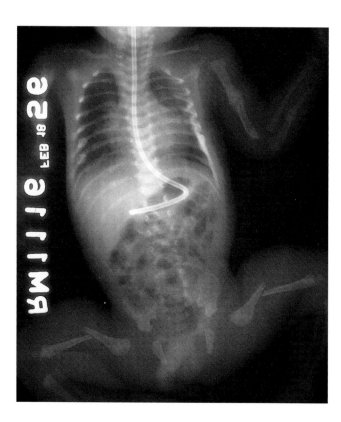

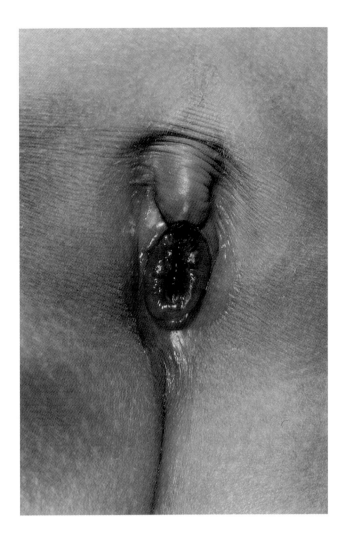

FIGURE 2–41. Urethral prolapse in a 5-year-old girl presenting with a complaint of "vaginal bleeding." A doughnut-shaped mass with erythema and edema representing a complete circular prolapse of the urethral mucosa is seen at the introitus. At the center of the doughnut is the urethral meatus, which shows gangrenous changes.

Infectious Diseases

Teresita A. Laude, M.D. and Binita R. Shah, M.D.

Varicella

SYNONYM   Chickenpox

DEFINITION

Varicella is an acute, highly contagious exanthematous illness caused by the varicella-zoster virus.

ETIOLOGY

Varicella-zoster virus, a member of the herpesvirus group.

EPIDEMIOLOGY

1. In temperate countries, varicella is a disease of childhood that occurs primarily in preschool and school children; in tropical and subtropical countries, it is more common in older children and adults.
2. Varicella is most commonly seen during late winter and early spring.
3. In the United States, an estimated 2.8 million cases occur annually.
4. Newborn infants may develop varicella if the mother contracted varicella within 5 days of delivery.

BOX 3–1   *Congenital Varicella Syndrome*

Seen in 2% of pregnancies when mother contracts varicella in the first trimester of pregnancy
Rarely seen after maternal zoster
Clinical features
   Hypoplasia of a limb
   Skin defect (zosteriform skin scarring)
   CNS abnormalities
      Cortical atrophy
      Mental retardation
   Ocular abnormalities
      Microphthalmia
      Cataract
      Chorioretinitis

PATHOGENESIS

1. Varicella is highly contagious. Secondary cases occur in 98% of susceptible persons exposed to an index case.
2. Primary infection occurs in the nasopharynx through droplet inoculation.
3. Local replication occurs in the nasopharynx.
4. Viremia and dissemination occur by circulating mononuclear cells.

CLINICAL FEATURES (see Table 3–1)

1. The incubation period is 14 to 16 days.
2. The disease is characterized by mild fever and constitutional symptoms in children.
3. It is more severe in adults and immunocompromised individuals.

LABORATORY

1. Tzanck test
   a. Procedure
      (1) Unroof a new vesicle.
      (2) Using the blunt end of a scalpel, scrape the base of the vesicle onto a glass slide.
      (3) Fix with alcohol by squeezing an alcohol swab onto the slide.
      (4) Air dry.
      (5) Stain with Giemsa or Wright reagent.
   b. Tzanck test is positive if:
      (1) It shows multinucleated giant cells with nuclei molded onto one another and balloon degeneration of epithelial cells.
      (2) It is not specific for varicella-zoster virus.
      (3) It is also positive in herpes simplex viral infection. The two cannot be differentiated by the Tzanck test.
2. Viral culture from a new vesicle

DIFFERENTIAL DIAGNOSIS

1. Herpes zoster with dissemination
2. Hand-foot-mouth disease
3. Eczema herpeticum
4. Mucha-Habermann disease

TREATMENT

1. Acyclovir is recommended for normal individuals 13 years old and older and for immunocompromised hosts.
2. To relieve pruritus and discomfort, colloidal oatmeal baths may be prescribed, as well as antipruritic lotions such as pramoxine.
3. Children with varicella should *not* receive salicylates because of their association with Reye syndrome.

PREVENTION

1. Active immunization
   a. Varicella vaccine (live attenuated vaccine)
   b. Now recommended for routine immunization
      (1) For healthy children 12 months to 13 years: a single dose
      (2) For persons over 13 years of age: two doses given 4 to 8 weeks apart
2. Passive immunoprophylaxis
   a. Varicella-zoster immune globulin (VZIG)
   b. Given to susceptible persons at risk of developing severe varicella. Examples include
      (1) Immunocompromised children
      (2) Neonates whose mothers experienced onset of varicella 5 days or less before delivery or within 48 hours after delivery
   c. Given as soon as possible after exposure (within 96 hours)

PROGNOSIS

In healthy children, varicella is a benign, self-limiting disease with a low rate of complications.

KEY POINTS

Varicella

- Varicella is more severe in individuals over 13 years of age.
- Infected varicella lesions may become the portal of entry for group A beta-hemolytic streptococcus (GABS), resulting in GABS invasive disease or streptococcal toxic shock syndrome, necrotizing fasciitis, or purpura fulminans.

TABLE 3–1
Clinical Features of Varicella

Skin Eruption

Centripetal distribution (more lesions are found on torso than on face and extremities)
Lesions also seen on scalp and mucous membranes
Lesions go through several stages:
  Papules
  Vesicles
  Pustules
  Followed by crusting
Classic lesion: a vesicle surrounded by erythema described as "a dew drop on a rose petal"
Different types of lesions may be seen together in the same anatomic area
Varying degrees of pruritus
Eruption lasts 5–7 days

Infectivity

Most contagious 1–2 days before and shortly after onset of rash
Lesions are infectious until they have turned into dried crusts

---

TABLE 3–2
Complications of Varicella

Most Common Complications

Secondary skin infection
  Examples: cellulitis, subcutaneous abscesses
  Pathogens: *Staphylococcus aureus;* group A beta-hemolytic *Streptococcus* (GABS)
Bronchopneumonia (more common in adults)

Other Less Common Complications

Lymphadenitis
Meningoencephalitis
Cerebellar ataxia
Reye syndrome
Reactive arthritis
Hemorrhagic chickenpox
Acute thrombocytopenia
Hepatitis
Myocarditis, pericarditis
Nephritis/nephrotic syndrome
Streptococcal toxic shock syndrome
Necrotizing fasciitis
Purpura fulminans

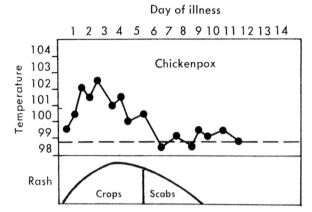

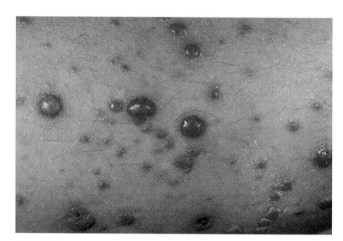

FIGURE 3-1. Schematic diagram illustrating the clinical course of a typical case of chickenpox. Crops of lesions appear and progress rapidly from macule to papule to vesicle to scabs. (From Katz SL et al (eds): Krugman's Infectious Diseases of Children, 10th ed. St. Louis, Mosby–Year Book, 1998.)

FIGURE 3-3. Centripetal distribution of varicella.

CHICKENPOX

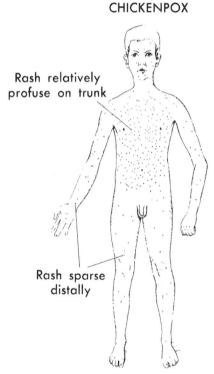

Rash relatively profuse on trunk

Rash sparse distally

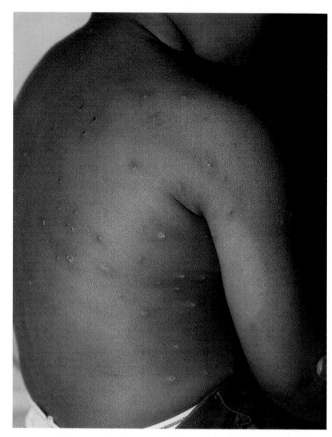

FIGURE 3-2. Schematic drawing illustrating the typical distribution of the rash of chickenpox. (From Katz SL et al (eds): Krugman's Infectious Diseases of Children, 10th ed. St. Louis, Mosby–Year Book, 1998.)

FIGURE 3-4. Lesions in different stages: papule, vesicle, pustule, crusted lesion.

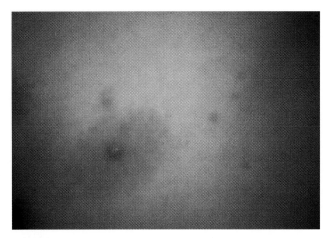

FIGURE 3–5. Classic varicella lesion: a "dew drop on a rose petal."

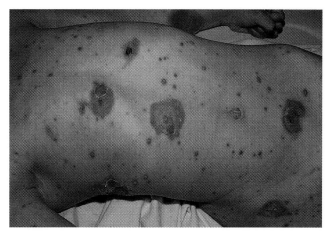

FIGURE 3–8. Bullous varicella resulting from secondary infection with *Staphylococcus aureus.*

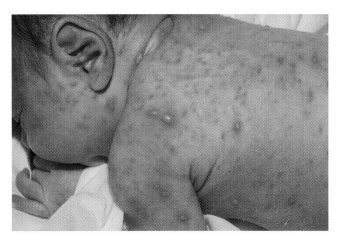

FIGURE 3–6. A 12-day-old newborn whose mother developed varicella 2 days before delivery.

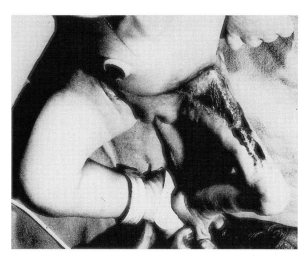

FIGURE 3–9. Congenital varicella syndrome illustrating cicatricial skin lesions and hypotrophic left lower limb. (From Srabstein JC, et al: Is there a congenital varicella syndrome? Pediatr 84:239, 1974.)

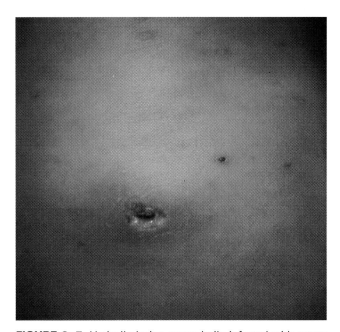

FIGURE 3–7. Varicella lesion secondarily infected with group A beta hemolytic Streptococcus (GABS) resulting in cellulitis.

Herpes Zoster

SYNONYM   Shingles

DEFINITION
An acute vesiculopustular eruption that occurs in a dermatomal distribution.

ETIOLOGY
The causative agent is varicella-zoster virus, a herpesvirus.

EPIDEMIOLOGY
It is more common in adults and immunocompromised hosts.

PATHOGENESIS
1. Herpes zoster is the localized recurrence of a varicella-zoster virus infection.
2. There is invariably a past history of varicella.
3. The virus is reactivated after lying dormant in a sensory ganglion.
4. Precipitating factors include:
   a. Lowered host immunity
   b. Radiation therapy
   c. Physical trauma
5. A young infant may develop herpes zoster if the mother had varicella during pregnancy.

INFECTIVITY
1. Between 1 and 3 weeks
2. A susceptible individual may contract varicella after exposure to a person with herpes zoster.

LABORATORY
1. Tzanck test (see p. 50)
2. Viral culture from a new vesicle

TABLE 3–3
Clinical Features of Herpes Zoster

Skin Lesions

Grouped vesicles on an erythematous base
Linear distribution
Site: along one or two dermatomes supplied by a spinal or cranial nerve
Lesions do *not* cross the midline of the body
Lesions may disseminate in immunocompromised individuals

Most Commonly Involved Dermatomes

Those supplied by thoracic spinal nerves (thorax)
Ophthalmic branch of the trigeminal nerve (forehead)

Pain

Minimal in children
Eruption may be preceded by tingling and hyperesthesia in adults

---

COMPLICATIONS
Postherpetic neuralgia (extremely rare in children).

BOX 3–2	*Ramsay Hunt Syndrome*

Herpes zoster affecting geniculate ganglion of otic nerve
Sites of eruption
  Pinna
  Auditory canal
  Anterior two thirds of tongue
Symptoms
  Bell's palsy
  Tinnitus
  Deafness
  Vertigo
  Decreased taste and hearing

TREATMENT
Acyclovir is indicated in immunocompromised individuals with herpes zoster.

KEY POINTS

Herpes Zoster
- The skin lesions consist of grouped vesicles in a unilateral dermatomal distribution.
- Herpes zoster may occur in a young infant if the mother had varicella during pregnancy.

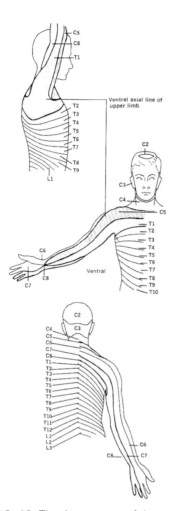

FIGURE 3–10. The dermatomes of the upper limb.

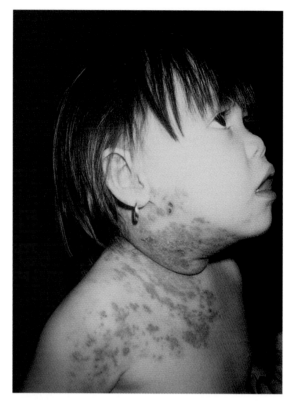

FIGURE 3–12. A 2-year-old girl with herpes zoster on C4 and C5 dermatomes. Her 7-month-old sibling contracted varicella from her.

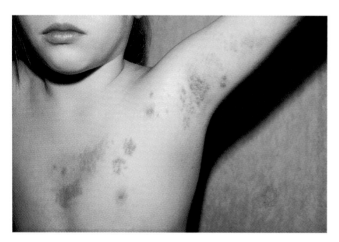

FIGURE 3–11. Herpes zoster involving the T1 dermatome. Lesions do not cross the midline.

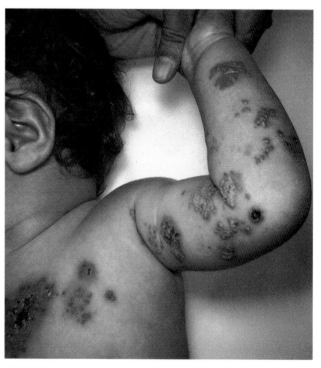

FIGURE 3–13. An 8-month-old infant with herpes zoster on C5 and C6 dermatomes. His mother had had varicella during the sixth month of pregnancy.

Herpes Simplex Infections

DEFINITION

Infections caused by herpes simplex virus that have a tendency to recur.

ETIOLOGY

The causative agent is *Herpesvirus hominis*, which consists of two closely related viruses:

1. Herpes simplex virus type 1 (HSV-1)
2. Herpes simplex virus type 2 (HSV-2)

EPIDEMIOLOGY

1. The disease may be seen in children of all age groups.
2. Recurrent orofacial herpes (fever blisters, cold sores) affects 25% to 40% of the American population.

PATHOGENESIS

Recurrence in HSV is explained by the following facts:

1. After an initial infection, the virus may remain quiescent in a sensory ganglion.
2. Reactivation resulting in clinical disease may follow a local rise in temperature such as that occurring during a febrile illness, sun exposure, or debilitating activities.

CLINICAL FEATURES

1. Most infections in children are subclinical.
2. The following are the forms of primary clinical infections:
   a. Herpetic gingivostomatitis (see Table 3–4)
   b. Herpetic dermatitis
      (1) Grouped vesicles on any skin surface
      (2) May invade the eye if the vesicles are periorbital, producing dendritic corneal ulcer.
      (3) Herpetic whitlow (on the fat pad of the digits)
      (4) May recur in the same site
      (5) Usually caused by HSV-1
   c. Herpetic vulvovaginitis
      (1) Painful ulcers on the skin and mucous membranes of the genitalia
      (2) May result from sexual abuse
      (3) Usually caused by HSV-2
   d. Eczema herpeticum (Kaposi varicelliform eruption; see p. 166)
      (1) Disseminated HSV infection on atopic dermatitis
      (2) Usually caused by HSV-1

LABORATORY

1. Tzanck test
   a. A rapid test that may be positive in 80% of herpes simplex infections
   b. Procedure
      (1) Unroof a new vesicle.
      (2) Using the blunt end of a scalpel, scrape the base of the vesicle onto a glass slide.
      (3) Fix with alcohol by squeezing an alcohol swab onto the slide.
      (4) Air dry.
      (5) Stain with Giemsa or Wright reagent.
   c. A positive test shows multinucleated giant cells with the nuclei molded onto each other and balloon degeneration of the epithelial cells.
2. Viral culture is more definitive.

TREATMENT

1. Herpetic gingivostomatitis
   a. Supportive therapy that includes antipyretics and dietary modifications (e.g., cool drinks, Popsicles, and soft diet)
   b. Oral anesthetic agents (e.g., lidocaine viscus) should *not* be used because they may be absorbed from the oral mucosa and carry a subsequent risk of toxicity.
2. Acyclovir given orally or intravenously for severe primary infections and in immunocompromised hosts.
3. Suppressive lower dose of acyclovir may be given in patients with frequently recurring infections.
4. Ophthalmologic consultation and/or prophylactic use of idoxuridine or trifluridine ophthalmic drops is recommended when the lesions are near the eye.

PROGNOSIS

Self-limiting in normal children

KEY POINTS

Herpes Simplex Infections

- The lesions are grouped vesicles.
- Tzanck test is a rapid test that may be positive in 80% of children with herpes simplex infections.

TABLE 3–4

Clinical Features of Acute Herpetic Gingivostomatitis

Usually caused by HSV-1
Most common form of HSV primary infection in children
Most common age: children 1–3 years of age
Lesions begin as vesicles, rapidly break down, and form
    shallow ulcers
  Ulcers: extremely painful, friable, and bleed easily
Sites: lips, tongue, buccal mucosa, gums, palate
Fever (often very high—up to 40°C)
Foul breath
Submaxillary lymphadenopathy
Inability to eat or drink
Self-limited illness; usually resolves in 4–7 days

Differential Diagnosis

Herpangina (coxsackievirus)
Acute tonsillopharyngitis (*Streptococcus pyogenes*)

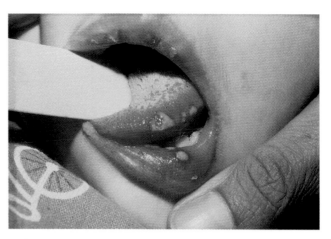

FIGURE 3–14. Herpetic gingivostomatitis.

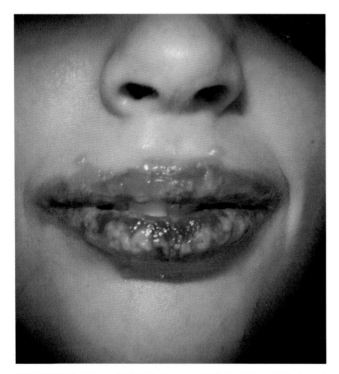

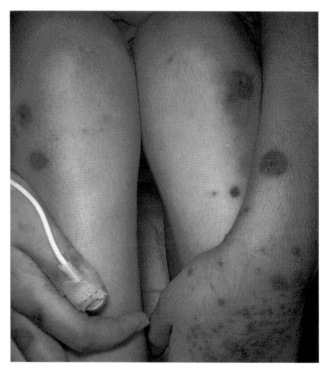

FIGURES 3–15 and 3–16. Herpes labialis. The child also developed erythema multiforme minor
(HSV is the most common cause of erythema multiforme).

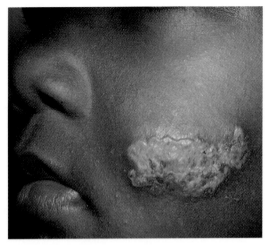

FIGURE 3–17. Herpetic vesicopustules that have become confluent.

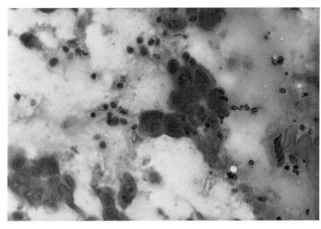

FIGURE 3–19. Positive Tzanck smear showing multinucleated giant cells with molding of the nuclei and ballooning of the epithelial cells. (Courtesy of Ed Heilman, M.D., State University of New York, Brooklyn, NY.)

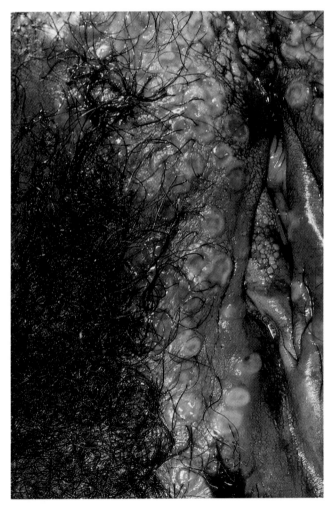

FIGURE 3–18. Herpetic vulvovaginitis in a sexually active adolescent.

Measles

SYNONYM   Rubeola

DEFINITION

A highly contagious disease characterized by an exanthem and an enanthem caused by the paramyxovirus.

ETIOLOGY

The causative agent is a paramyxovirus, an RNA virus.

BOX 3-3 *Koplik Spots*

Pathognomonic enanthem of measles

Seen 2 days before and 2 days after the rash appears

Absence does not exclude diagnosis (transient nature)

Common site: opposite lower molars; may spread to the rest of the mouth

Seen as white papular dots on an erythematous buccal mucosa

  Looks like: "salt grains sprinkled on a red background"

EPIDEMIOLOGY

1. Measles is now rare in developed countries because of successful universal immunization.
2. However, it still occurs in epidemics in developing countries, where it may be fatal in severely malnourished children.
3. The last outbreak in the United States occurred in 1990. In 1997, a total of 137 cases was reported, the lowest ever.

PATHOGENESIS

1. The organism is transmitted via respiratory droplets.
2. It replicates in the upper respiratory tract.
3. Viremia follows.

LABORATORY

1. Diagnosis is usually made from a typical clinical presentation.
2. Complete blood count shows leukopenia with a relative lymphocytosis.
3. A rise in measles antibody titers in samples drawn during the acute and convalescent stages may be demonstrated.
4. Cerebrospinal fluid examination in children in whom encephalitis is suspected shows
   a. Increased protein
   b. Normal glucose
   c. Mild pleocytosis with a predominance of lymphocytes

TREATMENT

1. Treatment is purely supportive.

BOX 3-4 *Measles and Vitamin A Therapy*

Currently recommended for children
  In developing countries
  In impoverished areas of developed countries
  Between 6 and 24 months of age who are hospitalized with measles-related complications
  With any of the following factors:
    Immunodeficiency
    Ophthalmologic evidence of vitamin A deficiency
    Impaired intestinal absorption
    Moderate to severe malnutrition including that associated with eating disorders
    Recent immigration from areas where there are high mortality rates for measles
Dose of vitamin A
  Single oral dose
    200,000 IU (age >1 year)
    100,000 IU (age 6–12 months)
  If there is ophthalmologic evidence of vitamin A deficiency
    Repeat dose next day
    Repeat dose at 4 weeks

---

2. Vitamin A therapy (see Box 3–4) in children with measles has been associated with a reduction in morbidity and mortality.

PREVENTION

1. Measles vaccine is given routinely (usually as measles-mumps-rubella [MMR] vaccine).
   a. First dose is given to healthy infants on or after their first birthday.
   b. Second dose is given at school entry (between 4 and 6 years of age).
2. Immune globulin (IG)
   a. IG is given to prevent or modify measles in susceptible persons.
      (1) Immunocompromised persons
      (2) Infants 6 months to 1 year of age
      (3) Infants less than 6 months (born to mothers without measles immunity)
      (4) Pregnant women
   b. IG should be given within 6 days of exposure.

PROGNOSIS

1. Self-limiting in normal children
2. May be fatal in malnourished children
3. Overall case-fatality rate in the United States has been less than 0.1% for many years.

KEY POINTS

Measles

- Measles is characterized by prominent prodromal symptoms of cough, coryza, and conjunctivitis (the three Cs).
- Confluence of the erythematous papules (morbilliform) is a significant feature of the eruption.

TABLE 3-5
Clinical Features of Measles

Incubation period: 10–12 days
Prominent prodrome
  Fever
  Three C's
    (1) Cough
    (2) Coryza
    (3) Conjunctivitis: exudative conjunctivitis, significant
      photophobia

Exanthem

Erythematous papular lesions
Start along hairline and proceed downward
Peak of eruption occurs on 3rd day (coincides with peak of
  fever/constitutional symptoms)
Rash is confluent in upper part of body
Rash resolves by 5th or 6th day
Branny desquamation and brown staining of skin follow

TABLE 3-6
Complications of Measles

Common Complications

Otitis media
Pneumonia
  Interstitial pneumonitis (measles virus)
  Bronchopneumonia (secondary bacterial infection)
Encephalomyelitis (incidence: 1 to 2 in 1000 cases of measles)
Laryngotracheobronchitis
Exacerbation of tuberculosis
Transient loss of hypersensitivity in tuberculin skin test

Rare Complications

Black measles (hemorrhagic measles)
Purpura fulminans
Disseminated intravascular coagulation
Subacute sclerosing panencephalitis

TABLE 3-7
Differential Diagnosis of Measles

Kawasaki disease
Scarlet fever
Drug eruptions
Meningococcemia
Rickettsial infections
Other viral exanthems
  Rubella
  Infectious mononucleosis
  Enteroviruses (coxsackievirus, echovirus)
  Roseola infantum

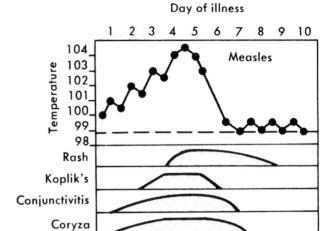

FIGURE 3-20. Schematic diagram of the clinical course of a typical case of measles. The rash appears 3 to 4 days after onset of the fever, conjunctivitis, coryza, and cough. Koplik spots develop 2 days before the rash. (From Katz SL et al (eds): Krugman's Infectious Diseases of Children, 10th ed. St. Louis, Mosby–Year Book, 1998.)

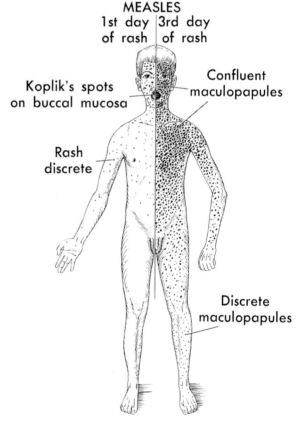

FIGURE 3-21. Schematic drawing of the development and distributin of measles rash. (From Katz SL et al (eds): Krugman's Infectious Diseases of Children, 10th ed. St. Louis, Mosby–Year Book 1998.)

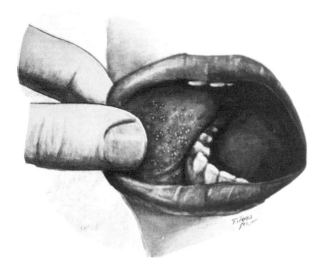

FIGURE 3-22. Koplik spots. (From Zahorsky J, Zahorsky TS: Synopsis of Pediatrics. St. Louis, CU Mosby, 1953.)

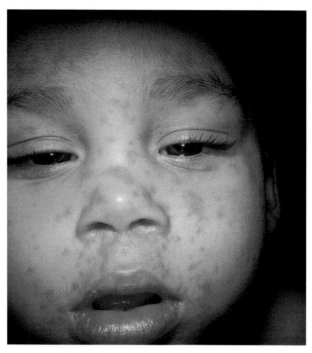

FIGURE 3-23. An 8-month-old child with fever, photophobia, coryza, conjunctivitis, and beginning rash of measles.

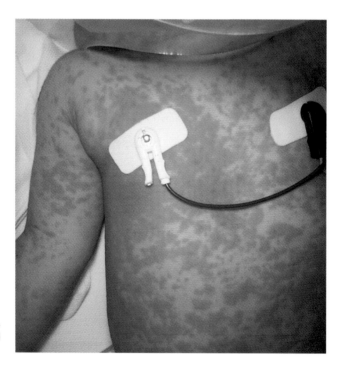

FIGURE 3-24. Morbilliform eruption (confluent, erythematous papules) on the torso and face. This child developed measles bronchopneumonia.

Rubella

SYNONYM   German Measles

DEFINITION

Rubella is a benign exanthematous infection with potentially devastating complications.

BOX 3–5   *Congenital Rubella Syndrome*

If a pregnant woman contracts rubella in the 1st trimester of pregnancy, there is a 20% chance that the baby may have congenital rubella syndrome.

FEATURES INCLUDE

Eye defects (cataract, glaucoma, microphthalmia, retinopathy; see Fig. 4–7 and Fig. 4–14)
Cardiac defects (patent ductus arteriosus, ventricular septal defect, pulmonic stenosis)
Deafness
Central nervous system (psychomotor retardation, microcephaly, mental retardation)
Bone lesions
Hepatosplenomegaly
Thrombocytopenia
Blueberry muffin lesions (represent sites of extramedullary hematopoiesis)
Interstitial pneumonitis

ETIOLOGY

The causative agent is a togavirus, an RNA virus.

EPIDEMIOLOGY

1. The incidence of rubella has declined dramatically because of successful vaccination, but outbreaks have occurred among unimmunized young adults.

2. Recent surveys have shown that 10% of young adults are susceptible to rubella.

PATHOGENESIS

1. The organism is acquired from infected respiratory droplets.
2. It replicates in the respiratory tract.
3. Viremia follows.

LABORATORY

1. Isolation of the virus from the nasopharynx in appropriate tissue culture
2. Serologic studies
   a. Demonstration of rubella-specific IgM
   b. Fourfold rise in IgG antibody titer from the acute phase to convalescence
      (1) Enzyme-linked immunosorbent assay (ELISA)
      (2) Hemagglutinin inhibition (HAI)
      (3) Complement fixation (CF)
      (4) Neutralization

TREATMENT

Supportive

PREVENTION

Rubella vaccine (incorporated in the MMR vaccine) is given to children between 12 and 15 months of age and repeated at 4 to 6 years of age.

PROGNOSIS

Recovery with no sequelae is common in uncomplicated postnatal rubella.

KEY POINTS

Rubella

- Rubella is a nondescript infection that can easily be missed.
- Prominent enlargement of the postauricular, posterior cervical, and suboccipital lymph nodes occurs.

TABLE 3–8
Clinical Features of Rubella

Incubation period: 14–21 days
Prodromal symptoms
  Absent in children
  In adolescents/adults: low-grade fever and malaise (1–4 days)
Exanthem
  Pink maculopapules
  Start on face and neck, progress to trunk and extremities
  Eruption becomes generalized within 24–48 hours
  Lesions are discrete
  By 3rd day
    Rash on face has disappeared
    Only extremities may be involved
  Eruption may be resolved by end of the 3rd day
  No desquamation
Pathognomonic sign
  Enlargement of lymph nodes
    Postauricular
    Posterior cervical
    Suboccipital

TABLE 3–9
Complications of Postnatal Rubella

Arthritis

More common in adolescents, adults
Incidence: 15% to 30%
One or more large or small joints are involved
Spontaneously resolves within 5–10 days

Encephalitis

Extremely rare
Incidence: 1 in 6000 cases

Purpura

May be thrombocytopenic or nonthrombocytopenic

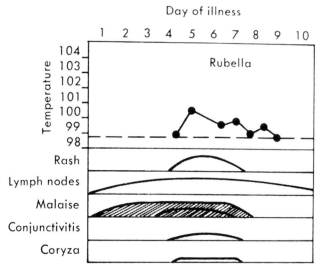

FIGURE 3-25. Schematic diagram illustrating the typical course of rubella in children and adults. Lymph nodes begin to enlarge 3 to 4 days before the rash appears. Prodromal symptoms (malaise) are minimal in children (*shaded area*). In adults there may be a 3- to 4-day prodrome (*hatched area*). Conjunctivitis and coryza, if present, are usually minimal and accompany the rash. (From Katz SL et al (eds): Krugman's Infectious Diseases of Children, 10th ed. St. Louis, Mosby–Year Book, 1998.)

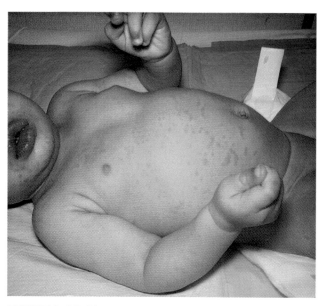

FIGURE 3-27. Discrete erythematous papules.

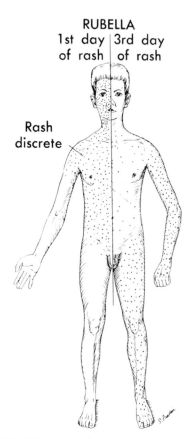

FIGURE 3-26. Schematic drawing illustrating the development and distribution of rubella rash. (From Katz SL et al (eds): Krugman's Infectious Diseases of Children, 10th ed. St. Louis, Mosby–Year Book, 1998.)

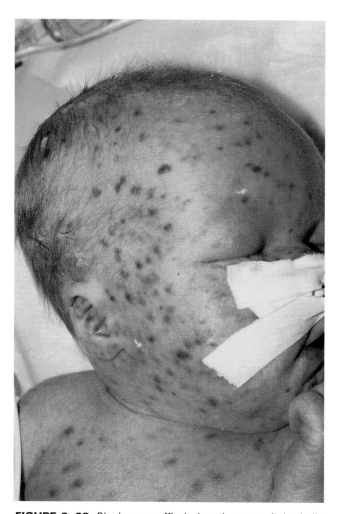

FIGURE 3-28. Blueberry muffin lesions in congenital rubella syndrome. They represent extramedullary sites of hematopoiesis. (Courtesy of Nathan Rudolph, M.D. State University of New York, Brooklyn, NY.)

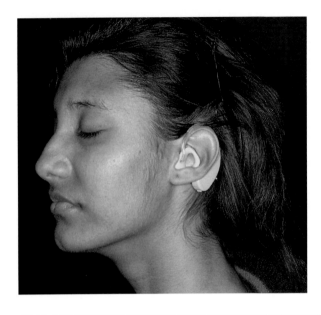

FIGURE 3-29. Microcephaly and deafness in a girl with congenital rubella syndrome.

Mumps

SYNONYM   Epidemic Parotitis

DEFINITION

Mumps is a systemic disease characterized by swelling of the salivary glands, particularly the parotid glands.

ETIOLOGY

A paramyxovirus

EPIDEMIOLOGY

1. It occurs throughout childhood.
2. The incidence of mumps has declined remarkably because of successful vaccination.

PATHOGENESIS

1. Humans are the only known natural hosts for this virus.
2. It is acquired by direct contact with the saliva of an infected person.
3. Viremia occurs with localization to the salivary glands.

CLINICAL FEATURES

1. Incubation period: 16 to 18 days
2. Painful tender swelling of the parotid glands
3. Although the disease involves both parotids (and other salivary glands), a unilateral presentation is not uncommon.
4. Inflammation of the opening of the Stensen ducts in the buccal mucosa.
5. Petechial eruption of the lower extremities and presternal edema have been reported in severe cases.
6. Communicability: From 1 to 2 days before to 9 days after the onset of parotid swelling.

LABORATORY

1. Isolation of the virus in tissue culture from the saliva, urine, or spinal fluid

2. Serologic antibody testing: complement fixation test
3. Elevation of serum amylase levels
   a. Abnormal in about 70% of cases of parotitis
   b. Peak values are seen during the 1st week of illness
   c. Values return to normal by the 2nd to 3rd weeks

COMPLICATIONS

1. Orchitis and epididymitis occur in adolescents and young adults (14% to 35%); sterility is rare.
2. Other rare complications
   a. Arthritis
   b. Encephalitis
   c. Pancreatitis
   d. Myocarditis
   e. Deafness
   f. Nephritis
   g. Thyroiditis

TREATMENT

Supportive

PREVENTION

Mumps vaccine is given to children between 12 and 15 months of age and repeated at 4 to 6 years of age. It is incorporated usually in the MMR vaccine.

PROGNOSIS

Good

KEY POINTS

Mumps

- Mumps presents as tender parotid swelling.
- Orchitis and epididymitis may be a complication in adolescent and young adult males.

TABLE 3–10
Differential Diagnosis of Mumps

Anterior cervical adenitis
Preauricular adenitis
Suppurative parotitis (e.g., *Staphylococcus aureus*)
Parotitis caused by other viruses
    Human immunodeficiency virus
    Parainfluenza virus
    Enteroviruses
Other causes of parotid swelling
    Sarcoidosis
    Sjögren syndrome
    Parotid duct stone
    Chronic wind instrument use

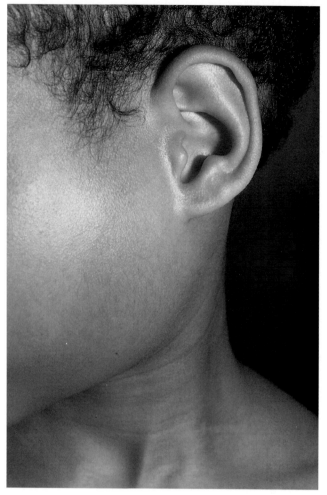

FIGURE 3–30. Parotid swelling of mumps.

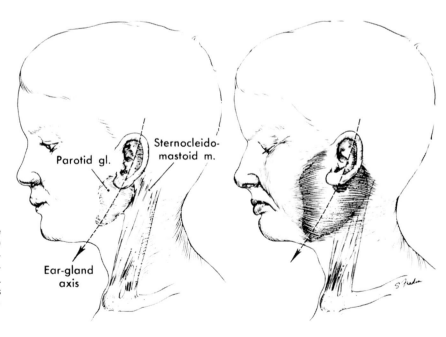

FIGURE 3–31. Schematic drawing of the parotid gland infected with mumps (*right*) compared with normal gland (*left*). Enlarged cervical lymph node is usually posterior to the imaginary line. (From Katz SL et al (eds): Krugman's Infectious Diseases of Children, 10th ed. St. Louis, Mosby–Year Book, 1998.)

Infectious Mononucleosis (IM)

DEFINITION

Infectious mononucleosis is a self-limited lymphoproliferative disease caused by the Epstein-Barr virus (EBV).

ETIOLOGY

Epstein-Barr virus, a DNA virus, belongs to the herpes group of viruses.

BOX 3-6	*Differential Diagnosis of Infectious Mononucleosis*

Streptococcal pharyngitis
Infectious mononucleosis-like illness caused by cytomegalovirus
Diphtheria
Leukemia
Other viral exanthems (e.g., rubella)
Viral hepatitis
Acquired toxoplasmosis
Kawasaki disease

EPIDEMIOLOGY

1. It occurs in all age groups but is usually unrecognized in infants and young children.
2. It presents in a more classic way in adolescents and young adults.
3. Period of communicability: indeterminate

LABORATORY

1. Atypical lymphocytosis on peripheral smears
   a. Very characteristic finding
   b. IM: High number (>10%) of atypical lymphocytes
   c. Other viral infections (e.g., rubella, hepatitis): less than 10% of atypical lymphocytes
2. Monospot test (heterophile) is negative in young children less than 4 years of age
3. Serology (see Table 3–12)

TREATMENT

1. Supportive therapy; self-limited illness in the majority of children
2. For upper airway obstruction (as indicated)
   a. Nasopharyngeal airway
   b. Prednisone
3. Corticosteroid therapy may be indicated for severe disease
   a. Hematologic complications
   b. Neurologic complications
   c. Cardiac complications
4. Family and patient education
   a. Avoid contact sports until spleen size has returned to normal.
   b. Seek immediate medical attention if the following occur:
      (1) Sudden onset of left-sided abdominal pain
      (2) Signs of peritoneal irritation (e.g., vomiting, pain)
      (3) Signs of hemorrhage (e.g., pallor, lethargy, fatigue)

KEY POINTS

Infectious Mononucleosis

- Triad of fever, exudative pharyngitis, and cervical adenitis
- In young children, IM may be vague in presentation, and the Monospot test may be negative.

TABLE 3–11
Clinical Features of Infectious Mononucleosis

Incubation period: 30–50 days
Fever
Sore throat
Exudative pharyngitis (>50% of cases)
Associated GABS pharyngitis (about 25% of cases)
Cervical lymphadenopathy
Hepatomegaly, icteric hepatitis
Splenomegaly: Moderate enlargement (about 50% of cases)
Skin rash
  Seen in 10% to 15% of cases
  Increased to 40% if penicillin or its derivatives is given inadvertently
  Morbilliform or scarlatiniform
Periorbital eyelid edema
Palatal petechiae
Central nervous system manifestations (see Table 3–14)

TABLE 3–12
Serum EBV Antibodies in EBV Infection

Infection	Anti-VCA IgG	Anti-VCA IgM	Anti-EA (D)	Anti-EBNA
No previous infection	0	0	0	0
Acute infection	+	+	+/0	0
Recent infection	+	+/0	+/0	+/0
Past infection	+	0	0	0

VCA, Viral capsid antigen; EA (D), early antigen diffuse staining; EBNA, Epstein-Barr nuclear antigen
From American Academy of Pediatrics: 1997 Red Book. American Academy of Pediatrics, Elk Grove Village, IL. 24th ed, p. 201.

TABLE 3–13
Complications of Infectious Mononucleosis

Upper airway obstruction
Splenic rupture → hemorrhage → shock → death
Hematologic
   Thrombocytopenia
   Agranulocytosis
   Hemolytic anemia
   Aplastic anemia
Disseminated lymphoproliferative disease
Chronic fatigue syndrome

TABLE 3–14
Infectious Mononucleosis: Central Nervous System Features

Encephalitis
Aseptic meningitis
Guillain-Barré syndrome
"Alice in Wonderland" syndrome
Transverse myelitis
Acute cerebellar ataxia
Cranial nerve palsies
Optic neuritis
Acute hemiplegia
Peripheral neuropathy

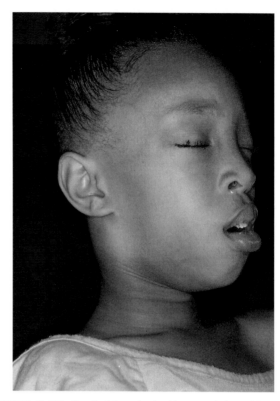

FIGURE 3–33. Cervical lymphadenitis, mouth breathing, and periorbital swelling.

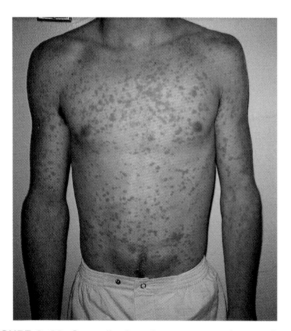

FIGURE 3–32. Generalized erythematous papular eruption of infectious mononucleosis precipitated by oral penicillin intake.

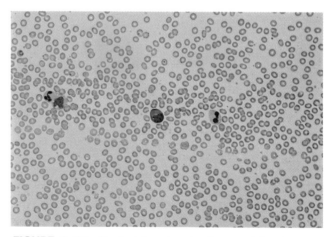

FIGURE 3–34. Atypical lymphocytes in a peripheral smear from a patient with infectious mononucleosis. Atypical lymphocytes are large and have abundant cytoplasm and varying nuclear shapes; some may show vacuoles. Indentation of the cytoplasm by a red blood cell is also seen.

Gianotti-Crosti Syndrome

SYNONYM   Papular Acrodermatitis of
                        Childhood

DEFINITION

Gianotti-Crosti syndrome is a benign disorder characterized by a distinct skin eruption.

EPIDEMIOLOGY

1. Affects infants and young children
2. Seen primarily in late summer to early fall

BOX 3-7   *Etiology of Gianotti-Crosti Syndrome*

Europe and Japan: Most common agent: hepatitis B virus
United States: Most common agents: Epstein-Barr virus, coxsackievirus

---

PATHOGENESIS

Unknown

LABORATORY

1. There may be mildly abnormal results on liver function tests.
2. Viral studies
    a. Hepatitis B virus (HBV) surface antigen
    b. EBV antibodies (see Table 3–12)

c. Culture from rectal and nasopharyngeal swabs for coxsackievirus

DIFFERENTIAL DIAGNOSIS

1. Papular urticaria
2. Other viral exanthems (e.g., coxsackie virus, echovirus)
3. Contact dermatitis

TREATMENT

None

KEY POINT

Gianotti-Crosti Syndrome

- The eruption is distinct, consisting of dense lentil-shaped, flesh-colored to slightly erythematous papules (2 to 4 mm in diameter) distributed over the face and extremities, with sparing of the trunk.

TABLE 3–15
Clinical Features of Gianotti-Crosti Syndrome

Skin lesions
   Distinct eruption
   Flesh-colored to slightly erythematous papules
   Dense, lentil-shaped
   Size: 2–4 mm
   Distribution: acral parts of body
      Face
      Upper and lower extremities
      Sparing of torso
   Eruption may last 2–6 weeks
Child otherwise asymptomatic

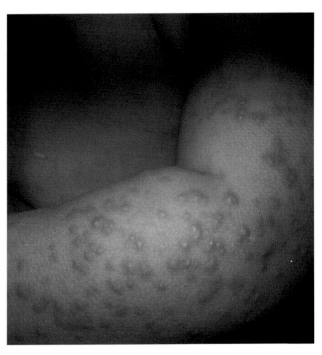 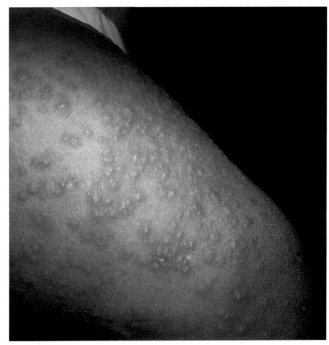

FIGURES 3–35 and 3–36. Dense lentil-shaped papules on the arms and legs of a child with Gianotti-Crosti syndrome. The torso was spared.

Roseola Infantum

SYNONYMS   Exanthem Subitum
              Sixth Disease

DEFINITION

An acute infection of infants characterized by a rash that appears after 3 to 4 days of high fever.

BOX 3-8	*Roseola Infantum*

Affects infants between 6 and 24 months of age
Appearance of a rash with defervescence

ETIOLOGY

1. The most common etiologic agent is human herpesvirus-6 (HHV-6).
2. Some cases are caused by human herpesvirus-7 (HHV-7).

EPIDEMIOLOGY

Infants 6 to 24 months of age are most commonly affected.

LABORATORY

1. Serology: Anti-HHV-6 immunoglobulin M (IgM), anti-HHV-7 IgM; IgG seroconversion
2. Polymerase chain reaction (PCR) demonstration of HHV-6 DNA

COMPLICATIONS

1. Febrile seizure during the prodromal stage (8%)
2. Encephalitis (very rare)

TREATMENT

Symptomatic

PROGNOSIS

Excellent

KEY POINT

Roseola Infantum

- A distinct sequence of 3 to 4 days of high fever followed by a nondescript eruption that lasts briefly.

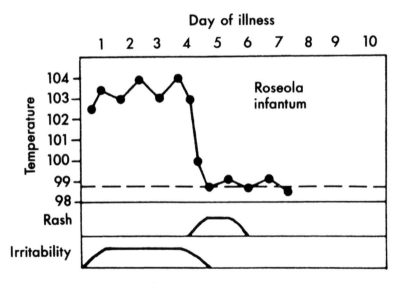

FIGURE 3-37. Schematic diagram illustrating the typical clinical course of roseola infantum. Between the third and fourth day, the temperature drops to normal, and a maculopapular eruption appears. (From Krugman PR: Infectious Diseases of Children, 9th ed. St. Louis, Mosby–Year Book, 1992.)

TABLE 3–16
Clinical Features of Roseola Infantum

Incubation period: 7–15 days
Prodrome
  High, unremitting fever for 3–6 days
  Infant looks well
  Bulging anterior fontanel (26%)
  Lymphadenopathy (cervical, occipital)
Rash
  Appears after temperature drops precipitously on 4th to 5th
    day. Rarely, rash appears before fever has subsided
    completely or not until after 1 afebrile day
  Discrete
  Pink
  Maculopapules
  Distribution
    Trunk
    Neck
    Few on extremities
    Lasts several hours to 2 days
  Clears completely without pigmentation or desquamation

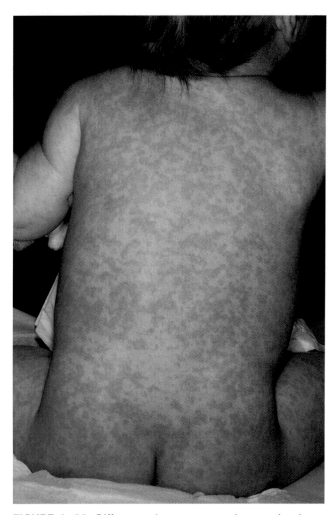

FIGURE 3–39. Diffuse erythematous papular eruption in an 11-month-old infant after 3 days of high fever.

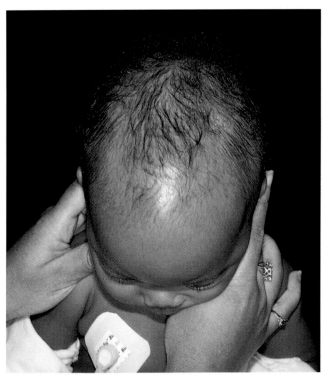

FIGURE 3–38. Bulging fontanel in an infant who was highly febrile and later developed a rash.

Erythema Infectiosum

SYNONYM   Fifth Disease

DEFINITION

A childhood exanthematous disease occurring in patients with primary human parvovirus (HPV) B19 infection.

ETIOLOGY

Human parvovirus B19, a DNA virus

EPIDEMIOLOGY

1. It can occur in children of all ages but is more common in school children.
2. Adults who are exposed to children, such as teachers and pediatricians, are at risk also.

3. Rare in African-American children
4. More common in late winter and early spring

PATHOGENESIS

Infection is spread by respiratory droplets during the prodrome.

CLINICAL FEATURES (see Box 3-9)

1. Constitutional symptoms (fever, coryza, malaise) are absent or very minimal.
2. Adults may present with no rash or an atypical rash and with or without recurrent arthralgia or arthritis.
3. Papular-purpuric "gloves and socks" (see Fig. 3-42) syndrome, a rare syndrome seen in older children and adolescents, is characterized by petechiae on the hands and feet that appear in a distinct gloves and socks distribution.

LABORATORY

1. Anti-HPV B19 IgM antibodies
2. IgG seroconversion

TREATMENT

Supportive

PROGNOSIS

Excellent

BOX 3-9	*Erythema Infectiosum*

Three stages of rash
1. Slapped cheek appearance (1 to 4 days)
2. Erythematous papular eruption over upper and lower extremities spreading to trunk; assumes a lace-like or reticulated appearance as it fades
3. Recurrent evanescent stage (for weeks or sometimes months) is precipitated by a variety of skin irritants such as:
   Sunlight
   Vigorous exercise
   Hot showers

KEY POINTS

Erythema Infectiosum

- Distinct eruption starts with a "slapped cheek" appearance followed by a lacy exanthem on the torso and extremities.
- Hydrops fetalis may be an outcome of maternal human parvovirus B19 infection. The virus is not teratogenic.

TABLE 3-17
Complications of Erythema Infectiosum

Infection during pregnancy leads to intrauterine infection of fetus
    May result in fetal wastage
    May result in hydrops fetalis
    Risk is <10%
    Can be diagnosed by serial ultrasound examinations
Aplastic crisis (see p. 260)
    Occurs in patients with sickle cell disease
    Occurs with other forms of congenital hemolytic anemia

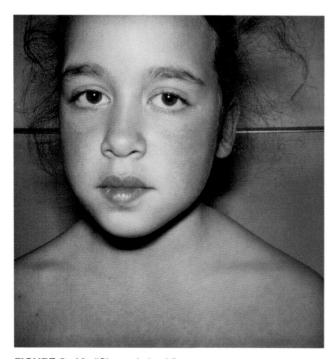

FIGURE 3-40. "Slapped cheek" appearance.

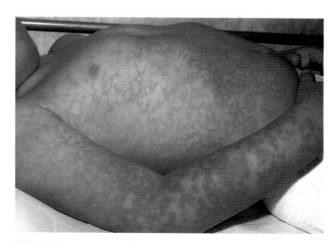

FIGURE 3-41. Reticulated erythematous papular eruption.

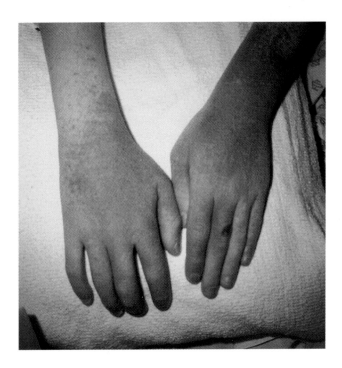

FIGURE 3–42. Papular-purpuric "gloves and socks" syndrome in a 10-year-old child. IgM antibodies to human parvovirus B19 were found.

Hand-Foot-Mouth Disease

DEFINITION
A childhood infection caused by coxsackievirus that is commonly seen during late summer or early fall.

ETIOLOGY
Coxsackie viruses A16, A5, A6, and A10

EPIDEMIOLOGY
1. More common in children during late summer and early fall
2. May occur in outbreaks

PATHOGENESIS
Route of infection is gastrointestinal.

CLINICAL FEATURES (see Box 3–10)
1. Incubation period: 7 days
2. Very mild constitutional symptoms: fever, malaise, diarrhea

LABORATORY
1. Viral culture from the vesicle, oropharyngeal and rectal swabs
2. Rise in neutralizing antibody titer

TREATMENT
Symptomatic

BOX 3–10	*Hand-Foot-Mouth Disease*

SKIN LESIONS

Oval gray-roofed vesicles with erythematous rims

Distributed bilaterally and symmetrically

On the sides of the feet, soles, hands, palms, and mouth (buccal mucosa, tongue, lips)

These three anatomic areas need *not all* be affected

Lesions last 7–10 days

In young infants, nonvesicular papular lesions may also be seen on the buttocks, upper thighs, and knees.

PROGNOSIS
Excellent

KEY POINT

Hand-Foot-Mouth Disease

■ Although lesions are commonly distributed over the hands, feet, and mouth, they may also occur outside those areas, especially in young infants.

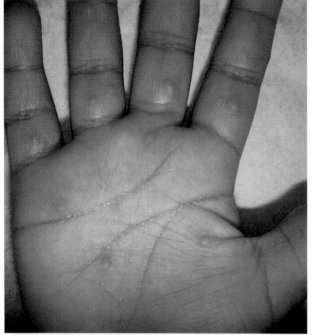

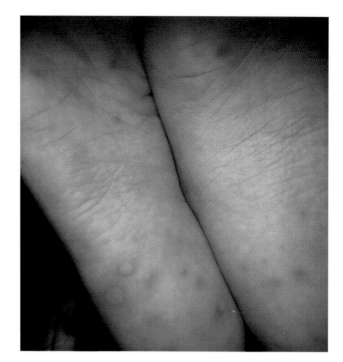

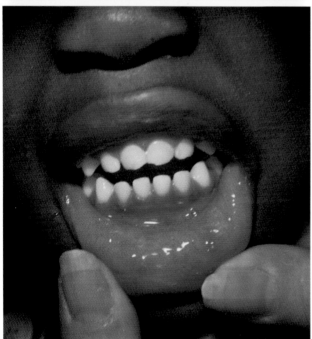

FIGURES 3–43, 3–44, and 3–45. Hand-foot-mouth disease. Vesicles on the hands, feet, and mouth.

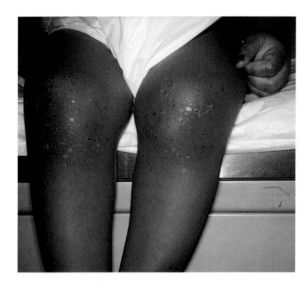

FIGURE 3–46. Hand-foot-mouth disease. A young infant with papules on the knees as well as vesicles on the hands, feet, and mouth.

Herpangina

DEFINITION

A characteristic enanthem produced by several enteroviruses

ETIOLOGY

Coxsackieviruses A1 through A10, A16, and A22, coxsackieviruses B1 through B5, echoviruses 3, 9, 16, 17, 25, and 30

EPIDEMIOLOGY

1. Children between 3 and 10 years are commonly affected.
2. Seen during summer or early fall.

LABORATORY

1. Viral culture: nasopharyngeal and rectal swabs
2. Serologic antibody testing

TREATMENT

Symptomatic

PROGNOSIS

Excellent

KEY POINT

Herpangina

- Lesions are microvesicles seen on the posterior part of the mouth.

TABLE 3–18
Clinical Features of Herpangina

Constitutional symptoms
  Fever, vomiting, sore throat, dysphagia
Lesions
  Tiny vesicles and/or ulcers
  Most common sites
    Posterior part of mouth
    Soft palate
    Uvula
    Anterior tonsillar pillars
  Occasionally
    Tonsils
    Posterior pharynx
    Buccal mucosa
Lesions last 1 week

TABLE 3–19
Differential Diagnosis of Herpangina

Herpetic gingivostomatitis
  Lesions consist of shallow ulcers
  Sites: tongue, gums, buccal mucosa, *anterior part of mouth*
Hand-foot-mouth disease
  Vesicles on hands, feet, mouth

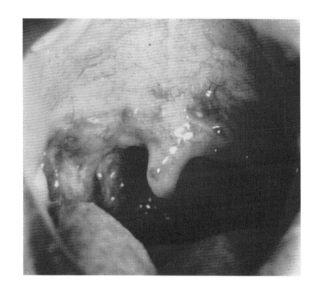

FIGURE 3-47. Herpangina. Tiny vesicles on the soft palate, uvula, and anterior tonsillar pillars. (Courtesy of Guinter Kahn, M.D., Miami, FL.)

Molluscum Contagiosum

DEFINITION

Intraepidermal tumors of the skin caused by infection with the molluscum contagiosum virus

ETIOLOGY

Molluscum contagiosum virus is a pox (DNA) virus.

EPIDEMIOLOGY

1. More common in children
2. Mildly contagious by direct contact

LABORATORY

Microscopic examination of the material squeezed out of the delling or umbilication, stained with Wright or Giemsa stain, shows intracytoplasmic inclusion (molluscum) bodies.

DIFFERENTIAL DIAGNOSIS

1. Milia: pinpoint white papules on sites of previous skin injury
2. Flat warts: flat-topped multiple papules commonly seen on the face

TREATMENT

1. Depending on the number and size of lesions, the age of the patient, and the availability of treatment, any of the following may be used:

   a. Conservative: no treatment for lesions around the eye
   b. Tretinoin gel or solution for small individual lesions
   c. Cantharone solution (a vesicant) for individual lesions
   d. Manual curettage of big lesions preceded by eutectic mixture of local anesthetics (EMLA) cream
   e. Cryotherapy with liquid nitrogen
2. Procedures c–e above are reserved for older children and are performed in a dermatologist's office.
3. In a dark-skinned child, postinflammatory hypopigmentation may result.

PROGNOSIS

Self-limiting in 2 to 3 years

KEY POINTS

Molluscum Contagiosum

- A benign infection of the skin that may be self-limiting
- Disseminated lesions may herald immune deficiency
- Painful treatment (manual curettage, cryotherapy) should be reserved for older children

TABLE 3–20
Clinical Features of Molluscum Contagiosum

Skin Lesions

Asymptomatic papules
Size: 2–5 mm
Papules with central umbilication (may be absent in small
  lesions)
Multiple
Dome-shaped
Discrete
Flesh-colored
Waxy

Most Common Distribution

Face
Neck
Upper torso

Other Features

Conjunctivitis with lesions located on or near the eyelids
Disseminated form may be seen in HIV infection
Genital lesions may be acquired from sexual activity
Lesions involute faster after they are irritated

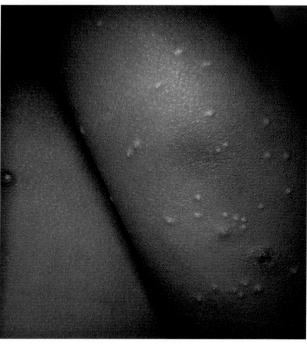

FIGURE 3–49. Numerous small lesions.

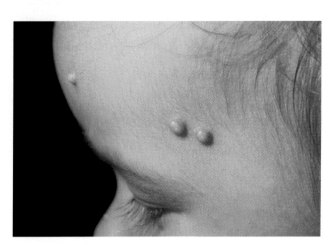

FIGURE 3–48. Large lesions of molluscum contagiosum.

Warts

SYNONYM   Verrucae

DEFINITION

Warts are intraepidermal tumors of the skin caused
by infection with the human papilloma virus (HPV).

ETIOLOGY

1. HPV, a DNA virus
2. Specific strains are trophic to regional areas.

EPIDEMIOLOGY

Except for condyloma acuminata, warts are more
common in children.

PATHOGENESIS

Virus may be spread by direct contact or autoinoculation.

CLINICAL FEATURES

1. Incubation period: 2 to 3 months
2. Clinical variants (see Table 3–21)

LABORATORY

HPV typing by in situ hybridization is not practical.

TREATMENT

1. Conservative—no treatment; spontaneous involution of most warts occurs within 2 years.
2. Preparations containing salicylic acid and lactic
   acid are applied either as a solution or as patches.
3. Tretinoin gel is applied nightly and washed in the
   morning (for flat warts).
4. Oral cimetidine 30 mg/kg/day in three divided
   doses for 3 months can be used for recalcitrant
   warts.

5. Twenty percent podophyllin in tincture of benzoin applied weekly can be used for anogenital warts. This agent must be washed off after 3 to 6 hours in a young child.
6. Refer to a dermatologist for any of the following:
   a. Cryotherapy with liquid nitrogen
   b. Electrodesiccation
7. Refer to a child protective agency if child abuse is suspected.

PROGNOSIS

Good

TABLE 3–21
Clinical Features of Warts

Clinical Variants
　Common wart (verruca vulgaris)
　　Discrete
　　Flesh-colored
　　Single or multiple papules with a rough surface
　　More common on the hands but may occur anywhere
　Flat wart (verruca plana)
　　Grouped, flat-topped
　　Flesh-colored or pigmented papules with smooth surface
　　Common on the face
　Anogenital wart (condyloma acuminata)
　　Cauliflowerlike, or
　　Pink filiform sessile papules with a rough surface
　　May be acquired from birth canal
　　May result from sexual abuse
　Plantar wart
　　Painful
　　Grows inward into sole of foot
　Periungual wart
　　Around the nail

KEY POINTS

Warts

- Warts are a benign infection of the skin, self-limiting in many cases.
- Condyloma acuminata may be acquired either perinatally from the maternal birth canal or from sexual abuse.
- Cimetidine given orally for 3 months may be useful for recalcitrant multiple warts.

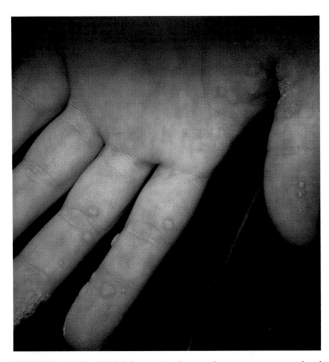

FIGURE 3–51. Multiple warts in an immunocompromised child.

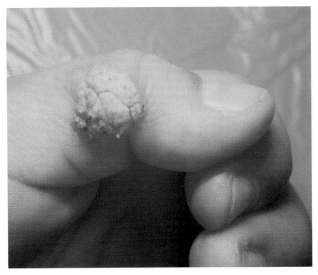

FIGURE 3–50. Verruca vulgaris (common wart) on the thumb of a child.

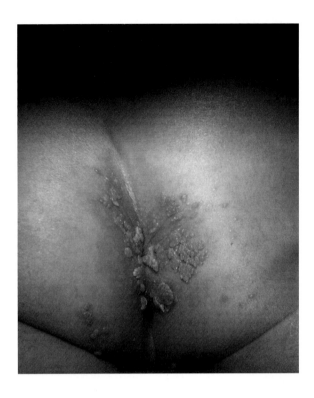

FIGURE 3–52. Condylomata acuminata in a 2-year-old child (see also Fig. 2–19).

Human Immunodeficiency Virus (HIV) Infection

DEFINITION

HIV infection is a disease that has a broad spectrum of clinical manifestations and a varied clinical course.

ETIOLOGY/PATHOGENESIS

1. It is caused by the human immunodeficiency virus, type 1 (HIV-1), a retrovirus.
2. Less commonly caused by HIV-2 (uncommon in the United States; more common in West Africa)
3. The predominant modes of transmission of infection are:
   a. Sexual contact
   b. Intravenous (from contaminated needles)
   c. Perinatal (maternal-infant transmission)
   d. Breastfeeding

EPIDEMIOLOGY

1. Acquired immunodeficiency syndrome (AIDS) in children accounts for 2% of all AIDS cases in the United States. This figure is increasing.
2. One or both parents of most infected children are infected themselves.
3. A few cases of pediatric HIV infection have resulted from sexual abuse.
4. The risk of infection for an infant born to an HIV-seropositive mother is estimated to be 15% to 20%. This figure is much less if the mother received antiretroviral therapy.

CLINICAL FEATURES

The incubation period is months to years—3 years for perinatally infected children (see also Tables 3–22 and 3–23).

LABORATORY

1. Screening: enzyme-linked immunosorbent assay (ELISA) serologic testing
2. If ELISA is positive, confirm with Western blot test
3. Both of above tests may be positive in the first 18 months of life because of maternally acquired antibodies. In young infants, the following are more reliable:
   a. HIV culture
   b. HIV polymerase chain reaction (PCR)
   c. HIV antigen (p24) detection assay
4. Serial CD4 + T-lymphocyte count is used to follow the state of immune deficiency.

DIFFERENTIAL DIAGNOSIS

1. Congenital immunodeficiency syndromes
2. HIV infection must be considered in any child
   a. Who presents with the findings listed in Tables 3–22 and 3–23 that cannot be readily explained
   b. Who presents with an opportunistic infection
   c. Who presents with a skin rash that is:
      (1) Atypical
      (2) Severe
      (3) Recurrent
      (4) Difficult to treat

TREATMENT

1. Antiretroviral therapy
   a. Azidothymidine (AZT)
   b. Dideoxyinosine (DDI)
   c. Dideoxycytidine (DDC)
2. Protease inhibitors
3. IV gamma globulin
4. Prophylaxis against *Pneumocystis carinii* pneumonia: trimethoprim-sulfamethoxazole
   a. All infants up to 12 months old who are HIV-infected
   b. HIV-infected children 1 to 5 years of age in whom the CD4 + T-lymphocyte count is less than 500 cells/uL
   c. HIV-infected children over 5 years of age in whom the CD4 + T-lymphocyte count is less than 200 cells/uL

5. Specific therapy for coexisting infections—e.g., acyclovir for herpes simplex virus infection
6. Supportive

PROGNOSIS

With the newer antiretroviral drugs and protease inhibitors, more children with perinatally acquired HIV infection are surviving infancy.

KEY POINTS

HIV Infection

- The rash in HIV may present in one of four ways: (1) atypical, (2) severe, (3) recurrent, or (4) difficult to treat.
- Opportunistic and nonopportunistic infections are common.

TABLE 3–22
Clinical Features of HIV Infection

Most common findings
   Failure to thrive
   Generalized lymphadenopathy
   Hepatosplenomegaly
   Anemia
   Developmental delay
   Oral candidiasis
   Parotitis
   Recurrent bacterial infections
   Opportunistic infections
   Lymphoid interstitital pneumonitis

TABLE 3–23
Skin Manifestations of HIV Infection

Seborrheic dermatitis
Disseminated molluscum contagiosum
Herpes simplex infections
Varicella-zoster infections
Crusted scabies
Onychomycosis
Bacillary angiomatosis

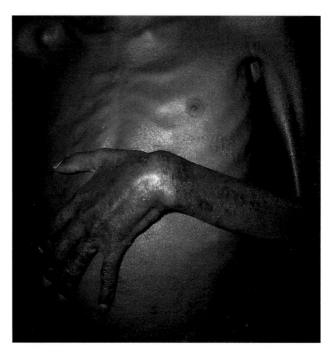

FIGURE 3–53. Severe wasting in a child with AIDS.

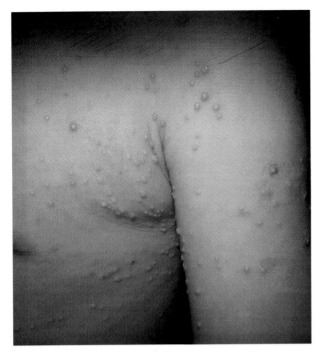

FIGURE 3-54. HIV infection. Disseminated molluscum contagiosum

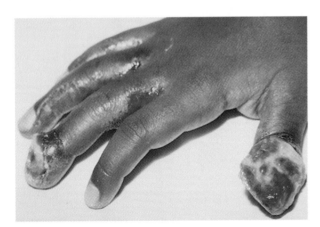

FIGURE 3-55. HIV infection. Herpes simplex viral infection in a 5-year-old child presenting as recurrent bouts of severe purulent erosions of the digits with destruction of the nails.

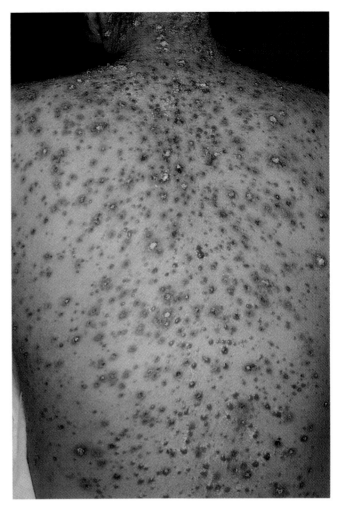

FIGURE 3-56. HIV infection. Severe generalized varicella.

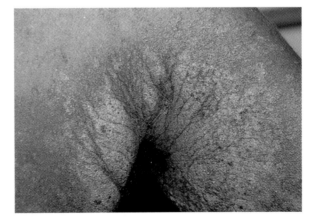

FIGURE 3-57. HIV infection. Crusted (Norwegian) scabies, psoriasiform scales and crusts of the axillae, hands, back, genitalia, and subungual areas.

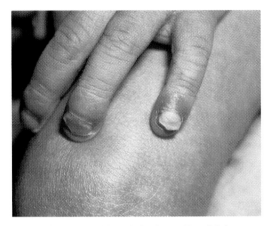

FIGURE 3–58. HIV infection. Candidal paronychia and onychomycosis.

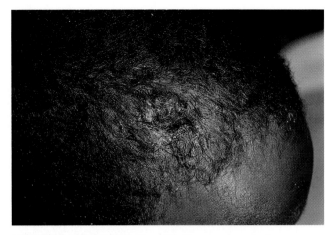

FIGURE 3–59. HIV infection. Bacillary angiomatosis, a vascular tumor, on the scalp of a 3-year-old boy with a CD4 count of 11. HIV PCR and electron microscopy confirmed the diagnosis. He had three other similar lesions on the back and arms.

Rocky Mountain Spotted Fever (RMSF)

DEFINITION

An acute systemic febrile illness with significant constitutional symptoms and a characteristic rash.

ETIOLOGY

The causative organism is a rickettsia, *Rickettsia rickettsii*, which is transmitted by any of the following vectors:

1. Dog tick, *Dermacentor variabilis*
2. Wood tick, *Dermacentor andersoni*
3. Lone star tick, *Amblyomma americanum*

EPIDEMIOLOGY

1. In the United States the disease is endemic in the southeastern states, central states, and Rocky Mountain states.
2. RMSF is more common in children.
3. It is more common in summer.

LABORATORY

1. Complete blood count (CBC)
   a. White blood count (WBC) normal or low (first 4 to 5 days) followed by leukocytosis (secondary bacterial infection)
   b. Thrombocytopenia
   c. Bandemia
   d. Anemia
2. Hyponatremia, hypoalbuminemia
3. Serum values of creatine phosphokinase (CPK) elevated
4. Immunofluorescent staining of skin biopsy material
   a. Rapid test
   b. Immunofluorescent *Rickettsia* from the skin rash can be seen usually between 4 and 8 days

5. Polymerase chain reaction (PCR) in blood and biopsy specimens (not widely available)
6. Specific serologic antibody titers demonstrate a rise late in the illness. Examples include:
   a. Indirect fluorescent antibody (most sensitive and specific)
   b. Indirect hemagglutination (most sensitive and specific)
   c. Complement fixation (highly specific, lacks sensitivity)
   d. Microagglutination (highly specific, lacks sensitivity)
7. Weil-Felix serologic test
   a. *Proteus* OX-19 and OX-2 agglutinins (+)
   b. Test becomes positive 10 to 14 days after onset of illness.
   c. Nonspecific and insensitive; thus *not* recommended
   d. Many false-positive results (e.g., *Proteus* infections, leptospirosis)

DIFFERENTIAL DIAGNOSIS

1. Ehrlichiosis
2. Atypical measles
3. Echoviral illness
4. Papular-purpuric glove and sock syndrome

TREATMENT

1. Early initiation of treatment based on clinical and epidemiologic data is mandatory.
2. Doxycycline
   a. May be used in all age groups.
   b. Dental staining is not a problem with one course of doxycycline.
   c. Dose: 4.4 mg/kg/day given orally or IV in two doses on day 1; then 2.2 mg/kg/day given orally or IV in two doses for 7 to 10 days (max dose: 200 mg/day).

3. Tetracycline
   a. For patients over 8 years of age
   b. Dose: 30 to 40 mg/kg/day given orally or IV in four doses for 7 to 10 days (max dose: 2 g/day).
4. Chloramphenicol is an alternate drug.

PROGNOSIS

1. Mortality rate is 4%.
2. Delay in initiation of treatment beyond day 6 of illness due to misdiagnosis is the major factor in most deaths.

KEY POINTS

Rocky Mountain Spotted Fever

- Treatment must be started early based on clinical and epidemiologic data alone.
- The characteristic erythematous papular and sometimes petechial rash starts on the distal extremities and spreads toward the center of the body.

TABLE 3–24
Clinical Features of Rocky Mountain Spotted Fever

Incubation period: 1 week
Tick bite: painless and often unrecognized
Prominent symptoms
    Fever
    Headache
    Myalgia
    Abdominal pain
Rash
    Starts from wrists, palms, and soles
    Within hours spreads centrally toward trunk
    Erythematous papular in nature
    May become petechial
    Rash may be absent ("spotless RMSF") in a few cases

TABLE 3–25
Complications of Rocky Mountain Spotted Fever

Disseminated intravascular coagulation
Peripheral gangrene
Multiorgan dysfunction
    Adult respiratory distress syndrome
    Renal failure
Neurologic sequelae
    Paralysis
    Blindness
    Deafness
    Intellectual impairment

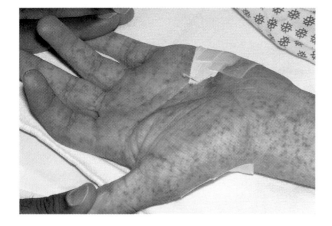

FIGURE 3–60. Petechial eruption of Rocky Mountain spotted fever starting in the distal extremities.

Erysipelas

SYNONYM   St. Anthony's Fire

DEFINITION

A distinctive type of infection of the skin (dermis and uppermost portions of the subcutaneous tissue) caused by group A beta-hemolytic streptococcus (GABS)

BOX 3–11   *Erysipelas*

Ability of infection to spread rapidly like a fire to involve very large areas of skin is the reason for its descriptive name, St. Anthony's fire.

ETIOLOGY

Group A beta-hemolytic streptococcus

EPIDEMIOLOGY

1. Uncommon
2. More frequent in the
   a. Very young
   b. Aged
   c. Debilitated
3. Lymphedema, other local lymphatic dysfunctions, and chronic ulcer of the skin may be predisposing factors.

PATHOGENESIS

1. The organism gains access to the deeper layers of the skin.
2. Preceding lesions: abrasions, lacerations, wounds, chronic ulcers or other skin breaks

LABORATORY

1. High WBC count with a shift to the left
2. GABS may be cultured from
   a. Blood
   b. Aspirate from the advancing margin of the lesion
   c. Oropharynx
3. Antistreptolysin-O (ASO) titer or streptozyme

DIFFERENTIAL DIAGNOSIS

1. Cellulitis
   a. Ill-defined borders
   b. Deeper tissue involvement
   c. Slow spread

   d. May be caused by other organisms such as *Staphylococcus aureus, Hemophilus influenzae*
2. Erisepelas-like presentation due to other bacteria
   a. Other streptococci (groups G, B, and C)
   b. *Streptococcus pneumoniae*
   c. *Staphylococcus aureus*
   d. *Yersinia enterocolitica*

TREATMENT

1. Hospitalization for intravenous antibiotics for 48 to 72 hours
2. Penicillin
3. Erythromycin, clindamycin, or cephalexin if patient is allergic to penicillin
4. Rest, immobilization, and elevation of affected part
5. Cool, wet dressings

PROGNOSIS

1. Good with early institution of antibiotic therapy
2. Recurrences are not uncommon and frequently occur at the same site.
3. Lymphatic channels are damaged with each recurrence of the infection, leading to lymphedema, which predisposes to further infections.

KEY POINTS

Erysipelas

- Group A beta-hemolytic streptococci are almost always the cause.
- A rapidly spreading, fiery red or crimson plaque with a sharp advancing border.

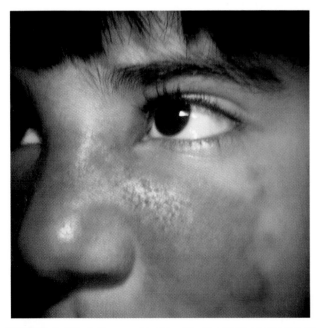

FIGURE 3–61. A 7-year-old girl with recurrent erysipelas on the cheeks. The lesion on the face created a "butterfly" appearance, involving both cheeks and the bridge of the nose. The lesion, a sharply demarcated fiery red plaque, was painful and tender.

TABLE 3–26
Clinical Features of Erysipelas

Well-circumscribed lesion
Fiery red plaque
Spreads peripherally at a rate of 2–10 cm/day
Lesion is hot and tender
Common sites: face and extremities
May occur anywhere
Constitutional symptoms: fever, chills, malaise, headache

Scarlet Fever

SYNONYM   Scarlatina

DEFINITION

Scarlet fever consists of a specific toxic and erythematous exanthem and enanthem.

ETIOLOGY

Group A beta-hemolytic streptococcus (*Streptococcus pyogenes*) strains that produce erythrogenic toxin

EPIDEMIOLOGY

1. Most cases occur in children between 2 and 8 years of age.
2. Most cases are seen in winter and early spring.

PATHOGENESIS

1. The oropharynx is the portal of entry.
2. Occasionally, a surgical wound may be the portal of entry (surgical scarlet fever).
3. The rash is produced by the erythrogenic toxin.
4. At least three immunologically distinct erythrogenic toxins have been identified. This explains recurrent episodes of scarlet fever in the same patient.

CLINICAL FEATURES

1. Average incubation period: 2 to 4 days (range 1 to 7 days)
2. Constitutional symptoms: sore throat, headache, malaise, fever
3. Occasionally, vomiting and abdominal pain occur.
4. Rash
   a. Punctiform erythematous papular rash produces a sandpaper texture.
   b. Blanches prominently when pressure is applied
   c. Generalized distribution
   d. More prominent in the intertriginous areas
5. Pastia sign: red streaks on the skin fold
6. Strawberry tongue
   a. White strawberry tongue: edematous red papillae project through the white-coated tongue in the first 2 days
   b. Red strawberry tongue: occurs when the white coating disappears and the red lingual papillae stand out
7. Petechiae on the palate

8. Tonsillopharyngitis
   a. Tonsils: erythematous, enlarged with patches of exudates
   b. Pharynx: beefy red
   c. Mild cases of scarlet fever: absence of exudate
   d. Surgical scarlet fever: pharyngeal and tonsillar involvement are absent
9. Marked desquamation 7 to 10 days later

BOX 3–12   *Desquamation and Scarlet Fever*

One of the most characteristic features

Extent and duration of desquamation are directly related to intensity of rash

Seen at end of first week

Appears as large areas of skin peeling off, giving rise to a "punch hole" appearance

Desquamation of hands and feet may be a presenting sign (if initial acute phase is mild and overlooked)

Desquamation is complete in most cases in 2 to 3 weeks

COMPLICATIONS

1. Acute glomerulonephritis
2. Rheumatic fever

TREATMENT

1. Penicillin parenterally or orally for 10 days
2. Erythromycin or clindamycin if patient is allergic to penicillin

PROGNOSIS

Excellent with early treatment

KEY POINTS

Scarlet Fever

- The rash consists of a generalized erythematous punctiform papular eruption with a sandpaper texture.
- Desquamation is prominent, especially in the hands and feet.

TABLE 3–27
Differential Diagnosis of Scarlatiniform Rash

Drug eruption
Arcanobacterium hemolyticum infection
Viral exanthem (e.g., hepatitis B virus, coxsackie virus)
Kawasaki disease
Infectious mononucleosis
Staphylococcal scarlatina
Toxic shock syndrome
Severe sunburn

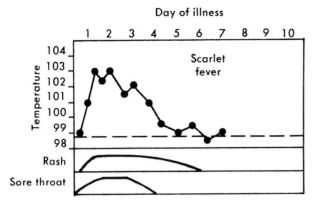

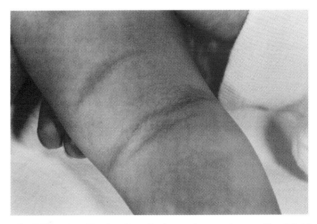

FIGURE 3–62. Schematic diagram of a typical case of un-treated uncomplicated scarlet fever. The rash usually appears within 24 hours of the onset of fever and sore throat. (From Katz SL et al (eds): Krugman's Infectious Diseases of Children, 10th ed. St. Louis, Mosby–Year Book, 1998.)

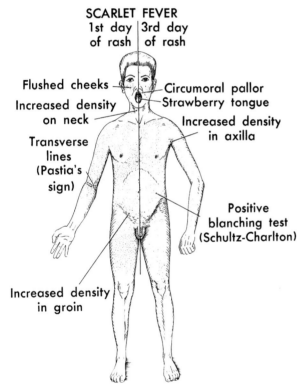

FIGURE 3–63. Schematic drawing illustrating the development and distribution of the scarlet fever rash. (From Katz SL et al (eds): Krugman's Infectious Diseases of Children, 10th ed. St. Louis, Mosby–Year Book, 1998.)

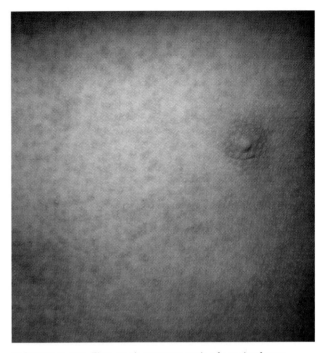

FIGURE 3–64. Fine erythematous rash of scarlet fever.

FIGURE 3–65. Pastia sign. Red streaks on the popliteal fold. (Courtesy of Guinter Kahn, M.D., Miami, FL.)

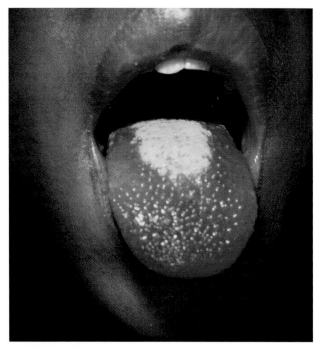

FIGURE 3-66. Scarlet fever. Red strawberry tongue (with white coating).

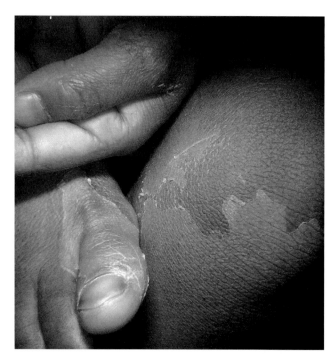

FIGURE 3-68. Scarlet fever. Desquamation of the knee, hand, and foot.

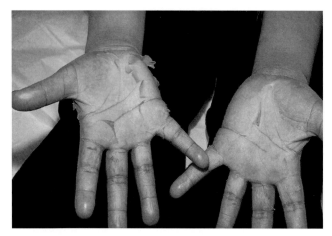

FIGURE 3-67. Scarlet fever. Desquamation of the hands.

Localized Streptococcal Skin Infections

ETIOLOGY

Group A beta-hemolytic streptococcus

A. Impetigo Contagiosa

1. More common in summer
2. Children of all ages affected except newborns
3. May be preceded by minor skin trauma, insect bites, underlying eczema
4. Lesions are vesicopustules with a yellow-gold or honey-colored crust surrounded by a rim of erythema.
5. Common distribution: exposed areas of the body

6. May be associated with regional lymphadenopathy
7. Both streptococci and staphylococci are commonly cultured from the lesions.
8. Complication: acute glomerulonephritis
9. Differential diagnosis: staphylococcal impetigo
   a. More common in young infants
   b. Occurs year round
   c. Flaccid bullous lesions
   d. More common on unexposed areas of the body
   e. No associated lymphadenopathy
10. Treatment
    a. Beta-lactam antibiotics (e.g., dicloxacillin)

b. Erythromycin or clindamycin if patient is allergic to penicillin

c. Topical mupirocin

B. Ecthyma

1. More common in summer
2. Children of all ages affected except newborns
3. May be preceded by minor skin trauma, insect bites
4. Skin lesions
   a. Discrete and round
   b. Surmounted by a dark crust
   c. Surrounded by a rim of shallow ulcer
   d. Involve the deeper layer of the skin (dermis) and may heal with scarring
5. Pure streptococci in culture
6. Differential diagnosis
   a. Cigarette burns (child abuse)
   b. Ecthyma gangrenosum (caused by *Pseudomonas aeruginosa*)
7. Treatment
   a. Penicillin
   b. Erythromycin or clindamycin if patient is allergic to penicillin
   c. Topical mupirocin

C. Cellulitis

1. May affect any age group
2. May be preceded by trauma to the skin, insect bite, or eczema
3. More common on exposed areas of the body
4. The lesion is a painful, erythematous, tender plaque with an ill-defined border.
5. Diagnosis: Culture from aspirate taken from the lesion
6. Differential diagnosis
   a. Cellulitis
      (1) Caused by other organisms such as *Staphylococcus aureus, Haemophilus influenzae, Pneumococcus*
      (2) Cultures may differentiate them
   b. Erysipelas
      (1) Well-defined margin
      (2) Expands rapidly
7. Treatment
   a. Beta-lactam antibiotics parenterally or orally depending on severity of illness (e.g., oxacillin or cephalosporin)
   b. Warm soaks

D. Perianal Dermatitis/Cellulitis

1. More common in infants and younger children
2. More common in boys
3. Perianal erythema, swelling, irritation
4. Symptoms: pain, pruritus
5. Culture perianally and specifically ask the laboratory to look for group A beta-hemolytic streptococcus
6. Differential diagnosis
   a. Candidiasis
   b. Child abuse
   c. Inflammatory bowel disease
   d. Psoriasis
7. Treatment
   a. Penicillin (erythromycin for patients with penicillin allergy)
   b. Topical mupirocin

E. Blistering Distal Dactylitis

1. More common in school-age children; less common in preschoolers
2. Lesions are tender blisters over the anterior fat pad of the thumb or fingers.
3. Organism may be cultured from the blisters.
4. A third of patients may have streptococcal pharyngitis.
5. Differential diagnosis
   a. Herpetic whitlow
   b. Contact dermatitis
   c. Dyshidrotic eczema
   d. Child abuse
6. Treatment
   a. Penicillin (erythromycin for patients with penicillin allergy)
   b. Warm soaks
   c. Topical mupirocin

KEY POINTS

Localized Streptococcal Skin Infections

- Impetigo contagiosa: The lesions have a honey-colored crust.
- Ecthyma: The lesions are discrete, round with a dark crust, and surrounded by a rim of shallow ulcer.
- Streptococcal cellulitis: The lesion is a painful tender erythematous swelling with an ill-defined border.
- Perianal dermatitis/cellulitis: The lesion consists of a vivid perianal erythema with pain and swelling.
- Blistering distal dactylitis: The lesions are tender blisters over the anterior fat pad of the thumb or fingers.

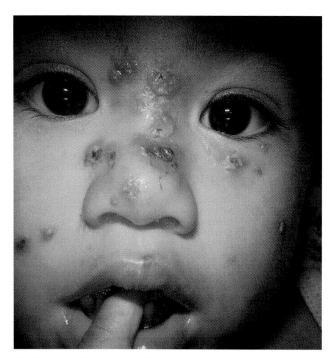

FIGURE 3–69. Lesions of impetigo contagiosa on the face, showing the honey-colored crust.

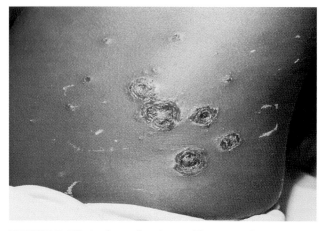

FIGURE 3–70. Lesions of ecthyma. These are discrete round lesions with a dark crust in the center surrounded by a rim of shallow ulcer.

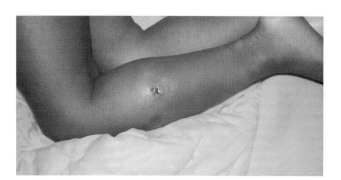

FIGURE 3–71. Streptococcal cellulitis showing erythematous swelling with an ill-defined border. A wound on the leg was the portal of entry of the organism.

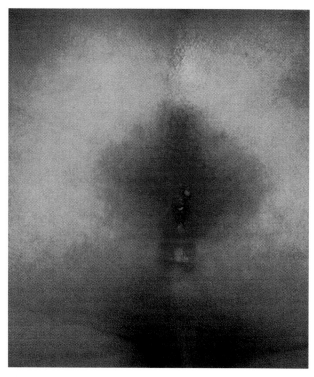

FIGURE 3–72. Perianal cellulitis showing vivid erythema perianally.

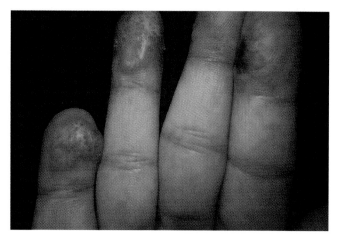

FIGURE 3–73. Blistering distal dactylitis involving several digits.

Streptococcal Toxic Shock Syndrome

SYNONYM   Group A Streptococcal Invasive Disease

DEFINITION

This is a life-threatening infection that is diagnosed by meeting a set of criteria (see Table 3–28).

ETIOLOGY

Group A beta-hemolytic streptococcus (GABS) M types 1 and 3 producing streptococcal pyrogenic exotoxin A (SPEA)

EPIDEMIOLOGY

1. More common in adults than children
2. Equal sex distribution
3. No seasonal prevalence
4. In children, varicella may be the initiating event.

PATHOGENESIS

1. Initial skin and soft tissue infection—e.g., varicella may lead to secondary infection with M type GABS
2. SPEA acts as a superantigen leading to production of proinflammatory cytokines (e.g., tumor necrosis factor-alpha, interleukin 1-beta, interleukin 6).
3. These cytokines produce shock and tissue injury.

CLINICAL FEATURES

1. Generalized scarlatiniform rash in addition to a localized infected portal of entry
2. Severe systemic symptoms
   a. Fever
   b. Chills
   c. Myalgia
   d. Vomiting
   e. Diarrhea
   f. Delirium
3. Findings on physical examination
   a. Shock
   b. Hypotension
   c. Signs of multiple organ dysfunction
4. Desquamation occurs 1 to 2 weeks later

LABORATORY

1. Cultures from the blood, skin, and soft tissue
2. Complete blood count
3. Serum chemistries and electrolytes
4. Appropriate radiologic studies

COMPLICATIONS

1. Acute renal failure
2. Adult respiratory distress syndrome
3. Overwhelming sepsis
4. Death

BOX 3-13   *Differential Diagnosis of Streptococcal Toxic Shock Syndrome*

Staphylococcal toxic shock syndrome (see Table 3–28)
Gram-negative sepsis
Rocky Mountain spotted fever
Heat stroke
Staphylococcal scalded skin syndrome
Kawasaki disease

TREATMENT

1. Hospitalization and stabilization of vital signs
   a. ABCs of resuscitation, cardiac and pulse oximetry monitoring
   b. Fluid resuscitation for septic shock
2. Systemic antibiotics: Provide coverage for both GABS and *Staphylococcus aureus* pending culture results. Once GABS is identified, penicillin G with or without clindamycin IV for 2 weeks or longer
3. Pressor agents (e.g., dopamine)
4. Surgical exploration may be indicated for soft tissue infection.

PROGNOSIS

Despite optimal care, mortality rate is 30%.

KEY POINTS

Streptococcal Toxic Shock Syndrome

- In children, a varicella lesion may be the portal of entry for GABS invasive disease.
- This is a life-threatening disease with multiorgan dysfunction.

TABLE 3–28
Differential Diagnosis: Staphylococcal Versus Streptococcal Toxic Shock Syndrome

Clinical Features	Staphylococcal TSS	Streptococcal TSS
Age (years)	15–35	20–50
Sex	More women	Either
Severe pain in skin	Rare	Common
Hypotension	100%	100%
Erythroderma	Very common	Less common
Bacteremia	Uncommon	60%
Tissue necrosis	Rare	Common
Predisposing factors	Tampons	Skin trauma
	Nasal packing	Varicella
Mortality	<30%	30% to 70%

TABLE 3–29
Proposed Case Definition for the Streptococcal Toxic Shock Syndrome

1. Isolation of group A streptococci
   A. From a normally sterile site (e.g., blood, cerebrospinal fluid, peritoneal fluid, tissue biopsy, surgical wound, etc.)
   B. From a nonsterile site (e.g., throat, superficial skin lesion, sputum, vagina)
2. Clinical signs of severity
   A. Hypotension; systolic blood pressure ≤90 mmHg in adults or <5th percentile for age in children
      and
   B. Two or more of the following signs:
      (1) Renal impairment: creatinine ≥2 mg/dL for adults or greater than or equal to twice the upper limit of normal for age
      (2) Coagulopathy: platelets ≤100,000/mm³ or disseminated intravascular coagulation
      (3) Liver involvement: serum alanine aminotransferase (SGPT), aspartate aminotransferase (SGOT), or total bilirubin concentrations greater than or equal to twice the upper limit of normal for age
      (4) Adult respiratory distress syndrome
      (5) Generalized erythematous macular rash that may desquamate
      (6) Soft tissue necrosis, including necrotizing fasciitis or myositis, or gangrene

An illness fulfilling criteria 1A and 2 (A and B) can be defined as a *definite* case. An illness fulfilling criteria 1B and 2 (A and B) can be defined as a *probable* case if no other etiology for the illness is identified.

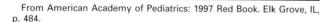

From American Academy of Pediatrics: 1997 Red Book. Elk Grove, IL, p. 484.

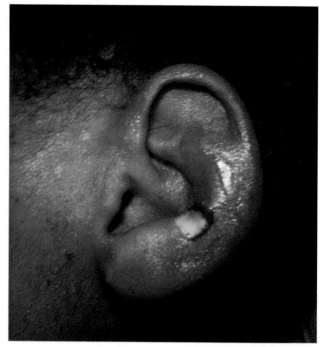

FIGURE 3–74. A 6-year-old boy admitted with group A streptococcal invasive disease had an infected varicella lesion on the ear, which was the portal of entry for GABS.

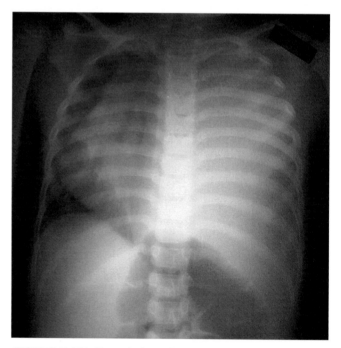

FIGURE 3–75. Frontal view of the chest in the same patient showing a complete opacification of the left lung field and mediastinal shift to the right. About 700 ml of pus, which later grew GABS, was drained from the pleural cavity.

Necrotizing Fasciitis (NF)

SYNONYMS Streptococcal Gangrene
"Flesh-Eating Bacteria"
Hospital Gangrene

DEFINITION

NF is a life-threatening infection of the fascia and adjoining tissues.

EPIDEMIOLOGY

1. Risk factors for children include:
   a. Varicella (a notable initiating event)
   b. Trauma
   c. Contamination of a surgical wound
   d. Infection of umbilical stump
2. Risk factors for adults include:
   a. Diabetes mellitus
   b. Peripheral vascular disease
   c. Intravenous drug abuse
   d. Immunodeficiency
   e. Malnutrition
   f. Surgery

PATHOGENESIS

1. Vascular injury and thrombosis result in widespread necrosis of the fascia and adjoining tissues.
2. Streptococcal toxin acting as a superantigen may be the direct cause of the necrosis.

LABORATORY

1. Complete blood count
2. Cultures (both aerobic and anaerobic) from the blood and soft tissues
3. Serum electrolytes, chemistries
4. Radiograph of the involved area may show subcutaneous gas.
5. Frozen-section biopsy
   a. Allows rapid evaluation of the pathology to confirm the diagnosis
   b. Allows identification of pathogens underlying the intact skin

COMPLICATIONS

1. Multiorgan failure
2. Fluid and electrolyte disturbances (extravasation of intravascular fluid into tissue)

DIFFERENTIAL DIAGNOSIS

1. Cellulitis
2. Purpura fulminans

TREATMENT

1. Hospitalization and surgical consultation
2. Immediate surgical exploration and debridement
3. Aggressive empiric intravenous antibiotics: clindamycin, penicillin, and an aminoglycoside for 2 weeks or longer
4. Repeat debridement within 24 to 48 hours may be necessary because of continued dissection of the infection into the surrounding tissues.
5. Hyperbaric oxygen may help in some cases.
6. Full-thickness skin grafting

PROGNOSIS

1. Mortality is 20%.
2. Delay in diagnosis and delay in surgical exploration are the major causes of death.

KEY POINTS

Necrotizing Fasciitis

- In children, an infected varicella lesion may be the portal of entry for GABS.
- Immediate surgical exploration and debridement may save the patient's life.

TABLE 3–30
Etiology of Necrotizing Fasciitis

GABS M types 1 and 3 producing proteases and pyrogenic toxins
Staphylococcus aureus
Pseudomonas aeruginosa
Anaerobes (e.g., *Bacteroides, Peptostreptococcus, Clostridium* sp.)
Mixed organisms (gram-negative bacilli and anaerobic bacteria)

TABLE 3–31
Clinical Features of Necrotizing Fasciitis

May involve any area of the body
Begins as an erythematous, painful, tender, ill-defined plaque (may be mistaken for cellulitis)
Duskiness, vesiculation may appear in center of affected area
Crepitance may be present over affected area
Soft tissue involvement expands rapidly
Signs of toxicity (high fever, malaise, altered sensorium)
Concurrent lesions of varicella in some cases

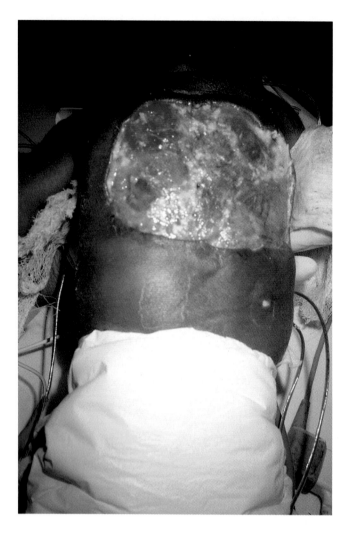

FIGURE 3–76. A 9-day-old male infant with necrotizing fasciitis from *Staphylococcus aureus*. This picture was taken on postoperative day 1.

Localized Staphylococcal Skin Infections

DEFINITION

A suppurative infection localized to the skin and soft tissue

ETIOLOGY

Coagulase-positive *Staphylococcus aureus*

EPIDEMIOLOGY

1. Transmission occurs from person to person via the hands and nasal discharge.
2. Organisms colonize the anterior nares and moist body areas in 30% of humans.
3. Asymptomatic carriers may be the source of infection.

A. Bullous Impetigo

1. This is an infection of infants and young children.
2. The lesions are flaccid blisters containing pus.
3. Rupture of the blisters leaves a narrow rim of scale at the edge of a shallow moist erosion.

4. Most common distribution is on the trunk, perineum, and covered areas.
5. Differential diagnosis includes
   a. Streptococcal impetigo
   b. Bullous arthropod bite
   c. Autoimmune blistering disease (e.g., pemphigus, linear IgA dermatosis)
   d. Epidermolysis bullosa
6. Treatment
   a. Topical mupirocin for solitary stable lesion
   b. Oral beta lactamase-resistant antibiotics for multiple and extensive lesions (e.g., dicloxacillin or cephalexin)

B. Folliculitis, Furunculosis, Carbunculosis

1. Folliculitis (Bockhart impetigo)—scattered small pustules involving hair follicles
2. Furuncle—a tender deep-seated nodule around a hair follicle with signs of "pointing"
3. Carbuncle—several confluent furuncles with openings on the surface
4. Laboratory diagnosis
   a. Culture of the lesions

b. Culture of the nasopharynx or perineum in a *Staphylococcus* carrier

c. Work-up for immunodeficiency in patients with recurrent furunculosis

5. Treatment

a. Beta lactamase-resistant antibiotic (e.g., dicloxacillin or cephalexin)

b. Incision and drainage

c. Antibacterial wash

d. Nasal mupirocin for 5 days for *Staphylococcus* carrier; or oral rifampin

C. Cellulitis

1. May be preceded by minor skin trauma

2. Involved area is ill-defined, tender, swollen, and erythematous.

3. Laboratory diagnosis: culture from aspirate from the lesion, and blood culture

4. Treatment: Beta lactamase-resistant antibiotic parenterally or orally depending on severity of illness (e.g., oxacillin or dicloxacillin).

KEY POINTS

Localized Staphylococcal Skin Infections

■ Recurrent staphylococcal furunculosis may occur in patients with immunodeficiency disorders.

■ Recurrent staphylococcal infections may mean that a *Staphylococcus* carrier is present in the household.

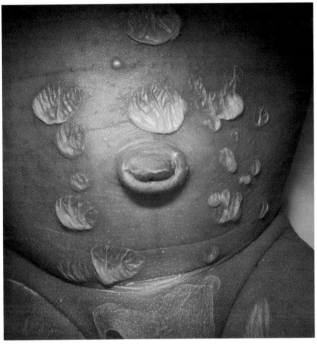

FIGURE 3–77. Bullous impetigo in an infant. Flaccid bullae are filled with purulent material.

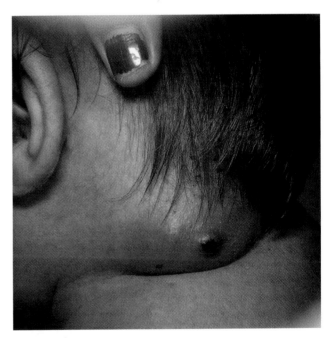

FIGURE 3–79. A furuncle on the posterior neck.

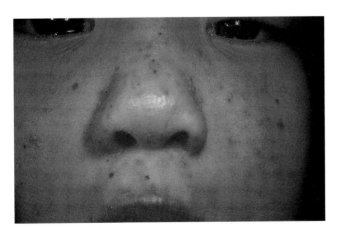

FIGURE 3–78. A 3-year-old boy with recurrent staphylococcal pustulosis of the face.

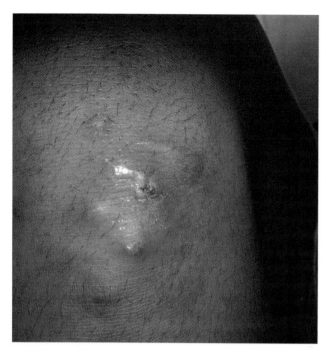

FIGURE 3–80. A carbuncle.

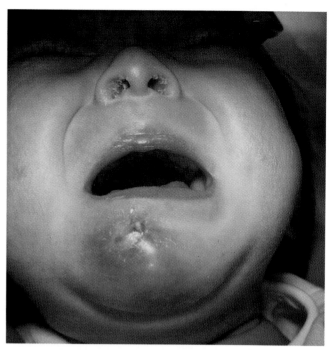

FIGURE 3–81. Staphylococcal cellulitis.

Staphylococcal Scalded Skin Syndrome (SSSS)

SYNONYMS   Ritter Disease (SSSS of the Newborn)

DEFINITION
This is a potentially serious but highly treatable toxin-mediated manifestation of a localized infection with certain strains of staphylococci.

ETIOLOGY
1. *Staphylococcus aureus* phage II, types 71 and 55
2. The organism produces an epidermolytic toxin called exfoliatin.

EPIDEMIOLOGY
1. Most commonly affected persons are infants and children less than 5 years of age because of their renal immaturity and inability to excrete the toxin.
2. Older children and adults may develop SSSS if they have renal impairment.
3. The full-blown picture is rare in African-American children.

PATHOGENESIS
1. The organism colonizes the mucous membranes of the nasopharynx, eyes, and selected areas (e.g., umbilical stump, circumcision sites), producing a localized infection.
2. The toxin is produced from that vantage point.

3. The toxin circulates and attaches to the cells of the epidermis, disrupting the latter.

CLINICAL FEATURES
1. Sudden onset of fever and irritability
2. Prominent crusting around the eyes and mouth occurs early.
3. Rash
   a. Generalized tenderness and erythema (staphylococcal scarlatina)
   b. Within 24 to 48 hours, flaccid blisters develop and then exfoliate in sheets, leaving a scalded-looking surface.
   c. The borders of the exfoliating skin are rolled like wet tissue paper.
4. Some cases do not progress beyond the staphylococcal scarlatina stage (forme fruste of SSSS).

LABORATORY
1. Culture from colonized sites such as the mucous membranes of the nasopharynx or conjunctiva may be positive.
2. Blood culture, if done, is usually negative.
3. Histologic examination of the exfoliated skin shows a partial split of the upper epidermis.

DIFFERENTIAL DIAGNOSIS
1. Scarlet fever during the initial stage of generalized erythema
2. Toxic epidermal necrolysis (TEN; see Table 3–32)

TREATMENT

1. Hospitalization and dermatology consultation
2. IV beta lactamase-resistant antibiotic (e.g., oxacillin or vancomycin)
3. Monitoring and replacing of fluid and electrolyte deficits.

KEY POINTS

Staphylococcal Scalded Skin Syndrome

- SSSS is a disease of infants and young children.
- Periorificial crusting is early and prominent.

> **BOX 3-14** *Nikolsky Sign*
>
> Positive sign: Slight rubbing of normal-looking adjacent skin results in blistering
> Conditions with a positive Nikolsky sign
>   Staphylococcal scalded skin syndrome
>   Toxic epidermal necrolysis
>   Stevens-Johnson syndrome
>   Pemphigus vulgaris

TABLE 3-32
Differential Diagnosis of Staphylococcal Scalded Skin Syndrome and Toxic Epidermal Necrolysis

	SSSS	TEN
Age	Infants	Older children, adults
Etiology	Staphylococcus aureus	Drugs
Skin tenderness	Present	May be absent
Exfoliating skin	White	Necrotic
Level of split	Upper epidermis	Full-thickness epidermis
Mortality	Nil	30%

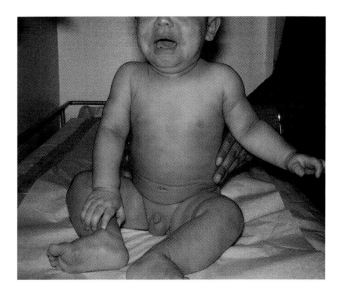

FIGURE 3-83. Staphylococcal scarlatina.

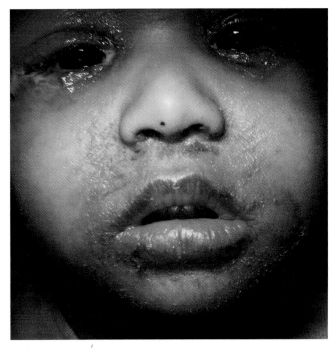

FIGURE 3-82. Perioral and periorbital crusting in staphylococcal scalded skin syndrome.

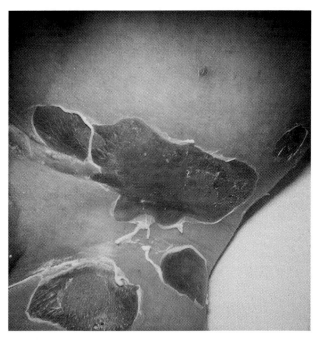

FIGURE 3-84. The borders of the exfoliating skin look like rolled wet tissue paper.

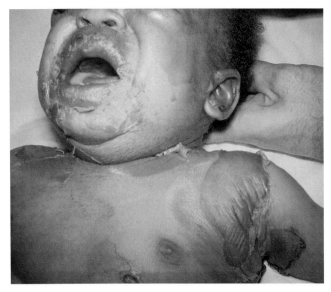

FIGURE 3-85. SSSS in a 1-year-old infant. On the third day of illness, the epidermis was already regenerating.

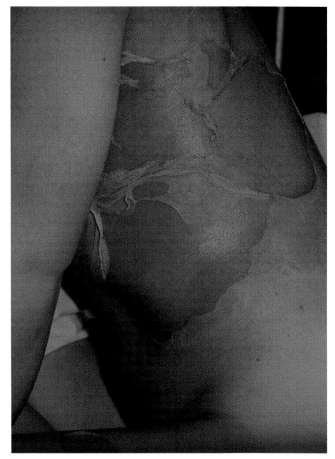

FIGURE 3-86. SSSS in a 9-year-old child with kidney failure.

Staphylococcal Toxic Shock Syndrome

DEFINITION
This is a potentially life-threatening infection caused by toxin-producing strains of staphylococci.

ETIOLOGY
Staphylococcus aureus phage II, which produces an enterotoxin, TSS toxin-1.

EPIDEMIOLOGY
1. Seen in all age groups, though more common in adults
2. Predisposing factors
   a. Use of tampons and contraceptive barriers
   b. Surgical wound
   c. Nasal packings
   d. Central venous lines

PATHOGENESIS
1. The organisms colonize selected sites, where they produce the toxin.
2. TSS toxin-1 acts as a superantigen, releasing cytokines such as tumor necrosis factor-alpha and interleukins 1 and 6, which are responsible for tissue injury and multiorgan failure.

CLINICAL FEATURES
1. Fever
2. Diffuse macular or scarlatiniform skin eruption
3. Hypotension
4. Involvement of three or more organ systems
   a. Gastrointestinal—vomiting and diarrhea
   b. Muscular—myalgia
   c. Mucous membranes—erythema
   d. Renal
   e. Hepatic
   f. Hematologic—platelets less than 100,000/mm^3
   g. Central nervous system
5. Desquamation occurs 1 to 2 weeks after onset of illness

LABORATORY
1. Cultures from infected sites
2. CBC including platelet count
3. Chemistries to monitor organ dysfunction
4. Appropriate radiologic studies

COMPLICATIONS

1. Disseminated intravascular coagulation
2. Organ failure
3. Death

DIFFERENTIAL DIAGNOSIS

1. Streptococcal toxic shock syndrome (see Table 3–29)
2. Kawasaki disease
3. Rocky Mountain spotted fever
4. Leptospirosis

TREATMENT

1. Hospitalization and stabilization of vital signs
2. Cardiovascular and respiratory support
3. Fluids and electrolytes

4. Removal of foreign bodies, drainage of infected sites
5. Beta-lactam antibiotic given intravenously (e.g., oxacillin or vancomycin).

PROGNOSIS

Staphylococcal toxic shock syndrome has a 15% mortality.

KEY POINTS

Staphylococcal Toxic Shock Syndrome

- Hypotension and multiorgan dysfunction are prominent.
- Rash is a diffuse scarlatiniform eruption.

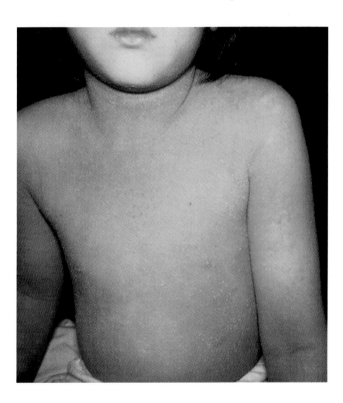

FIGURE 3–87. Diffuse scarlatiniform eruption in a child with staphylococcal toxic shock syndrome.

Erythrasma

DEFINITION

A mild, chronic, localized, superficial infection of the body folds and clefts characterized by areas of discolored, scaly patches.

ETIOLOGY

Corynebacterium minutissimum, a normal skin flora

EPIDEMIOLOGY

1. More common in tropical and subtropical geographic areas
2. More frequent in adults than children

PATHOGENESIS

1. Unknown
2. Diabetes may be a predisposing factor in adults

BOX 3–15 | *Differential Diagnosis of Erythrasma*

Contact dermatitis
Tinea cruris
Tinea pedis
Candidiasis

LABORATORY

Wood lamp examination: coral red fluorescence

TREATMENT

1. Oral erythromycin for 5 days
2. Topical erythromycin or clindamycin

PROGNOSIS

Persists indefinitely without treatment

KEY POINTS

Erythrasma

- Affects intertriginous areas
- Coral red fluorescence on Wood lamp examination

TABLE 3–33
Clinical Features of Erythrasma

Skin Lesions

Appear as asymptomatic dry scaly patches
Color: pink to brown
Older lesions show wrinkling of skin
Common distribution
    Axillae
    Toe webs
    Groin
    Intergluteal fold
    Inframammary area
    Periumbilical areas

Wood Lamp Examination: Coral red fluorescence

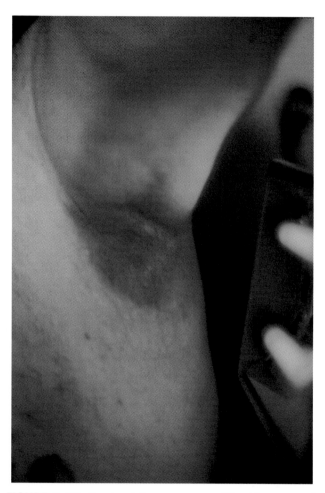

FIGURE 3–89. Coral red fluorescence on Wood lamp examination.

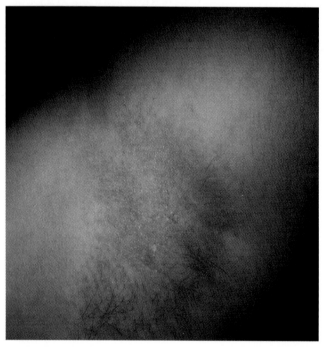

FIGURE 3–88. A 10-year-old girl with hypothyroidism showing erythrasma on the axilla.

Ecthyma Gangrenosum

DEFINITION

A cutaneous manifestation of *Pseudomonas septicemia*

ETIOLOGY

The causative organism is *Pseudomonas aeruginosa.*

LABORATORY

1. Culture of skin lesions and blood
2. Skin biopsy shows a necrotizing vasculitis

BOX 3–16 *Predisposing Factors for Pseudomonas Septicemia*

Individuals with immunosuppression for a variety of reasons
Debilitated preterm newborns
Patients with cystic fibrosis
Patients with congenital immune disorders
Malnourished infants, especially in impoverished countries
Patients with severe thermal burns
Hospitalized patients undergoing intensive antibiotic treatment or those with indwelling urinary, arterial, or venous catheters

---

COMPLICATIONS

Scarring of the affected areas may result in anal strictures.

TREATMENT

1. Hospitalization; surgical and dermatological consultations
2. Any of the following antibiotics may be given intravenously: cefotaxime, gentamicin, amikacin, piperacillin.
3. Appropriate wound care
4. Skin grafting as necessary

KEY POINTS

Ecthyma Gangrenosum

- The characteristic skin lesions are ulcers with a black eschar surrounded by erythema.
- Seen in immunosuppressed individuals

TABLE 3–34
Clinical Features of Ecthyma Gangrenosum

Skin Lesions

Bullae and hemorrhagic pustules that evolve into necrotic ulcers surrounded by an erythematous halo
Characteristic black eschar in center of lesion
Common distribution
    Perineal (anogenital) area
    Intertriginous areas

Other Features

Majority associated with septicemia

TABLE 3–35
Differential Diagnosis of Ecthyma Gangrenosum

Ecthyma caused by *Streptococcus*
Thermal burns
Purpura fulminans
Staphylococcal furunculosis
Pyoderma gangrenosum

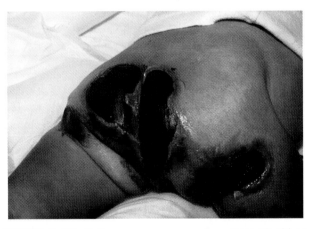

FIGURE 3–90. Ecthyma gangrenosum in a 7-month-old severely malnourished infant. Ulcers with black eschar surrounded by a rim of erythema are visible here.

Pertussis

SYNONYM   Whooping Cough

DEFINITION

A preventable respiratory infection that can occur in all age groups

ETIOLOGY

The causative organism is *Bordetella pertussis,* a gram-negative pleomorphic bacillus.

EPIDEMIOLOGY

Infants and young children are frequently infected by respiratory droplets from older siblings and adults who have a mild or atypical illness such as an upper respiratory infection or chronic cough.

LABORATORY

1. Culture of nasopharyngeal swab sample in Bordet-Gengou media
   a. Best recovery of organisms occurs during the catarrhal stage.
   b. Organisms may be recovered for up to 2 to 3 weeks during the paroxysmal stage.
2. Rapid test: direct immunofluorescent assay of nasopharyngeal secretions
3. Absolute lymphocytosis
   a. Seen at the beginning of the paroxysmal stage
   b. Persists for 3 to 4 weeks
   c. May *not* be present in young infants

BOX 3-17   *Differential Diagnosis of Pertussis*

Pertussis-like syndrome may be caused by
- Adenovirus
- *Bordetella parapertussis*
- *Chlamydia trachomatis*
- Respiratory syncytial virus

TABLE 3-36
Complications of Pertussis

Respiratory
    Bronchopneumonia
    Atelectasis
Central nervous system
    Seizures
    Encephalopathy
      Anoxia
      Cerebral hemorrhages
Otitis media
Hemorrhagic
    Subconjunctival bleeding
    Petechiae
    Epistaxis
Death

TREATMENT

1. Hospitalize young infants; cardiac and pulse oximetry monitoring.
2. Respiratory isolation is necessary, since this is a highly contagious disease.
3. Supportive therapy
   a. Suctioning of secretions
   b. Humidified oxygen (as indicated)
   c. Maintenance of adequate hydration and nutrition
4. Erythromycin
   a. Given orally for 14 days
   b. If started early during the catarrhal stage, it may abort or modify the course of the disease.
   c. Eradicates *B. pertussis* from the upper respiratory tract.
   d. It does not have any effect on the clinical course of a fully established illness.
5. Cough suppressants are not used.

PREVENTION

1. Erythromycin given as soon as possible to exposed persons, preferably during the incubation period, will prevent or modify the course of the disease.
2. Routine immunization with pertussis vaccine consists of a total of five doses given at 2, 4, 6, and 15 to 18 months and a booster given at 4 to 6 years of age.

PROGNOSIS

Guarded in the very young infant.

KEY POINTS

Pertussis

- Pertussis is a life-threatening infection in very young infants.
- A common source of infection is an adult with vague respiratory complaints.

TABLE 3-37
Clinical Features of Pertussis

Incubation period: 7–13 days.
Three stages (each lasting 2 weeks)
1. Catarrhal
2. Paroxysmal
3. Convalescent

Catarrhal Stage

URI symptoms (fever absent or low grade, mild coryza, cough)

Paroxysmal Stage

Series of coughs ending with an inspiratory whoop
Whoop may be absent in young infants
Apnea (in infants <6 months of age)
Petechiae, subconjunctival hemorrhage (during paroxysms of cough)

Convalescent Stage

Waning of symptoms

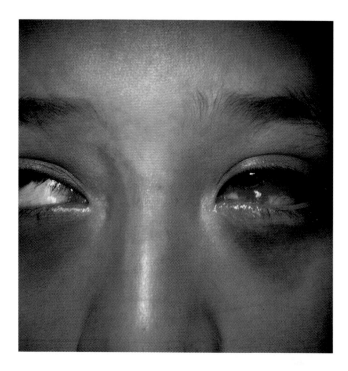

FIGURE 3–91. Ecchymoses and conjunctival hemorrhage in a 6-year-old unimmunized child with pertussis.

Buccal Cellulitis

DEFINITION

Buccal cellulitis is a bacterial infection of the dermis and subcutaneous tissues of the cheek.

ETIOLOGY

Hematogenous dissemination

1. *Streptococcus pneumoniae*
2. *Haemophilus influenzae,* type b (with the use of *H. influenzae* vaccine, incidence is vanishing)

EPIDEMIOLOGY

1. Most common age at presentation is between 3 months and 4 years.
2. Peak incidence occurs at around 9 months.

PATHOGENESIS

1. Observed tendency of these bacterial pathogens to cause cheek infection is not clear.
2. When buccal cellulitis is associated with otitis media, it has been suggested that the cheek infection results from extension of the middle ear infection through lymphatic channels to the buccinator nodes.

LABORATORY

1. Leukocytosis is usually present
2. Blood culture
3. Aspiration of the infected area for Gram stain and culture
   a. Site to aspirate: most inflamed central area (not the advancing border)

BOX 3–18 *Differential Diagnosis of Buccal Cellulitis*

Popsicle panniculitis (see p. 176)
   An acute cold injury to the fat of the cheeks
   Red, indurated, ill-defined nodule
   Lesion is close to the corner of the mouth
   Well-appearing infant
   May be unilateral or bilateral
   Presents during hot summer months
   History of sucking on a cold object about 1 to 3 days earlier (an important clue)
Cellulitis from other causes (e.g., following trauma)
   Staphylococcus aureus
   Group A beta-hemolytic streptococci
Trauma (e.g., child abuse)
Angioedema from insect stings

---

   b. Advancing border is most likely to contain the organism in erysipelas. In cellulitis the advancing border is indistinct and probably represents extension of edema from the more centrally inflamed area.
   c. Aspiration can be done with a No. 22 needle on a 3-mL syringe with or without prior injection of 0.1 mL of sterile water or a nonbacteriostatic sterile saline solution into the subcutaneous tissue. Fluid can be recovered by exerting a negative pressure on the syringe.
4. Cerebrospinal fluid examination, if indicated

COMPLICATIONS

1. Metastatic distant infection from associated bacteremia (e.g., meningitis, arthritis)
2. Intracranial extension (e.g., cavernous sinus thrombosis)

TREATMENT

1. Hospitalization
2. Parenteral antibiotic therapy (pending culture results) until patient shows clinical signs of improvement
   a. In infants and children coverage for *S. pneumoniae* and *H. influenzae* (especially in children <5 years of age who have not been immunized adequately): cephalosporin (e.g., ceftriaxone or cefotaxime)
   b. Penicillinase-resistant penicillin, if clinically indicated (e.g., following trauma; oxacillin for *S. aureus* and group A beta-hemolytic streptococci)
   c. Cefuroxime alone is another alternative. It covers Gram-positive bacteria including *S. aureus* and *H. influenzae.*
3. After clinical improvement occurs, an orally administered antibiotic (e.g., amoxicillin/clavulanate or cefuroxime) is usually continued to complete a 7- to 10-day course.

PROGNOSIS

Excellent with prompt treatment

KEY POINTS

Buccal Cellulitis

- Presents as salmon pink to violaceous (purplish) discoloration of the cheek in a febrile infant
- Purplish blue discoloration is not pathognomonic of any bacterial pathogen; it can be seen either with *H. influenzae* or *S. pneumoniae.*

TABLE 3–38
Clinical Features of Buccal Cellulitis

Sudden onset of fever (rarely patient may be afebrile)
Signs of inflammation: tenderness, warmth, and coin-shaped discoloration of cheek
Discoloration
　Salmon pink to violaceous (purplish) hue
　Not a pathognomonic sign of any particular bacterial pathogen
Laterality
　Almost always unilateral
　Bilateral involvement is extremely rare
Concomitant middle ear infection
　Seen in 75% of patients
　If unilateral, always ipsilateral to the cellulitis
Concomitant meningitis
　May be present especially in young infants (in absence of clinical signs of meningeal involvement)

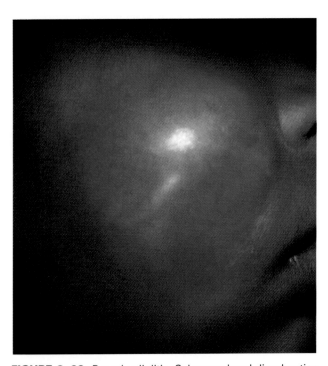

FIGURE 3–92. Buccal cellulitis. Salmon-colored discoloration of the cheek in a 3-year-old highly febrile child with ipsilateral otitis media. Blood culture was positive for *S. pneumoniae.*

Gonococcal Infections

DEFINITION

This is an infection caused by *Neisseria gonorrhoeae*, and often seen in children under certain circumstances.

ETIOLOGY

Neisseria gonorrhoeae, a gram-negative diplococcus, is the causative agent.

EPIDEMIOLOGY

1. There is an increasing incidence of penicillinase-producing *N. gonorrhoeae* (about 30% of the isolates seen in the United States).
2. This infection may be seen in the following groups of children:
   a. Newborn infants—acquired from the maternal birth canal
   b. Prepubertal children—as a result of sexual abuse

c. Adolescents—as a result of sexual abuse or voluntary sexual activity

CLINICAL FEATURES (see also Table 3–40)

1. Incubation period is 2 to 7 days.
2. Newborns: ophthalmia neonatorum (see p. 127)
   a. Copious purulent discharge from both eyes
   b. Inflammation of the eyelids and conjunctivae
3. Sexually abused children
   a. Copious purulent discharge from the vagina (vulvovaginitis) or penis
   b. Other sites that may be involved are the rectum and throat.
4. Disseminated gonococcal infection (DGI; see Box 3–19)

BOX 3–19 *Disseminated Gonococcal Infection*

Results from gonococcal bacteremia
Seen in 0.5% to 3% of patients with gonorrhea
Site of primary infection (any of the following)
   Cervix
   Urethra
   Anal canal
   Conjunctiva
   Pharynx
High-risk groups
   Female adolescents
   Menstruating women
   Pregnant women
   Those with pharyngeal gonorrhea
   Those with deficiency of terminal component of complement C5, C6, C7, or C8

LABORATORY

1. Gram stain of appropriate specimen: gram-negative intracellular paired organisms
2. Culture in Thayer-Martin chocolate agar of specimens taken from the eyes, vagina, cervix, penis, anus, and throat

---

TABLE 3–39
Complications of Gonococcal Infections

Blindness
Meningitis
Infective endocarditis
Osteomyelitis
Pelvic inflammatory disease
Sterility
Severe psychological trauma

---

3. blood culture or synovial fluid culture is positive in about 50% of patients with DGI.

DIFFERENTIAL DIAGNOSIS

1. Meningococcemia
2. Arthritis from other causes (e.g., infectious, inflammatory, or collagen diseases)

TREATMENT

1. For ophthalmia neonatorum:
   a. Ceftriaxone 25 to 50 mg/kg/day IV or IM (not to exceed 125 mg) given once
   b. Local eye care with saline irrigation at frequent intervals
2. For nondisseminated gonococcal infection:
   a. Ceftriaxone 125 mg IM in a single dose *and*
   b. Erythromycin or azithromycin for prepubertal children and doxycyclin or azithromycin for children older than 8 years of age (for the presumption that patient has concomitant *Chlamydia trachomatis*)
   c. Rule out other sexually transmitted diseases (STDs)
3. For DGI:
   a. Hospitalization
   b. Ceftriaxone 50 mg/kg/day IV or IM once a day for 7 days (maximum/1g/day) *and*
   c. Erythromycin, tetracycline, doxycycline, or azithromycin given orally (for the presumption that patient has concomitant *C. trachomatis*)
   d. Spectinomycin or ciprofloxacin for patients allergic to β-lactam drugs
   e. Rule out other STDs
4. Refer patient to social service and child protection agencies.

KEY POINT

Gonococcal Infections

■ Most gonococcal infections in children are a result of sexual abuse.

TABLE 3–40
Clinical Features of Disseminated Gonococcal Infection Arthritis-Dermatitis Syndrome

Rash

Seen in 50% to 75% of cases
Hemorrhagic pustules or vesicles at times with a necrotic base
Few in number
Distributed on the distal extremities
Lesions represent septic emboli

Arthritis

Seen in >90% of cases
May be migratory
Associated pain and swelling of big joints (most common: knees, ankles, wrists, elbows)
Uncommon in small joints of hands and feet
Tenosynovitis common

Other Features

Fever, chills, malaise, signs of septicemia

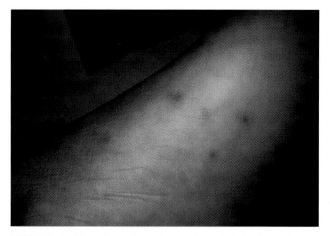

FIGURE 3-93. Disseminated gonococcal infection. Hemorrhagic pustules on the distal extremity of a 16-year-old sexually active girl. She had fever and swelling of the hands, knees, and wrists.

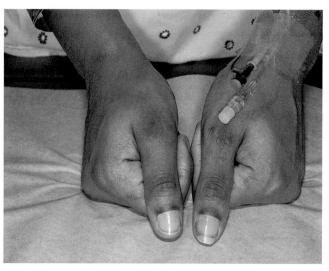

FIGURE 3-94. Swelling of the phalanges of the right thumb and hemorrhagic rash in disseminated gonococcal infection.

Meningococcemia

DEFINITION

Meningococcal infections are characterized by fever and petechial eruption; meningitis may accompany the septicemia.

ETIOLOGY

1. *Neisseria meningitidis*, an aerobic, fastidious gram-negative diplococcus.
2. There are eight pathogenic serogroups: A, B, C, X, Y, Z, W-135, and L.

EPIDEMIOLOGY

1. In the United States more than half the cases are due to serogroup B.
2. Most common age
   a. Primarily affects young children
   b. Peak age incidence: 6 to 12 months
3. Male-to-female ratio is 2 to 3:1.
4. More commonly seen in winter and spring
5. At risk are individuals with
   a. Inherited or acquired terminal complement deficiencies (C5-9)
   b. Properdin deficiency
   c. Immunoglobulin deficiency
   d. Asplenia

PATHOGENESIS

1. Asymptomatic colonization of the respiratory tract provides the focus for the spread of the organisms.
2. Transmission occurs from person to person through droplets of respiratory tract secretions.
3. Bacteremia leads to sepsis.

LABORATORY

1. Cultures from blood, skin lesions, and cerebrospinal fluid in all patients with suspected meningococcemia
2. Cultures of synovial fluid (if indicated)
3. Gram stain of smears from petechial skin lesions
4. Ancillary tests
   a. Complete blood count
   b. Sedimentation rate
   c. Coagulation profile
   d. Serum electrolytes including urea nitrogen and creatinine

---

BOX 3-20   *Differential Diagnosis of Meningococcemia*

PETECHIAL/PURPURIC LESIONS
Gonococcemia
Echoviral infection
Subacute bacterial endocarditis
Henoch-Schönlein purpura

TREATMENT

1. Hospitalization and stabilization of vital signs
   a. ABCs of resuscitation, cardiac and pulse oximetry monitoring
   b. Fluid resuscitation for septic shock
2. Antibiotic therapy
   a. Penicillin G intravenously 300,000 units/kg/day (given every 4 to 6 hours) up to 24 million units/day for 7 days

b. Cefotaxime or ceftriaxone are acceptable alternatives

c. Chloramphenicol (if patient is allergic to penicillin)

3. Rifampin to index case (after the course of penicillin has been completed)

a. Adults: 600 mg every 12 hours for 2 days

b. Children: 10 mg/kg (maximum 600 mg) every 12 hours for 2 days

PREVENTION

1. Close contacts of an index case are at an increased risk for invasive meningococcal disease.

a. Prophylactic rifampin (dose as mentioned above)

b. Given to all close contacts.

(1) Household, child care center, and nursery school contacts

(2) Any person who had contact with patient's oral secretions within 7 days prior to onset of disease

2. Meningococcal vaccine (a serogroup-specific quadrivalent vaccine [serotypes A, C, Y, W-135]) is approved for use in children over 2 years old.

3. Screening for complement deficiency in patients diagnosed with meningococcal disease

KEY POINTS

Meningococcemia

■ Petechial lesions are seen in patients with meningococcal bacteremia.

■ Purpura fulminans is a manifestation of disseminated intravascular coagulation, a complication of meningococcemia.

TABLE 3–41
Clinical Features of Meningococcemia

Incubation period: 1–10 days
Systemic symptoms
  Fever
  Chills
  Hypotension
  Meningitis
  Arthritis
Skin lesions
  Initially may be urticarial, maculopapular, or petechial
  Petechiae may progress to ecchymosis and ischemic necrosis
  Common sites: trunk and extremities

TABLE 3–42
Complications of Meningococcemia

Disseminated intravascular coagulation → purpura fulminans
Neurologic sequelae from meningitis
Waterhouse-Friderichsen syndrome
  Bleeding into adrenals
  Shock → coma → death

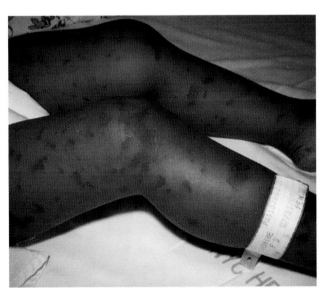

FIGURE 3–96. Purpura fulminans in meningococcemia.

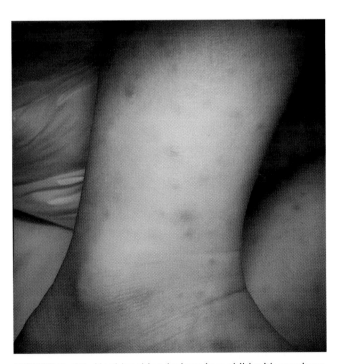

FIGURE 3–95. Nonblanching lesions in a child with meningococcemia.

Acquired Syphilis

SYNONYM   Lues

DEFINITION

An infectious disease that if untreated becomes a chronic systemic infection that passes through different stages.

ETIOLOGY

Treponema pallidum, a spirochete

EPIDEMIOLOGY

1. The general incidence of acquired syphilis in the United States is rising.
2. The incidence is higher in urban areas.
3. Occurs in sexually active adolescents and adults.
4. May result from sexual abuse in children.

CLINICAL FEATURES

1. Incubation period: approximately 3 weeks
2. Primary stage: chancre lasting 1 to 6 weeks
   a. Solitary, painless, indurated, eroded lesion on the genitalia
   b. This lesion represents the site of inoculation.
   c. It may not be recognizable in a girl if it is located in the cervix.
3. Secondary stage: secondary syphilis, appearing 2 to 10 weeks later
   a. Fever, malaise, chills
   b. Lymphadenopathy
   c. Arthralgia
   d. Rash
      (1) Discrete erythematous papulosquamous lesions on the torso, palms, and soles
      (2) Nonpruritic
   e. Condyloma lata
      (1) Flat-topped papules that coalesce to form small plaques
      (2) Distributed on the anogenital area
   f. Moth-eaten alopecia
   g. Mucous patches on the tongue and mouth
4. Subclinical latent stage: diagnosable only by the presence of a reactive serologic test; lasts 1 to 40 years or more.

5. Late stage: seen in approximately one third of individuals. Characterized by cutaneous, visceral, cardiovascular, and CNS lesions that can lead to debilitation and death.

LABORATORY

1. Screening tests: nontreponemal tests
   a. VDRL (Venereal Disease Research Laboratory) test
   b. RPR (rapid plasma reagin) test
2. Confirmatory test: treponemal test FTA-ABS (fluorescent treponemal antibody absorption) test
3. Dark-field microscopy of smears taken from lesions from moist skin or mucous membranes
4. Rule out other STDs including HIV infection.
5. Cerebrospinal fluid examination in children (to detect asymptomatic neurosyphilis)

TREATMENT

1. Early acquired syphilis (primary, secondary, latent syphilis of <1 year duration)
   a. Benzathine penicillin G
   b. Dose: 50,000 units/kg (up to adult dose of 2.4 million units) IM in a single dose
2. Late-latent syphilis (>1 year duration except neurosyphilis)
   a. Benzathine penicillin G as above
   b. Three consecutive weekly injections
3. For children allergic to penicillin
   a. Erythromycin *or*
   b. Tetracycline (>8 years of age) *or*
   c. Doxycycline (>8 years of age) *or*
3. Refer patient to a child protection agency (if indicated).

KEY POINTS

Acquired Syphilis

- Syphilis may be acquired from sexual abuse.
- It must be considered in the differential diagnosis of an illness occurring in a sexually active adolescent.

TABLE 3–43
Differential Diagnosis of Acquired Syphilis

Primary Chancre

Herpes progenitalis
Lymphogranuloma venereum
Behçet disease
Chancroid
Granuloma inguinale
Reiter syndrome

Secondary Syphilis

Pityriasis rosea
Guttate psoriasis
Lichen planus
Scabies
Drug eruption
Id reaction
Condyloma acuminata

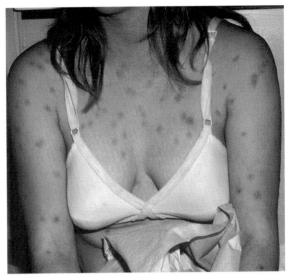

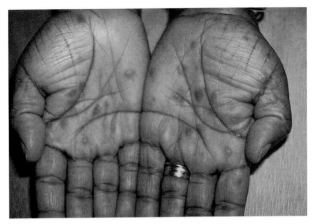

FIGURE 3–98. The palms and soles are common sites of secondary syphilis eruptions (see also Fig. 2–21).

FIGURE 3–97. Secondary syphilis, showing diffuse papulosquamous lesions.

Congenital Syphilis

DEFINITION

An intrauterine infection acquired by the fetus from a mother infected with *Treponema pallidum*.

ETIOLOGY

Treponema pallidum, a spirochete

EPIDEMIOLOGY

1. The incidence of congenital syphilis in the United States is rising.
2. It is associated with lack of maternal prenatal care and illicit drug use.

LABORATORY

1. Screening tests: nontreponemal tests on cord blood
   a. VDRL (Venereal Disease Research Laboratory) test
   b. RPR (rapid plasma reagin) test

2. Confirmatory test: treponemal test FTA-ABS (fluorescent treponemal antibody absorption) test
3. Dark-field microscopy of lesions from moist skin or mucous membranes
4. Radiograph of the long bones
5. Cerebrospinal fluid examination looking for:
   a. Pleocytosis
   b. Increased protein
   c. VDRL test positive

COMPLICATIONS

1. Stillbirth
2. Blindness
3. Deformities such as saddle nose, saber shin

BOX 3–22   *Hutchinson Triad*

Interstitial keratitis
Hutchinson teeth
Eighth nerve deafness

DIFFERENTIAL DIAGNOSIS

1. Congenital rubella syndrome
2. Congenital toxoplasmosis
3. Congenital cytomegalovirus infection

TREATMENT

1. Penicillin
   a. Aqueous crystalline penicillin G
      (1) Dose: 100,000 to 150,000 U/kg/day IV (given every 8 to 12 hours)
      (2) Duration: 10 to 14 days *or*

BOX 3–21   *Cutaneous Eruptions of Early Congenital Syphilis*

Skin lesions
Macules or papules or papulosquamous lesions
  Round or oval in shape
  Erythematous
  Lesions fade to coppery brown color
Vesicobullous hemorrhagic lesions
  Rare but highly diagnostic
Palmoplantar scaling

b. Procaine penicillin G
   (1) Dose: 50,000 units/kg IM daily
   (2) Duration: 10 to 14 days
c. Duration of treatment is 3 weeks when there is CNS involvement.
2. Follow serology at 1, 2, 4, and 6-month intervals until results are negative.

KEY POINTS

Congenital Syphilis

- Congenital syphilis has varied manifestations.
- Untreated or inadequately treated early congenital syphilis may result in manifestations of late congenital syphilis.

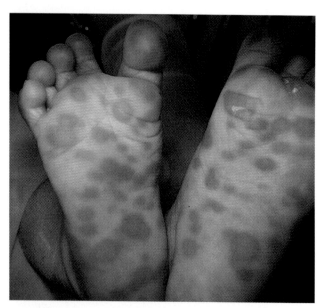

FIGURE 3–99. Copper-colored macules on the palms and soles.

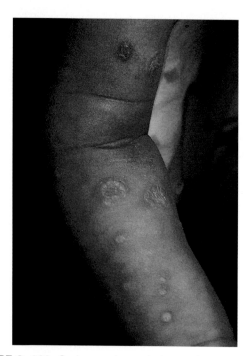

FIGURE 3–100. Scaly papules and plaques in a 3-month-old infant with congenital syphilis.

TABLE 3–44
Clinical Features of Early Congenital Syphilis (<2 Years of Age)

Clinical signs may be absent or minimal
Rhinitis (snuffles)
    Profuse mucopurulent discharge
    May result in rhagades or fissure around mouth
Cutaneous eruptions (see Box 3–21)
Mucous membrane lesions
    Round, slightly raised, pale, moist patches on lips or mouth
    Moist wart-like lesions in anogenital area
Hepatosplenomegaly
Lymphadenopathy
Long bones
    Osteochondritis, periostitis
    Pathologic fractures
    Pseudoparalysis of Parrot

TABLE 3–45
Clinical Features of Late Congenital Syphilis (>2 Years of Age)

Interstitial keratitis
    Appearing between 6 and 14 years
    Corneal opacity
    Pain, photophobia, lacrimation
Hutchinson teeth
    Notching of biting surface of permanent upper central incisors
Eighth nerve deafness
Mulberry or Moon molar
Saber shins
Higoumenaki sign (unilateral thickening of inner clavicle)
Syphilitic arthritis (Clutton joints—age 8–15 years)
Paroxysmal cold hemoglobinuria
Gummas in bones
Other ocular changes (choroiditis, retinitis, optic atrophy)

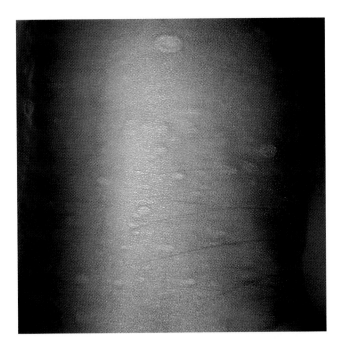

FIGURE 3–101. Congenital syphilis. Scattered lesions on the torso.

Infant Botulism

DEFINITION

A neuroparalytic disorder caused by *Clostridium botulinum* in infants

ETIOLOGY

1. *C. botulinum*, a gram-positive, spore-forming, toxin-elaborating anaerobic bacillus is found most commonly in soil, water, agricultural products, and honey.
2. Seven distinct serotypes (A to G) and specific neurotoxins of the serotypes of *C. botulinum* have been identified.
3. Serotypes A and B cause more than 90% of cases of infant botulism.

EPIDEMIOLOGY

1. In the United States, between 60 and 90 cases of infant botulism are reported annually to the Centers for Disease Control and Prevention (CDC); nearly half the cases occur in California.
2. Clustering of cases is related to either higher concentrations of *C. botulinum* spores in the soil (California, southern Pennsylvania, Utah, Hawaii) or ingestion of honey in religious practices (following Jewish New Year celebration).
3. Most common age
   a. Infants less than 1 year of age
   b. Range: 7 to 351 days
   c. About 95% of cases occur in the first 4 months of life.
4. Incubation period is estimated at 3 to 30 days from exposure to spore-containing soil or honey.
5. No sex predilection

PATHOGENESIS (see Fig. 3–102)

1. Infant botulism results when the ingested spores of *C. botulinum* germinate in the gastrointestinal tract and release a neurotoxin, which is responsible for the illness. (Food-borne botulism results after ingestion of food contaminated by one of the *preformed* toxins.)
2. In normal nerve conduction, release of acetylcholine from the motor end plates in response to depolarization is required.
3. Clostridial neurotoxin causes neuromuscular paralysis by binding irreversibly to nerve terminals and blocking the presynaptic release of acetylcholine at all postganglionic parasympathetic nerve terminals, some postganglionic cholinergic sympathetic nerve terminals, and the motor end plates.
4. Formation of new motor end plates is necessary for recovery (this may require several weeks).

PREDISPOSING FACTORS

1. Honey
2. Aminoglycosides (e.g., gentamicin) can worsen the clinical signs of botulism because they prevent the presynaptic release of acetylcholine.

CLINICAL FEATURES (see also Tables 3–46 and 3–47)

1. Clinical presentation may range from mild disease to sudden unexpected death.
2. The onset can be insidious or fulminant.
3. Infant botulism may be one of the causes of sudden infant death syndrome.

LABORATORY

1. Identification of *C. botulinum* organisms or toxin in the stool, gastric aspirate, or foods such as

honey can be accomplished with the help of the local health department or the CDC, Atlanta.

2. An enema (using sterile, nonbacteriostatic water) may be necessary to obtain a stool specimen.
3. In the majority of the cases, the source of spores remains unknown.
4. Rarely, toxin has been demonstrated in serum (about 1% of infants).
5. Chest and abdominal radiographs may suggest intercostal paralysis (bell-shaped thorax) and show signs of paralytic ileus (dilated intestinal loops, fecal impaction).
6. Electromyography
   a. Used to assess the integrity of neuromuscular transmission
   b. Example: Electromyography of the ulnar nerve showing an incremental or "staircase" response in a compound motor action potential to high rates of repetitive stimulation (20 and 50 Hz) is diagnostic.

COMPLICATIONS

1. Respiratory failure requiring assisted ventilation
2. Complications related to prolonged hospitalization
3. Secondary infections (pneumonia, otitis media, urinary tract infections)

DIFFERENTIAL DIAGNOSIS

1. Conditions usually considered at the initial presentation (admission diagnosis):
   a. Sepsis
   b. Meningitis/encephalitis
   c. Dehydration
   d. Viral syndrome
2. Subsequent usual working diagnoses:
   a. Poliomyelitis
   b. Viral polyneuritis
   c. Inborn error of metabolism
   d. Hypothyroidism
   e. Metabolic encephalopathy
   f. Poisoning (drug or chemical—e.g., organophosphate poisoning)
   g. Myasthenia gravis
   h. Guillain-Barré syndrome
   i. Brain stem encephalitis
   j. Hirschsprung disease
   k. Wernig-Hoffmann disease

TREATMENT

1. Hospitalization (intensive care unit) for meticulous supportive care
2. Respiratory support: if required, an endotracheal tube is used to maintain and protect the airway; mechanical ventilation may be needed.
3. Nutritional support is given until the infant has an adequate gag reflex and sucking and swallowing capabilities (preferably with nasogastric or nasojejunal feeding). Parenteral hyperalimentation (poses risk of infection) may be used for patients with absence of normal bowel motility.
4. Specific treatment
   a. Human-derived botulinum antitoxin (also called botulism immune globulin [BIG])
   b. Treatment is begun as early in the illness as possible.
   c. In the United States, BIG can be obtained from the California Department of Health Services, Infant Botulism Prevention Program (telephone: 510-540-2646).
5. Antibiotics may increase the release of neurotoxin into the gut by lysis of *C. botulinum* and exacerbate the illness. They should be used only to treat secondary infections.
6. Equine botulinum antitoxin is *not* recommended in infants for the following reasons:
   a. The circulating concentration of toxin in infants is believed to be at a very low level.
   b. There is a risk of anaphylaxis and of life-long hypersensitivity.
   c. There is no evidence of its effect on the toxin-producing organisms in the gut.
7. Anticholinesterase drugs are generally of no value.

PREVENTION

1. Honey should not be given to infants less than 1 year of age.
2. Breastfeeding may modify the severity of illness or rapidity of onset. Reported infants with the fulminant variety who died at home were all formula-fed, whereas 70% of infants admitted to the hospital with botulism were breastfed.
3. Currently, evidence that corn syrup (both light and dark) may be a potential source of botulinum spores is lacking.
4. Infant botulism is not transmitted from person to person.

PROGNOSIS

1. Gradual improvement with complete recovery occurs in the majority of the patients over a period of time (range, 10 days to 8 weeks).
2. Rarely, patients may experience relapse.
3. In the United States, the case-fatality rate among hospitalized patients is less than 1%.

KEY POINTS

Infant Botulism

- Most common form of botulism seen today
- Diagnosis must be considered in any infant presenting with constipation, hypotonia, poor feeding, or lethargy.
- Diagnosis must be considered in any infant (typically afebrile) who presents with signs or symptoms suggestive of sepsis but has negative results on blood, urine, and cerebrospinal fluid cultures.
- Progressive, symmetrical, descending, flaccid paralysis of the bulbar musculature and cranial nerve palsies occur first, followed by involvement of the somatic musculature.
- In food-borne botulism a preformed toxin is ingested, whereas in infant botulism a toxin is produced in the gut after *C. botulinum* spores have been ingested.

TABLE 3–46
Clinical Symptoms of Infant Botulism

Constipation
 Usually the first clinical symptom
 May precede other symptoms/signs by few weeks
Lethargy
Decreased activity
Poor suck, slow feeding
Pooling of secretions
Poor cry
Floppiness
Weakness
Loss of head control

TABLE 3–47
Clinical Signs of Infant Botulism

Progressive, symmetrical, descending, flaccid paralysis of
 bulbar musculature and cranial nerve palsies, followed by
 involvement of somatic musculature
 Generalized hypotonia, poor head control
 Ptosis
 Facial weakness/lack of facial movements
 Dilated nonreactive or poorly reactive pupils
 Ophthalmoplegia, diplopia
 Decreased or absent gag reflex
 Dysphasia
 Absence of sensory deficits (in majority of patients)
 Deep tendon reflexes usually present (unless involved
  muscles are very weak)
 Paralysis of respiratory muscles, respiratory arrest
Autonomic dysfunction
 Paralytic ileus
 Gastric dilatation
 Urinary retention
 Impaired gastrointestinal motility (constipation)
 Hypotension

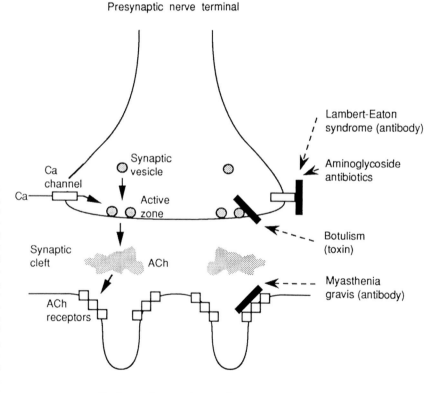

FIGURE 3–102. Sites of involvement in disorders of neuromuscular transmission. *Left,* Normal transmission involves depolarization-induced calcium (Ca) through voltage-gated channels. This stimulates release of acetylcholine (Ach) from synaptic vesicles at the active zone and into the synaptic cleft. Ach binds to Ach receptors and depolarizes the postsynaptic muscle membrane. *Right,* Disorders of neuromuscular transmission result from blockage of Ca channels (Lambert-Eaton syndrome or aminoglycoside antibiotics), impairment of Ca-mediated Ach release (botulinum toxin), or antibody-induced internalization and degradation of Ach receptors (myasthenia gravis). (From Aminoff MJ, Greenberg DA, Simon RP (eds): Clinical Neurology, 3rd ed. E. Norwalk, Appleton and Lange, 1996.)

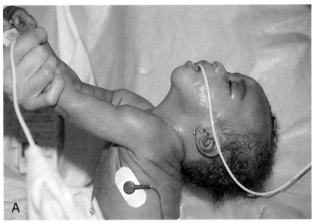

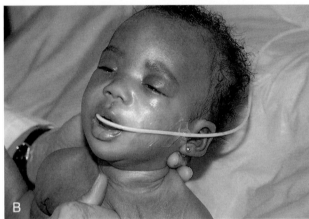

FIGURE 3–103. *A,* Infant botulism. A 12-week-old infant with hypotonia and a head lag. *Clostridium botulinum* organisms and type B neurotoxin were identified in her stool. No source of exposure to *C. botulinum* spores was identified. *B,* Ptosis and expressionless face are seen despite painful stimulus applied to the chest. The infant required hospitalization for 6 weeks, mainly for nutritional support, but she recovered completely in 8 weeks.

Tinea Capitis

SYNONYM   Ringworm of the Scalp

DEFINITION

Tinea capitis is a common, highly contagious fungal infection of the scalp that is seen in school children.

ETIOLOGY

1. The prevalent dermatophyte that causes this infection in the United States is *Trichophyton tonsurans.*
2. The other organisms are:
   a. *Microsporum canis*
   b. *Trichophyton violaceum*
   c. *Trichophyton verrucosum*
   d. *Microsporum audouinii*

EPIDEMIOLOGY

1. It is more common among African-American children in urban areas.
2. The peak age incidence is 2 to 6 years.
3. Rarely seen in adults

PATHOGENESIS

1. Tinea capitis due to *T. tonsurans, T. violaceum,* and *M. audouinii* is transmitted from person to person (anthropophilic).

2. *M. canis* and *T. verrucosum* are acquired from infected animals: cats, dogs, and cattle (zoophilic).
3. Other sources of infection are asymptomatic classmates and asymptomatic household members.

LABORATORY

1. Potassium hydroxide (KOH) preparation of a diseased hair (for technique, see next section on Tinea Corporis)
   a. *T. tonsurans* tinea capitis (endothrix): The fungal spores are inside the hair shaft.
   b. *Microsporum* species (ectothrix): The fungal spores are outside the hair shaft.

BOX 3–23	*Tinea Capitis and "Id" Hypersensitivity Reaction*

May be seen in children with kerions
Presents as an acute papular eruption on the face, neck, and trunk
Commonly mistaken for griseofulvin allergy (because it frequently coincides with the start of griseofulvin treatment)
A true delayed hypersensitivity; trichophytin skin test is positive

2. Fungal culture is performed using dermatophyte test media (DTM), Mycosel, or Sabouraud media.
3. Wood lamp examination
   a. *T. tonsurans* tinea capitis does not fluoresce.
   b. *Microsporum* tinea fluoresces with apple green color.

COMPLICATION

Permanent scarring in severe untreated tinea capitis

TREATMENT

1. Griseofulvin
   a. Dose: 15 to 20 mg/kg/day (maximum 1 g/day) given once or twice daily
   b. Administration: with milk or fatty meal
   c. Duration of treatment: 6 weeks
   d. Laboratory monitoring is not necessary in a healthy child.
2. Newer antifungals
   a. Itraconazole, fluconazole, terbinafine
   b. Any of these may be used if the organism is resistant to griseofulvin.
   c. Caution must be used because they interact with other drugs.

3. Prednisone
   a. Dose: 1 mg/kg/day (maximum 40 mg/day) for 5 days
   b. Can dramatically resolve the severe inflammation of a kerion.
   c. No tapering is necessary.
4. Shampoo: selenium sulfide or ketoconazole shampoo is used twice a week.
5. The child is advised to use his own towels, hairbrush, comb, and hats.
6. The child may go back to school after treatment has been started.

KEY POINTS

Tinea Capitis

- The three clinical variants of tinea capitis are noninflammatory, inflammatory (kerion), and seborrheic. The latter is commonly mistaken for dandruff.
- "Id" reaction may be seen with inflammatory tinea capitis. It is commonly misdiagnosed as a griseofulvin allergic reaction.

TABLE 3–48
Clinical Forms and Features of Tinea Capitis

Noninflammatory Tinea

Single or multiple lesions
Patchy or well-circumscribed areas of hair loss
Scaliness or stubs of broken hairs ("black dot tinea")

Inflammatory Tinea (Kerion)

Boggy, painful, tender mass with follicular pustules
Often associated with secondary regional lymphadenopathy

Seborrheic Tinea

Diffuse crusting and scaling with minimal hair loss
More common among girls

TABLE 3–49
Differential Diagnosis of Tinea Capitis

Alopecia areata
Trichotillomania
Scalp furunculosis
Psoriasis of scalp
Seborrheic dermatitis
Pityriasis rubra pilaris

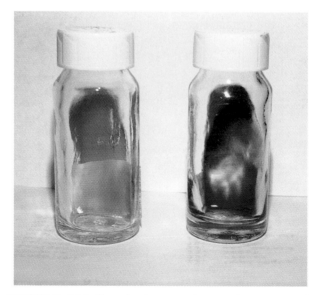

FIGURE 3–104. Fungal culture on dermatophyte test media (DTM). The original agar is yellow. It changes color to red when it becomes positive in 2 to 3 weeks.

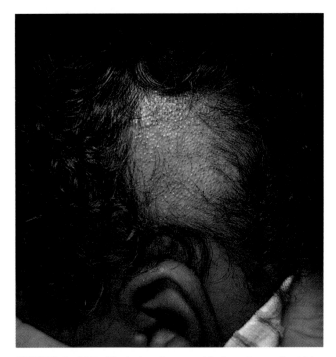

FIGURE 3–105. Black dot tinea capitis in a 1-month-old infant.

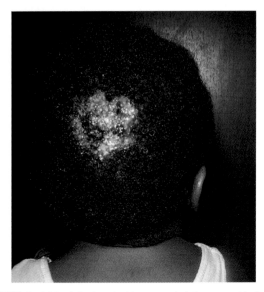

FIGURE 3–106. A kerion (a boggy, painful mass with follicular pustules).

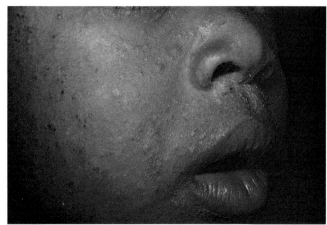

FIGURE 3–107. Id reaction in the child in Figure 3–106; it was thought by the mother to be a reaction to griseofulvin.

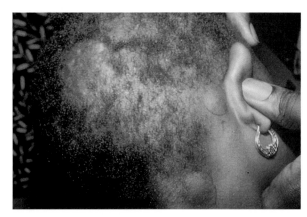

FIGURE 3–108. Prominent postauricular and cervical lymphadenopathy in a child with tinea capitis (seen here as patchy areas of hair loss).

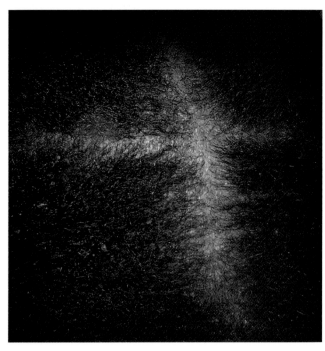

FIGURE 3–109. Seborrheic tinea capitis.

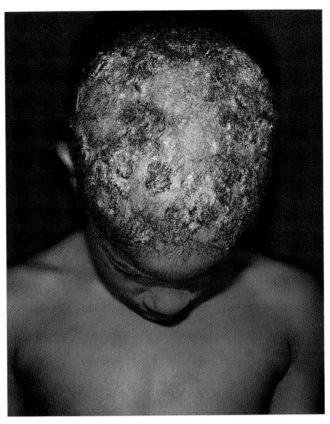

FIGURE 3-110. Tinea capitis involving the whole scalp.

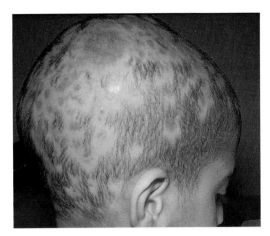

FIGURE 3-111. Scarring in severe tinea capitis.

Tinea Corporis

SYNONYMS   Ringworm of the Smooth Skin
            Tinea Circinata

DEFINITION

Tinea corporis is an infection of the skin caused by certain fungi.

ETIOLOGY

The causative organisms belong to one of three major genera:

1. *Trichophyton*
2. *Microsporum*
3. *Epidermophyton*

EPIDEMIOLOGY

1. Seen in all age groups
2. May be concurrent with tinea capitis

PATHOGENESIS

Transmitted by infected scales or materials shed from skin lesions in an infected person, animal, or fomites.

LABORATORY

1. Potassium hydroxide (KOH) preparation—technique:

   a. Put a scraping from the lesion on a glass slide.
   b. Add one drop of 10% KOH or Chlorazol Black.
   c. Pass briefly over a flame.
   d. Examine under a microscope and look for hyphae and spores.
2. Fungal culture using dermatophyte test media (DTM), Mycosel, or Sabouraud media

DIFFERENTIAL DIAGNOSIS

1. Herald patch of pityriasis rosea
2. Granuloma annulare
3. Nummular eczema.

TREATMENT

1. Topical antifungal (imidazoles, allylamines) twice daily for 10 to 14 days
2. Griseofulvin for 1 week for extensive tinea corporis at a dose of 15 to 20 mg/kg/day given with food.

KEY POINT

Tinea Corporis

- Tinea corporis consists of a scaly annular lesion with an active advancing border and a clear space in the center.

TABLE 3–50
Clinical Features of Tinea Corporis

Affects any exposed areas such as
  Face (tinea faciei)
  Extremities
  Body (tinea corporis)
Skin lesions
  Annular
  Solitary or multiple
  Varying size
  Active scaly, raised, erythematous, papulovesicular border,
    with central clearing
  One or two rings within a bigger ring may be seen
Tinea incognito
  Results from treatment with topical steroids, which
    suppress inflammation but not infection

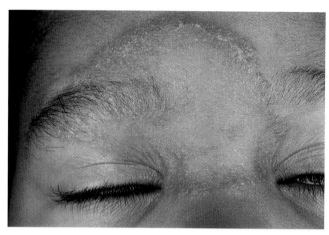

FIGURE 3–113. Tinea faciei. Lesion has an active scaly advancing border and clearing in the center.

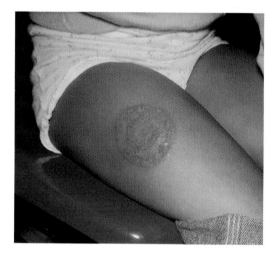

FIGURE 3–114. Tinea corporis with a ring within a ring.

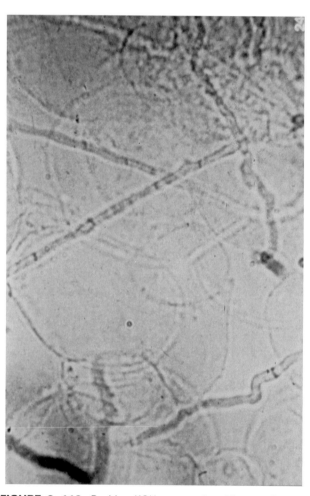

FIGURE 3–112. Positive KOH preparation. Elongated structures are hyphae.

Other Dermatophyte Infections

A. Tinea Pedis

1. Synonym: athlete's foot
2. It is more common in adolescents and young adults; it is uncommon but not rare in young children whose parents are also infected.
3. Most common organisms
   a. *Trichophyton rubrum*
   b. *T. mentagrophytes*

4. Lesions consist of
   a. Odoriferous pruritic scaly fissures and maceration of moist skin
   b. Sites: between toes and sides of both feet
5. Laboratory diagnosis
   a. KOH preparation
   b. Fungal culture
6. Treatment
   a. Terbinafine cream twice daily for 14 days
   b. Short course of griseofulvin.

B. Tinea Manum

1. Synonym: ringworm of the hand
2. Presents as
   a. Diffuse dry scaliness of one palm, or
   b. A well-circumscribed plaque of varying size on the dorsum of one hand
3. There may be associated bilateral tinea pedis (one hand–two feet disease).
4. Laboratory diagnosis
   a. KOH preparation
   b. Fungal culture
5. Treatment: topical antifungal

C. Tinea Cruris

1. Synonym: jock itch
2. More common in adolescents and young adults
3. Most common organisms
   a. *Trichophyton rubrum*
   b. *T. mentagrophytes*
   c. *Epidermophyton floccosum*
4. Predisposing factors
   a. Obesity
   b. Tight underwear
5. Eruption consists of
   a. Pruritic erythematous scaly lesions with active border
   b. Sites: groin and upper thighs

6. Laboratory diagnosis
   a. KOH preparation
   b. Fungal culture
7. Treatment
   a. Imidazole cream twice daily for 2 to 4 weeks
   b. Do not use preparations combined with high-potency topical steroids
   c. Short course of griseofulvin in severe cases
   d. Loose-fitting underwear

D. Onychomycosis

1. Synonym: tinea unguium, ringworm of the nail
2. Uncommon but may be seen in healthy children whose parents have tinea pedis or tinea of the nails
3. Most common organisms
   a. *T. rubrum*
   b. *T. mentagrophytes*
4. Affected nails are discolored and dystrophic with subungual debris.
5. Laboratory diagnosis
   a. KOH preparation
   b. Periodic acid-Schiff (PAS) stain, microscopy of pulverized nail
   c. Fungal culture
6. Treatment: pulse dosing with itraconazole 50 to 200 mg bid for 1 week for 2 to 3 months

KEY POINTS

Other Dermatophyte Infections

- Tinea pedis, tinea cruris, and onychomycosis are rare in children except in those whose parents are also infected.
- Do not use preparations combining a topical antifungal with a high-potency topical steroid.
- Treat onychomycosis with a systemic antifungal agent.

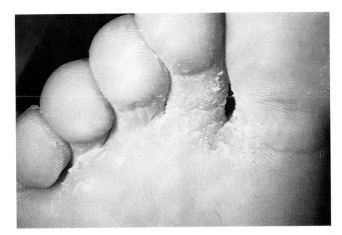

FIGURE 3–115. Tinea pedis in a child whose father also had tinea pedis.

TABLE 3–51
Differential Diagnosis of Tinea Pedis

Juvenile Plantar Dermatosis
Synonyms: "wet foot, dry foot" syndrome; soggy sock dermatitis
Chafing of skin results from change from wet to dry environment
Affects the plantar surfaces of the forefeet; interdigital areas are spared
Bilateral
Dry, glazed appearance with fissures
Seen more commonly in children with history of atopy
Treatment: Apply hydrophilic petrolatum on the forefeet immediately after being wet

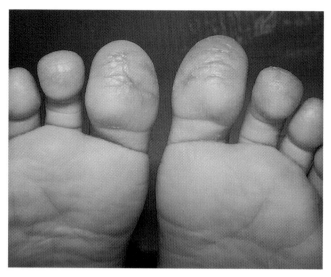

FIGURE 3-116. Juvenile plantar dermatosis mistakenly treated as tinea pedis.

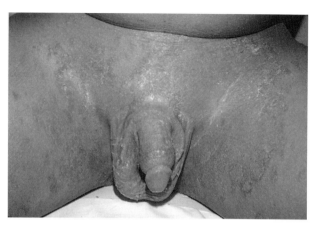

FIGURE 3-118. Tinea cruris.

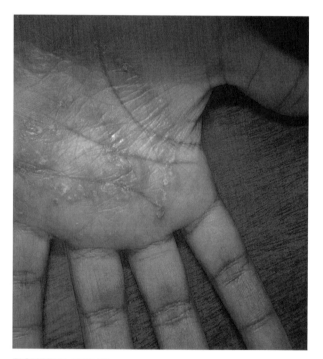

FIGURE 3-117. Tinea manum.

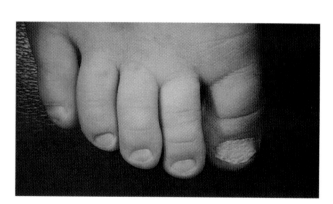

FIGURE 3-119. Onychomycosis.

Tinea Versicolor

SYNONYM   Pityriasis Versicolor

DEFINITION

This is a skin infection caused by a yeast-like organism.

ETIOLOGY

Malassezia furfur, also known as *Pityrosporum orbiculare* or *Pityrosporum ovale*

EPIDEMIOLOGY

1. More common in the tropics

2. In temperate countries, it is seen more often during the summer months.
3. More common in adolescents and young adults

LABORATORY

1. Wood lamp examination shows a yellow fluorescence, and this maps out the involved areas.
2. KOH preparation demonstrates hyphae and spores ("spaghetti and meatballs")

DIFFERENTIAL DIAGNOSIS

1. Postinflammatory hypopigmentation
2. Confluent and reticulated papillomatosis
3. Epidermodysplasia verruciformis

TREATMENT

1. Selenium sulfide 2.5% lotion
   a. Apply over the affected areas and wash off after 30 minutes
   b. Apply daily for 1 week, then less often
2. Terbinafine spray twice daily for 1 week
3. Imidazole cream or lotion bid for 2 weeks
4. Ketoconazole
   a. In older children and adolescents
   b. 200 mg once daily orally for 5 days
   c. Contraindicated in those with hepatic dysfunction
5. Selenium sulfide or ketoconazole shampoo on scalp twice weekly

KEY POINTS

Tinea Versicolor

- Lesions of tinea versicolor may be either hypopigmented or fawn-colored scaly macules that become confluent.
- There is a high rate of recurrence despite adequate treatment.

TABLE 3–52
Clinical Features of Tinea Versicolor

Skin Lesions

Active lesions may be either hypopigmented or tan-colored macules with scales
Lesions tend to become confluent
Common distribution
    Upper chest
    Back
    Shoulder
    Neck
    Upper arms
Recurrence is common
Hypopigmentation resolves slowly

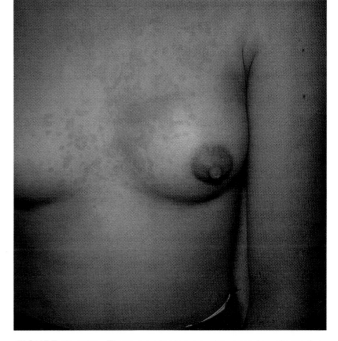

FIGURE 3–121. Tinea versicolor on the anterior chest. Lesions are slightly scaly, hyperpigmented confluent papules.

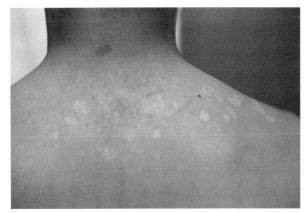

FIGURE 3–120. Tinea versicolor on the shoulder. Lesions are slightly scaly, hypopigmented, confluent papules.

Candidiasis

SYNONYM   Moniliasis

DEFINITION

An infection with *Candida albicans* that results in a spectrum of illnesses

ETIOLOGY

The organism is *Candida albicans,* a ubiquitous yeast.

EPIDEMIOLOGY

1. Newborns can acquire the infection from the maternal birth canal.
2. Oral antibiotic use may be a predisposing factor.
3. Invasive disease or severe recurrent mucocutaneous disease may be seen in immunodeficient individuals or those suffering from endocrinologic disorders.

CLINICAL FEATURES

The different clinical forms include:

1. Oral thrush—white plaques on the buccal mucosa and dorsal surface of the tongue
2. Candidal diaper dermatitis (see Box 3–24)

BOX 3–24   *Candidal Diaper Dermatitis*

Beefy red eruption
Sharp border
Satellite lesions
Scaling, especially along the border
Sites
  Perineum
  Scrotum and labia (always involved)
  Upper thighs
  Buttocks

---

3. Candidal intertrigo
   a. Moist erythema
   b. Sites
      (1) Neck
      (2) Axillae
      (3) Inframammary areas in obese adolescents
4. Congenital cutaneous candidiasis
   a. Results from ascending maternal infection
   b. Generalized eruption
   c. Scaly papulovesicles
   d. Benign course
5. Candidal paronychia with or without candidal onychomycosis
6. Chronic mucocutaneous candidiasis (candidal granuloma) is seen in patients with immunologic defects.

LABORATORY

1. KOH preparation shows pseudohyphae and spores
2. Culture

DIFFERENTIAL DIAGNOSIS

1. Milk particles
2. Oral lichen planus
3. Contact irritant diaper dermatitis
4. Erosive intertrigo of histiocytosis X
5. Dermatophyte onychomycosis

TREATMENT

1. Nystatin cream, imidazole cream, or allylamine cream
2. Nystatin suspension
3. Parenteral ketoconazole, fluconazole, itraconazole, or amphotericin B for severe invasive disease

KEY POINTS

Candidiasis

- Mucocutaneous infection may be seen in normal healthy newborns.
- Severe recurrent mucocutaneous infection may herald an underlying immunodeficiency.

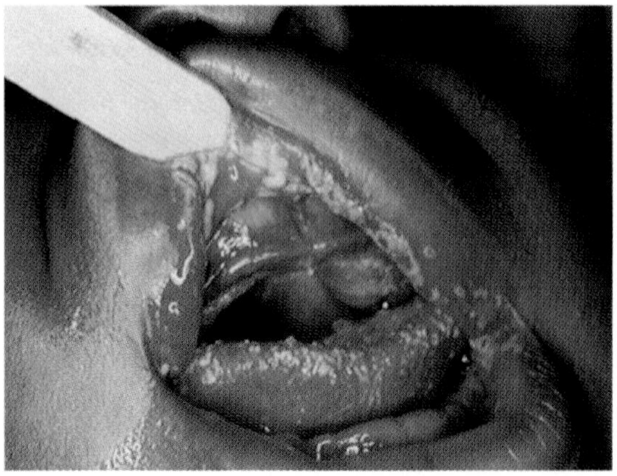

FIGURE 3–122. Oral candidiasis. (From Hurwitz S: Clinical Pediatric Dermatology, 2nd ed. Philadelphia, W.B. Saunders, 1993.)

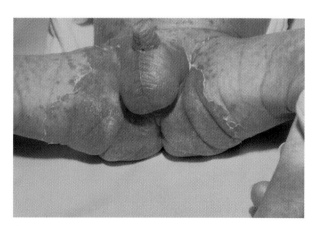

FIGURE 3–123. Candidal diaper dermatitis. There is scaling at the periphery and satellite lesions outside the border. In a male infant the scrotal skin is always involved.

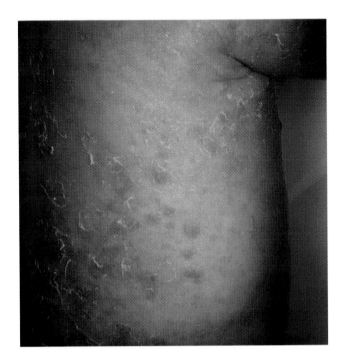

FIGURE 3–124. Congenital cutaneous candidiasis in a newborn. Generalized scaly papulovesicles. The mother had heavy candidal vaginitis and premature rupture of the membranes.

Scabies

DEFINITION
Scabies is an infestation of the skin with a mite.

ETIOLOGY
1. The organism is a mite, an acarus, *Sarcoptes scabiei* var *hominus.*
2. It is an obligate human parasite.
3. It dies within 48 hours when not on the human body.

EPIDEMIOLOGY
1. In the United States 1 million cases are reported annually.
2. It is more common in crowded living quarters and nursing homes.
3. It is a highly contagious disease transmitted by close personal contact.

> **BOX 3–25**   *Scabies*
>
> Common contacts are household members, babysitters, and playmates.
> Treat all contacts.

PATHOGENESIS
1. The female mite invades the upper layer of the skin and produces a burrow.
2. It deposits two eggs daily for 4 to 5 weeks, the mite's life span.
3. Only 10% of the eggs develop into adult mites.
4. The infested person has an average of 12 mites on the skin.
5. The signs and symptoms are a result of a delayed hypersensitivity, cell-mediated immune response.

CLINICAL FEATURES (see Table 3–53)
1. Incubation period is 4 to 6 weeks.
2. Norwegian or crusted scabies
   a. Consists of thick psoriasiform crusted lesions
   b. It is seen in persons with Down syndrome, immunocompromised hosts, or institutionalized individuals.
   c. The lesions teem with mites.
3. Scabies incognito is undiagnosed scabies resulting from the use of topical steroids.

LABORATORY
Light microscopic examination of skin scrapings from the burrow or a new unexcoriated lesion demonstrates the mite, egg, or excretions (67% yield). A negative scraping does not rule out scabies.

COMPLICATIONS
1. Secondary infection with *Staphylococcus aureus or Streptococcus pyogenes* may occur.
2. With *S. pyogenes,* acute glomerulonephritis may ensue.

DIFFERENTIAL DIAGNOSIS
1. Papular urticaria
2. Drug eruption
3. Other arthropod bites
4. Crusted (Norwegian) scabies may be mistaken for psoriasis.

TREATMENT

1. Permethrin 5% cream
   a. Apply from the neck down and leave overnight.
   b. Change all the clothes and bedsheets the following morning.
   c. Repeat 1 week later for best results.
2. Alternate preparations for school-age children
   a. Gamma benzene hexachloride (lindane 1%) cream or lotion used as described for permethrin
   b. Caution: If used improperly and a significant amount is systemically absorbed, it may be neurotoxic.
3. Treat all contacts.
4. Pruritus may remain for 3 to 4 weeks after treatment.
5. For crusted or Norwegian scabies
   a. Isolate the patient.
   b. Apply several or sequential courses of topical permethrin or gamma benzene hexachloride.
   c. Oral ivermectin at a single dose of 200 μg/kg

KEY POINTS

Scabies

- The papular eruption is intensely pruritic and generalized.
- Interdigital web lesions are less commonly seen in children.
- Young infants may have hyperpigmented nodular lesions, especially along the axillary line.

TABLE 3–53
Clinical Features of Scabies

Skin Eruption

Consists of intensely pruritic papular lesions
Excoriations are common
Pruritus is worse at night
Distribution
   Generalized, but more numerous on:
   Waist
   Male genitalia
   Interdigital webs
   Wrists
   Axillae
   Areolae of breasts
   Face and scalp spared except in infants and immunocompromised hosts
Burrows may not always be evident, especially in children
Eruption may become eczematized from chronic scratching

Scabies in Babies

Palms, soles, face, and scalp may be involved
Lesions may include bullae and vesicles
Hyperpigmented nodules may be seen along the axillary line

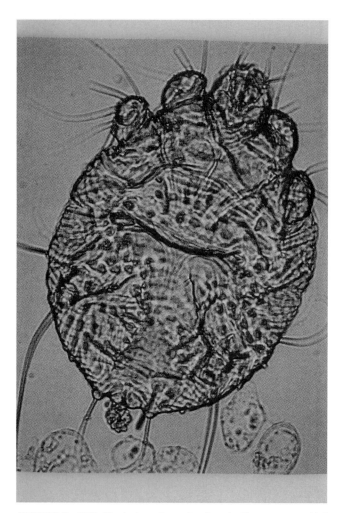

FIGURE 3–125. Ventral surface of a female *Sarcoptes scabiei* organism.

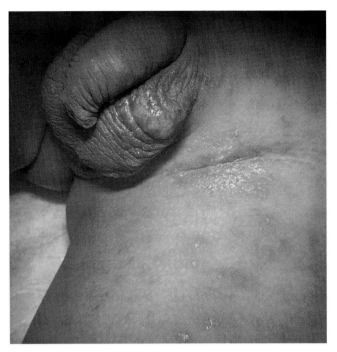

FIGURE 3–126. Scabies lesions on the genitalia.

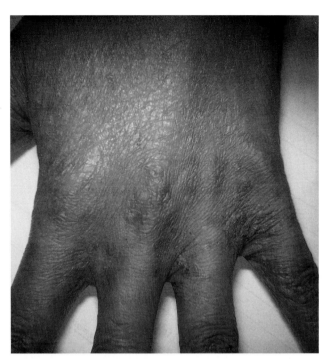

FIGURE 3–127. Scabies. Interdigital involvement.

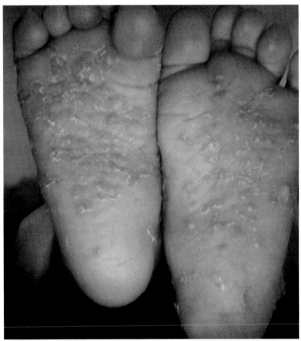

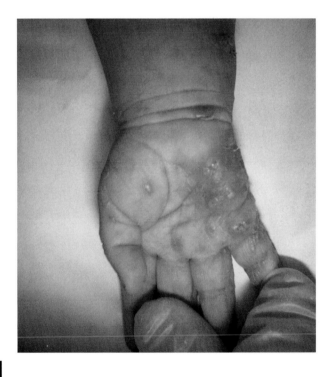

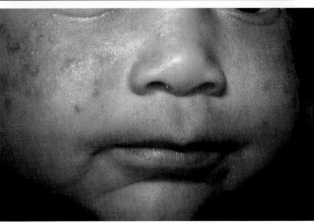

FIGURES 3–128, 3–129, 3–130. An infant with scabies lesions on the soles, palm, and face.

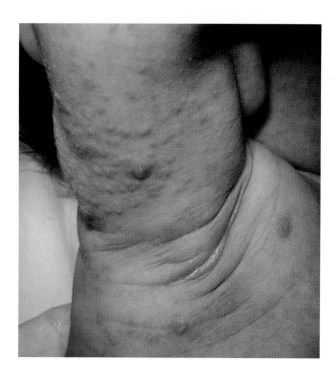

FIGURE 3–131. Scabies. Hyperpigmented nodules on the upper arm and axilla of an infant.

Pediculosis Capitis

DEFINITION

Pediculosis is scalp infestation with lice.

ETIOLOGY

1. The organism is *Pediculus humanus* var *capitis.*
2. It is a blood-sucking wingless insect.
3. It is an obligate human parasite.

EPIDEMIOLOGY

1. The highest incidence occurs among school children.
2. Outbreaks occur in schools and crowded living quarters.
3. It is exceedingly rare in African-Americans.
4. There seems to be an increasing incidence of permethrin- and lindane-resistant pediculosis.

CLINICAL FEATURES

1. Intensely itchy scalp
2. Lice and nits attached to hairs may be visible.
3. A papular dermatitis of the neck and back of the ears may occur.
4. Cervical and occipital lymphadenopathy may be seen.
5. Nits of *Phthirus pubis* (crab or pubic louse) may attach to eyelashes; this may result from sexual abuse.

DIFFERENTIAL DIAGNOSIS

1. Hair casts
2. Impetigo of the scalp

TREATMENT

1. Permethrin 1% cream rinse: Apply for 10 minutes, then rinse off *or*
2. Gamma benzene hexachloride (1% lindane) shampoo: Apply for 10 minutes, then rinse off.
3. Nits and lice on scalp hair may be removed with fine-toothed comb.
4. Nits on the eyelashes may be treated with petrolatum and then removed manually.
5. For recalcitrant cases of pediculosis, the following may be tried:
   a. Apply thick petrolatum, 30 to 40 g, all over the scalp, put a shower cap on the head, and leave overnight. Wash off the following morning.
   b. Apply 5% permethrin cream every 8 hours.
   c. Give sulfamethoxasole-trimethoprim orally at the usual dose for 3 days. Repeat 1 week later. This works on the bacteria that live symbiotically in the louse's gut.
   d. Single oral dose of ivermectin 200 μg/kg.

KEY POINTS

Pediculosis Capitis

- Pediculosis is highly communicable.
- Nits of *Phthirus pubis* on the eyelashes may result from sexual abuse.

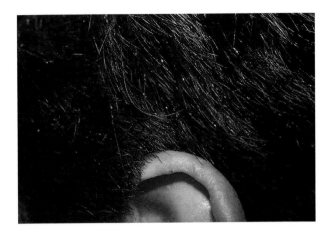

FIGURE 3–132. Pediculosis capitis. Nits of *Pediculus humanus* var *capitis* attached to the scalp hair.

Cutaneous Larva Migrans

SYNONYM   Creeping Eruption

DEFINITION

An infestation of the skin with the larvae of the dog or cat hookworm.

ETIOLOGY

1. Larva of the dog or cat hookworm *Ancylostoma braziliense*
2. Larva of other less common parasites
   a. *Ancylostoma caninum*
   b. *Ancylostoma duodenale*
   c. *Necatur americanus*
   d. *Strongyloides stercoralis*

EPIDEMIOLOGY

1. The following are endemic regions:
   a. Southeastern United States
   b. Caribbean
   c. Central America
   d. South America
   e. Southeast Asia
2. Common in moist, sandy areas

CLINICAL FEATURES

1. Lesion consists of an intensely pruritic, serpiginous mobile track in the upper epidermis.
2. Common distribution: foot, buttock, hand

DIFFERENTIAL DIAGNOSIS

Tinea infections, contact dermatitis, granuloma annulare

TREATMENT

1. Topical application of thiabendazole suspension to the advancing edge of the track twice daily for 10 days.
2. Thiabendazole orally 25 to 50 mg/kg/day in two divided doses for 2 to 4 days

KEY POINTS

Cutaneous Larva Migrans

- The lesion is serpiginous and mobile.
- It is acquired most commonly by walking barefoot in endemic areas.

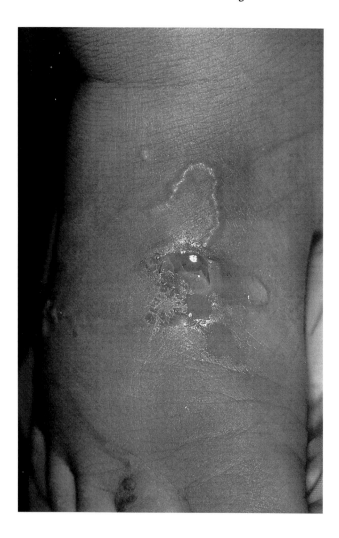

FIGURE 3–133. Cutaneous larva migrans. Foot of an infant who visited a relative in Florida with nine cats. A bulla overlies the serpiginous lesion.

4

Ophthalmology

Binita R. Shah, M.D.

Ophthalmia Neonatorum

SYNONYMS   Neonatal Conjunctivitis
Neonatal Blennorrhea

DEFINITION
Ophthalmia neonatorum is an inflammation of the conjunctiva within the first 4 weeks of life.

EPIDEMIOLOGY
1. Ophthalmia neonatorum is the most common infection in the first month of life.
2. Major causes of ophthalmia neonatorum (in decreasing order) are:
   a. Chemical (most common cause in hospitals using silver nitrate prophylaxis)
   b. Chlamydial (see p. 129)
   c. Bacterial
      (1) Gonococcal
      (2) Bacterial conjunctivitis (due to other bacteria)
   d. Viral (herpes simplex [predominantly type 20])

BOX 4–1 *Gonococcal Conjunctivitis*

Incubation period: 2 to 5 days
May present at birth (premature rupture of membranes)
May be delayed beyond 5 days of life (partially suppressed by ocular prophylaxis)
Must be considered in any infant less than 2 to 3 weeks of age with conjunctivitis
Eye findings
   Bilateral involvement
   Intense lid edema, marked conjunctival injection, and chemosis
   May start as mild conjunctivitis with watery or serosanguineous discharge at first
   Discharge rapidly becomes thick, mucopurulent, and copious
   May be associated with other distant foci of infection (meningitis, arthritis, anorectal infection)

---

3. In the United States, the incidence of gonococcal ophthalmia is 0.3% in 1000 live births, and the incidence of ophthalmia due to *Chlamydia trachomatis* is 8.2 in 1000 live births.

PATHOGENESIS
1. Direct inoculation of the neonate's conjunctival sac by the organism during passage through an infected birth canal
2. With premature rupture of the membranes, transmission of maternal genital organisms can occur before birth.
3. The risk of chlamydial conjunctivitis in an infant born to an infected mother ranges from 20% to 50%.

CLINICAL FEATURES
1. Gonococcal conjunctivitis (see Box 4–1).
2. Chemical conjunctivitis
   a. Occurs in about 10% of neonates after instillation of 1% silver nitrate drops
   b. Bilateral hyperemia and edema of the conjunctiva *within* the first 24 hours of life
   c. Typically mild inflammation, absence of purulence, and spontaneous resolution in 1 to 3 days with no therapy.
   d. Gram stain reveals only a few white blood cells and no bacteria.

LABORATORY
1. To exclude gonococcal ophthalmia
   a. Gram stain of the purulent discharge material (gram-negative intracellular diplococci)
   b. Culture/sensitivities of ocular discharge, blood, and cerebrospinal fluid (to exclude distant foci)
      (1) *Neisseria gonorrhoeae* is extremely sensitive to drying and temperature changes.
      (2) Culture specimen should be inoculated immediately onto a selective medium such as Thayer-Martin chocolate agar and incubated at 35° to 37°C in an atmosphere of 5% to 10% CO_2.
2. To exclude *C. trachomatis* infection (see p. 130)
3. To exclude other organisms
   a. Gram stain (e.g., gram-negative rods [*Pseudo-*

monas aeruginosa], gram-positive cocci [*Staphylococcus aureus*])

b. Cultures for aerobic and anaerobic nongonococcal bacteria

c. Viral culture

4. Normal inhabitants of the skin and mucous membranes (e.g., staphylococci, *Neisseria* species) may contaminate exudate. Thus, the presence of bacteria on a Gram-stained smear may not be related etiologically to conjunctivitis.

DIFFERENTIAL DIAGNOSIS (see also Table 4–1)

1. Dacryocystitis
   a. A complication of dacryostenosis (congenital obstruction of the nasolacrimal duct)
   b. Pain, redness, edema around the lacrimal sac, persistent tearing, and conjunctivitis
   c. Usually unilateral
   d. Bacteria causing infection most frequently are *S. aureus* and *Streptococcus pneumoniae.*
2. Conjunctival hyperemia from other causes
   a. Corneal abrasion due to eye trauma (e.g., during delivery or by fingernails)
   b. Neonatal glaucoma

TREATMENT

1. Gonococcal conjunctivitis
   a. If Gram stain of the purulent material shows gram-negative intracellular diplococci, infant must be hospitalized with a presumptive diagnosis to receive the treatment.
   b. Patient is isolated with standard precautions (contact) until effective systemic antibiotic therapy has been given for at least 24 hours. Exudate is highly contagious.
   c. Systemic antibiotic therapy
      (1) A single dose of ceftriaxone 25 to 50 mg/kg (maximum 125 mg) given intravenously or intramuscularly *or*
      (2) A single dose of cefotaxime 100 mg/kg given IV or IM
   d. Adjunctive therapy: Immediate irrigation of eyes with saline followed by irrigation several times a day until the purulent discharge subsides.
   e. Topical antibiotic therapy alone is not adequate

and is not necessary once the patient has received systemic antibiotic therapy.
   f. Suspect co-infection with *C. trachomatis* if patient fails to respond satisfactorily despite adequate therapy.
   g. Mother and her sexual partner(s) must be evaluated for sexually transmitted diseases (STDs) including *C. trachomatis,* and treated appropriately.
2. Chemical conjunctivitis: No therapy required; this is a self-limited entity.
3. Herpes simplex virus conjunctivitis: Systemic acyclovir as well as topical therapy (see p. 56).

PREVENTION

1. Neonatal ocular prophylaxis
   a. Recommended for prevention of gonococcal ophthalmia in all infants born vaginally and by cesarean section; it is required by law in most of the United States.
   b. Most commonly used agents (a single-use ampule or tube) include either
      (1) Silver nitrate 1% aqueous solution *or*
      (2) Erythromycin 0.5% ophthalmic ointment *or*
      (3) Tetracycline 1% ophthalmic ointment
   c. Prophylactic agent should be given immediately after birth and definitely within 1 hour after delivery.
2. Neonates born to mothers who have gonorrhea at the time of delivery should receive a single dose of parenteral antibiotic (as mentioned above) in addition to the ocular prophylaxis.

KEY POINTS

Ophthalmia Neonatonem

- Gonococcal ophthalmia is a potentially blinding condition.
- *N. gonorrhoeae* or *P. aeruginosa* can penetrate an intact cornea leading to ulceration, perforation, and endophthalmitis within hours of infection.
- Traditional method of differentiating ophthalmia by the age at presentation is helpful but *not* absolutely reliable as a diagnostic clue; laboratory studies *must* be used to distinguish the various etiologies.

TABLE 4–1
Etiology of Ophthalmia Neonatorum

Bacterial
Most Common

Chlamydia trachomatis

Common

Neisseria gonorrhoeae
Staphylococcus aureus
Hemophilus species
Streptococcus pneumoniae

Occasional

Pseudomonas aeruginosa
Group B streptococci
Escherichia coli
Neisseria meningitidis
Moraxella catarrhalis
Mixed (gonococcal and chlamydial)

Chemical (common)

Silver nitrate instillation

Viral (rare)

Herpes simplex type 2
Coxsackievirus A9
Echovirus
Adenovirus
Cytomegalovirus

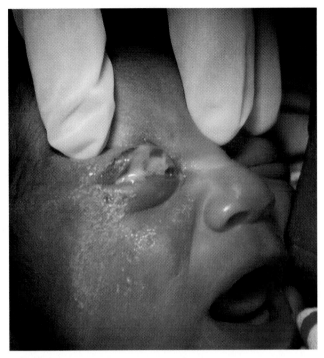

FIGURE 4–1. Gonococcal ophthalmia. A 4-day-old neonate with copious, grossly purulent discharge and involvement of both eyes. Both Gram stain and culture were positive for *N. gonorrhoeae.*

TABLE 4–2
Complications of Gonococcal Ophthalmia

Ocular	Systemic
Corneal ulceration	Meningitis
Corneal/globe perforation	Septicemia
Iridocyclitis	Arthritis
Flat anterior chamber	Endocarditis
Secondary glaucoma	Death
Panophthalmitis	
Blindness	

Chlamydial Ophthalmia

SYNONYM   Inclusion Blennorrhea
Neonatal Inclusion Conjunctivitis

DEFINITION

Ophthalmia neonatorum is an inflammation of the conjunctiva within the first 4 weeks of life. Conjunctivitis due to *Chlamydia* is referred to as inclusion blennorrhea or chlamydial ophthalmia.

ETIOLOGY

Chlamydia trachomatis

EPIDEMIOLOGY

1. About 50% of infants born vaginally of infected mothers acquire chlamydia during delivery.
2. The infant may become infected at one or more anatomic sites including
   a. Conjunctiva
   b. Nasopharynx
   c. Rectum
   d. Vagina
3. The most frequent disease that results is neonatal inclusion conjunctivitis.
4. Of infants acquiring *C. trachomatis:*

| BOX 4-2 | *Clinical Features of Chlamydial Ophthalmia* |

Incubation period: 5 to 14 days
Bilateral; however, in early stages, one eye may appear more infected than the other
Mild to moderate hyperemia of conjunctiva
Swelling of lids, chemosis
Greater involvement of palpebral than bulbar conjunctiva
Mild to copious mucopurulent discharge
Pseudomembrane formation
Cornea rarely affected
Usual duration of conjunctivitis: about 1 to 2 weeks (occasionally much longer)

    a. Risk of conjunctivitis is 25% to 50%
    b. Risk of pneumonia is 5% to 20%

LABORATORY AND DIFFERENTIAL DIAGNOSIS

1. To exclude other causes of conjunctivitis, most importantly gonococcal ophthalmia, see p. 127 and Table 4–1.
2. For diagnosis of chlamydial ophthalmia any of the following methods may be used:
    a. Giemsa stain of the conjunctival scraping
        (1) Identifies characteristic intracytoplasmic inclusion bodies that may be present in the epithelial cells of the conjunctiva
        (2) Polymorphonuclear cells present in the discharge do not contain inclusion bodies.
    b. Direct fluorescent antibody (DFA) staining for elementary bodies in clinical specimens
    c. Enzyme immunoassay (EIA) is rapid, sensitive, and specific.
    d. Nucleic acid amplification methods (polymerase chain reaction [PCR])
    e. Isolation of *C. trachomatis* in tissue culture

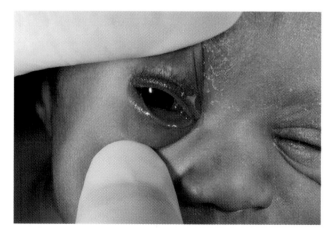

FIGURE 4–2. Chlamydial conjunctivitis in a 2-week-old neonate presenting with mild mucopurulent eye discharge with hyperemia of the palpebral conjunctiva involving both eyes. Direct fluorescent antibody staining for elementary bodies was positive, and both Gram stain and culture were negative for *N. gonorrhoeae.*

TREATMENT

1. No hospitalization is required; patient is treated as an outpatient.
2. Topical therapy alone is inadequate (does not eliminate infection at other sites).
3. Systemic therapy eliminates infection in eyes as well as in other infected sites.
    a. Erythromycin estolate or erythromycin ethylsuccinate
    b. Dose: 50 mg/kg/day for a total of 10 to 14 days
    c. With systemic therapy, there is no need to use topical therapy.
4. Co-infection with *C. trachomatis* and *N. gonorrhoeae*
    a. May be present in some neonates
    b. May be difficult to differentiate the two clinically
    c. Chlamydial infection should be suspected when conjunctivitis persists despite appropriate therapy for gonococcal infection.
5. Mother and her sexual partner(s) must be evaluated for sexually transmitted diseases (STDs) and treated appropriately.
6. Without treatment, acute inflammation continues for several weeks and then enters a subacute stage of mild conjunctival infection with minimal purulent discharge.

PREVENTION

1. Prophylactic regimen used for prevention of gonococcal ophthalmia (see p. 128) is *not* effective for prevention of chlamydial ophthalmia.
2. Neonates born to mothers with untreated chlamydial infection at the time of delivery should be treated with oral erythromycin (see treatment section) for 14 days.

KEY POINT

Chlamydial Ophthamia

■ Most common cause of conjunctivitis in the neonatal period

TABLE 4–3
Complications of Neonatal Chlamydial Infections

Ocular	Systemic
Corneal scarring (of varying degree) Vision usually not affected	Pharyngitis Otitis media Pneumonia

Acute Conjunctivitis

SYNONYM   "Red Eye"

DEFINITION

Acute conjunctivitis is an inflammation of the conjunctiva, usually as a result of infection or allergy.

EPIDEMIOLOGY

1. Viral conjunctivitis is most commonly seen during the fall and winter months.
2. Gonococcal and chlamydial conjunctivitis is seen in the following age groups:
   a. Neonates delivered through an infected birth passage (see pp. 127–130)
   b. Sexually active adolescents

PATHOGENESIS

1. Conjunctiva is sterile at birth but rapidly becomes colonized with surface bacteria.
2. Despite the constant presence of bacteria, the conjunctiva rarely becomes infected because of:
   a. Constant bathing by tears and mechanical wiping provided by blinking
   b. Antibacterial substances in tear film (lysozyme, IgA, lactoferrin, B lysin)
3. Routes by which conjunctiva becomes infected:
   a. Direct inoculation by contaminated fingers or fomites (most frequent)
   b. Droplet infection
   c. Swimming pools
   d. Infected contiguous areas (e.g., eyelids, lacrimal duct)
4. Viral conjunctivitis occurs as a part of viral upper respiratory tract infection (URI).

LABORATORY

1. Acute conjunctivitis is usually a clinical diagnosis based on the history and physical examination.

2. Gram stain, culture, and sensitivity of scraping of conjunctiva
   a. Are usually not required (neither practical nor economically feasible)
   b. *Must* be done in all cases of ophthalmia neonatorum (see p. 127) or in cases with hyperacute purulent conjunctivitis
   c. For conjunctival culture:
      (1) First wipe away any discharge; it should not be used for culture (invariably contaminated).
      (2) Evert the lower lid and wipe a moistened cotton-tip applicator along the entire cul-de-sac, directly streaking the material onto an agar plate.

DIFFERENTIAL DIAGNOSIS

1. Traumatic corneal abrasions
2. Infectious corneal ulceration
3. Acute iritis
4. Acute glaucoma

TREATMENT

1. Bacterial conjunctivitis
   a. Topical antibiotic eye ointment or drops
      (1) Ointment preferred (stays longer in conjunctival sac)
      (2) Drops are quickly diluted by tears or washed out of eyes
   b. Initial drug of choice: sulfacetamide or erythromycin
   c. Neomycin-containing preparations are *not* preferred (high prevalence of neomycin sensitivity; patient may experience worsening of symptoms)
   d. Conjunctivitis usually improves within 5 to 7 days (regardless of treatment)
2. Adenovirus conjunctivitis
   a. Cool compresses
   b. Artificial tears

BOX 4-3   *Etiology of Acute Conjunctivitis*

INFECTIOUS

Bacterial
Haemophilus influenzae
Streptococcus pneumoniae
Staphylococcus aureus
Neisseria gonorrhoeae
Chlamydia trachomatis

Viral
Adenovirus
Herpes virus (HSV type 1; HSV-2 [neonates])
Varicella

NONINFECTIOUS
Allergic
Traumatic (e.g., foreign body, corneal abrasion)
Chemical (e.g., alkali burn)
Glaucoma
Uveitis

SYSTEMIC DISEASES
Kawasaki disease (see pp. 410–413)
Stevens-Johnson syndrome (see pp. 181–183)
Toxic shock syndrome (see pp. 89–90)

c. Isolation precautions including hand washing after contact with eyes
3. Allergic conjunctivitis
   a. Vasoconstricting, decongestant eye drops in majority of cases
   b. Steroid eye drops in severe cases
   c. Cromolyn sodium drops for vernal conjunctivitis
4. Ophthalmology consultation and slit-lamp examination
   a. Immediate for all patients with suspected herpes simplex or zoster conjunctivitis
   b. Immediate for all cases of hyperacute conjunctivitis
   c. If conjunctivitis is unresponsive after 3 to 7 days of palliative care
   d. If intense pain or decreased vision is present and if corneal or uveal involvement is suspected

KEY POINTS

Acute conjunctivitis

- Most common viral cause of acute conjunctivitis is adenovirus.
- Most common identifiable cause of bacterial conjunctivitis is *Hemophilus influenzae*.
- Most prominent symptom of allergic conjunctivitis is bilateral itching.
- Neisseria conjunctivitis is a vision-threatening ophthalmic emergency.
- Consult ophthalmologist *before* using topical steroids to treat acute conjunctivitis.

TABLE 4–4
Clinical Features of Bacterial Conjunctivitis

History of exposure	Absence of pain
Often bilateral disease	Absence of photophobia
Purulent exudate (moderate to copious)	Absence of preauricular adenopathy
Conjunctiva: marked hyperemia, chemosis	Absence of URI signs/symptoms
Cornea normal	Concurrent otitis media ($\pm$)
Vision, ocular movements normal	Culture (+) for causative bacteria
Pupillary size and reaction normal	

TABLE 4–7
Clinical Features of Allergic Conjunctivitis

Recurrent history of similar illness	Bilateral involvement
Seasonal exacerbations (spring, summer, fall)	Itching (hallmark of allergic eye disease)
History of atopy (allergic rhinitis, asthma, eczema)	Watery to mucoid eye discharge
	Conjunctiva: diffuse injection
Concurrent allergic rhinitis/rhinosinusitis	Palpebral conjunctiva: papillary hypertrophy
Concurrent signs of atopy	Vision, ocular movements normal
	Pupillary size and reaction normal

TABLE 4–5
Clinical Features of Hyperacute Conjunctivitis
(see Fig. 2–22)

Often bilateral	Conjunctiva: markedly injected, chemosis
Copious mucopurulent discharge	Corneal perforation (about 10% of cases)
Sexually active adolescents	Culture (+): *Neisseria gonorrhoeae* or *N. meningitides*
Gram stain: gram-negative intracellular diplococci	

TABLE 4–8
Clinical Features of Vernal Conjunctivitis

More severe form of allergic conjunctivitis
Age at onset: 3 to 12 years
Palpebral conjunctiva: giant papillae ("cobblestone appearance")
Tissue infiltration with eosinophils and basophils
Giemsa-stained smear: intact eosinophils
Tear and serum immunoglobulin E level: elevated

TABLE 4–6
Clinical Features of Herpes Keratoconjunctivitis

Primary Infection	**Recurrent Infection**
Eyelids may be clear	Unilateral
Vesicles on erythematous base	Mucoid discharge
Conjunctivitis	Conjunctiva: injected follicles
Cornea: usually clear	Cornea: dendrite ulcer; fluorescein stain (+)
Vision ($\pm$)	Decreased corneal sensation
	Burning, intense foreign body sensation

TABLE 4–9
Clinical Features of Adenoviral Conjunctivitis

Adenoviral Syndromes

Acute follicular conjunctivitis
Pharyngoconjunctival fever
Epidemic keratoconjunctivitis
Acute hemorrhagic conjunctivitis

Findings

History of URI
History of exposure
Incubation period: 5–14 days
Foreign body sensation
Photophobia
Blepharospasm (lid
  squeezing in response to
  light)
Preauricular
  lymphadenopathy
Concurrent pharyngitis
Involvement: unilateral 50%;
  bilateral 50%

Intense redness, edematous
  lids
Watery discharge
Conjunctiva: chemosis,
  injected follicles
Pinpoint or larger
  subconjunctival
  hemorrhage
Cornea: punctate keratopathy
Vision often decreased
Pupillary size and reactions
  normal
Ocular movements normal

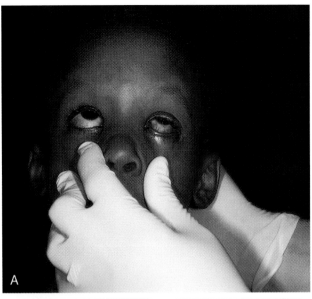

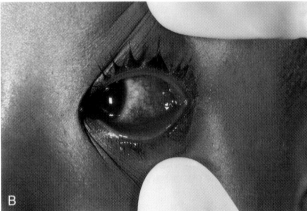

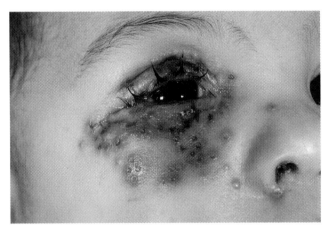

FIGURE 4–3. Herpes keratoconjunctivitis. Primary infection by herpes simplex in a 9-month-old infant. Multiple vesicles were present that quickly progressed to pustular and scab formations. The cornea was not involved. Herpes simplex type 1 was cultured from the vesicle (ocular infections are usually caused by HSV-1 except in newborns, in whom HSV-2 predominates).

FIGURE 4–4. *A* and *B,* Adenoviral conjunctivitis. Bilateral eye involvement with intense bulbar and palpebral conjunctival injection and hemorrhage. Patient also had marked pharyngeal injection and a high fever (pharyngoconjunctival fever); he had been exposed to a classmate with similar "red eyes."

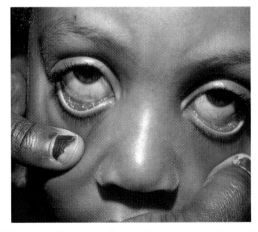

FIGURE 4–5. Vernal conjunctivitis demonstrating palpebral conjunctiva with giant papillae ("cobblestone appearance").

Infantile Glaucoma

SYNONYM   Congenital Glaucoma

DEFINITION

Glaucoma is a condition characterized by an increase in intraocular pressure in the anterior chamber that leads to damage to the optic nerve head.

1. Infantile or congenital glaucoma occurs during the first 3 years of life.
2. Juvenile glaucoma occurs after the age of 3 years.

ETIOLOGY/PATHOGENESIS (see Table 4–10)

1. The anterior chamber is an aqueous fluid-filled space between the cornea and the iris diaphragm.
2. Aqueous humor is produced by the ciliary body at the posterior base of the iris. It passes through the pupil and exits through the trabecular meshwork and Schlemm's canal, which is located at the junction of the cornea and the iris anteriorly (iridocorneal angle) (see Fig. 4–8).
3. Blockage of the outflow of aqueous humor for any reason causes a rise in intraocular pressure.

EPIDEMIOLOGY

1. The incidence of primary infantile glaucoma is 1 to 2 in 10,000 live births.
2. Male-to-female ratio is 2:1.
3. Age at diagnosis
   a. At birth (about 25%)
   b. Before 1 year of age (about 80%)
4. Bilateral eye involvement occurs in about 58% to 80% of patients.
5. Bilateral involvement is seen in 90% of infants, especially those presenting before 3 months of age.

INHERITANCE

1. Sporadic occurrence: about 90% of cases
2. The inheritance of infantile glaucoma is multifactorial.
   a. An affected parent has about a 5% chance of having an affected child.
   b. Parents of an affected child have a 5% chance of having another child with glaucoma.

CLINICAL FEATURES (see also Table 4–11)

1. Epiphora (excessive tearing)
   a. Results from irritation of corneal nerve endings secondary to stretching of the cornea
   b. Secondary to breakdown of epithelium with resultant irritation
2. Photophobia (light sensitivity may be severe enough to cause infants to bury their faces to avoid the light)
3. Blepharospasm (voluntary eyelid closure)
   a. Secondary to iritis or corneal epithelial breaks
   b. Results from glare caused by corneal edema
4. Corneal haze results from corneal epithelial and stromal edema.
5. "Haab striae"
   a. Visible as horizontal lines crossing the central cornea
   b. Secondary to tears in Descemet's membrane caused by stretching of the cornea
6. Megalocornea (see Box 4–5)
7. Buphthalmos or "ox-eye"
   a. Immaturity of scleral and corneal collagen permits the increased intraocular pressure to distend the globe in patients under 3 years of age.
   b. Buphthalmos develops as the overall size of the eye increases.
8. "Red eye"
   a. Secondary to injected conjunctival blood vessels
   b. May mimic conjunctivitis or red eye from other causes
9. "Blue sclera": Expansion of the sclera results in thinning, which allows increased visibility of the choroid giving a bluish appearance.

BOX 4-4   *Intraocular Pressure*

- Intraocular pressure for infants and children is same as that of adults
- Average intraocular pressure: about 16.5 mmHg (normal range 10–20)
- Intraocular pressure of >25 mmHg strongly suggests glaucoma

---

BOX 4-5   *Infantile Glaucoma*

"CLASSIC TRIAD"

- Epiphora
- Blepharospasm
- Photophobia

MEGALOCORNEA

- A corneal diameter of >10 mm in a term infant or >12 mm in an infant at 1 year

NORMAL CORNEAL DIAMETER

- 10 mm at birth in a full-term infant
- 11.8 mm at 1 year of age
- 12 mm (adult size) by 2 years of age

LABORATORY

1. Evaluation of anterior chamber angle with gonioscopy
2. Intraocular pressure measurement
   a. Preferably performed in an awake infant in a room with low light. Patient should be comforted with a bottle or breastfeeding.
   b. In infants, anesthesia (light sedation) may be required to measure the pressure.
3. Evaluation for refractory errors

COMPLICATIONS

1. Visual field loss and diminished visual acuity result from
   a. Optic nerve damage
   b. Deprivation amblyopia
   c. Corneal opacities
   d. Corneal scarring
2. High degree of myopia, astigmatism (secondary to increased axial length of globe)

DIFFERENTIAL DIAGNOSIS

1. Excess tearing
   a. Nasolacrimal duct obstruction
      (1) An affected infant presents with pooling of tears onto the lower lid and cheeks.
      (2) When infant cries, tears fail to arrive at the external nares; thus rhinorrhea is absent.
   b. Corneal abrasion
   c. Foreign body
   d. Ocular inflammation (e.g., iritis)
2. Corneal haziness
   a. Birth trauma (e.g., forceps injury)
   b. Congenital infections (e.g., herpes simplex virus)
3. Congenital megalocornea

TREATMENT

1. Prompt referral to an ophthalmologist for evaluation and treatment.
2. Treatment is primarily surgical.
   a. Goal of surgery is to improve the aqueous outflow from the eye, thus reducing the ocular tension and subsequent damage to the optic nerve and cornea.
   b. Various procedures used include either goniotomy, goniopuncture, trabeculotomy, trabeculectomy, cyclocryotherapy, cyclodiathermy, and laser treatment.
3. Medical therapy may be used either prior to or after surgery to keep intraocular pressure low. Commonly used agents include carbonic anhydrase inhibitors, beta blockers, and miotics.

PROGNOSIS

1. The earlier the onset of glaucoma, the poorer the visual prognosis.
2. Legally blind (visual acuity 20/200 or worse)
   a. If glaucoma is present at birth: over 50% of eyes
   b. If glaucoma occurs later: only 20% of eyes

KEY POINTS

Infantile Glaucoma

- Epiphora, blepharospasm, and photophobia are the "classic triad"; however, these symptoms are present in only about one third of affected patients at the time of diagnosis.
- Mean horizontal corneal diameter is 10 mm in a full-term infant, 11.8 mm at 1 year, and 12 mm (adult size) by 2 years of age.
- Infantile glaucoma must be excluded in any infant with a corneal diameter of over 12 mm.
- Infantile glaucoma results in blindness if left untreated or not treated promptly.

TABLE 4–10
Etiology of Infantile Glaucoma

Primary Glaucoma

About 50% of cases
An isolated developmental defect of drainage apparatus in anterior chamber angle
Absence of any systemic or other ocular disease

Secondary Glaucoma

About 50% of cases
Glaucoma associated with systemic or ocular disease
Trauma (hyphema—interferes with aqueous homor outflow)
Congenital rubella syndrome (glaucoma, cataracts)
Sturge-Weber syndrome (glaucoma [30%], unilateral, occurs ipsilateral to skin lesion)
Neurofibromatosis (tumor involvement of angle structures)
Lowe syndrome (glaucoma [60%], bilateral cataracts [75%])
Marfan syndrome (ectopia lentis, glaucoma)
Aniridia (glaucoma [75%], cataracts [50% to 85%])
Homocystinuria (secondary to lens dislocation)
Pierre Robin syndrome
Persistent hyperplastic primary vitreous
Retinopathy of prematurity
Chromosomal abnormalities (e.g., Down syndrome)
Uveitis (e.g., juvenile rheumatoid arthritis)
Tumors (retinoblastoma, neuroblastoma, xanthogranuloma)

TABLE 4–11
Clinical Features of Infantile Glaucoma

Epiphora	Corneal asymmetry
Photophobia	Corneal haziness (corneal edema)
Blepharospasm	Dulled red fundus reflex (corneal edema)
Buphthalmos or "ox-eye"	Haab striae (horizontal lines crossing central cornea)
"Blue sclera"	Megalocornea
"Red eye"	Cupping of optic nerve head

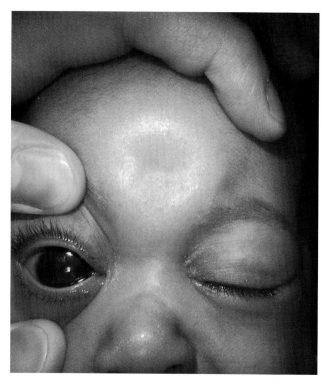

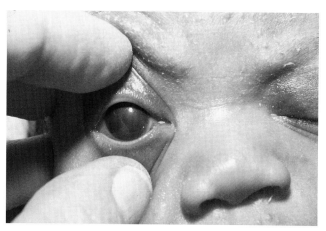

FIGURE 4–7. Congenital glaucoma in a patient with congenital rubella syndrome. Congenital glaucoma occurs in about 10% of patients with congenital rubella. Glaucoma develops because of abnormal angle development. When this is present at birth, it causes an enlarged, hazy cornea as seen in this patient. (A cloudy, edematous or white cornea, however, also may be found in patients with normal intraocular pressure as part of rubella embryopathy.)

FIGURE 4–6. Infantile glaucoma with megalocornea (note that you can hardly see any sclera) in a 3-month-old infant. In a patient with unilateral eye involvement which allows comparison with the normal eye, the diagnosis of megalocornea is readily made. Diagnosis is often delayed in patients with bilateral involvement. Diagnosis is especially difficult in absence of corneal cloudiness or when bilateral corneal enlargement is symmetrical.

Hyphema

DEFINITION

Presence of blood in the anterior chamber of the eye

EPIDEMIOLOGY

1. Traumatic hyphema is more common in children than in adults.
2. Traumatic hyphema occurs more often in males than in females.

3. BB gun injuries are the single most common cause of significant traumatic visual loss in children.

PATHOGENESIS (see Figure 4–8)

1. The anterior chamber is a space between the iris (posteriorly) and the cornea (anteriorly). It is filled with aqueous humor, a clear fluid produced by the highly vascular ciliary body. The ciliary body is attached to the iris and is located immediately posterior to it.

BOX 4–6 *Etiology of Hyphema*

TRAUMATIC HYPHEMA (MOST COMMON)	NONTRAUMATIC HYPHEMA (LESS COMMON)
Blunt or penetrating injury to the globe	Sickle cell disease
Examples	Leukemia
Injuries by ball, BB pellet, stick, pencil	Retinoblastoma
Projectile toys, stones, blow by fist	Hemophilia
Child abuse, birth trauma	Juvenile xanthogranuloma

2. Any object striking the globe with sufficient kinetic force may rupture a blood vessel in the ciliary body or iris leading to bleeding, which accumulates as hyphema.
3. Hyphema resolves as blood exits through the trabecular meshwork (located circumferentially in the angle of the anterior chamber at the junction of the iris and the cornea).

CLINICAL FEATURES/EVALUATION

1. Pain, blurred vision, history of trauma (mechanism of injury, nature of object, and time of injury must be documented for both medical and legal reasons)
2. Measurements of visual acuity and intraocular pressure (IOP)
3. Exclude other injuries (e.g., lens dislocation, vitreous hemorrhage). If a ruptured globe is suspected, no further examination should be carried out. A protective eye shield is applied, and further evaluation is performed by an ophthalmologist under general anesthesia.
4. Somnolence (reasons unknown); if marked somnolence is present, exclude intracranial injury.
5. If the hyphema has layered out (settled by gravity) in the anterior chamber, it can be graded by its volume relative to that of the anterior chamber:
   a. Grade 1: blood filling less than one third of anterior chamber
   b. Grade 2: blood filling one third to less than one half of anterior chamber
   c. Grade 3: blood filling one half to less than total space of anterior chamber
   d. Grade 4: blood filling the entire anterior chamber
6. Microhyphema
   a. No blood seen on gross examination
   b. Suspended RBCs seen on slit-lamp examination
7. Diffuse hyphema
   a. Occurs initially when blood has spread throughout the anterior chamber but before it layers out or settles
   b. Aqueous humor appears turbid.

LABORATORY

1. Sickle cell preparation and hemoglobin electrophoresis in all African-American or Hispanic patients or those of Mediterranean descent
2. Complete blood count, platelet count, bleeding time, prothrombin time, and partial thromboplastin time for patients with nontraumatic hyphema

TREATMENT

1. Controversy exists about the ideal treatment plan (e.g., hospitalization, bed rest, eye patching, various drug regimens, and surgical procedures).
2. Hospitalization is preferred, with a prompt ophthalmology consultation.
3. Strict bed rest with only bathroom privileges permitted.
4. Elevate the head of the bed to 30 to 45 degrees to promote settling and reabsorption of blood.
5. Shield the involved eye *at all times* to prevent further trauma, particularly rubbing.
6. To prevent rebleeding:
   a. Cycloplegic eye drops (e.g., atropine): dilate the pupil and relax the injured ciliary body
   b. Antifibrinolytic agents (aminocaproic acid or tranexamic acid): reduce lysis of the initial clot until the ruptured blood vessels heal.
   c. For pain, avoid aspirin or nonsteroidal anti-inflammatory drugs.
7. Corticosteroid eye drops or systemic steroids decrease intraocular inflammation and prevent formation of synechiae in the angle of the anterior chamber.
8. For elevated IOP use a topical beta blocker; if required, oral acetazolamide or methazolamide
9. Surgical evacuation: with significant decrease in vision, corneal blood staining, persistence of substantial clot or "black ball" hyphema, or elevated IOP despite medical therapy
10. Gonioscopy examination in 4 weeks; a mirrored contact lens is used to allow inspection of the angle of the anterior chamber to determine any damage to the trabecular meshwork.

PROGNOSIS

1. Excellent in uncomplicated hyphema, which usually resolves within 4 to 6 days.
2. In 90% of patients the prognosis for vision is 20/40 or better in the absence of rebleeding.
3. After rebleeding only 40% to 60% of patients will have 20/40 vision or better.

KEY POINTS

Hyphema

- Prompt evaluation by an ophthalmologist to exclude more extensive injury to the internal and more posterior structures in all patients with traumatic hyphema
- Rebleeding occurs 3 to 5 days after the initial hemorrhage (~30% of patients) and is a poor prognostic sign
- Sickle cell disease or trait is associated with increased risk of complications of hyphema

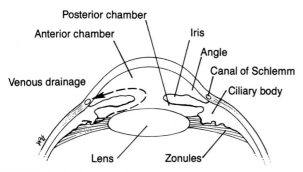

FIGURE 4-8. Cross-section of the normal angle structures, showing the flow of aqueous humor. (From Swartz MH: Textbook of Physical Diagnosis, 2nd ed. Philadelphia, WB Saunders, 1994, p. 119.)

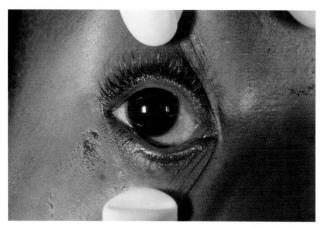

FIGURE 4-9. Grade 2 hyphema in a 12-year-old male following blunt trauma (hit in the eye by a ball).

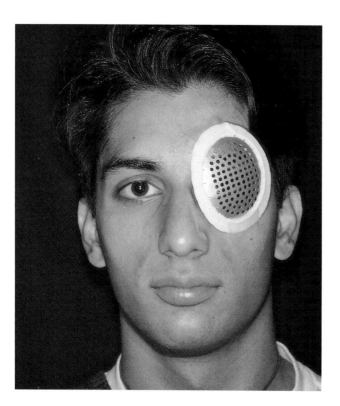

TABLE 4-12
Complications of Hyphema

Immediate Risks

Rebleeding (up to 30% of patients)
    Usually occurs within first 6 days (most often between 3rd and 5th days)
    Results from lysis or retraction of clot at site of ruptured blood vessel
Elevation of IOP
    Transient or persistent glaucoma (blockage of trabecular meshwork)
Bloodstaining of cornea
Sickle cell hyphema
    Circulating RBCs lead to sickling in acidic, hypoxic environment of anterior chamber
    Sickle cells have difficulty passing through outflow system, resulting in precipitate acute rise in IOP

Long-Term Risks

Loss of vision or deprivation amblyopia (optic nerve atrophy resulting from persistent IOP)
Traumatic cataract
Retinal detachment
Chronic glaucoma

FIGURE 4-10. Fox metal shield that fits entirely over the bony orbit and completely encases the eye is applied over the involved eye. An eye patch is not used (unless corneal pathology is present) because it prevents recognition of a sudden visual loss in the event of a re-bleed.

Hordeolum

SYNONYM Stye

DEFINITION

1. External hordeolum: an acute suppurative infection of the glands of Zeis or Moll
2. Internal hordeolum: an acute suppurative infection of the meibomian gland

ETIOLOGY

Staphylococcus aureus

PATHOGENESIS

1. The glands of Zeis are sebaceous glands attached to the hair follicles along the lid margin.
2. The meibomian glands are sebaceous glands located within the tarsal plates.
3. Obstruction of sebaceous glands is followed by infection.

PREDISPOSING FACTORS

Recurrences are frequently seen in patients with

1. Chronic staphylococcal blepharitis or seborrhea
2. Immunocompromised states
3. Underlying allergy causing itching

LABORATORY

Clinical diagnosis; no laboratory tests are required.

COMPLICATIONS

1. Progression of infection to the lid (preseptal cellulitis) or orbit (orbital cellulitis)
2. Lid scarring and contraction with recurrent infections

DIFFERENTIAL DIAGNOSIS

1. Chalazion
2. Preseptal cellulitis

a. Eyelid erythema, edema, and warmth
b. Post-traumatic: periorbital skin abrasion, laceration
c. Associated with bacteremia or sinusitis: fever, signs of sinusitis
3. Pyogenic granuloma
a. Deep red pedunculated lesion
b. May develop after trauma or surgery to the conjunctiva or skin

TREATMENT

1. Warm moist compresses for 15 to 20 minutes several times a day. Hordeolum either resolves or drains spontaneously after this treatment.
2. Topical antibiotic (e.g., bacitracin or sulfacetamide ointment) may be tried; however, topical antibiotics do not appear to alter the course.
3. Patients with recurrent difficult hordeolum: a systemic antistaphylococcal antibiotic may be used to reduce the indigenous flora.
4. Surgical incision and drainage: usually not indicated in the majority of cases

PREVENTION/PROGNOSIS

1. Recurrences are common (possibly due to reinfection through contaminated hands or altered secretions that tend to plug the ducts, predisposing to infection).
2. Eyelash scrubs: baby shampoo applied to a clean washcloth and used to scrub the base of eyelashes once or twice daily may help.

KEY POINTS

Hordeolum

- A purulent staphylococcal infection of the sebaceous glands

---

TABLE 4–13
Clinical Features of Hordeolum

Hordeolum
  Either external or internal
  Signs of inflammation: warm, tender, erythema
  Usual size: 5–10 mm in diameter
  Purulent drainage if spontaneously ruptured
  Usually single lesion
  May be multiple or bilateral
  Associated findings: palpable preauricular node or blepharitis
  Recurrent hordeolum: several lesions in various stages of resolution or evolution
External hordeolum
  A small, circumscribed superficial abscess
  Located at lid margin
  Tends to point to the skin surface
Internal hordeolum
  A larger circumscribed abscess
  Located on conjunctival surface of the lid
  May point to skin or to palpebral conjunctival surface

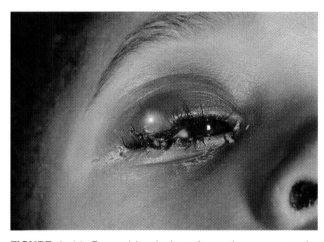

FIGURE 4–11. External hordeolum. An erythematous, tender swelling at the lid margin points externally.

Chalazion

DEFINITION

A lipogranuloma of the meibomian gland within the tarsal plate

ETIOLOGY/PATHOGENESIS

1. A lipogranuloma in an obstructed meibomian gland
2. May represent a residual of a resolved internal hordeolum

LABORATORY

1. Chalazion is a clinical diagnosis.
2. Slit-lamp examination may aid in evaluation of meibomian glands; eversion of the involved eyelid may allow better visualization of the nodule.

COMPLICATIONS

1. Large chalazion: distortion of the vision (astigmatism results from pressure exerted on the globe)
2. Secondary infection of the surrounding tissue may develop with subsequent swelling of entire lid.

DIFFERENTIAL DIAGNOSIS

1. Internal hordeolum (see p. 139)
2. Pyogenic granuloma
   a. Deep red pedunculated lesion
   b. May develop after trauma or surgery to the conjunctiva or skin

TREATMENT

1. If there is any evidence of chronic inflammation, use warm moist compresses for 15 to 20 minutes several times a day.
2. Consider a topical antibiotic (e.g., bacitracin or erythromycin ointment)
3. Light massage over the lesion several times a day may help.
4. Ophthalmology consultation for large chalazion
5. If chalazion does not disappear after 3 to 4 weeks of appropriate medical therapy, and if the patient wants it removed for cosmetic reasons:
   a. Incision and curettage
   b. Rarely, injection into and around chalazion of steroids (e.g., triamcinolone acetonide). *Caution:* This form of therapy can lead to permanent depigmentation of the skin at the injection site.

PROGNOSIS

1. Small chalazion: spontaneously disappears over many weeks to months in some patients.
2. Recurrences are common.
3. Tear deficiency and lid scarring may result from multiple excisions of chalazia.

KEY POINTS

Chalazion

- A lipogranuloma of the meibomian gland
- A slowly growing, firm, round, mobile, nontender tarsal mass

---

TABLE 4–14
Clinical Features of Chalazion

Common presenting complaint: eyelid lump
Chronic lesion
Slowly growing nodule (swelling)
Located within the substance of the lid (midportion of the tarsus)
May occur on lid margin if opening of the duct is involved
Located more often in the upper lid than in the lower lid
Firm
Well localized
Usual size: 2–10 mm in diameter or more
Usually single; may be multiple
Absence of signs of acute inflammation
   Nontender
   Nonerythematous

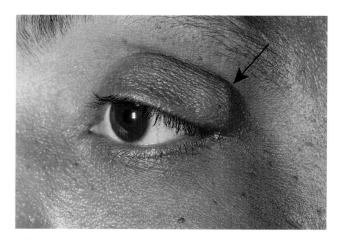

FIGURE 4–12. Chalazion. A pea-sized, mobile, painless, noninflamed nodule is seen within the body of the eyelid.

Cataract

DEFINITION

Any opacity of the crystalline lens is called a cataract. The degree of opacity varies from a small dot to total clouding of the lens.

CLASSIFICATION AND ETIOLOGY (see Box 4–7 and Box 4–8)

1. Laterality: unilateral (monocular) or bilateral
   a. Most bilateral cataracts are genetic or metabolic in origin.

BOX 4-7	*Etiology of Cataracts: Intrauterine Infections*

- TORCH
  *T*oxoplasmosis, *O*thers (varicella-zoster), *Ru*bella, *C*ytomegalovirus, *H*erpes simplex
- Rubeola

b. The contrary is usually not true of unilateral cataracts.
2. Degree of opacity
   a. Complete cataract (totally opaque)
   b. Partial cataract (only a portion of the lens has lost its transparency). Examples include:
      (1) Anterior or posterior polar cataract (opacity localized just to anterior or posterior pole of the lens)
      (2) Nuclear (opacity in center of the lens)
      (3) Zonular or lamellar (only a zone or lamella of the lens is opaque)
      (4) Posterior subcapsular (opacity located just anterior to the posterior pole of the lens; seen with long-term steroid use, uveitis due to juvenile rheumatoid arthritis, neurofibromatosis [type II])
      (5) Anterior subcapsular (e.g., atopic dermatitis)
      (6) Anterior lenticonus (Alport syndrome)

EPIDEMIOLOGY

1. One in every 250 newborns (0.4%) has some form of congenital cataract.
2. Pediatric cataracts account for an estimated 15% to 20% of childhood blindness in the industrialized countries.
3. Congenital cataracts
   a. Idiopathic: about 50% to 60% of cases
   b. Secondary: about 40% to 50% of cases

INHERITANCE

1. Approximately 8% to 33% of isolated congenital cataracts are hereditary.
2. Modes of inheritance
   a. Most common: autosomal dominant with variable penetrance
   b. Autosomal recessive: seen in families with high rates of consanguinity
   c. X-linked recessive (e.g., Lowe or Alport syndrome)

DIAGNOSIS/LABORATORY

1. Various modalities for the evaluation of the cataract and its effect on the vision include:
   a. Slit-lamp examination
   b. Retinoscopy
   c. Fundoscopy
   d. Ultrasonograpy
2. Analysis of red blood cell galactose kinase should be done in any patient with a cataract without an identifiable cause.
3. If clinically indicated, investigate:
   a. TORCH titers (toxoplasmosis, rubella, cytomegalovirus, herpes simplex, syphilis)
   b. Serum calcium and phosphorus

COMPLICATIONS

1. Irreversible deprivation amblyopia
2. Complications in the aphakic eye (following surgical removal of cataract) include
   a. Glaucoma
   b. Early retinal detachment

DIFFERENTIAL DIAGNOSIS

Conditions associated with leukokoria (see also Table 4–19)

1. Retinoblastoma
2. Retinopathy of prematurity
3. Persistent hyperplastic primary vitreous
4. Retinal detachment
5. Severe uveitis

BOX 4-8	*Etiology of Cataracts*

METABOLIC DISORDERS
Galactosemia
    Galactokinase deficiency
    Galactose-1-phosphate uridyl transferase
      deficiency
Diabetes mellitus
Hypoglycemia
Hypoparathyroidism
Pseudohypoparathyroidism
Alport syndrome
Lowe syndrome

CHROMOSOMAL DISORDERS
Trisomy 21, 13, 18

MENDELIAN INHERITANCE
Autosomal dominant
Autosomal recessive
X-linked

OTHER CONDITIONS
Atopic dermatitis
Congenital ichthyosis
Ectodermal dysplasia
Crouzon syndrome
Microphthalmia
Aniridia
Coloboma
Trauma (e.g., child abuse)

TREATMENT

1. Ophthalmology consultation
2. Surgical removal is indicated for visually significant cataract
   a. Must be treated as soon as possible (often within days of birth)
   b. Risk of irreversible deprivation amblyopia if not treated early
3. Postoperatively
   a. Optical correction of aphakic eye (eye without a lens)
   b. Options for optical correction include spectacles, contact lens
4. Genetic counseling and examination of parents and siblings as indicated (e.g., in patents with isolated congenital cataracts)

PROGNOSIS

With no treatment, progressive visual loss is the natural course of a visually significant cataract in children because of sensory deprivation.

KEY POINTS

Cataract

- Red reflex should be examined by direct ophthalmoscopy in newborns and at each of the infant's regularly scheduled visits in the first years of life.
- Infants with a monocular cataract should be treated as soon as possible, often within days of birth, and no later than 17 weeks of age.
- The only sign of galactose kinase deficiency may be a cataract.
- Exclude child abuse or occult trauma in children presenting with cataracts (especially when complete) as an isolated finding.

TABLE 4–15
Clinical Features of Cataract

Most Frequent Signs	Other Signs/Symptoms
Leukokoria (white pupillary reflex)	Infants: visual inattentiveness (bilateral cataracts)
Unequal or poor red fundus reflex	Older children: deprivation amblyopia
Strabismus	Noticed by parents (anterior polar cataract)
Nystagmus	Microphthalmia (monocular cataract)

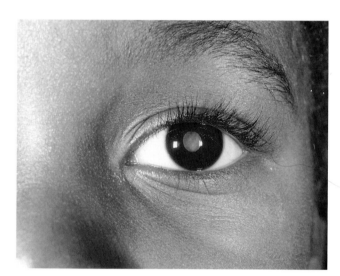

FIGURE 4–14. Congenital rubella syndrome with a nuclear cataract. Cataracts are present in about 20% of infants born with congenital rubella syndrome. The opacification may be nuclear (confined to the center of the lens) or complete (involving all layers of the lens). Other eye findings include glaucoma, anterior uveitis, and micro-ophthalmia. Rubella virus has been cultured from a central nuclear portion of the lens years after birth.

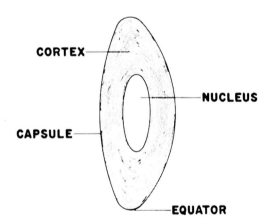

FIGURE 4–13. Basic lens anatomy. (From Potter WS: Pediatric cataracts. Pediatr Clin North Am 40: 842, 1993.)

Retinoblastoma

DEFINITION

A malignant neuroectodermal tumor arising from the nuclear layer of the retina.

ETIOLOGY/INHERITANCE

1. Retinoblastoma gene is a recessive suppressor gene (also called an anti-oncogene or recessive oncogene) located on the long arm of chromosome 13.
2. Retinoblastoma results from loss of both copies of a recessive oncogene.
3. Three recognized patterns of retinoblastoma are seen (see Table 4–16).
   a. Hereditary (30% to 40%)
      (1) Hereditary and bilateral: 25%
      (2) Hereditary and unilateral: 15%
   b. Nonhereditary (sporadic) and unilateral (60%)
   c. Chromosomal deletion (6%)
4. About 25% to 30% of patients with multifocal tumors have a negative family history (new germinal mutations)
5. Chromosomal deletion (13q) syndrome: Other findings include mental retardation, microcephaly, and cardiac, eye, and skeletal defects.

BOX 4–9   *Cardinal Signs Suggestive of Ocular Tumors*

Leukokoria
Strabismus
Poor fixation on a visual target by one or both eyes
Poor following of a visual target by one or both eyes
More strenuous objection to covering better-seeing eye than covering visually more impaired eye
Redness of eye
Visible abnormal appearance of one or both eyes

EPIDEMIOLOGY

1. Incidence: 1 in 18,000 to 20,000 live births
2. No predilection for sex or race
3. Mean age at diagnosis
   a. Unilateral disease (21 months)
   b. Bilateral disease (12 months)
   c. About 80% of cases are diagnosed before age 3 to 4 years; median age at diagnosis is 2 years.
   d. Rarely, diagnosis is made at birth, during adolescence, or in adulthood.
4. Laterality
   a. Unilateral disease (65% to 75%)
   b. Bilateral disease (25% to 35%)
5. All bilateral cases are assumed to be hereditary (germinal mutation).

CLINICAL FEATURES (see also Table 4–17 and Table 4–18)

1. Leukokoria (white pupillary reflex or "cat's eye" reflex)
   a. Most frequent presenting sign (about 60% of cases)
   b. Seen because of reflection of light from the surface of the white tumor
2. Strabismus
   a. Second most frequent sign (about 20% of cases)
   b. Either esotropia (eyes turning in) or exotropia (eyes turning out)
   c. Whereas esotropia is common in the general pediatric population, exotropia is extremely rare. Thus, the presence of exotropia in an infant should arouse a strong suspicion of retinoblastoma.
3. Retinoblastoma may be detected on routine examination.
4. Trilateral retinoblastoma syndrome
   a. Bilateral retinoblastoma
   b. Lesions in the vestigial photoreceptor tissue of the pineal region (the "third eye")

LABORATORY

1. Complete blood count (exclude bone marrow involvement)
2. Chromosome analysis
3. Funduscopy and slit-lamp examination to exclude cataract
4. Radiographs of the orbit or skull
   a. *Not* indicated
   b. Intratumoral calcification is pathognomonic of retinoblastoma.
5. Ultrasonography and computed tomography of the orbit
   a. More sensitive to the presence of calcification
   b. Provide information about extent of tumor including involvement of optic nerve
6. Magnetic resonance imaging (better visualization of optic nerve)
7. Confirmation of diagnosis by indirect ophthalmoscopy under general anesthesia (nerve and bony structures)
8. Blood samples of patient, siblings, parents, and grandparents for identification of germinal mutation
9. Aqueous humor analysis
   a. Values of lactate dehydrogenase and phosphoglucose isomerase are elevated in most patients.
   b. Usually *not* done; requires needle aspiration, and safety is unknown.
10. Patients with disseminated disease beyond the globe (as indicated)
    a. Bone scan
    b. Skeletal series
    c. Bone marrow aspiration
    d. Lumber puncture

DIFFERENTIAL DIAGNOSIS (see Table 4–19)

1. Coat's disease
   a. Telangiectasia in peripheral portion of retina, leading to intraretinal and subretinal exudation and retinal detachment
   b. Seen in male children at an average age of 6 years
   c. Absence of calcification on ultrasound
2. Persistent hyperplastic primary vitreous
   a. Failure of embryonic hyaloid system (primary vitreous) to reabsorb, producing a white pupil at birth or shortly thereafter
   b. Occurs in term infants
   c. Almost always unilateral

TREATMENT

1. Hospitalization and prompt referral to an ophthalmologist for confirmation of the diagnosis
2. Multidisciplinary approach including ophthalmologist, pediatric oncologist, radiation oncologist, and geneticist
3. Treatment is individualized depending on the size, location, and number of tumors.
4. Therapeutic options include
   a. Enucleation
   b. External beam radiation
   c. Photocoagulation
   d. Cryotherapy
   e. Systemic chemotherapy (for orbital spread or distant metastasis)
5. All family members should be examined by an ophthalmologist.

PROGNOSIS

1. Overall cure rate for retinoblastoma itself is over 90%.
2. Prognosis for vision depends on size and location of tumor at initiation of treatment.

3. Second nonocular tumors
   a. Seen in patients with hereditary form of retinoblastoma
   b. Usually appear 5 years after the diagnosis of retinoblastoma
   c. Can occur at an irradiated or nonirradiated site
   d. Nonocular tumors include
      (1) Osteosarcoma (most common)
      (2) Malignant melanoma
      (3) Pinealoma, pinealoblastoma
      (4) Sarcoma

PREVENTION

1. Genetic counseling for the patient and family with hereditary form of retinoblastoma
2. Prenatal diagnosis for the retinoblastoma genome.
3. If a germinal mutation is confirmed, periodic examination of the opposite eye is indicated.

KEY POINTS

Retinoblastoma

- Most common primary malignant intraocular tumor of childhood
- Presence of leukokoria should be considered presumptive evidence of retinoblastoma until proven otherwise
- "Cat's eye" reflex is often noted in flash photographs; red reflex is normal, white reflex is abnormal
- Every child with strabismus must have a funduscopic examination after pupillary dilatation to rule out intraocular tumor.
- Retinoblastoma must be considered in a child who does not respond to medical therapy for orbital cellulitis.

TABLE 4–16
Comparison of Hereditary and Sporadic Retinoblastoma

Hereditary Retinoblastoma	Sporadic Retinoblastoma
About 30% to 40% of all cases	About 60% of all cases
Positive family history (5% to 10% of cases)	None
New germline mutation (90% to 95% of cases)	No germline mutation
Autosomal dominant inheritance with complete penetrance	Nonheritable
Increased risk of retinoblastoma in offspring	No increased risk in offspring
Mean age at diagnosis: 12 months	Mean age at diagnosis: 21 months
Bilateral >80% of cases (at diagnosis)	Always unilateral
Unilateral: 15% of cases (very young age, multifocal)	Usually unifocal
Increased risk of second nonocular tumor	No increased risk of second tumor

---

TABLE 4–17
Clinical Features of Retinoblastoma

Most Frequent Signs

Leukokoria (white pupillary reflex or "cat's eye" reflex)
Abnormal or absent red reflex
Strabismus

TABLE 4–18
Clinical Features of Retinoblastoma

Less Frequent Signs

Clouding of cornea
Poor vision
Glaucoma
Watering of eye
Red eye
Orbital cellulitis with proptosis
Heterochromia
Anisocoria

Pain (with secondary glaucoma or inflammation)
Tumor extension into anterior chamber leading to
   Hyphema (bleeding)
   Pseudohypopyon (inferior layering of tumor cells)
Metastatic spread
   Hematogenous (bone/bone marrow/liver/lymph nodes)
   Through optic nerve (brain, ↑ intracranial pressure)
   Through optic nerve sheath (cerebrospinal fluid)

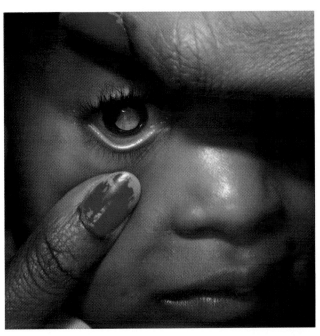

FIGURE 4–15. White pupillary reflex instead of red reflex in a 2-year-old child with retinoblastoma presenting with a history of white pupil for 4 months.

TABLE 4–19
Differential Diagnosis of White Pupillary Reflex

Retinoblastoma
Coat disease (exudative
   retinopathy)
Cataract
Vitreous hemorrhage
Endophthalmitis
Ocular larva migrans (*Toxocara
   canis*)
Toxoplasmosis
Uveitis
Phakomatosis

Persistent hyperplastic
   primary vitreous
Retinopathy of prematurity
Congenital retinal folds
Retinal coloboma
Retinal detachment
Retinal dysplasia
Hematoma
Hemangioma
Medulloepithelioma

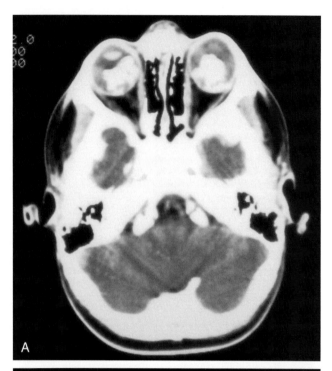

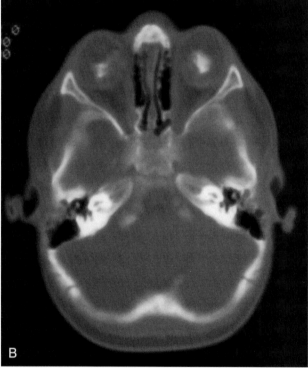

FIGURE 4–16. Bilateral retinoblastoma. Axial CT scan of the head. *A,* Soft tissue window demonstrates bilateral large calcified intraorbital masses. *B,* Bone window delineates dense calcifications within the masses.

5

Otolaryngology

Binita R. Shah, M.D.

Preseptal Cellulitis

SYNONYM   Periorbital Cellulitis

DEFINITION

An infection and inflammation involving the eyelid and the surrounding tissues *anterior* to the orbital septum (without involvement of the eye or orbital contents) (see Fig. 5–3)

ETIOLOGY/PATHOGENESIS

1. Nontraumatic
   a. Associated with bacteremia
      (1) *Streptococcus pneumoniae* (most common in United States)
      (2) *Haemophilus influenzae* type b (in developing countries [due to lack of vaccination])
   b. Associated with sinusitis (antecedent upper respiratory tract infections)
      (1) Bacterial: *S. pneumoniae*, nontypable *H. influenzae*, *Moraxella catarrhalis*
      (2) Viral: Adenovirus, parainfluenza virus
   c. Associated with local infections of lid or periorbital region
      (1) Bacterial (hordeolum, dacryocystitis, impetigo): *Staphylococcus aureus*, *Streptococcus pyogenes*
      (2) Viral: herpes simplex, varicella-zoster virus
2. Post-traumatic: puncture wounds, lacerations, blunt trauma, animal or human bites
   a. *S. aureus* or *S. pyogenes* (most common)
   b. Anaerobic bacteria (*Peptococcus, Peptostreptococcus, Bacteroides*)

EPIDEMIOLOGY

More common during winter months

CLINICAL FEATURES

1. Almost always unilateral involvement (about 95% of cases)
2. Bilateral involvement in viral etiology
3. Signs of inflammation: erythema, tenderness, warmth, swelling of eyelids
4. Eye itself is not involved.
5. Systemic signs: fever, irritability (toxicity unusual except in patients with bacteremia)
6. Inflammation extends over the superior orbital rim onto the brow in preseptal cellulitis, whereas in orbital cellulitis the attachment of the orbital septum to the superior orbital rim prevents edema from extending over the brow.

LABORATORY

1. Leukocytosis may be present.
2. Blood culture
3. Gram stain and culture (aerobic, anaerobic) of material aspirated from an abscess
4. Computed tomography: indications (any of the following):
   a. When eyeball cannot be examined adequately
   b. With suspected orbital cellulitis
   c. With suspected orbital fracture
   d. With suspected retained foreign body
5. Cerebrospinal fluid examination (in young infants with suspected *H. influenza* bacteremia or in any patient with meningeal signs)

DIFFERENTIAL DIAGNOSIS

1. Orbital cellulitis (see Table 5–1)
2. Conjunctivitis with secondary inflammation and edema of the lids (see pp. 131–133)
   a. Adenoviral
      (1) Copious serous discharge
      (2) Intense conjunctival hyperemia
      (3) Photophobia
      (4) Preauricular lymphadenopathy
      (5) May have concurrent pharyngitis
      (6) History of exposure to others with similar illness
   b. Bacterial (*S. pneumoniae, S. pyogenes, H. influenzae, S. aureus*)
      (1) Mucopurulent discharge
      (2) May have concurrent otitis media
3. Angioedema involving eyelids (see p. 389)
   a. With its rich supply of mast cells, eyelids are a common site of angioedema and urticarial reactions.
   b. Abrupt onset
   c. Pruritic, swelling lasting 24 to 72 hours

d. Presence of urticaria and recurrent episodes are important clues.

4. Sympathetic periorbital edema (not an actual infection, but swelling caused by impedance of local venous drainage secondary to paranasal sinusitis)

TREATMENT

1. Hospitalize: younger children (<5 years old) or children with signs of sepsis, absence of immunization, obvious trauma, or noncompliant family
2. Parenteral antibiotic therapy (pending culture results and until patient shows clinical improvement)
   a. Coverage for *S. pneumoniae* and *H. influenzae* (in children <5 years old, particulary those who have not been immunized adequately: cephalosporin [e.g., cefotaxime or ceftriaxone])
   b. Penicillinase-resistant penicillin (e.g., oxacillin) for *S. aureus* and other gram-positive bacteria if clinically indicated (e.g., in patients with hordeolum and cellulitis)
   c. Cefuroxime is another alternative if the possibility of meningitis has been excluded. It covers gram-positive bacteria including *S. aureus* and *H. influenzae.*
   d. Parenteral antibiotic therapy is continued until clinical improvement is noted and patient has remained afebrile for at least 24 to 48 hours.
   e. Oral antibiotic therapy (e.g., amoxicillin/clavu-lanate acid) is continued for an additional 7 to 10 days after discharge from the hospital.
3. Ophthalmology and/or otolaryngology consultations: whenever orbital involvement cannot be excluded
4. Incision and drainage of eyelid or periorbital abscess: if fluctuation is present
5. In patients who are not admitted:
   a. Oral antibiotics (10 to 14 days): Dicloxacillin, amoxicillin/clavulanate acid, or cefaclor
   b. Daily follow-up
   c. Hospitalize if patient is not improving after 48 hours of oral antibiotic therapy.

KEY POINTS

Preseptal Cellulitis

- Signs of orbital involvement (proptosis, decreased vision, decreased ocular motility, and pain on eye movement) are *absent* in preseptal cellulitis.
- An "apparent case" of preseptal cellulitis may be an initial manifestation of a developing orbital cellulitis.

TABLE 5-1

Cardinal Differentiating Signs: Preseptal Cellulitis Versus Orbital Cellulitis

Clinical Findings	Preseptal Cellulitis	Orbital Cellulitis
Proptosis	Absent	Present
Ocular motility	Normal	Limited
Pain on eye movement	None	Present
Vision	Normal	Often decreased
Chemosis	Usually none	Common
Pupillary reaction	Normal	Often abnormal
Corneal sensation	Normal	Often reduced

Modified from Steinkuller PG, Edmond JC, Chen RM: Ocular infections. *In* Feigin RD, Cherry JD (eds): Textbook of Pediatric Infectious Diseases, 4th ed. Philadelphia, W.B. Saunders, 1998, p. 788.

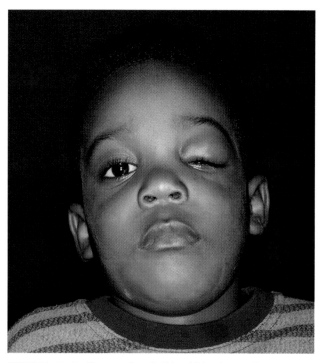

FIGURE 5-1. Preseptal cellulitis. Lid edema, intense erythema, and tenderness were present in the left eye in this child with no clinical signs of orbital involvement. CT scan showed ethmoid and maxillary sinusitis but no proptosis or involvement of the orbital contents.

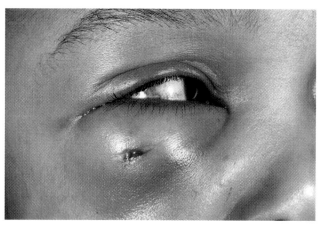

FIGURE 5-2. Post-traumatic preseptal cellulitis. An erythematous, tender periorbital swelling was seen following a dog bite (abrasion at the site of the bite and bulbar conjunctival injection are visible).

Orbital Cellulitis

DEFINITION

An infection and inflammation of the tissues of the orbit *posterior* to the orbital septum. Infection may involve all orbital structures including the extraocular muscles, sensory and motor nerves, and the optic nerve (see Fig. 5–3).

EPIDEMIOLOGY

1. Median age of children admitted for orbital cellulitis due to sinusitis is 7 years.
2. More common during winter months, when the frequency of upper respiratory tract infections and sinusitis increases.

ANATOMY/PATHOGENESIS (see Fig. 5–3)

1. Orbital septum: a fascial layer extending vertically from the periosteum of the orbital rim to the tarsal plates within the lids. It separates the subcutaneous lid structures from the orbit and acts as an anatomic barrier against the passage of infection.

BOX 5–1 | *Clinical Features of Orbital Cellulitis* (see also Table 5–1)

Almost always unilateral (characteristic)
Eyelids: erythema, edema, tenderness, warmth
Proptosis
Chemosis (edema of the conjunctivae)
Impaired vision
Ophthalmoplegia or decreased eye movements
Pain on movement of the globe
Orbital and retro-orbital pain
Elevated intraocular pressure
Systemic signs (more pronounced than in preseptal cellulitis)
 Fever
 Headache
 Septic appearance

BOX 5–2 | *Differential Diagnosis of Inflammatory Proptosis*

Infection
 Orbital cellulitis
 Cavernous sinus thrombosis
Intraocular inflammatory tumors
 Primary (e.g., retinoblastoma)
 Metastatic (e.g., neuroblastoma, rhabdomyosarcoma, Burkitt lymphoma, leukemia)
 Sarcoidosis
 Letterer-Siwe disease (histiocytosis X)
Endocrine
 Exopthalmos

---

2. Preceding or concurrent acute paranasal sinusitis leading to orbital cellulitis
 a. Occurs in about 75% to 90% of cases
 b. Most commonly involved sinuses: ethmoid, followed by maxillary and frontal
 c. Orbit is bordered on three sides by sinuses and thus is susceptible to contiguous infection.
 d. Orbital cavity is separated from the ethmoid air cells by the thinnest orbital bone-lamina papyracea. Congenital bony dehiscences are commonly found in the lamina, through which sinus infection can easily spread into the orbit.
3. Ophthalmic venous system has no valves. Thus, venous and lymphoid communications between the face, nasal cavity, sinuses, and pterygoid region allow free flow in either direction. These channels also connect directly with the cavernous sinus.
4. Trauma (penetrating ocular injury) or intraorbital surgery
5. Dental infections and dental surgery

LABORATORY

1. Leukocytosis is usually present.
2. Blood, nasal, and nasopharyngeal cultures: usually negative or noncontributory
3. Funduscopy with pupils dilated: excludes intraocular tumor
4. Computed tomography (CT) of the orbit
 a. Determines the extent of infection (helps in deciding whether surgical drainage is needed)
 b. Excludes intraocular tumor
5. Gram stain and culture (aerobic, anaerobic) of material aspirated from either the sinuses or the surgically drained abscess
6. Lumbar puncture (in patients with meningeal and/or cerebral signs)

TREATMENT

1. Hospitalization and prompt otolaryngology and ophthalmology consultations (neurosurgical consultation is needed if intracranial complication is suspected)
2. A decision on whether immediate surgery is indicated or should wait until the initial response to antimicrobial therapy is known depends on clinical examination as well as findings on CT scan of the orbit.
3. Intravenous antibiotic therapy (pending culture results) should provide coverage for
 a. Pathogens most commonly seen with sinusitis: *S. pneumoniae,* nontypable *H. influenzae, Moraxella, S. aureus,* other *Streptococcus* species and gram-negative organisms as well as anaerobes (see Table 5–5)
 b. A third-generation cephalosporin (e.g., ceftriaxone or cefotaxime) *and* oxacillin
 c. Metronidazole or clindamycin is added when anaerobic infection is suspected.
 d. Therapy can be narrowed following culture and sensitivity results obtained from surgical specimen or blood.

e. Mean hospital stay is between 10 and 14 days. With clinical improvement, patient can be discharged home and antibiotic therapy continued orally for an additional 7 to 14 days. Patient is reevaluated by close follow-up appointments.

4. Surgical drainage (endonasal endoscopic surgery): some indications:

a. Orbital abscess or subperiosteal abscess

b. Vision decreased or decreasing

c. Proptosis severe or progressing despite appropriate intravenous antibiotics

d. Clinical response to treatment is not prompt or CT scan shows no improvement after 48 to 72 hours of appropriate intravenous antibiotics.

KEY POINTS

Orbital Cellulitis

- A vision-threatening and potentially life-threatening emergency
- Cardinal signs are proptosis, chemosis, decreased vision, and decreased ocular motility.
- Most frequent and serious complication of acute sinusitis
- Most common intraocular tumor that may mimic orbital cellulitis is retinoblastoma

---

TABLE 5–2
Etiology of Orbital Cellulitis

Neonates: *S. aureus*, gram-negative bacilli
Children (most common pathogens)
  S. aureus, Steptococcus species
  S. pneumoniae, nontypable *Haemophilus influenzae*
  Polymicrobial infection common
Anaerobes: *Peptostreptococcus, Bacteroides, Fusobacterium*
  may also be involved
Immunodeficient or diabetic states: fungi (*Aspergillus, Mucor* species)
Trauma (penetrating ocular injury) or intraorbital surgery:
  S. aureus
Skin infection: *S. aureus, Streptococcus* species

TABLE 5–3
Complications of Orbital Cellulitis

Orbital Complications

Subperiosteal and orbital abscess
Endophthalmitis
Septic uveitis
Retinitis
Exudative retinal detachment
Optic neuropathy (either direct infection or aseptic optic neuritis)
  Decreased vision and color perception
  Afferent pupillary defect (Marcus Gunn sign)
Proptosis causing corneal opacification (secondary to exposure)
Secondary glaucoma

Intracranial Complications

Meningitis
Brain abscess
Epidural or subdural empyema
Cavernous sinus thrombosis (abnormalities of cranial nerves III, IV, V, and VI)

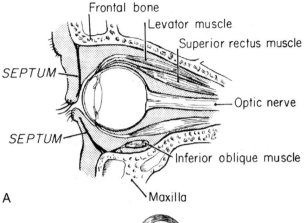

A

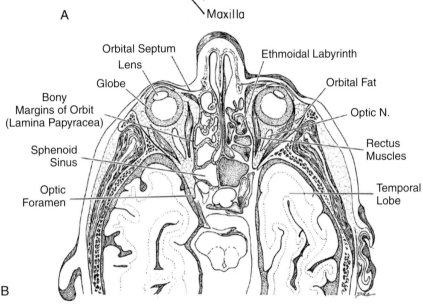

B

FIGURE 5–3. *A,* Sagittal view of the orbit illustrating position of the orbital septum. The orbital septum is an extension of the orbital periosteum to the tarsal plate in both upper and lower eyelids and acts as a physical barrier to preseptal infection, thus preventing spread of infection to the orbital contents. (Reproduced with permission from Smith TF, O'Day D, Wright PF: Clinical Implications of Preseptal Cellulitis in Childhood. Pediatrics 62: 1007, 1978.) *B,* Schematic drawing of structures important in computed tomographic evaluation of preseptal and orbital cellulitis. (Reproduced with permission from Goldberg F, Berne AS, Oski FA: Differentiation of Orbital Cellulitis from Preseptal Cellulitis by Computed Tomography. Pediatrics 62:1001, 1978.)

TABLE 5–4
Classification of Orbital Cellulitis

Stage

I	Inflammatory edema	Edema in medial or lateral upper eye lid
		Usually nontender, minimal skin changes
		No induration, visual impairment, or limitation of occular motility
II	Orbital cellulitis	Edema of orbital contents with varying degree of proptosis, chemosis, limited ocular motility and/or visual loss
III	Subperiosteal abscess	Proptosis down and out with severe signs of orbital cellulitis
		Abscess beneath the periosteum of ethmoid, frontal, or maxillary bone (in that order of frequency)
IV	Orbital abscess	Abscess within fat or muscle cone in posterior orbit
		Severe chemosis, proptosis (globe displaced forward or down and out)
		Complete ophthalmoplegia, moderate to severe visual loss
V	Cavernous sinus thrombosis	Proptosis, globe fixation, severe loss of visual acuity
		Prostration, signs of meningitis
		Proptosis, chemosis, and visual loss in contralateral eye
		Bilateral cranial nerve (III, IV, V, VI) palsies

Modified from Wald ER, Pang D, Milmore G, Schramm VL. Sinusitis and its complications in the pediatric patient. *In* Pediatric Otolaryngology, PCNA. Philadelphia, WB Saunders, 1981, page 787.

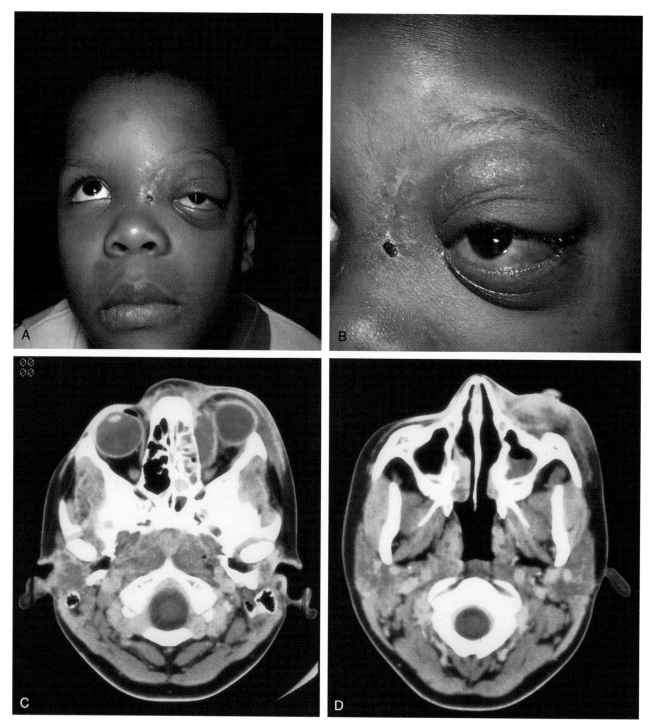

FIGURE 5–4. *A,* Orbital cellulitis of the left eye in a 9-year-old child who presented with unilateral eye involvement with marked proptosis (outward and inferior displacement of the globe) and impaired extraocular movement. He also had exquisite tenderness over the ethmoid and maxillary sinuses. *B,* Close-up showing chemosis, lid erythema, and proptosis. *C* and *D* Axial CT scan at the level of the sinuses and orbit. *C,* Left-sided exophthalmus. In addition, there is ethmoid and sphenoid opacification with extraconal extension (subperiosteal abscess) adjacent to the medial rectus muscle. *D,* Fluid in the left maxillary sinus and mucus in both nasal cavities.

Acute Bacterial Sinusitis

DEFINITION

1. Sinusitis is an inflammation of the mucosal lining of one or more of the paranasal sinuses.
2. Sinusitis is arbitrarily categorized by duration of symptoms as:
   a. Acute sinusitis: symptoms lasting 10 to 30 days
   b. Subacute sinusitis: symptoms lasting 30 days to 3 months
   c. Chronic sinusitis: symptoms lasting over 3 months

EPIDEMIOLOGY

1. Most children have an average of three to eight viral URIs annually; 10% to 15% of children (e.g., day care attendees) have about 12 episodes annually.
2. Approximately 0.5% to 5% of URIs are complicated by acute bacterial sinusitis.

ANATOMY/PATHOGENESIS

1. Paranasal sinuses consist of four paired structures (see Box 5–3)

BOX 5–3   *Paranasal Sinuses*

FOUR PAIRED STRUCTURES

Maxillary: Aerated soon after birth
Ethmoid: Aerated soon after birth
Sphenoid: Aerated between 3rd and 5th year of life
Frontal: Aerated between 6th and 10th year of life
          May be absent or asymmerical

---

2. The inferior, middle, superior turbinates, each with a corresponding meatus underneath, are situated along the lateral wall of the nasal cavity. The maxillary, frontal, anterior ethmoid sinuses open into the middle meatus; the posterior ethmoid and sphenoid sinuses open into the superior meatus.
3. The patency of the sinus ostia, function of the ciliary apparatus, and quality of secretions are important to the normal physiology of the sinuses.
4. Causes of ostial obstruction (examples):
   a. Viral upper respiratory infection (URI) and allergic inflammation (most frequent)
   b. Cystic fibrosis
   c. Asthma
   d. Immotile cilia
   e. Immune disorder
   f. Nasal polyp
   g. Deviated septum

CLINICAL FEATURES

1. Common cold (rhinosinusitis and/or cough) persisting without improvement for more than 10 to 14 days
   a. Nasal discharge of any color (yellow, green, or white)
   b. Nasal discharge of any quality (clear or thick)
   c. Daytime cough (dry or wet, may be worse at night); cough occurring only at night is a common residual symptom of uncomplicated URI.
2. Classic signs/symptoms (seen in older children and adults but *almost never* in young children)
   a. Periorbital edema
      (1) Edema may involve upper or lower lid
      (2) Usually develops gradually (hours to days)
      (3) Usually most obvious in early morning after awakening; edema may decrease and actually disappear during the day.
   b. Facial pain
   c. High fever ($>39°C$)
   d. Tooth pain
   e. Tenderness or facial swelling overlying the maxillary, ethmoid, or frontal sinus
   f. Headache (feeling of "fullnes," dull ache in either the supraorbital or retro-orbital area)
3. Helitosis, especially in the absence of pharyngitis, tooth decay, or a nasal foreign body

LABORATORY

1. Sinusitis is usually a clinical diagnosis.
2. Transillumination (for maxillary or frontal sinus)
   a. In adolescents and adults: useful if light transmission is either normal or absent
   b. Unequal or poor transmission of light through the involved sinuses is the basis for a clinical diagnosis; however, this correlates poorly with the illness.
3. Sinus aspirate is the gold standard for a definitive diagnosis.
4. Nasopharyngeal or throat cultures are not useful for predicting the sinus pathogen.
5. Radiography of sinuses
   a. Indicated in patients with complications or recurrent or severe infections, when diagnosis is uncertain, or when sinus surgery is being contemplated.
   b. Findings on plain radiographs, CT scans, or magnetic resonance imaging (MRI) include any of the following:
      (1) Air-fluid levels
      (2) Complete opacification
      (3) Mucosal thickening of more than 4 mm
   c. No radiographic findings alone confirms a diagnosis of acute bacterial sinusitis.
   d. Abnormal radiographs reflect the presence of inflammation; cause of the inflammation (bacterial, viral, or allergic) *must* be correlated with clinical findings.
   e. Plain "sinus series": Normal findings make a diagnosis of sinusitis highly unlikely, but abnormal findings are only moderately helpful be-

cause an uncomplicated viral URI also results in abnormal radiographic signs.

    f. Plain sinus series includes:

      (1) Waters' view (occipitomental) for maxillary sinuses

      (2) Caldwell view (anteroposterior) for ethmoid and frontal sinuses

      (3) Submentovertex and lateral views for sphenoid sinuses

DIFFERENTIAL DIAGNOSIS

1. Viral URI and acute bacterial sinusitis
   a. May be indistinguishable on the basis of clinical findings alone
   b. The *duration* of the signs/symptoms rather than their *mere presence* is the most important feature distinguishing the two.
2. Nasal foreign body
   a. Unilateral nasal discharge
   b. Purulent, bloody, or foul-smelling discharge
3. Streptococcosis
   a. Group A streptococcal infection in children under 3 years old
   b. Throat culture positive
4. Adenoiditis
   a. Normal sinus radiographs
   b. Persistent mucopurulent discharge lasting more than 10 days

TREATMENT

1. Antimicrobial therapy: usually a 10- to 14-day course (for at least 7 days past the point of substantial improvement or resolution of signs/symptoms) with
   a. Amoxicillin (usually initial drug of choice)
   b. For treatment failures or in areas with a high prevalence of beta-lactamase strains: amoxicillin-clavulanate or second- or third-generation cephalosporin (cefaclor, cefuroxime)
2. Decongestants and antihistamines are *not* helpful.
3. Hospitalization, parenteral antibiotics, and otolaryngology consultation are needed for
   a. Patients with orbital or intracranial complications
   b. Indications for sinus drainage and irrigation
      (1) Intense pain
      (2) Treatment failure
      (3) Suppurative complications
      (4) Immunocompromised status

KEY POINTS

Acute Bacterial Sinusitis

- Should be suspected when viral URI lingers without improvement for more than 10 to 14 days or when an acute severe URI presents with fever of more than 39°C, facial pain, or swelling
- Mucopurulent nasal discharge occurs frequently in viral URI. It is *not* an indication for antimicrobial therapy unless it persists *without* improvement for more than 10 to 14 days.
- Frontal sinusitis causes most intracranial complications, meningitis being the most common.

TABLE 5–5
Etiology of Acute Bacterial Sinusitis

Immunocompetent Host

S. pneumoniae (25% to 30%)
Nontypable *H. influenzae* (15% to 20%)
M. catarrhalis (15% to 20%)
Streptococcus pyogenes (2% to 5%)
Viral (7% to 10%; adenovirus, rhinovirus, or parainfluenza virus)
Anaerobes (2% to 5%)
Sterile (20% to 35%)

Immunocompromised Host

S. aureus (cystic fibrosis, defect in white blood cell function)
Fungi and *Pneumocystis* (acquired immunodeficiency syndrome)

Modified from Wald E: Sinusitis in children. Pediatr Infect Dis J 7: 449, 1988.

TABLE 5–6
Complications of Acute Bacterial Sinusitis

Orbital Complications (Most Frequent)

Facial cellulitis
Periorbital or orbital cellulitis
Orbital subperiosteal or orbital abscess
Optic neuritis

Cranial and Intracranial Complications (Second Most Common)

Meningitis (most common; seen with ethmoiditis, sphenoiditis, or frontal sinusitis)
Epidural abscess (second most common; seen with frontal sinusitis)
Potts puffy tumor or osteomyelitis (seen with frontal sinusitis)
Brain abscess
Subdural empyema
Cavernous sinus thrombosis (seen with sphenoiditis)
Osteomyelitis of maxilla

Pulmonary

Asthma and/or bronchitis (bronchopulmonary tree contaminated by nasal/sinus secretions)

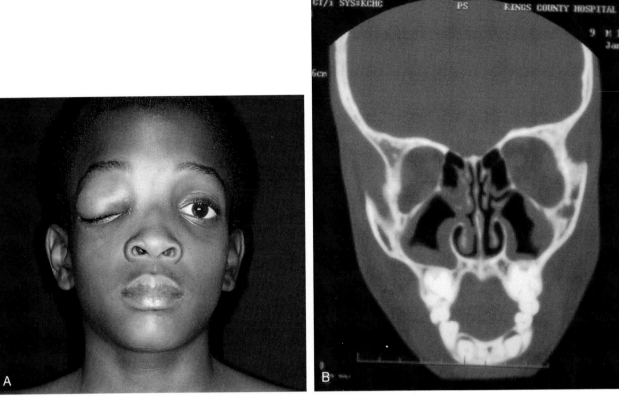

FIGURE 5–5. *A,* Acute bacterial sinusitis presenting with periorbital edema. Periorbital edema may involve the upper or lower lid. It usually develops gradually (over hours to days). Edema is most obvious in the early morning after awakening and may decrease and actually disappear during the day. *B,* Coronal CT scan of the sinuses viewed at soft tissue and bone windows demonstrates fluid in the nasal cavity and ethmoid sinuses. There is significant mucosal thickening in both maxillary sinuses.

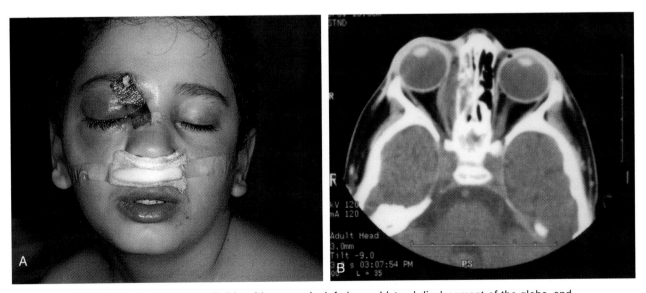

FIGURE 5–6. *A,* Orbital cellulitis with proptosis, inferior and lateral displacement of the globe, and impaired extraocular movement in an 8-year-old child. *B,* Axial CT scan of the orbits shows exophthalmos of the right globe. In addition, there is fluid in the right ethmoid sinus with extraconal extension adjacent to the right medial rectus muscle (subperiosteal abscess). Orbital cellulitis is the most frequent serious complication of acute sinusitis and usually follows ethmoiditis or frontal sinusitis.

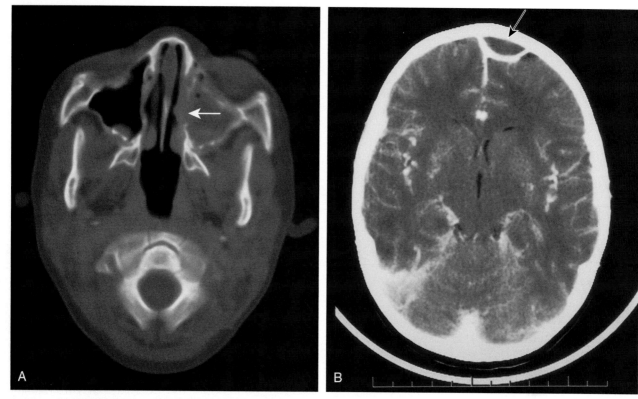

FIGURE 5–7. *A,* Sinusitis with epidural abscess in a 5-year-old child presenting with high fever and severe headache. Axial CT scan at the level of the sinuses viewed at a bone window demonstrates opacification of the left maxillary sinus causing erosion of the medial wall *(arrow). B,* Same CT scan at the level of the brain viewed at soft tissue window shows a lenticular, peripherally enhancing mass adjacent to the inner table of the skull that represents an epidural abscess *(arrow).*

Acute Mastoiditis

DEFINITION

Mastoiditis is an infection within the mastoid air cells. It is classified as acute or chronic. Acute mastoiditis is further subdivided according to the pathologic stage of involvement.

1. Acute mastoiditis (without periosteitis or osteitis)
2. Acute mastoiditis with periosteitis: Infection involves the periosteum covering the mastoid process.
3. Acute coalescent mastoiditis (acute mastoid osteitis, acute suppurative mastoiditis)
   a. Extensive suppuration fills the mastoid air cells and causes an osteitis that destroys the bony trabeculae that separate the air cells.
   b. This results in coalescence of the air cells; hence it is descriptively termed acute coalescent mastoiditis.

ETIOLOGY

1. Despite its relation to middle ear disease, organisms causing acute mastoiditis occur in different proportions than in acute otitis media (AOM).
2. The most common aerobes are:

   a. *Streptococcus pneumoniae* (most common)
   b. *S. pyogenes* (second most common)
   c. *Staphylococcus aureus* (third most common)
   d. *Haemophilus influenzae* (less common)
3. Mixed cultures of aerobes (*Pseudomonas* sp) and anaerobes (gram-negative cocci, gram-positive bacilli, and gram-negative bacilli) are occasionally isolated; however, they are common in subacute or chronic mastoiditis.

PATHOGENESIS

1. The mastoid antrum connects directly to the middle ear cavity via a narrow channel, the aditus ad antrum. The mucous membrane that lines the mastoid air cells is continuous with that of the mastoid antrum, aditus, and the middle ear cavity. Easy movement of air, secretions, and microorganisms is facilitated among these structures.
2. Blockage of the aditus ad antrum by an inflammatory process results in sequestration and poor drainage of the mastoid antrum.

LABORATORY

1. Gram stain and bacterial culture (aerobic and anaerobic) of the middle ear cavity aspirate or subperiosteal abscess and mastoid mucosa

BOX 5-4 — *Clinical Features of Acute Mastoid Osteitis*

Most commonly preceded by acute otitis media (AOM)

Absence of a prior history of AOM does not exclude acute mastoid osteitis

Erythema, tenderness, and swelling over the mastoid bone

Pinna displaced outward and downward

Fluctuance in periauricular tissues (usually indicates subperiosteal abscess)

Purulent otorrhea may be present filling the ear canal

Narrowing of external auditory canal ("sagging" of the skin of the posterosuperior canal due to a subperiosteal abscess)

Systemic signs: fever

BOX 5-5 — *Clinical Features of Acute Mastoiditis (Without Periosteitis or Osteitis)*

Almost all patients with AOM have inflammation of mastoid air cells

Occurs as a natural extension or part of the pathologic process of AOM

Most common pathologic stage of acute mastoiditis

Signs or symptoms related to AOM are present

No clinical signs of mastoiditis are present

CT scan

"Cloudy mastoids" suggestive of general inflammation

No evidence of either periosteitis or osteitis

Usually resolves as middle ear–mastoid inflammation subsides (as a natural process or as a result of treatment)

Failure to resolve leads to acute mastoiditis with either periosteitis or osteitis or to chronic mastoiditis

BOX 5-6 — *Clinical Features of Acute Mastoiditis with Periosteitis*

Tenderness and erythema over the mastoid process

No destruction of bony trabeculae on CT scan

2. Blood culture (expectation of bacterial recovery should be low)
3. Leukocytosis (often present but is of no consequence in diagnosis or management)

4. CT scan of the temporal bone has superseded plain radiographs of the mastoid. Any of the following (if present) can be readily demonstrated:
   a. A fluid-filled middle ear cavity and mastoid
   b. Demineralization of the bony trabeculae of the mastoid
   c. Evidence of intracranial complications
5. Lumbar puncture in any infant with clinical signs or symptoms of meningitis

DIFFERENTIAL DIAGNOSIS

1. Retroauricular lymphadenitis
2. Periauricular cellulitis
3. Parotitis (e.g., mumps, enterovirus) causing displacement of the pinna
4. Angioedema (e.g., insect bites)
5. Leukemia
6. Lymphoma
7. Benign and malignant tumors of the mastoid

TREATMENT

1. Acute mastoiditis (without periosteitis or osteitis) can be treated like AOM with oral antimicrobial therapy.
2. For patients with acute mastoiditis with either periosteitis or osteitis:
   a. Hospitalization and otolaryngology consultation
   b. Antibiotics (pending culture results)
      (1) Parenteral cefotaxime and oxacillin (to cover the most common pathogens [*S. pneumoniae*, *S. pyogenes*, *S. aureus*, and *H. influenzae*])
      (2) Oral antibiotics should be continued to complete a 14- to 21-day course after discharge from the hospital. A longer duration of antibiotics may be required for patients with complications or no clinical response.
   c. Myringotomy with insertion of a tympanostomy tube for drainage in patients with mastoiditis and periosteitis. If patient does not show improvement in 24 to 48 hours, a simple mastoidectomy should be performed.
   d. Cortical mastoidectomy is performed in patients with mastoiditis and osteitis.

PROGNOSIS

1. Good, if treated early
2. Intracranial complications can lead to neurologic deficits and death.

PREVENTION

Appropriate early treatment of otitis media will prevent mastoiditis.

KEY POINT

Acute Mastoiditis

- Mastoiditis should be considered in a patient with otitis media that is unresponsive to antibiotic therapy.

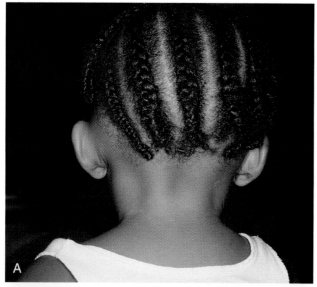

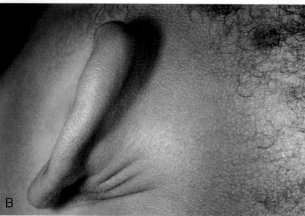

FIGURE 5–8. *A,* Acute mastoid osteitis in a 14-month-old infant with downward and lateral (outward) displacement of the auricle. She also had purulent otorrhea. *B,* Close-up showing erythema and swelling over the mastoid bone.

TABLE 5–7
Complications of Mastoiditis

Complications Depend on Direction in Which the Suppurative Process Extends:

Laterally
  Subperiosteal abscess (most common extracranial complication)
Superiorly
  Epidural abscess
  Subdural empyema
  Brain abscess
  Meningitis
  Venous sinus thrombophlebitis
Medially
  Petrositis
  Facial nerve palsy
  Bezold abscess
    (infection through mastoid tip invades planes of neck leading anterior to sternocleidomastoid muscle)
Posteriorly
  Occipital osteomyelitis

Facial Palsy With Acute Otitis Media

DEFINITION

Acute otitis media (AOM) complicated by facial palsy

EPIDEMIOLOGY

1. Before the introduction of antibiotics, facial palsy occurred in 0.6% of patients owing to AOM and in 2.3% of patients owing to chronic otitis media.
2. With antibiotic usage for the treatment of otitis media, the rate of facial palsy has decreased significantly.
3. Facial palsy due to AOM constitutes about 9% of all facial palsies in children and between 3% and 5% all facial palsies in adults.

PATHOGENESIS

1. The facial nerve is an important component of the middle ear cavity. On the medial wall of the

BOX 5–7   *Facial Palsy with Acute Otitis Media*

PERIPHERAL FACIAL PALSY

Flaccid paralysis of *all* facial muscles on affected side
Nasolabial fold remains flat on affected side
Unable to wrinkle forehead on affected side
Unable to close the eye on affected side
Drooping of corner of the mouth on affected side
Facial weakness when asked to puff out cheeks against resistance
Difficulty in eating and drinking with dribbling of liquids from weak corner of mouth (may or may not be present)
Impairment of lacrimation on the affected side (may or may not be present)

middle ear cavity, the facial nerve courses horizontally across the middle ear cleft just above the oval window.
2. A thin layer of bone usually covers the facial nerve. However, about one third of patients have an incomplete bony covering (congenital bony dehiscence) in the bony fallopian canal that permits entry of infectious agents.
3. Blood vessels supplying the facial nerve are interconnected with those of the middle ear and mastoid. Inflammation of these blood vessels results in vascular stasis, edema, and thrombosis, leading to compression of the facial nerve.

CLINICAL FEATURES

1. Facial palsy due to AOM occurs in children within 2 to 3 days of the onset of the illness.
2. Facial palsy is peripheral, and its features are same as those of Bell's palsy (see Box 5–7)

LABORATORY

1. Complete blood count
2. Cultures of blood and aspirate from the middle ear (obtained through myringotomy)
3. If facial palsy does not improve following intravenous antibiotic therapy and myringotomy, a high-resolution computed tomography (CT) scan of the temporal bone is indicated to identify coalescence in the mastoid (suggestive of acute mastoiditis).

TREATMENT

1. Hospitalization; otolaryngology and neurology consultations
2. Intravenous antibiotics (e.g., second- or third-generation cephalosporin) to cover the most common pathogens (*Streptococcus pneumoniae, Haemophilus influenzae,* and *Moraxella catarrhalis*) causing AOM
3. Wide myringotomy (inferior quadrant), preferably with insertion of a tube to permit decompression of the middle ear cavity and yield fluid for culture
4. Indications for mastoidectomy: evidence of acute mastoiditis and failure to improve after antibiotics and myringotomy
5. Decompression of the bony fallopian canal
   a. Seldom indicated
   b. Opening the bony canal runs the risk of damaging the inflamed or friable facial nerve and disrupting the blood supply, leading to worsening ischemia.
6. Systemic corticosteroids are not effective in this form of facial palsy.

KEY POINT

Facial Palsy with Acute Otitis Media

■ Treatment of AOM complicated by facial palsy requires parenteral antibiotic therapy and wide myringotomy.

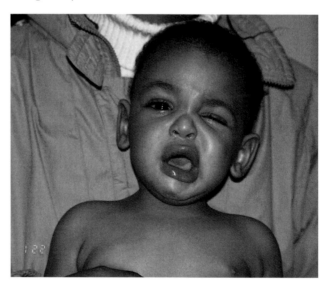

FIGURE 5–9. A 9-month-old infant with right-sided peripheral facial palsy and right acute otitis media. He was treated with parenteral antibiotics and myringotomy and showed complete recovery of facial palsy over a period of 6 months.

Obstructive Sleep Apnea

DEFINITION

1. Apnea is cessation of air flow at the level of nostrils and mouth lasting for at least 10 seconds (20 seconds in premature infants).
2. Hypopnea is reduced but not complete cessation of air flow.
3. Sleep apneas are classified as:
   a. Obstructive sleep apnea (OSA): cessation of air flow at the nose and mouth despite apparent, often vigorous, inspiratory efforts. These efforts are, however, ineffective owing to lack of airway patency. Usually a condition of partial obstruction with some degree of air flow is maintained (by increased effort) between periods of complete obstruction.

b. Central apnea: cessation of air flow with *no* apparent respiratory effort

c. Mixed apnea: both central and obstructive apnea occur without interruption by effective respiration

4. The spectrum of abnormalities ranging from obstructive hypoventilation (obstructive hypopnea) to OSA is known as obstructive sleep apnea syndrome.

EPIDEMIOLOGY

1. Central apnea is seen most commonly in neonatal period.
2. Obstructive apnea is seen most commonly in children.
3. Any child has the potential to develop OSA (presence of prominent tonsils and adenoids)
4. Most common cause of OSA in children is adenotonsillar hypertrophy.
5. Peak incidence of OSA in children is 2 to 6 years.
6. Prepubertal male and female children are equally affected. (Adults: males outnumber females.)

DIAGNOSIS

1. Hemogram/hematocrit (hypoxia causing polycythemia)
2. Serum electrolytes (compensatory metabolic alkalosis for hypoventilation)
3. Radiographs
   a. Lateral radiograph of neck for evaluation of pharyngeal obstruction
   b. Chest posteroanterior and lateral: for evaluation for pneumonia and/or atelectasis related to aspiration and for evaluation for cor pulmonale
4. Electrocardiogram and echocardiogram for evidence of cardiomegaly and cor pulmonale
5. Diagnosis of OSA is made by
   a. Episodes of partial or complete airway obstruction during sleep associated with hypoxia (SaO_2 <90%) and hypercarbia ($PaCO_2$ > 45 mmHg) during sleep
   b. Presence of significant consequences due to sleep-related asphyxia and sleep deprivation (e.g., cor pulmonale, failure to thrive)
6. Recording of breathing sounds during sleep on audiocassettes by parents. This recording can be heard and analyzed by a physician.
7. Sleep study (polysomnography)
   a. To confirm OSA
   b. To calculate apnea/hypopnea index
      (1) Number of apnea and hypopnea events per hour of sleep
      (2) Index over 5 is abnormal

TREATMENT

1. Patients with worsening of airway obstruction secondary to an acute illness may require hospitalization and continuous monitoring (cardiac and pulse oxymetry). Therapeutic interventions include

a. Nasopharyngeal airway to bypass the obstruction

b. Continuous positive airway pressure or biphasic positive airway pressure (BiPAP)

2. A short course of steroids given orally (prednisone 2 mg/kg/day for 5 days) may reduce pharyngeal lymphoid tissue that may worsen OSA (e.g., for infectious mononucleosis)
3. Antibiotic, if indicated for acute illness (e.g., for streptococcal pharyngitis)
4. Weight reduction for obese patients
5. Consultation with pediatric pulmonologist and otolaryngologist for operative interventions (as indicated)
   a. Tonsillectomy and adenoidectomy
      (1) For patients with hyperplasia of adenoids and tonsils leading to OSA and complications
      (2) Usually patients experience dramatic relief of symptoms of OSA.
   b. Uvulopalatopharyngoplasty (UPPP)
      (1) Rarely performed in children; more often done in adults
      (2) Indications: patients who fail to respond to adenotonsillectomy or patients with neuromuscular disorders
   c. Tracheostomy for the rare child who fails to respond to both adenotonsillectomy and UPPP

BOX 5–8   *Complications Related to Obstructive Sleep Apnea*

Pulmonary hypertension and cor pulmonale (repeated episodes of hypoxia or hypercarbia with respiratory acidosis constrict the pulmonary arterioles)
Systemic hypertension
Growth failure (poor caloric intake during day and hypermetabolic state at night)
Pectus deformity
Respiratory failure and death postanesthesia
Neurologic dysfunction
Asphyxial encephalopathy
Developmental delay
Behavioral disturbances
Hypersomnolence

KEY POINTS

Obstructive Sleep Apnea

■ The two most common presenting symptoms of OSA are snoring and sleep disturbances.

■ Physical signs of obstruction are often not present when the child is awake; a child with suspected OSA *must* be examined during sleep.

■ Presence of hypercarbia and hypoxia and evidence of long-term sequelae of airway obstruction are more important than an arbitrary duration of apneic episodes in the evaluation of a child with OSA.

TABLE 5-8
Predisposing Conditions for Obstructive Sleep Apnea

Adenotonsillar hyperplasia (most common)
Nasal polyps (respiratory allergies, cystic fibrosis)
Chronic rhinitis
Nasal septal deviation
Choanal stenosis
Obesity (pickwickian syndrome)
Mandibular hypoplasia
  Pierre Robin anomaly
  Treacher-Collins syndrome
Down syndrome
  Hypotonia (collapse of pharyngeal tissues to hypopharynx during sleep)
  Midface hypoplasia

TABLE 5-9
Clinical Features of Obstructive Sleep Apnea

Night symptoms
  Breathing difficulty or apnea during sleep
  Snoring
  Restlessness
  Enuresis
Daytime symptoms
  Excessive daytime somnolence
  Morning headaches
  Behavioral problems (e.g., excessive crankiness)
  Feeling of being tired during the day
  Learning problems, poor school performance
Difficulty in swallowing
Frequent upper respiratory tract and/or middle ear infections
Failure to thrive (child)
Obesity (pickwickian syndrome [adolescents/adults])
Mouth breathing
  Craniofacial developmental changes
  Orthodontic malformations
Aspiration of pharyngeal secretions during obstructive episodes
  Recurrent pneumonias
  Chronic nocturnal cough

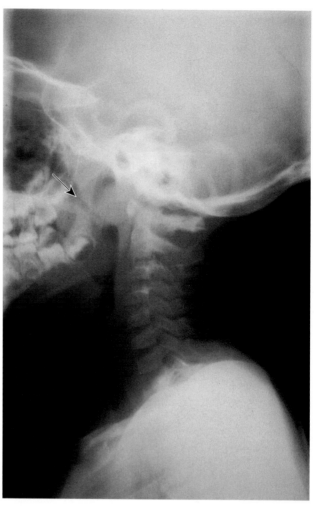

FIGURE 5-11. Lateral view of the airway in a boy with pronounced snoring. Note enlarged adenoids and tonsils causing significant narrowing of the nasopharynx and hypopharynx.

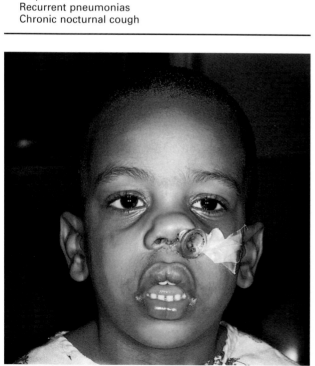

FIGURE 5-10. Obstructive sleep apnea resulting in significant oxygen desaturation (pulse oxymetry ~70% during sleep) in this child who had a long history of snoring. A nasopharyngeal airway was required to relieve the obstruction. A nasopharyngeal airway is well tolerated by children.

6

Dermatology

Teresita A. Laude, M.D.

Atopic Dermatitis (AD)

SYNONYM   Eczema

DEFINITION

A chronic or relapsing skin disorder characterized by dryness of the skin and pruritus.

ETIOLOGY

1. Unknown
2. There is a genetic predisposition.
3. Main trigger factors
   a. Irritants
   b. Heat and humidity
   c. Infections
      (1) *Staphylococcus aureus*
         (a) A major flare factor
         (b) The atopic skin is heavily colonized at all times.
         (c) The organism is believed to act as a superantigen and thus is responsible for the release of major inflammatory cytokines.
      (2) Herpes simplex virus (HSV), dermatophyte
   d. Allergens—housedust mites, pollens, molds
   e. Stress, anxiety, psychosocial problems
4. Food hypersensitivity
   a. Seen in 10% of children, mostly young infants
   b. Offenders: cow's milk protein, soy, wheat, eggs, peanuts

EPIDEMIOLOGY

1. Ten percent of the U.S. pediatric population has atopic dermatitis.
2. Onset occurs before 5 years of age in 85%; before 1 year of age in 60%.

PATHOGENESIS

1. Two hypotheses:
   a. Increased cyclic AMP-phosphodiesterase activity
   b. Diminished cell-mediated immunity
2. Both result in overactivity of the T helper 2 (TH2) subset of T lymphocytes and thus in significant inflammation.

CLINICAL FEATURES (see Table 6–1)

1. Severity of atopic dermatitis varies.
   a. Mild: less than 20% of body surface area involved
   b. Moderate: between 20% and 50% of body surface area involved
   c. Severe: more than 50% of body surface area involved
2. Nummular eczema
   a. Variant characterized by discoid, well-circumscribed, often oozing annular plaques
   b. Most common on the extremities
3. Personal or family history of asthma or allergic rhinitis
4. The presence of the following minor clinical features is helpful in diagnosing mild or atypical cases:
   a. Dennie-Morgan infraorbital fold
   b. Periorbital darkening
   c. Pityriasis alba
   d. Infra-auricular fissure
   e. Follicular accentuation
   f. Keratosis pilaris
   g. Hyperlinear palms
   h. Ichthyosis vulgaris
   i. Headlight sign
   j. White dermographism

LABORATORY

1. Most children have elevated serum IgE levels.
2. Those whose eczema is made worse by aeroallergens have positive results on skin tests for specific allergens.
3. The radioallergosorbent test (RAST) is not helpful in diagnosing food allergy unless the result is negative (food allergy excluded).

COMPLICATIONS

1. Eczema herpeticum (Kaposi varicelliform eruption) is seen in disseminated HSV infection
2. Generalized exfoliative dermatitis (erythroderma)

TREATMENT

1. Parental education: Establish realistic parental expectations.

BOX
6–1

BOX 6–1 · *Differential Diagnosis of Atopic Dermatitis*

Seborrheic dermatitis (see Table 6–3)
Contact dermatitis
Drug eruption
Fungal infections
Scabies
In severe intractable atopic dermatitis:
  Wiskott-Aldrich syndrome
  Job syndrome (hyper-IgE syndrome)
  Netherton syndrome
  Severe combined immunodeficiency syndrome
  Chronic granulomatous disease
  Infective dermatitis of human T-cell leukemia-lymphoma virus (HTLV-1) infection

2. Dry skin care
   a. Brief bath or shower lasting not more than 5 minutes
   b. Mild unscented soap or liquid cleanser
   c. Patting (not rubbing) the skin dry, leaving some moisture
   d. Use of emollients (moisturizers) as soon as the child leaves the bath or shower
      (1) Hydrophilic petrolatum for young infants during winter
      (2) Heavy creams in other age groups, used all year round
      (3) Used at minimum twice a day; optimally several times a day
3. Topical corticosteroids (see Table 6–2)
   a. Ointments work better than creams.
   b. Applied over the affected areas no more than twice a day (once a day for highly potent steroids)
   c. The steroid is applied first, then the emollient over it.
   d. Midpotency (classes 4 and 5) to high-potency (classes 2 and 3) steroid ointments are used for 3 to 7 days, followed by low-potency (classes 6 and 7) ointments for 1 to 2 weeks.
   e. Use only class 6 and 7 ointments on the face.
   f. Topical steroids are used only on active lesions and may be discontinued during periods of remissions.
4. Liberal use of systemic antibiotics
   a. For clinically infected lesions
   b. For severe and intractable flares regardless of clinical appearance
   c. Beta-lactam antibiotics
   d. Duration: 2 to 3 weeks
5. Antihistamines
   a. Best given at night at double the usual dose
   b. Hydroxyzine 1 mg/kg/day
   c. Diphenhydramine 5 mg/kg/day
   d. Doxepin for older children 10 mg at bedtime
   e. Low sedating antihistamines (e.g., loratadine, cetirizine) may be given to children who go to school.
6. Hospitalization may be indicated for patients with the following conditions:
   a. Eczema herpeticum (for intravenous acyclovir)
   b. Generalized erythroderma
   c. Severe flare unresponsive to conventional treatment
7. Severe intractable cases of atopic dermatitis must be referred to a dermatologist.
8. If allergy is a major triggering factor, an allergist must be consulted.
9. Emotional support and counseling is needed for families with many psychosocial problems.
10. Any of the following may be used by the dermatologist for treating intractable cases:
    a. Ultraviolet B phototherapy
    b. Tacrolimus (FK 506) ointment
    c. Cyclosporine orally

PROGNOSIS

In the majority of children, the disease improves with age.

KEY POINTS

Atopic Dermatitis

- Atopic dermatitis is a chronic multifactorial relapsing dermatitis.
- The most prominent clinical features are dryness of the skin and pruritus.
- Establishing realistic parental expectations is crucial in the treatment.

TABLE 6–1
Clinical Features of Atopic Dermatitis

Skin Lesions
Pruritus
Dry skin (xerosis)
Erythematous
Excoriated plaques
May be lichenified and hyperpigmented

Infantile Form
Onset at 6–8 weeks of age
Face commonly involved
Diaper area commonly spared
Distribution of lesions: more extensor than flexor
Process tends to be more exudative

Childhood Form
Flexural in distribution
Neck
Wrists
Antecubital areas
Popliteal areas

TABLE 6–2
Potency Ranking of Some Commonly Used Topical Steroids

Class	
1	Betamethasone dipropionate ointment
	Diflorasone diacetate ointment
	Clobetasol propionate cream
	Clobetasol propionate ointment
	Halobetasol propionate cream
	Halobetasol propionate ointment
2	Amcinonide ointment
	Betamethasone dipropionate cream
	Mometasone furoate ointment
	Diflorasone diacetate ointment
	Halcinonide cream
	Fluocinonide gel
	Fluocinonide ointment
	Desoximetasone cream
3	Triamcinolone acetonide ointment
	Fluticasone propionate ointment
	Diflorasone diacetate cream
	Halcinonide ointment
	Fluocinonide cream
4	Flurandrenolide ointment
	Mometasone cream
	Triamcinolone acetonide cream
	Fluocinolone acetonide ointment
	Hydrocortisone valerate ointment
5	Flurandrenolide cream
	Fluticasone propionate cream
	Triamcinolone acetonide lotion
	Hydrocortisone butyrate cream
	Fluocinolone acetonide cream
	Hydrocortisone valerate cream
6	Desonide ointment
	Desonide cream
	Desonide lotion
	Aldometasone dipropionate cream
	Aldometasone dipropionate ointment
	Fluocinolone acetonide solution
7	Hydrocortisone

Class 1 is the most potent, and potency descends with each class to class 7, which is least potent. There is no significant difference between agents within any given class.

TABLE 6–3
Differential Diagnosis of Infantile Atopic Dermatitis and Seborrheic Dermatitis

	Infantile Atopic Dermatitis	Seborrheic Dermatitis
Onset	6–8 weeks	First 3 weeks of life
Site of onset	Face, extensors of extremities	Scalp, face, eyebrows, ears
Lesions	Dry, papular, erythematous	Greasy, scaly papules
Family history of atopy	Positive	May or may not be positive

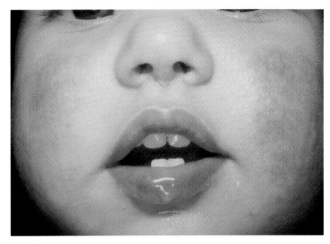

FIGURE 6–1. Infantile atopic dermatitis: involvement of the cheeks. The nose is spared (headlight sign).

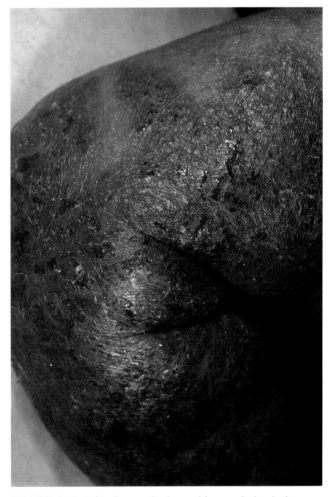

FIGURE 6–2. Infantile atopic dermatitis: exudative lesions on the lower extremity.

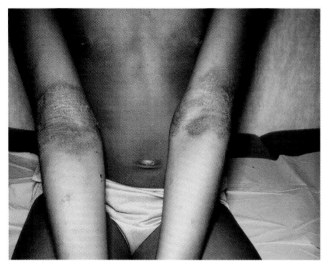

FIGURE 6-3. Atopic dermatitis. An older child with involvement of the antecubital areas.

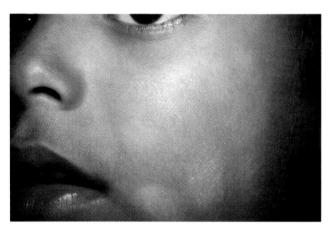

FIGURE 6-4. Pityriasis alba.

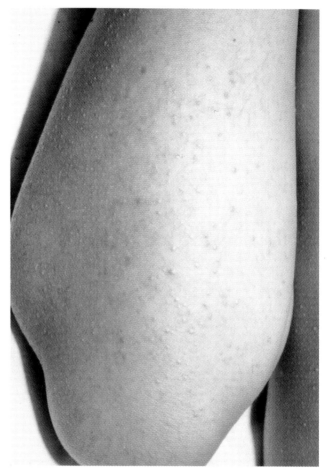

FIGURE 6-5. Keratosis pilaris.

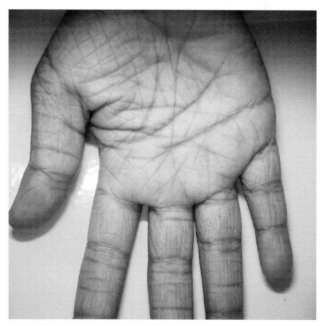

FIGURE 6-6. Hyperlinear palm.

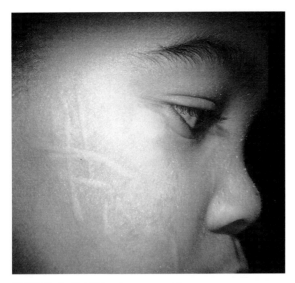

FIGURE 6–7. White dermographism.

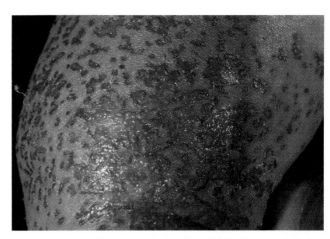

FIGURE 6–10. Close-up of Figure 6–9 showing both eroded areas and shallow ulcers caused by herpes simplex virus.

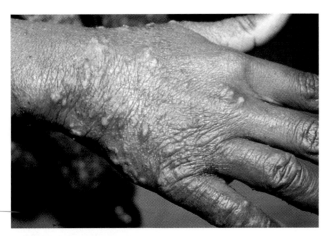

FIGURE 6–8. Atopic dermatitis. Secondarily infected lesion showing pustules of *Staphylococcus aureus.*

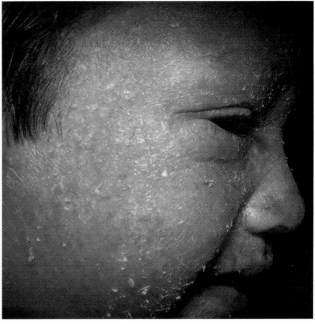

FIGURE 6–11. A child with atopic dermatitis who developed generalized erythroderma. The upper layer of the skin is exfoliating in pieces on a background of generalized erythema.

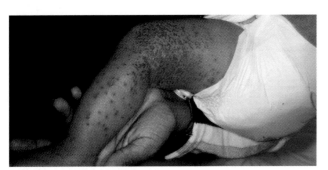

FIGURE 6–9. Eczema herpeticum: A young infant with atopic dermatitis exposed to a parent with herpes simplex labialis.

Postinflammatory Hyperpigmentation and Hypopigmentation

DEFINITION

Secondary skin changes often seen in dark-skinned individuals

PATHOGENESIS

1. Hyperpigmentation results from movement of melanin pigment into the dermis from the epidermis following vacuolar degeneration of the basal layer.
2. Hypopigmentation results from an inability of the keratinocytes (epidermal cells) to accept pigment granules from the melanocytes.

CLINICAL FEATURES

1. Postinflammatory hypopigmentation commonly follows an acute inflammatory process, whereas postinflammatory hyperpigmentation follows a chronic inflammatory process.
2. Lesions conform to the shape and size of the original eruption.
3. This is a cosmetic problem that sometimes worries the parents more than does the underlying original dermatitis.
4. Self-limiting

COMPLICATION

Cosmetic

TREATMENT

1. No treatment in the majority of cases
2. Parents must be reassured.
3. In postinflammatory hyperpigmentation, hydroquinone creams may be used.
4. In postinflammatory hypopigmentation camouflage make-up will cover the lesion.

KEY POINTS

Postinflammatory Hyperpigmentation and Hypopigmentation

- Postinflammatory hyperpigmentation and hypopigmentation are common secondary changes of any inflammatory disorder in dark-skinned individuals.
- These changes are self-limiting.

BOX 6-2	*Differential Diagnosis of Postinflammatory Hyperpigmentation and Hypopigmentation*

Café-au-lait spots
Pigmented nevus
Vitiligo
Pityriasis alba
Nevus depigmentosus

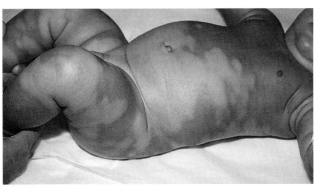

FIGURE 6-12. Generalized atopic dermatitis resulting in severe postinflammatory hypopigmentation.

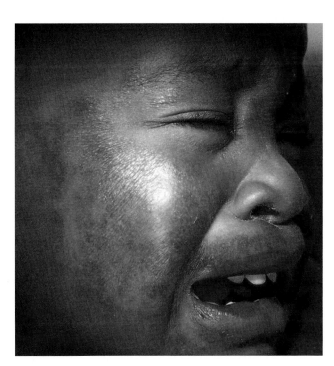

FIGURE 6-13. Chronic atopic dermatitis with postinflammatory hyperpigmentation.

Allergic Contact Dermatitis

DEFINITION

A form of delayed hypersensitivity reaction that results from exposure of a sensitized individual to a contact allergen.

EPIDEMIOLOGY

1. More common in children than infants
2. Poison ivy dermatitis is seen during the summer

PATHOGENESIS

In poison ivy dermatitis, the active substance uroshiol combines with an epidermal protein and is then presented by the Langerhans' cells to T lymphocytes, which become activated, releasing inflammatory cytokines.

CLINICAL FEATURES

1. Onset: The rash appears after a latent period of 5 to 14 days. In subsequent exposures, the latent period may be as short as 12 to 48 hours.
2. Erythema, oozing, vesicles, and papules occur in the area of the skin corresponding to contact with the allergen.
3. In poison ivy dermatitis the vesicles and bullae may be arranged in a linear manner.
4. There may be marked edema of the face and periorbital areas in severe poison ivy dermatitis.
5. Pruritus is prominent.
6. Allergy to poison ivy cross-reacts with poison sumac and poison oak.

LABORATORY

Skin patch testing

TREATMENT

1. Avoid exposure to allergic sensitizers if known.
2. Use a high or midpotency topical corticosteroid cream.
3. Refer to a dermatologist for patch testing.
4. Poison ivy dermatitis
   a. Compresses of Burow's solution (1:20 dilution) for patients with severe exudation
   b. Topical high or midpotency steroid cream twice a day
   c. In moderate to severe cases a course of oral prednisone 1 mg/kg/day may be used for 1 week; then taper the drug for another week.
   d. Provide a picture of the plant for patient and family education.

KEY POINTS

Allergic Contact Dermatitis

- Poison ivy, nickel, rubber and potassium dichromate in shoes, and neomycin are examples of common allergic contact sensitizers in children.
- Treat moderate or severe poison ivy dermatitis with a course of an oral corticosteroid.

BOX 6-3 *Etiology of Allergic Contact Dermatitis*

In children the most common offending contact allergens are:
   Plants (poison ivy, poison sumac, poison oak)
   Nickel (jewelry, metal wrist bands, snap buttons of trouser jeans)
   Shoes (rubber and leather)
   Topical medications containing neomycin or ethylenediamine

---

TABLE 6-4
Differential Diagnosis

	Allergic Contact Dermatitis	Irritant Contact Dermatitis
Examples	Poison ivy dermatitis, nickel dermatitis, shoe dermatitis	Diaper dermatitis, liplicking dermatitis, hand dermatitis
Pathogenesis	True immunologic reaction	Adequate exposure to irritating substances
Individuals affected	Selected individuals	All individuals of all age groups

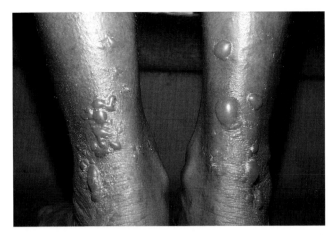

FIGURE 6-14. Poison ivy dermatitis: linear bullae on both lower legs.

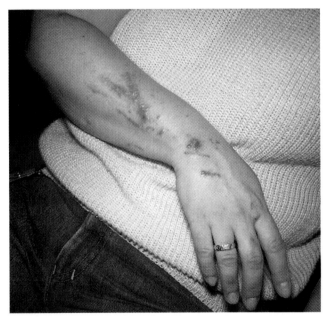

FIGURE 6-15. Poison ivy dermatitis: linear papules on the arm.

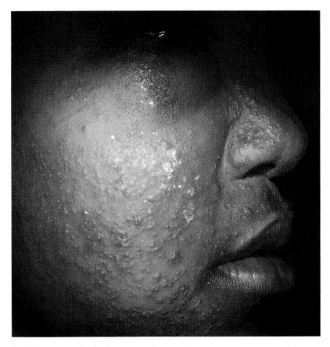

FIGURE 6-16. Poison ivy dermatitis: severe edema and oozing on the face.

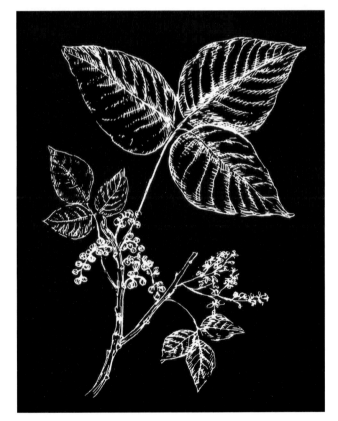

FIGURE 6-17. Poison ivy plant.

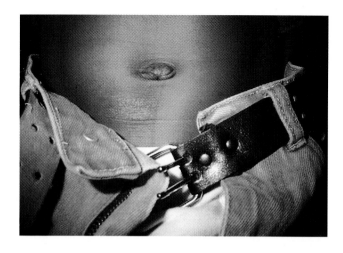

FIGURE 6–18. Nickel contact dermatitis resulting from the snap button of the jeans and buckle of the belt.

Diaper Dermatitis

SYNONYMS   Diaper Rash
Napkin Dermatitis

DEFINITION

An eruption in infants that is limited to the lower abdomen, upper thighs, and gluteal, perianal, and genitocrural areas. It results from prolonged contact with soiled diapers and is the best example of a contact irritant dermatitis.

ETIOLOGY

1. Prolonged contact with moisture, friction, and maceration
2. The concept that the ammonia in urine is the major etiologic factor has recently been challenged.
3. The role of *Candida albicans* is also unclear.

EPIDEMIOLOGY

1. General incidence: 10% to 20% of all infants
2. Most common in infants under 2 years of age
3. No sex difference
4. May occur in older patients with urinary and fecal incontinence

PATHOGENESIS

1. Prolonged contact with urine and feces macerates and destroys the epidermis and with it the normal barrier function of the skin.
2. Yeast infection may further complicate this dermatitis, resulting in persistent and severe inflammation.

CLINICAL FEATURES

1. Several morphologic subtypes
   a. Chafing and redness
   b. Papulopustular eruption
   c. Granulomatous reactions (pseudoverrucous papules and nodules, Jacquet granuloma)

2. Distribution
   a. Convex surfaces (i.e., buttocks, thighs, abdomen)
   b. Spares creases

BOX 6–4   *Differential Diagnosis of Diaper Dermatitis*

Seborrheic dermatitis
Napkin psoriasis
Histiocytosis X
Scabies
Miliaria
Jacquet granuloma has been misdiagnosed as condyloma acuminata

---

LABORATORY

None

COMPLICATIONS

1. Secondary candidal infection
2. Granuloma gluteale infantum

TREATMENT

1. Frequent diaper changes
2. Use of barrier creams or ointments—zinc oxide, hydrophilic petrolatum with every diaper change
3. Hydrocortisone cream twice a day for 3 days in the presence of severe inflammation
4. Nystatin cream for candidal infection
5. No need to change to cloth diapers because the new disposable diapers are superabsorbent.

KEY POINT

Diaper Dermatitis

■ Diaper dermatitis is a contact irritant dermatitis.

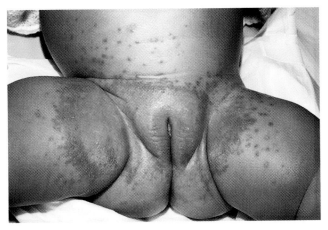

FIGURE 6-19. Diaper dermatitis with secondary candidal infection.

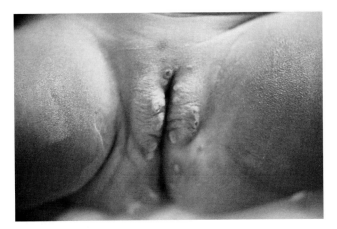

FIGURE 6-20. Jacquet granuloma.

Urticaria

SYNONYM   Hives

DEFINITIONS

1. Urticaria is an acute type I hypersensitivity reaction characterized by edematous skin lesions.
2. Angioedema is a giant, deeper urticaria involving the dependent parts of the body.
3. Acute urticaria has a total duration of less than 6 weeks.
4. Chronic urticaria lasts longer than 6 weeks.
5. If exposure to the offending agent is not stopped, acute urticaria may evolve into chronic urticaria.

EPIDEMIOLOGY

1. Uncertain incidence
2. By adolescence, 10% to 20% of the population has experienced at least one episode of acute urticaria.

PATHOGENESIS

1. Acute urticaria: An IgE-induced release of histamine results in increased capillary permeability and subsequent transudation of fluid into the dermal interstices.
2. Angioedema: Fluid accumulation involves the subcutaneous tissue.

LABORATORY

1. Diagnosis of urticaria is based on a very thorough history. If the history is unrevealing, laboratory tests may be performed.
2. Acute urticaria
   a. Throat culture, antistreptolysin-O (ASLO)
   b. Liver function tests, hepatitis serology
3. Chronic urticaria (to exclude connective tissue disease)
   a. Antinuclear antibodies (ANA)
   b. Sedimentation rate
   c. Other serologic tests depending on the results of the two screening tests (a and b)
   d. Skin biopsy

DIFFERENTIAL DIAGNOSIS

1. Erythema multiforme
2. Urticaria pigmentosa (mastocytosis)
3. Angioneurotic edema

TREATMENT

1. Discontinue or avoid offending agent if known.
2. Epinephrine 1:1000 aqueous solution 0.01 mL/kg subcutaneously for acute urticaria
3. Antihistamines
   a. Classes
      (1) H1 inhibitors: hydroxyzine, diphenhydramine, cyproheptadine, loratadine, cetirizine
      (2) H2 inhibitors: cimetidine
      (3) H1 and H2 inhibitors: doxepin
   b. Combinations within a class or combinations of different classes of antihistamines may be used if there is no response to single drug therapy.
4. Soothing colloidal baths
5. Lotions containing pramoxine and hydrocortisone
6. Systemic corticosteroids in severe cases
7. Refer patients with chronic urticaria to a dermatologist.

KEY POINTS

Urticaria

- A thorough history is necessary to identify the possible cause of acute urticaria.
- The older child must be asked directly what he or she thinks may be the cause.
- Empiric treatment with an antihistamine may be necessary in many cases.

TABLE 6–5
Causes of Acute Urticaria (5 I's)

Ingested Substances

Foods
  Nuts
  Milk products
  Eggs
  Shellfish, fish
  Chocolate
  Strawberries, citrus fruits
  Tartrazine, azo dyes, benzoates
Medications
  Antibiotics
  Aspirin
  Nonsteroidal anti-inflammatory agents
  Codeine

Injections

Antibiotics
Immunizations
Blood products

Infections

Streptococcus pyogenes
Mycoplasma pneumoniae
Hepatitis A, B, C

Insect Bite Reactions

Idiopathic (>50%)

TABLE 6–6
Causes of Chronic Urticaria

Collagen Vascular Diseases

Lupus erythematosus
Dermatomyositis
Juvenile rheumatoid arthritis

Occult Infections

Sinusitis
Dental abscesses

Physical Agents

Cold
Pressure
Solar
Water

Cholinergic Urticaria

Idiopathic (>50%)

TABLE 6–7
Clinical Features of Urticaria

Lesions of Acute Urticaria

Edematous
Ill-defined elevations
Pale in the center and erythematous at the periphery (flare)
Lesions vary in size and shapes
Individual lesions do not last >24 hours
Varying degrees of pruritus

Angioedema

Ill-defined
Asymmetrical
Common areas involved: eyelids, lips

Papular Urticaria

Reaction to arthropod assault
Lesions are small papules
Located mainly on the extremities

Urticarial Vasculitis

Urticaria of collagen vascular diseases
Individual lesions last >24 hours
Lesions are *not* pruritic

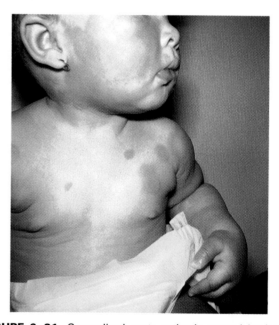

FIGURE 6–21. Generalized acute urticaria caused by ingestion of orange juice.

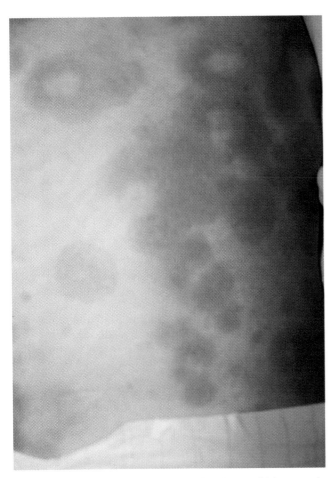

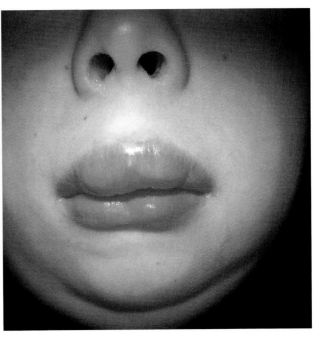

FIGURE 6–23. Angioedema of the lips after ingestion of aspirin.

FIGURE 6–22. Urticaria. Close-up of lesions, which are pale edematous plaques with irregular margins and a surrounding erythematous flare.

FIGURE 6–24. Acute urticaria: Lesions were outlined by a pen, and 24 hours later the outlined lesions were gone.

Arthropod Bites

SYNONYMS   Insect Bites
                        Bug Bites

DEFINITION

A localized skin reaction to the bite of an insect

ETIOLOGY

Many species of insects

EPIDEMIOLOGY

1. More common during summer because of outdoor activities

2. Some individuals are more attractive to insects than others. For example, in the same family, two children may be exposed, but only one child is bitten. The reason for this is poorly understood.

PATHOGENESIS

Arthropods produce their effects on the skin by a variety of mechanisms, more than one of which may be implicated simultaneously.

1. Mechanical trauma
2. Injection of directly injurious substances
3. Injection of normally harmless substances into a previously sensitized host
4. Secondary infection
5. Invasion of the host's tissue
6. Contact reactions
7. Reactions to retained mouthparts
8. Transmission of disease

BOX 6–5	*Differential Diagnosis of Arthropod Bites*

Staphylococcal furunculosis
Drug eruption
Acute urticaria
Molluscum contagiosum
Urticaria pigmentosa
Varicella

LABORATORY

None

TABLE 6–8
Clinical Features of Arthropod Bites

Flying insect bites
  Examples: mosquitoes, gnats, midges, flies, bees, wasps, hornets
  Lesions are on exposed parts of body
  Lesions are scattered (far apart)
Crawling insect bites
  Examples: bedbugs, ants
  Insect is trapped inside the clothing and attacks covered areas of the body.
  Lesions are close to each other: "breakfast-lunch-dinner bite."
Classic lesion
  An urticarial papule surmounted by a punctum surrounded by varying amounts of erythema and edema
Other features
  Lesion may become bullous.
  Intense pruritus
  Pain may be present.
  Angioedema of dependent areas may be seen.
  Cat flea bites
    Lesions are distributed on lower extremities (corresponding to the height to which fleas can jump)
Papular urticaria
  A hypersensitivity response to insect bites
  Lesions are numerous and commonly distributed on the extremities.

TREATMENT

1. Avoid further exposure.
2. Lotion containing pramoxine and hydrocortisone may be applied twice daily on the affected areas.
3. Oral antihistamines may be used for severe pruritus.
4. Individuals known to be allergic to Hymenoptera (bees, wasps, hornets) should carry a sublingual sympathomimetic drug such as isoprenaline 10 mg. Adrenaline should be readily available.

PREVENTION

1. Wear protective clothing.
2. Avoid wearing brightly colored clothes and flowery prints.
3. Personal insect repellent (diethyltoluamide [DEET]) applied to skin and clothes
  a. Repellents containing more than 10% DEET should not be used on children by spray or regular application.
  b. May use repellents containing citronella.
4. Avoid hair tonics, hair sprays, deodorants, perfumes, and scented soaps with strong odors that may attract bees.

PROGNOSIS

Most arthropod bites are self-limiting if exposure is broken.

KEY POINT

Arthropod Bites

- Arthropod bite reactions occur in individuals sensitized to injurious or normally harmless substances that have been previously injected by the insect into the skin.

TABLE 6–9
Complications of Arthropod Bites

Secondary infection
  Staphylococcus aureus
  Streptococcus pyogenes
Anaphylactic shock
  Unusual except after Hymenoptera (bee, wasp, hornet) stings
Prurigo nodularis
  Persistent, nodular, and hyperpigmented lesions resulting from chronic rubbing and picking

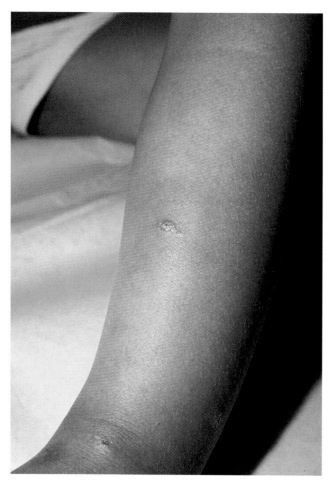

FIGURE 6–25. Mosquito bite reaction on the arm. The lesions are far apart.

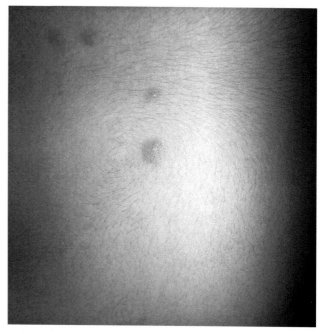

FIGURE 6–27. "Breakfast-lunch-dinner" bite reaction to a crawling insect trapped inside the shirt.

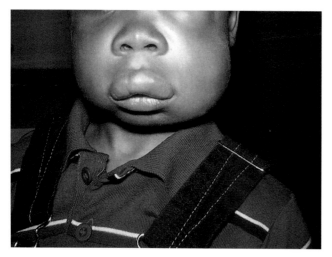

FIGURE 6–26. Bee sting reaction resulting in severe facial angioedema.

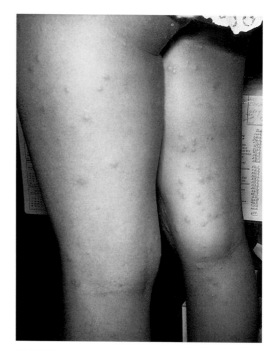

FIGURE 6–28. Papular urticaria.

Popsicle Panniculitis

DEFINITION
An inflammation of the perioral subcutaneous fat following cold exposure

ETIOLOGY
The cause is prolonged contact of the cold object (e.g., a Popsicle) with the tissue around the angle of the mouth.

EPIDEMIOLOGY
1. Seen in young infants who suck on the Popsicle but do not rotate it inside the mouth. As a result, the cold object remains in contact with the buccal fat for some time, causing cold injury.
2. Commonly seen in summer.

PATHOGENESIS
1. Vasoconstriction occurs on contact with a cold object, followed by vasodilatation.
2. Further cold exposure results in formation of ice crystals in the fat cells of the subcutaneous tissue.

LABORATORY
In cases in which the diagnosis is in doubt, a skin biopsy demonstrates lobular panniculitis with or without fat crystals.

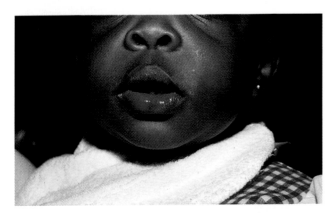

FIGURE 6–29. Popsicle panniculitis. A 1-year-old sucked on a Popsicle 2 days before erythematous indurated lesions appeared adjoining each side of the mouth. She was thought to have buccal cellulitis and was hospitalized unnecessarily.

TREATMENT
1. Condition is self-limiting.
2. There is no treatment.

KEY POINTS

Popsicle Panniculitis

- A history of exposure to the cold object is often not volunteered and therefore must be elicited.
- The lesions are adjacent to the angle of the infant's mouth.

BOX 6–6   *Differential Diagnosis of Popsicle Panniculitis*

BUCCAL CELLULITIS (see p. 101)
Bacterial infection (caused by any of the following pathogens)
  Staphylococcus aureus
  Streptococcus pyogenes
  Haemophilus influenzae type b
  Streptococcus pneumoniae
Lesion usually unilateral
Lesion not adjacent to the angle of the mouth
Signs of toxicity (fever, pain, tenderness of affected area)
Cultures from blood and lesion usually positive

TABLE 6–10
Clinical Features of Popsicle Panniculitis

Skin Lesions

Red
Indurated
Ill-defined nodules
Location: adjacent to the angles of the mouth
Unilateral or bilateral
May have minimal pain, burning, or itching

Important History

An interval of 1–2 days elapses between sucking a Popsicle or cold object and full development of clinical changes

---

Exfoliative Dermatitis

SYNONYM   Generalized Erythroderma

DEFINITION
A reactive condition that may occur as a presentation or as a complication of a primary skin disorder.

EPIDEMIOLOGY
More common in adults than in children

PATHOGENESIS
Unknown

LABORATORY
1. Serum protein electrophoresis may show a polyclonal increase in gamma globulins.
2. Skin biopsy: to determine the primary underlying skin disease

Primary skin disorders associated with exfoliative dermatitis
  Atopic dermatitis
  Psoriasis
  Seborrheic dermatitis
  Drug eruption
  Ichthyosis
  Pityriasis rubra pilaris
  Sarcoidosis
  Mycoses fungoides
Idiopathic in some patients

COMPLICATIONS

1. Dehydration
2. Severe protein loss
3. High-output cardiac failure
4. Sepsis

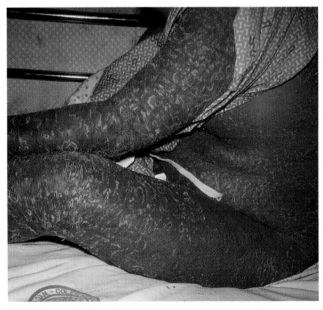

FIGURE 6-30. Exfoliative dermatitis in a boy with psoriasis. There is intense erythema of the skin, and fragments of the skin are exfoliating.

DIFFERENTIAL DIAGNOSIS

1. Staphylococcal scalded skin syndrome
2. Post–scarlet fever desquamation

TREATMENT

1. Hospitalization and dermatology consultation
2. Monitoring and maintenance of fluids and electrolytes
3. Hydrophilic petrolatum ointment applied topically to the skin twice a day
4. Low-potency topical steroid ointment (e.g., hydrocortisone 1%) applied to the skin twice a day
5. Treatment for the underlying skin disease

KEY POINTS

Exfoliative Dermatitis

- In the majority of instances, exfoliative dermatitis is associated with a primary skin disorder.
- Treatment must be gentle and conservative: bland emollients and low-potency topical steroids are used.

TABLE 6-11
Clinical Features of Exfoliative Dermatitis

Skin

Diffuse redness
Tenderness of the skin
Diffuse generalized desquamation
Fragments of scales fall off spontaneously or when scratched
Scales are found wherever the child is (e.g., on bedding, on chairs, on examining table)
Specific clinical findings of underlying skin disorder

Other Features

Fever and chills

Erythema Nodosum

DEFINITION

A reactive inflammatory disorder of the subcutaneous fat

EPIDEMIOLOGY

More common in older children

PATHOGENESIS

Unknown

LABORATORY

1. Culture and serology for *Streptococcus pyogenes*
2. Tuberculin skin test
3. In doubtful cases: skin biopsy (septal panniculitis)
4. Other tests depending on the suspected etiology

> **BOX 6-8**   *Etiology of Erythema Nodosum*
>
> Some of the known precipitating factors are:
>   *Streptococcus pyogenes* infections
>   Tuberculosis
>   Drugs: sulfonamides, oral contraceptives
>   Deep fungal infections: histoplasmosis, coccidi-
>   oidomycosis
>   Inflammatory bowel disease
>   *Yersinia enterocolitica* infections
>   Idiopathic (>30% of cases)

DIFFERENTIAL DIAGNOSIS

1. Cellulitis
2. Ecchymoses
3. Child abuse
4. Calcified hematoma

TREATMENT

1. Identify and treat the precipitating factor.
2. Oral nonsteroidal anti-inflammatory agents are used for symptomatic relief.

KEY POINTS

Erythema Nodosum

- In children, the most common precipitants are group A beta-hemolytic streptococcal and tuberculous infections.
- The lesions consist of red, painful, and tender nodules on the anterior aspects of the lower legs.

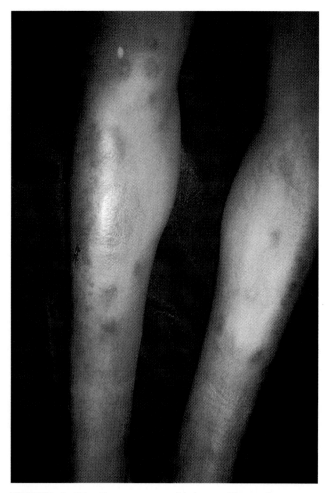

FIGURE 6-31. Fourteen-year-old boy with erythema nodosum caused by group A beta-hemolytic streptococcal infection.

TABLE 6-12
Clinical Features of Erythema Nodosum

Skin Lesions

Erythematous
Painful
Tender
Subcutaneous nodules
Overlying skin changes in color from red to blue to greenish-
  yellow and then fades
Common locations
  Symmetrically distributed
  On extensor surfaces such as shins

Other Features

Sudden onset
Symptoms last an average of 2 weeks

Drug Eruptions

DEFINITION
Adverse immunologic or nonimmunologic skin reactions to various systemic drugs

ETIOLOGY
Antibiotics are by far the most common causes of drug eruptions.

EPIDEMIOLOGY
1. Adverse drug reactions are less common in children than in adults for the following reasons:
   a. Fewer medications prescribed
   b. Less prior sensitization
   c. Differences in metabolism and pharmacokinetics
2. In a large study, 4.7% of children had definite or probable adverse drug events.
3. Cutaneous reactions comprise about 20% to 40% of adverse drug reactions.

PATHOGENESIS
1. Drug eruptions may be both immunologic (allergic) and nonimmunologic in nature.
2. Different drugs may produce different kinds of reactions at different times in the same patient.

CLINICAL FEATURES
1. Exanthematous or morbilliform drug eruption
   a. This is the most common form of drug eruption.
   b. The eruption appears within a week of starting the drug or a few days after the drug is discontinued.
   c. The lesions consist of erythematous papules in a generalized confluent (morbilliform) distribution.
   d. Pruritus varies.
2. Urticarial drug eruption
   a. This is an allergic type I immediate hypersensitivity (IgE-mediated) reaction.
   b. The hives may be accompanied by angioedema.
   c. Pruritus is prominent.
3. Serum sickness-like reaction
   a. Commonly associated with cefaclor.
   b. The lesions are urticarial.
   c. May be accompanied by arthralgia.
4. Fixed drug eruption (see Box 6–9)
5. Erythema multiforme minor
   a. May be caused by any drug
   b. Classic lesions consist of target or iris lesions, which are annular edematous plaques with necrotic centers.
   c. There may be involvement of one mucous membrane (e.g., mouth).
   d. The same picture may be caused by herpes simplex virus.

BOX 6–9 *Fixed Drug Eruption*

SKIN LESIONS
Solitary
Few or numerous
Annular erythema
Measures 1–3 cm
May become bullous
Erythema fades → dusky blue discoloration that can last for weeks
Pruritus varies
Location
   Any skin surface
   Occasionally on mucous membranes
Lesions recur on the same sites on re-exposure to the same drug

OTHER FEATURES
Pathogenesis unknown
Common offending agents
   Laxatives containing phenolphthalein
   Acetaminophen
   Antibiotics

---

6. Stevens-Johnson syndrome (erythema multiforme major) (see p. 181)
7. Toxic epidermal necrolysis (TEN) (see p. 183)

LABORATORY
There is no test that confirms suspicion of a drug eruption.

COMPLICATION
Anaphylaxis may occur with urticaria (type 1 hypersensitivity reaction).

DIFFERENTIAL DIAGNOSIS
1. Viral exanthem
2. Urticaria from other causes
3. Contact dermatitis

TREATMENT
1. Discontinue the offending drug.
2. Epinephrine 1:1000 aqueous solution 0.01 mL/kg subcutaneously for acute urticarial drug eruption
3. Oral antihistamines
4. Soothing colloidal baths
5. Hydrocortisone lotion 1% to 2.5% once or twice daily.

KEY POINTS
Drug Eruptions
- Not all drug eruptions are allergic in nature.
- Stevens-Johnson syndrome and toxic epidermal necrolysis are life-threatening forms of drug reaction.

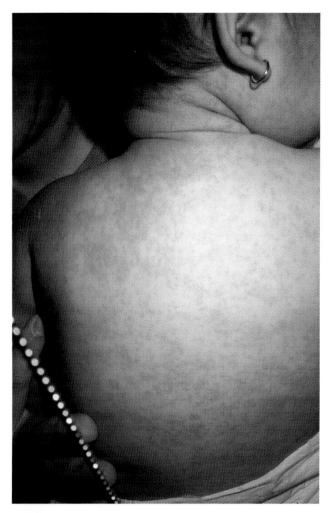

FIGURE 6–32. "Ampicillin rash," a morbilliform drug eruption commonly mistaken for a viral exanthem.

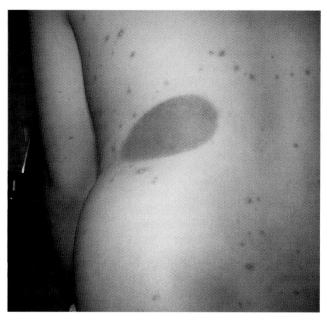

FIGURE 6–34. Acute fixed drug eruption in a boy with varicella who took acetaminophen.

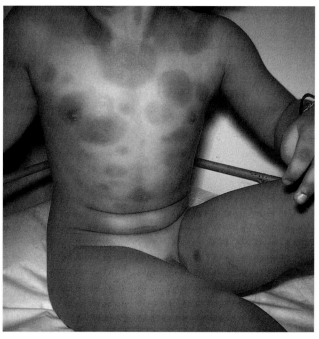

FIGURE 6–35. Multiple fixed drug eruptions secondary to acetaminophen.

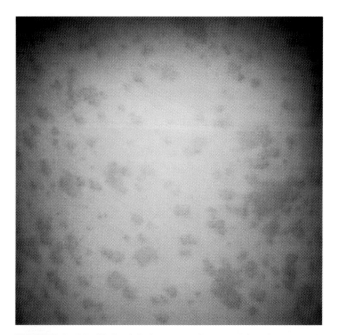

FIGURE 6–33. Urticarial drug eruption resulting from ampicillin.

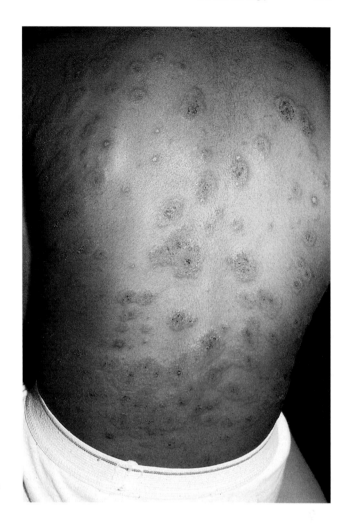

FIGURE 6–36. Erythema multiforme minor resulting from penicillin; numerous target or iris lesions are seen.

Stevens-Johnson Syndrome

SYNONYM   Erythema Multiforme Major

DEFINITION
A severe form of adverse drug reaction characterized by a distinct eruption and involvement of at least two mucous membranes.

EPIDEMIOLOGY
1. The exact incidence is unknown.
2. The peak incidence occurs in the second decade of life.

PATHOGENESIS
Unknown

LABORATORY
1. Cultures (to exclude treatable infectious causes)
2. Monitor electrolytes
3. Other tests (e.g., chest x-ray, liver function tests) depending on other organ involvement

---

BOX 6–10   *Etiology of Stevens-Johnson Syndrome*

MOST COMMON OFFENDING DRUGS

Anticonvulsants
  Barbiturates
  Diphenylhydantoin
  Carbamazepine
  Lamotrigene
Antibiotics
  Penicillins
  Sulfonamides (cotrimoxazole)
Nonsteroidal anti-inflammatory agents
  Ibuprofen
  Naprosyn

INFECTIOUS AGENT (INSIGNIFICANT ETIOLOGY)

Mycoplasma pneumoniae

COMPLICATIONS

1. Secondary bacterial infection
2. Fluid and electrolyte imbalance
3. Ocular sequelae
   a. Symblepharon
   b. Corneal ulceration
   c. Blindness
4. Severe pneumonia
5. Scarring of the skin

DIFFERENTIAL DIAGNOSIS

1. Kawasaki disease
2. Measles
3. Toxic epidermal necrolysis
4. Pemphigus vulgaris

TREATMENT

1. Hospitalization; dermatology and ophthalmology consultations
2. Discontinue offending drug.
3. Management of fluids, electrolytes, and nutrition
4. Periodic cultures of the skin, eyes, and mucosae

5. Skin care
   a. Warm tap water compresses and colloidal baths
   b. Petrolatum ointment over denuded areas
6. Systemic corticosteroids
   a. Use is controversial.
   b. If used
      (1) Use early
      (2) High dose of 2 mg/kg/day of prednisone
      (3) If no response, discontinue after 4 days

PROGNOSIS

1. Significant morbidity
2. Protracted course of 3 to 6 weeks
3. Mortality rate is 5% to 15%

KEY POINT

Stevens-Johnson Syndrome

■ Stevens-Johnson syndrome is characterized by prominent mucous membrane involvement and skin denudation involving less than 20% of body surface area.

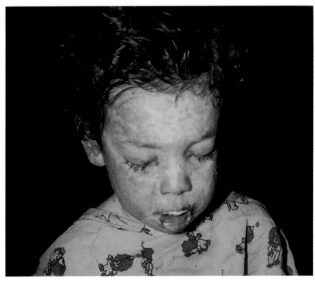

FIGURE 6–37. A 3-year-old boy with Stevens-Johnson syndrome caused by cotrimoxazole given for a urinary tract infection. He had severe stomatitis and conjunctivitis.

TABLE 6–13
Clinical Features of Stevens-Johnson Syndrome

Skin Lesions

Erythematous macules
Purpuric macules
Papules
Blisters leading to erosions
Target or iris lesions
Erosions involve <20% of body surface area
Individual erosions are <3 cm in diameter

Other Features

May be preceded by upper respiratory symptoms
Two or more mucous membranes are involved resulting in exudative or erosive stomatitis, conjunctivitis, or vulvovaginitis
Associated findings may include
  Arthritis/arthralgia
  Pneumonia
  Hepatitis

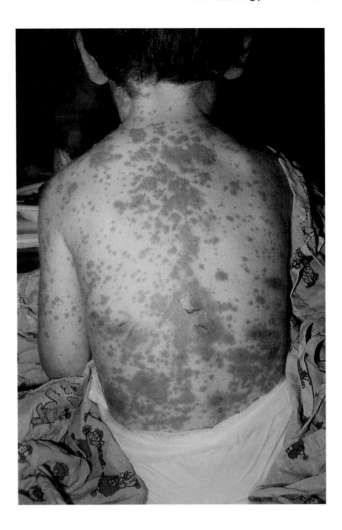

FIGURE 6-38. Stevens-Johnson syndrome. Same patient showing the skin eruption, which consisted of erythematous papules and some blisters that resulted in minimal denudation (less than 20% of body surface area).

Toxic Epidermal Necrolysis (TEN)

DEFINITION

1. TEN is a severe life-threatening form of adverse drug reaction involving the skin and mucous membranes.
2. It is considered by some to be a severe form of Stevens-Johnson syndrome, with blistering involving more than 30% of the body surface area.

EPIDEMIOLOGY

1. Exact incidence is unknown.
2. It is more common in adults than in children.
3. The incidence is increased in individuals infected with human immunodeficiency virus (HIV).

PATHOGENESIS

1. Exact pathogenesis is unknown.
2. Hypotheses include:
   a. Accumulation of toxic metabolites
   b. Slow acetylators in patients with sulfonamide toxicity
   c. Epoxide hydrolase deficiency in patients with anticonvulsant toxicity

---

BOX 6-11	*Etiology of Toxic Epidermal Necrolysis*

DRUGS
Anticonvulsants
  Barbiturates
  Diphenylhydantoin
  Carbamazepine
  Lamotrigene
Nonsteroidal anti-inflammatory agents
  Ibuprofen
Antibiotic
  Sulfonamides: cotrimoxazole

LABORATORY

1. Serum electrolytes
2. Cultures of the skin and mucosae
3. Hematoxylin and eosin staining of a frozen sample of exfoliating skin shows a full-thickness epidermis.

COMPLICATIONS

1. Blindness
2. Contractures

3. Esophageal strictures
4. Severe scarring of the skin

DIFFERENTIAL DIAGNOSIS

1. Severe burn
2. Staphylococcal scalded skin syndrome (SSSS) (see p. 95)
   a. In SSSS the split occurs in the superficial upper layer of the epidermis.
   b. In TEN it includes the full thickness of the epidermis.

TREATMENT

1. Hospitalization in a burn unit or intensive care unit (ICU); ophthalmology and dermatology consultations
2. Discontinue the offending drug.
3. Optimize fluids, electrolytes, and nutrition.
4. Monitor for infection (cultures of skin and mucosae).
5. Maintain meticulous skin care
   a. Wash skin with normal saline.
   b. Remove loose skin and blisters.
   c. Apply petrolatum to provide barrier for skin.
   d. Do not use silver sulfadiazine.
6. Use of systemic corticosteroids is controversial.

PROGNOSIS

Mortality rate is 30%.

KEY POINTS

Toxic Epidermal Necrolysis

- TEN shares many features with Stevens-Johnson syndrome.
- The most common offending drugs include anticonvulsants, sulfonamides, and nonsteroidal anti-inflammatory agents.
- The patient is best cared for in a burn unit.

TABLE 6–14
Clinical Features of Toxic Epidermal Necrolysis

Skin Lesions

Necrotic
Dark skin peels off in sheets measuring >3 cm
Bullae and erosions involve >30% of body surface area
Face and upper part of body are more prominently involved
Positive Nikolsky sign
  Not specific for TEN
  Rubbing the adjacent normal skin of a blister enlarges the erosion

Other Features

Mucous membrane involvement
  Exudative stomatitis
  Purulent conjunctivitis
  Vulvovaginitis
Explosive onset with full-blown picture occurring within 24 hours
Severe toxicity with fever and prostration

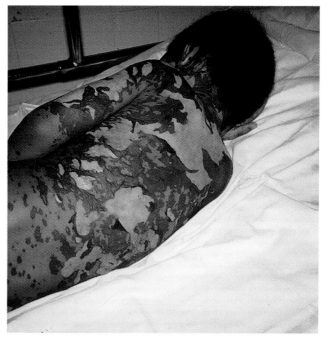

FIGURE 6–39. A 3-year-old boy who developed TEN a week after taking phenobarbital for a febrile seizure. Seventy percent of the body surface area was involved. Dark necrotic skin peeled off, leaving a raw dermis.

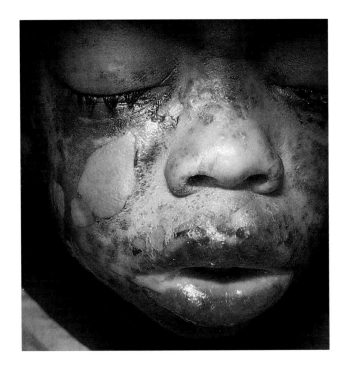

FIGURE 6–40. Severe involvement of the eyes and mouth in TEN.

Pyogenic Granuloma

DEFINITION

A reactive, noninfectious, vascular growth

PATHOGENESIS

1. Most probably occurs after minor occult trauma to the skin
2. May also be seen on port wine stains
3. May occur as a complication of oral retinoids

BOX 6–12	*Differential Diagnosis of Pyogenic Granuloma*

Small hemangioma
Spitz nevus in an African-American child
Pilomatricoma
Kaposi sarcoma (rare in children)
Bacillary angiomatosis in HIV infection (rare in children)

LABORATORY

A skin excision biopsy may be performed if the clinical diagnosis is uncertain.

TREATMENT

1. Refer the patient to a dermatologist.
2. Cryotherapy: freezing with liquid nitrogen
3. Shave excision and electrodesiccation of the base
4. Pulse dye laser excision

KEY POINTS

Pyogenic Granuloma

- Pyogenic granuloma is not pyogenic.
- The lesion is friable and tends to bleed.

TABLE 6–15
Clinical Features of Pyogenic Granuloma

Skin Lesions

Red
Soft
Friable
Exophytic mass
Average size 5–20 mm
More common on face, extremities, and upper part of body
Lesion tends to bleed on minor trauma
May be accompanied by satellite lesions

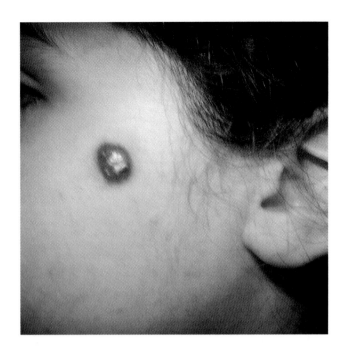

FIGURE 6–41. Pyogenic granuloma of 8 months' duration on the face.

Henoch-Schönlein Purpura (HSP)

SYNONYM   Anaphylactoid Purpura

DEFINITION

A hypersensitivity disorder characterized by cutaneous and systemic manifestations

ETIOLOGY

HSP may be precipitated by

1. Bacterial infection (group A beta-hemolytic streptococci)
2. Viral infection (human parvovirus B19)
3. Drugs (e.g., aminosalicylic acid, captopril, ciprofloxacin)
4. Insect bites (bee stings)
5. Unknown allergens

EPIDEMIOLOGY

1. More common in children between 5 and 15 years of age.
2. Rare in infants
3. Male-to-female ratio is 1.5:1.
4. Uncommon in African-American children

BOX 6–13   *Differential Diagnosis of Henoch-Schönlein Purpura*

Rocky Mountain spotted fever
Drug eruption
Enteroviral exanthem
Erythema multiforme
Meningococcemia
Gonococcemia
Child abuse
Acute glomerulonephritis

BOX 6–14   *Henoch-Schönlein Purpura in Infancy*

Atypical presentation
  Lesions may be urticarial
  Angioedema
    Scalp
    Periorbital regions
    Hands and feet
    Chest wall
Acute hemorrhagic edema (Finkelstein's disease)
  Variant of HSP in young infants
  No systemic involvement
  Lesions are big, cockade (medallionlike), erythematous, edematous, and acrally distributed

---

PATHOGENESIS

1. Circulating IgA macromolecules or immunocomplexes are deposited in the skin and affected organs, activating the alternate pathway of the complement system and leading to formation of the membrane attack complex of complement and chemotactic factors.
2. This results in an inflammatory reaction and leukocytoclastic vasculitis with depletion of factor XIII, which leads to further bleeding and fibrin deposition.

LABORATORY

1. Complete blood count is normal; there is no thrombocytopenia.
2. Urinalysis
3. Skin biopsy may be done in doubtful cases. The findings are those of leukocytoclastic vasculitis: capillary endothelial swelling, fibrin deposits, and perivascular neutrophilic fragments ("nuclear dusts").
4. On direct immunofluorescence of the skin lesion, IgA deposits on the capillary walls are seen. These are best seen in lesions less than 48 hours old.

TREATMENT

1. Bed rest
2. There is no specific treatment.
3. Nonsteroidal anti-inflammatory drugs are given for symptomatic relief of arthritis, edema, or fever.
4. Systemic corticosteroids
   a. May be used in children with severe gastrointestinal, renal, or CNS complications.
   b. Prednisone therapy (dose: 1 to 2 mg/kg/day) may produce dramatic improvement

PROGNOSIS

1. Majority of cases are self-limiting, and symptoms resolve in a few weeks.
2. Long-term morbidity and mortality is attributed almost exclusively to renal disease. Serial urinalyses and follow-up surveillance of renal function are recommended if the initial tests show any abnormality.

KEY POINTS

Henoch-Schönlein Purpura

- The skin lesions are characteristic palpable purpura in dependent parts of the body.
- In young infants, the lesions may consist of urticaria and angioedema.
- Gastrointestinal, joint, and renal symptoms may be present in varying degrees.
- Intussusception in children past infancy must raise the possibility of HSP (see p. 338).

TABLE 6–16
Clinical Features of Henoch-Schönlein Purpura

Typical Skin Lesions

Palpable purpura
Distribution
  From buttocks down the lower extremities
  Upper extremities may be involved
  Torso usually spared
  Brownish pigmentation may result from hemosiderin deposits
    on skin

Other Features

Preceding upper respiratory symptoms
Gastrointestinal symptoms (75% of cases)
  Colicky abdominal pain
  Vomiting
  Gross or occult blood in stool (>50% of cases)
  Hematemesis
Joint symptoms (60% of cases)
  Arthritis or arthralgia
  Most commonly involved joints: knees, ankles, other large
    joints
Renal involvement (25% to 50% of cases)
  Microscopic or macroscopic hematuria
  Proteinuria
Hypertension

TABLE 6–17
Complications of Henoch-Schönlein Purpura

Gastrointestinal
  Bowel obstruction or perforation
  Intussusception (vasculitis of bowel wall, necrosis;
    see p. 338)
Renal
  Nephrotic syndrome
  Azotemia, oliguria
  Hypertensive encephalopathy
  Chronic glomerulonephritis (5% of cases)
Pulmonary hemorrhage
Central nervous system
  Seizures
  Coma
  Paresis
Testicular torsion

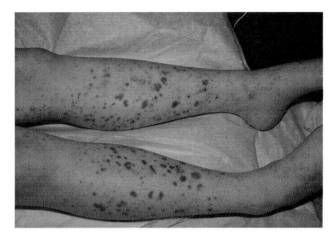

FIGURE 6-42. Skin lesions of Henoch-Schönlein purpura in its typical distribution—on the lower extremities.

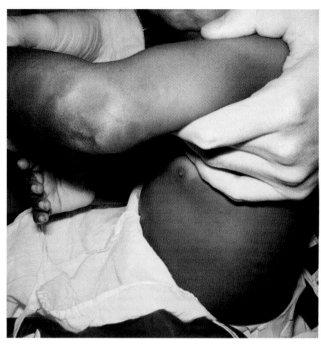

FIGURE 6-44. A young infant with Henoch-Schönlein purpura showing urticarial lesions on the upper extremities.

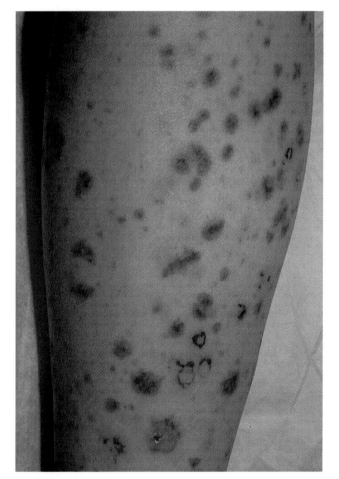

FIGURE 6-43. Close-up of patient in Figure 6-42 showing raised palpable purpura.

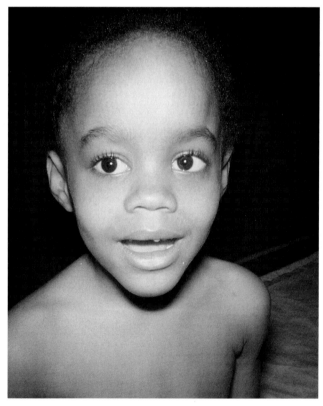

FIGURE 6-45. Same patient showing edema of the scalp and forehead.

Seborrheic Dermatitis

SYNONYMS   Cradle Cap
Dandruff

DEFINITION

A disorder of unknown etiology that is seen in the extreme edges of the pediatric age group.

ETIOLOGY

1. Unknown
2. *Pityrosporum orbiculare* has been implicated.

EPIDEMIOLOGY

1. More commonly seen in very young infants and adolescents
2. It is the most common rash in the first month of life.

PATHOGENESIS

1. It is believed that increased activity of the sebaceous glands occurs in individuals with seborrheic dermatitis.
2. There is increased epidermal cell turnover.

CLINICAL FEATURES

1. Onset usually occurs at age 2 to 6 weeks.
2. The lesions consist of greasy scales with erythema of the scalp.
3. The other areas involved are the eyebrows, central oval of the face, ears, neck, postauricular fold, and intertriginous areas, where the lesions appear as scaly papules.
4. In adolescents, seborrheic dermatitis appears as fine diffuse scales (dandruff) and scaly papules on the central oval of the face.
5. It may be severe in patients with HIV infection and in those with Leiner disease (complement 5 dysfunction).

BOX 6–15   *Differential Diagnosis of Seborrheic Dermatitis*

Atopic dermatitis
    Onset occurs after 6 weeks of age
    Lesions are dry
    Family history of atopy is present
Histiocytosis X
    Purpuric lesions are present
    Intertrigo is deep and erosive
    Hepatosplenomegaly
    Child does not look well
Psoriasis
    Lesions are well-circumscribed plaques with thick white scales
    Distributed over the extensors of the extremities

COMPLICATION

Secondary monilial infection

TREATMENT

1. Keratolytic shampoo
2. Warm mineral oil compresses over the scalp
3. Topical low to midpotency corticosteroid solution applied to the scalp, or cream applied to nonhairy areas
4. In severe cases, fluocinolone acetonide 0.01% topical oil may be prescribed.
5. Ketoconazole shampoo and cream can be used in adolescents.

KEY POINTS

Seborrheic Dermatitis

- Seborrheic dermatitis is the most common rash seen in the first month of life.
- The lesions consist of greasy scales and papules on the scalp and face.

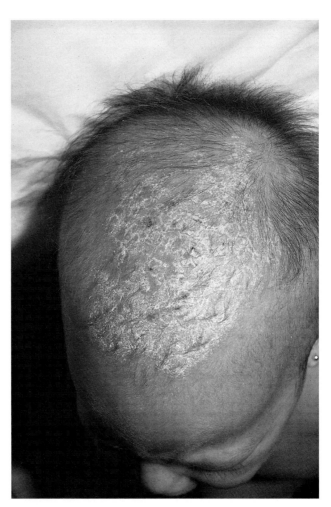

FIGURE 6–46. Scalp of a 2-week-old newborn with scaly lesions of seborrheic dermatitis.

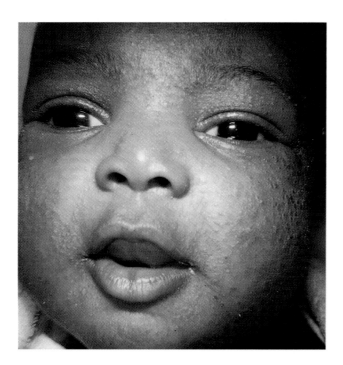

FIGURE 6–47. Seborrheic dermatitis. Greasy papular eruption on the face of a 3-week-old infant; scales could be scraped from the eyebrows. The ears were similarly involved.

Pityriasis Rosea

DEFINITION

A benign, self-limiting eruption with a distinct presentation

ETIOLOGY

1. Exact etiology is still unknown.
2. Cause is presumed to be viral, but no single virus has been consistently isolated.

EPIDEMIOLOGY

1. Pityriasis rosea is more commonly seen in spring and fall.
2. It is more common in children, adolescents, and young adults.
3. Rare in infants

PATHOGENESIS

Unknown

CLINICAL FEATURES

1. Herald patch
   a. Seen in 80% of patients
   b. Solitary, 2- to 6-cm round, erythematous scaly plaque
   c. May be seen anywhere on the skin surface
   d. Precedes the rest of the eruption by 5 to 10 days
   e. Commonly mistaken for tinea
2. The lesions are
   a. Multiple oval, pink, scaly papules 1 to 2 cm in size
   b. Distributed mostly on the trunk and upper arms but may also involve the face.
   c. The long axes of the lesions are parallel to the skin cleavage lines, resulting in a Christmas tree pattern.
   d. New eruption continues for 2 weeks.
   e. Eruption lasts 6 to 12 weeks.
3. There are varying degrees of pruritus.
4. There are less common atypical clinical variants
   a. Papular pityriasis rosea in African-American children
   b. Intensely irritated or inflamed edematous lesions
   c. Lesions limited to the buttocks and groin

BOX 6–16 | *Differential Diagnosis of Pityriasis Rosea*

Syphilis
Mucha-Habermann disease
Guttate psoriasis
"Id" reaction of fungal infection
Drug eruption
Herald patch may be mistaken for tinea corporis

LABORATORY

Serologic tests for syphilis must be performed in sexually active individuals because the rash of secondary syphilis may look identical to that of pityriasis rosea.

TREATMENT

1. Most patients do not need treatment.
2. Parents must be reassured and informed about the total duration of the eruption.
3. Symptomatic relief from pruritus may be obtained from
   a. Colloidal oatmeal baths
   b. A combination of pramoxine and hydrocortisone lotion, 1% or 2%
4. Severe extensive cases may benefit from short-term ultraviolet B phototherapy.

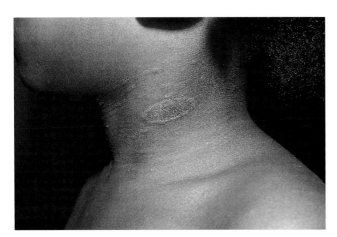

FIGURE 6–48. Herald patch on the neck.

KEY POINTS

Pityriasis Rosea

- Pityriasis rosea is self-limiting. The eruption may last 6 to 12 weeks.
- A herald patch is seen in 80% of cases. Its absence does not preclude a diagnosis of pityriasis rosea.

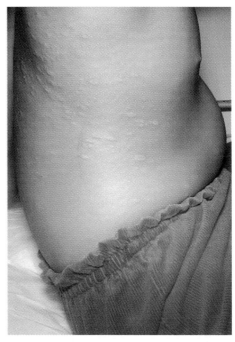

FIGURE 6–49. Oval papulosquamous lesions of pityriasis rosea follow the skin lines of cleavage. Most eruptions are truncal in distribution.

Lichen Striatus

DEFINITION

A self-limiting eruption, seen mostly in children, characterized by a unilateral linear distribution of lichenoid papules, usually over an extremity

ETIOLOGY

Unknown

EPIDEMIOLOGY

1. Uncommon
2. Seen predominantly in children between 5 and 10 years of age

LABORATORY

None

TREATMENT

Low-potency topical steroid may be tried for 2 to 3 weeks.

BOX 6–17 *Differential Diagnosis of Lichen Striatus*

Epidermal nevus
Contact dermatitis
Linear lichen planus
Linear psoriasis

PROGNOSIS

The lesion resolves after several months.

KEY POINT

Lichen Striatus

- Lichen striatus is a benign self-limiting, linear papular lesion commonly seen on the extremity of a child.

TABLE 6–18
Clinical Features of Lichen Striatus

Sudden onset
Closely set, small, discrete, lichenoid papules
Pink or flesh-colored
Lesions may be hypopigmented compared with adjacent skin, especially in African-Americans
A unilateral linear band is formed
Most common site: an extremity
Pruritus: mild to absent
Nail changes: when the lesion encroaches on a proximal nail fold

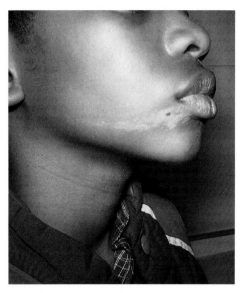

FIGURE 6–51. Lichen striatus on the side of the face.

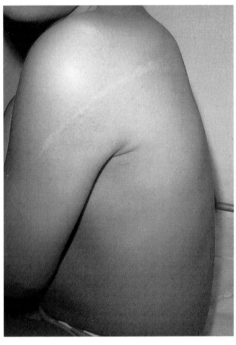

FIGURE 6–50. Lichen striatus on the shoulder that traveled down the arm.

Psoriasis

DEFINITION

A chronic skin disorder characterized by epidermal proliferation

ETIOLOGY

The exact cause is not known.

EPIDEMIOLOGY

1. It is more common in adults than in children.
2. A positive family history is found in 30% of patients.
3. Onset in children may occur as early as the first months of life.

PATHOGENESIS

1. The exact pathogenesis is unclear.
2. There is a rapid epidermal cell turnover. Whereas normally it takes 28 days for an epidermal cell (keratinocyte) to travel from the basal layer to the surface of the skin, in persons with psoriasis, this journey takes 3 to 4 days.

LABORATORY

1. Throat culture, perianal culture to rule out streptococcal infection
2. In cases in which the diagnosis is in doubt, skin biopsy

COMPLICATIONS

1. Generalized exfoliative dermatitis (erythroderma)
2. Psoriatic arthritis

Nummular eczema
Tinea corporis
Tinea capitis
Seborrheic dermatitis
Pityriasis rosea
Lichen planus

TREATMENT

1. Refer the patient to a dermatologist.
2. Medium to high potency topical corticosteroid
3. Tar bath and tar shampoo
4. Keratolytic agents such as salicylic acid in petrolatum may be applied topically.
5. If a streptococcal infection is present, a course of penicillin or erythromycin may be helpful.
6. If flares are precipitated by recurrent streptococcal infections, tonsillectomy or monthly injections of benzathine penicillin may be necessary.
7. Calcipotriene, a vitamin D analogue in a cream or ointment and scalp solution, may be tried.
8. Topical retinoid: tazarotene
9. A combination of all of the above.
10. In severe cases:
    a. Ultraviolet B phototherapy
    b. Oral acitretin
    c. PUVA (psoralen + UVA phototherapy)

PROGNOSIS

A chronic disease with relapses and remissions.

KEY POINTS

Psoriasis

- Guttate psoriasis is commonly precipitated by streptococcal infections in children.
- Treatment in children consists of topical agents in most instances. Systemic treatment is reserved for severe recalcitrant disease.

TABLE 6–19
Clinical Features of Psoriasis

Skin Lesions

Erythematous plaques
Location
  Symmetrically distributed on extensors of extremities
  Scalp
  Perianal area
  Umbilical region
  May be generalized
Pruritus in varying degrees
Thick silvery scales cover the plaques
Auspitz sign: Removal of scales reveals pinpoint bleeding sites

Other Features

Nail changes
  Pitting
  Oil spot sign—yellow-brown discoloration
  Subungual hyperkeratosis
Psoriatic arthritis
  More common in adults
  May precede cutaneous lesions

TABLE 6–20
Clinical Variants of Psoriasis

Guttate Psoriasis

More common in children
Acute onset
Small drop-like scaly plaques
Location: trunk and extremities
History of a preceding group A beta-hemolytic streptococcal
  infection may be elicited

Napkin Psoriasis

Presents in young infants
Very well circumscribed erythematous plaque
Scaling is minimal because of constant wetness of the area
Location: groin

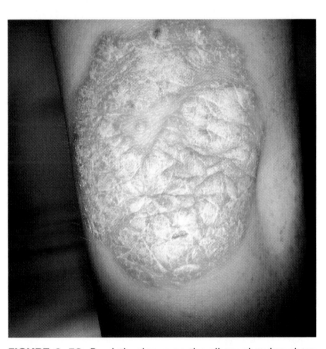

FIGURE 6–52. Psoriatic plaque on the elbow showing sharp demarcation, erythema, and thick silvery scales.

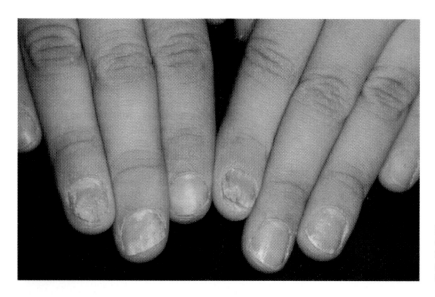

FIGURE 6–53. Psoriasis of the nail with dystrophy, discoloration, and crumbling of the nail plate. (From Hurwitz S: Clinical Pediatric Dermatology, 2nd ed. Philadelphia, WB Saunders, 1993.)

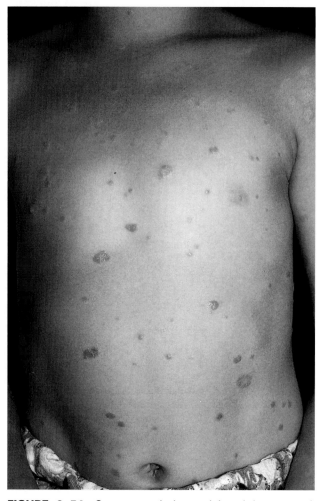

FIGURE 6–54. Guttate psoriasis precipitated by group A beta-hemolytic streptococcal pharyngitis. The lesions are small, scaly, and drop-like in shape.

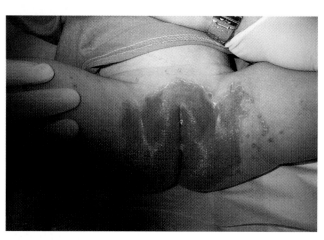

FIGURE 6–55. Napkin psoriasis.

Acne

SYNONYM   Acne Vulgaris

DEFINITION

Acne is a common multifactorial disorder of the pilosebaceous unit that begins during puberty.

ETIOLOGY

This is a result of increased levels of androgen.

EPIDEMIOLOGY

1. Acne is most common during the adolescent years.
2. Severe acne is more common in boys.

PATHOGENESIS

Four factors involved in the production of acne are:

1. Increased sebum production
2. Abnormal keratinization of the follicular epithelium
3. Proliferation of bacteria, the *Propionibacterium acnes*
4. Inflammation

BOX 6-19   *Differential Diagnosis of Acne*

Keratosis pilaris rubra faciei
Adenoma sebaceum
Milia
Staphylococcal pustulosis
Acneiform drug eruption
Follicular mucinosis

LABORATORY

Acne in prepubertal children requires the following work-up to rule out tumor or hyperplasia of the adrenal cortex and polycystic ovary:

1. Serum level of dehydroepiandrosterone (DHEAS)
2. Total and free plasma testosterone

3. Luteinizing hormone–follicular-stimulating hormone (LH-FSH) ratio
4. Pelvic sonogram

COMPLICATIONS

1. Severe untreated acne may result in scarring.
2. The adolescent with significant acne may become socially inhibited.

TREATMENT

1. Refer patients with moderately severe and severe acne to a dermatologist.
2. Tretinoin cream or gel 0.025%, 0.05%, or 0.1%; tretinoin gel microsphere 0.1%
3. Topical antibiotics (solution, lotion, gel, pledgets)
   a. Erythromycin
   b. Clindamycin
4. Benzoyl peroxide 5% or 10% cream or gel
5. Azelaic acid 20% cream
6. Adapalene gel 0.1%
7. The best treatment is a combination of the above topical agents, one used in the morning and the other at night.
8. Systemic antibiotics in the presence of many inflammatory lesions
   a. Tetracycline 250 to 500 mg twice daily
   b. Minocycline 50 to 100 mg twice daily
9. Oral antibiotics are given at a full dose for 1 month and then tapered accordingly.
10. Isotretinoin
    a. Indicated for severe and nodulocystic acne
    b. This is prescribed by a dermatologist, taking the necessary precautions, especially in female patients. It is teratogenic.

KEY POINTS

Acne

- Acne is the most common skin problem among adolescents.
- The lesions consist of comedones, papules, pustules, and, in severe cases, nodules and cysts.
- Combination topical therapy is the most effective form of treatment.

TABLE 6–21
Clinical Features of Acne

Primary noninflammatory lesions: comedones
  Open comedones (blackheads)
  Closed comedones (whiteheads)
Inflammatory lesions: inflamed papules and pustules
In a given patient: usually a combination of above
Most commonly involved areas
  Face
  Chest
  Shoulders
Nodulocystic acne
  Severe form, with nodules and cysts
  More common in males

TABLE 6–22
Other Variants of Acne

Acne Neonatorum/Infantile Acne

Self-limiting
Due to increased androgen
May be so severe that it leaves behind some scars (pits)
Such severe acne must be treated with topical agents
Congenital adrenal hyperplasia must be ruled out in severe
    infantile acne.

Pomade Acne

Lesions are exclusively distributed over forehead
Follows use of greasy grooming substances on scalp
May be aggravated by hair on the forehead ("bangs")

Steroid Acne

Complication of chronic use of corticosteroids (either systemic
    or high-potency topical agents)
Lesions are monomorphic
More common in adolescents

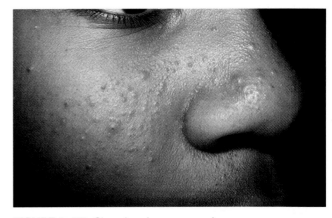

FIGURE 6–57. Closed and open comedones.

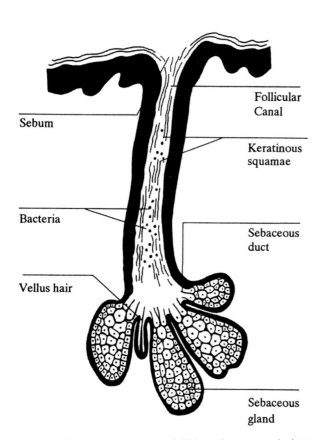

FIGURE 6–56. A sebaceous follicle, where acne lesions evolve.

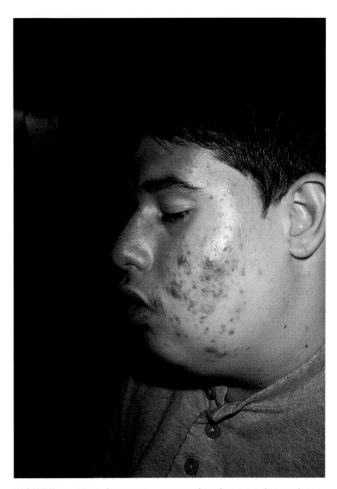

FIGURE 6–58. Inflammatory acne showing papules and pustules.

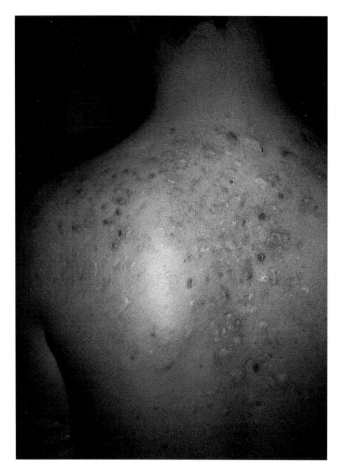

FIGURE 6-59. Nodulocystic acne on the back.

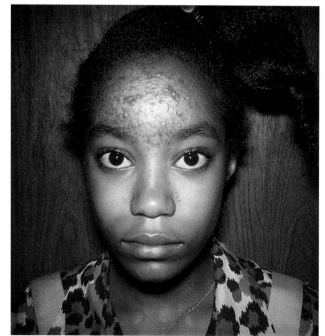

FIGURE 6-61. Pomade acne.

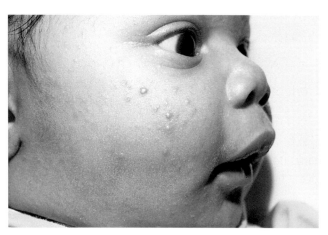

FIGURE 6-60. Acne neonatorum.

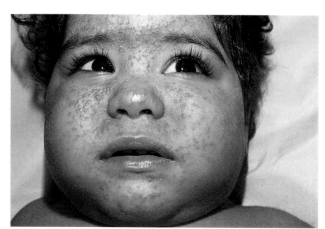

FIGURE 6-62. Steroid acne in an infant in whom infantile myoclonic seizures were treated with ACTH and prednisone. He had a Cushingoid appearance.

Infantile Acropustulosis

DEFINITION
A relatively uncommon, noninfectious, self-limiting disorder

ETIOLOGY
1. The exact cause is unknown.
2. A few patients have a preceding history of scabies.

EPIDEMIOLOGY
It is more common in African-American male infants.

PATHOGENESIS
Unknown

BOX 6-20	*Differential Diagnosis of Infantile Acropustulosis*
Scabies	
Dyshidrotic eczema	
Transient neonatal pustular melanosis	

LABORATORY
A skin biopsy, if performed, shows an intraepidermal collection of neutrophils.

COMPLICATIONS
Secondary infection may occur.

TREATMENT
1. Topical corticosteroids may be used during relapses.
2. Oral antihistamines may be used to alleviate the pruritus.

KEY POINTS

Infantile Acropustulosis

- The eruption consists of recurrent crops of tiny pruritic papules, vesicles, and pustules.
- It is a self-limiting disorder that is resolved by the age of 3 years.

TABLE 6-23
Clinical Features of Infantile Acropustulosis

Skin Eruption

Crops of tiny, pruritic papules, vesicles, and pustules
Distributed on the hands and feet (acral distribution); very rarely, there may be lesions on the scalp
Natural course
  Onset within first 3 months of life
  Lesions last 7–10 days, then resolve and recur 4–6 weeks later
  Intervals between episodes become longer
  Completely resolved by 3 years of age

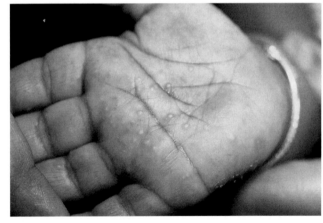

FIGURE 6-64. Infantile acropustulosis: tiny vesicles and pustules on the palm.

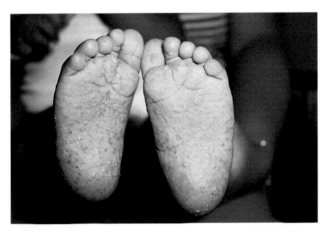

FIGURE 6-63. Infantile acropustulosis: tiny vesicles and pustules on the soles.

Granuloma Annulare

DEFINITION

A common self-limiting inflammatory disorder of unknown origin characterized by papules and nodules arranged in an annular configuration; histopathologically it is characterized by palisading granulomas.

ETIOLOGY

1. The exact cause is unknown.
2. It may be a reaction to trauma such as insect bites or sun exposure.
3. There is a purported association with diabetes mellitus in patients with extensive lesions of granuloma annulare.

EPIDEMIOLOGY

It is more common in children than in adults.

PATHOGENESIS

Unknown

CLINICAL FEATURES

There are four clinical variants:

1. Dermal granuloma annulare
   a. This is the most common form.
   b. The lesions may be solitary or multiple.
   c. They consist of asymptomatic, slightly erythematous or flesh-colored papules or nodules arranged in an annular configuration and measuring 1 to 5 cm.
   d. There is no surface change (e.g., scales).
   e. The lesions are commonly distributed on the distal extremities such as the dorsa of the feet and hands.
2. Subcutaneous granuloma annulare
   a. Seen exclusively in children
   b. The lesions are asymptomatic hard nodules.
   c. The most common distribution involves the extensor areas (e.g., the shins).
   d. May exist alone or in combination with classic dermal granuloma annulare
   e. It used to be referred to as pseudorheumatoid nodules.

BOX 6–21	*Differential Diagnosis of Granuloma Annulare*

Tinea corporis
Sarcoidosis
Figurate erythemas
Erythema multiforme
Lichen planus
Cutaneous larva migrans

3. Papular granuloma annulare
   a. The lesions consist of widespread 1- to 2-mm, flesh-colored papules.
   b. Commonly involve the trunk
4. Perforating granuloma annulare
   a. A rare variant
   b. The lesions are skin-colored crusted papules found on the distal part of the extremities.

LABORATORY

1. In severe cases, a glucose tolerance test may be performed.
2. Skin biopsy, if done, shows palisading granulomas.

TREATMENT

1. No treatment is necessary in the majority of cases.
2. Tapes impregnated with topical corticosteroid (flurandrenolide) can be applied over the lesion for 12 hours daily. Watch for side effect of skin atrophy.

PROGNOSIS

Most lesions of dermal granuloma annulare disappear within 1 to 2 years.

KEY POINTS

Granuloma Annulare

- Granuloma annulare is a benign self-limiting disorder.
- The most common lesions are skin-colored papules or nodules arranged in an annular configuration.
- They are most common over the dorsa of the hands and feet.

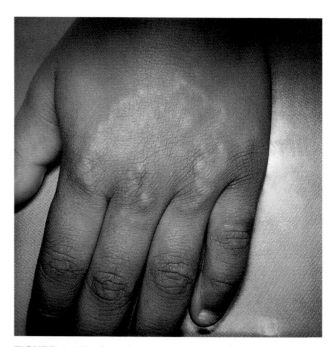

FIGURE 6–65. Granuloma annulare on the dorsum of the hand. The nodules are arranged in an annular configuration.

Perioral Granulomatous Dermatitis in Childhood

SYNONYMS   Gianotti-type Perioral Dermatitis
Rosacealike Eruption of Children
FACE (Facial Afro-Caribbean
Childhood Eruption)

DEFINITION

A distinctive granulomatous process of unknown cause with a benign course and no associated systemic manifestations.

ETIOLOGY

Unknown

EPIDEMIOLOGY

1. Uncommon but not rare
2. Median age: prepubertal (range: 7 months to 13 years)
3. Equal male-to-female ratio
4. Equal African-American–white ratio

PATHOGENESIS

It is thought that use of a topical fluorinated steroid on the face for a banal rash causes the rash to become worse, so more is used, resulting in perioral dermatitis; a rebound phenomenon then occurs when the topical steroid is discontinued.

BOX 6–22	*Differential Diagnosis of Perioral Granulomatous Dermatitis*

Contact dermatitis
Sarcoidosis
Lupus miliaris disseminatus faciei
Benign cephalic histiocytosis
Granulosis rubra nasi

TABLE 6–24
Clinical Features of Perioral Granulomatous Dermatitis

Skin Lesions

Dense, slightly scaly, 1- to 3-mm infiltrated papules or
    micronodules
Flesh colored to erythematous
Rarely, some pustules
Lesions closely spaced and may become confluent
Distribution
    Periorificial—perioral, perinasal, periorbital (especially on
        lower eyelid)
    Other areas (rare)—preauricular, neck, upper chest and back,
        perivulvar

Other Features

Pruritus variable
No systemic symptoms

LABORATORY

Skin biopsy is helpful in distinguishing this entity from other causes of perioral dermatitis. Findings: Sarcoidal granulomas in the dermis arranged in a perifollicular and interfollicular distribution.

COMPLICATION

Pitted scars

TREATMENT

1. Metronidazole cream or gel twice daily for 1 month, then once daily until skin is completely clear.
2. The following may be used as an adjunctive treatment:
    a. Oral tetracycline (for children >8 years): Dose: 250 to 500 mg/day
    b. Oral erythromycin (for children <8 years): Dose: 30 to 40 mg/kg/day in divided doses
    c. Class 6 or 7 topical steroid (desonide, hydrocortisone)

PROGNOSIS

Waxes and wanes for weeks and months

KEY POINTS

Perioral Granulomatous Dermatitis in Childhood

- Periorificial distribution of infiltrated papules and micronodules
- Probably represents a juvenile form of rosacea

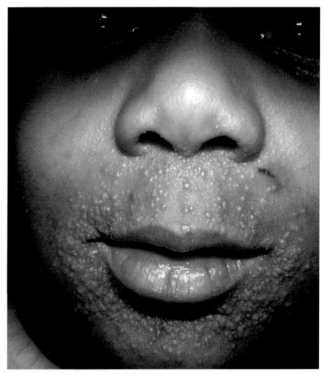

FIGURE 6–66. Perioral granulomatous dermatitis in a 3-year-old boy. Dense infiltrated papules are seen in a perioral and periorbital distribution.

Granuloma Gluteale Infantum

SYNONYMS   Kaposi Sarcomalike Granuloma
Granuloma Intertriginosum
Infantum

DEFINITION

A benign disorder of infants characterized by granulomatous reddish-blue nodules in the diaper area

ETIOLOGY

1. Unknown
2. The following have been suggested as possible causes:
   a. Use of fluorinated steroids
   b. Moniliasis
   c. Starch powder

BOX 6-23	*Differential Diagnosis of Granuloma Gluteale Infantum*
Lymphoma Sarcoma Hemangioma Nodules of scabies	

EPIDEMIOLOGY

Seen in infants who wear diapers

PATHOGENESIS

1. Unknown
2. May be a cutaneous response to local inflammation or maceration.

LABORATORY

Biopsy shows epidermal hyperplasia and a dense mixed inflammatory infiltrate in the dermis with hemorrhage and new capillary formations.

TREATMENT

Treat the underlying diaper dermatitis.

1. Frequent diaper changes
2. Nystatin cream for candidiasis

PROGNOSIS

Resolves spontaneously in several weeks or months

KEY POINTS

Granuloma Gluteale Infantum

- Granuloma gluteale infantum may look like lymphoma or sarcoma in the diaper area.
- It is a benign self-limiting condition.

TABLE 6-25
Clinical Features of Granuloma Gluteale Infantum

Skin Lesions
Reddish-purple granulomatous nodules
Lesions measure 0.5–4.0 cm
Distribution
Groin
Upper thigh
Inguinal area
Suprapubic area
Buttocks

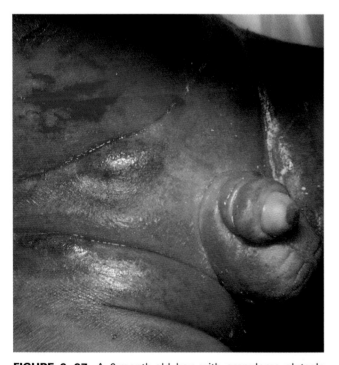

FIGURE 6-67. A 6-month-old boy with granuloma gluteale infantum.

Lichen Sclerosus et Atrophicus (LSA)

DEFINITION

A benign condition characterized by white lesions in the genitalia

ETIOLOGY

1. The cause is unknown.
2. *Borrelia burgdorferi* infection has been implicated in the past, but this theory is of limited value.

EPIDEMIOLOGY

1. It is less common in children than in adults.
2. Female-to-male ratio 9:1

PATHOGENESIS

Unknown

CLINICAL FEATURES

See Table 6–26

BOX 6–24	*Differential Diagnosis of Lichen Sclerosus et Atrophicus*

Vitiligo in the anogenital area (vitiligo has no signs of atrophy)
May be mistaken for sexual abuse

LABORATORY

Biopsy, if performed, shows:

1. Thinning of the epidermis
2. Edema of the dermis
3. Fibrosis of the collagen
4. Presence of inflammatory infiltrates
5. Follicular plugging

TREATMENT

A high-potency topical steroid cream applied twice daily for 3 to 4 months has been reported to result in significant improvement.

PROGNOSIS

The disorder is self-limiting and usually resolves with the onset of menarche.

KEY POINTS

Lichen Sclerosus et Atrophicus

- In girls, the lesions are atrophic depigmented plaques in the anogenital area in the shape of an hourglass.
- In boys, phimosis with an atrophic depigmented plaque at the tip of the penis is the most common presentation.

TABLE 6–26
Clinical Features of Lichen Sclerosus et Atrophicus

In girls
  Ivory-colored papules become confluent
  Form a porcelain-white plaque around the anus and vulva
  Anogenital lesions have a figure-of-8 or hourglass configuration
  Patient may have complaints of pruritus, burning, or constipation
In boys
  Phimosis is a common presentation
  Called balanitis xerotica obliterans
Extragenital lesions
  May be seen in 42% of cases
  Appear as atrophic depigmented patches with characteristic cigarette paperlike wrinkling of the surface

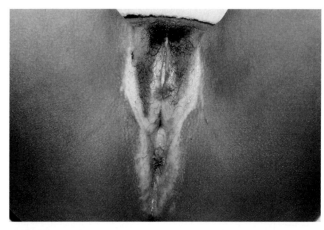

FIGURE 6–68. Lichen sclerosus et atrophicus in a girl showing the hourglass-shaped porcelain white atrophy in the anogenital area.

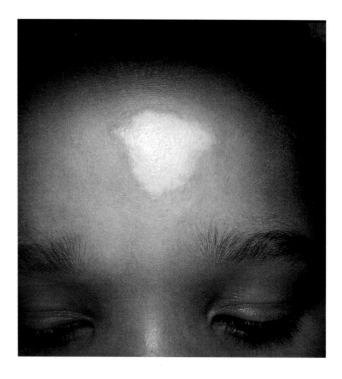

FIGURE 6–69. Lichen sclerosus et atrophicus on the forehead.

Linear IgA Disease of Childhood

SYNONYM   Benign Chronic Bullous
           Dermatosis of Childhood

DEFINITION

A rare nonhereditary blistering disorder characterized by distinctly grouped bullae

ETIOLOGY

1. The cause is unknown.
2. It is believed to be an autoimmune disorder.

EPIDEMIOLOGY

1. It is the most common of all nonhereditary bullous disorders of childhood.
2. Most cases begin in the first 3 years of life.

PATHOGENESIS

Unknown

LABORATORY

The clinical diagnosis must be confirmed by three laboratory tests:

1. A skin biopsy that shows a subepidermal blister
2. Direct immunofluorescence of perilesional skin tissue that shows linear IgA deposits in the basement membrane
3. Indirect immunofluorescence that shows circulating IgA anti–basement zone antibodies (seen in 70% of patients)

TREATMENT

1. Refer the patient to a dermatologist.

BOX 6–25	*Differential Diagnosis of Linear IgA Disease of Childhood*

Arthropod bite reaction
Dermatitis herpetiformis
Bullous pemphigoid
Pemphigus vulgaris
Bullous impetigo

2. The disease responds to any of the following systemic drugs:
   a. Dapsone
   b. Sulfapyridine
   c. Corticosteroids
3. These drugs work by their anti-inflammatory action.
4. In most cases, a significant response is seen at a full dose in 2 weeks.
5. The dose may then be tapered accordingly.

PROGNOSIS

Spontaneous complete remission by puberty.

KEY POINTS

Linear IgA Disease of Childhood

- Linear IgA disease is the most common of all nonhereditary blistering disorders.
- The characteristic lesions are oval sausage-shaped bullae and vesicles in a clustered rosette pattern.

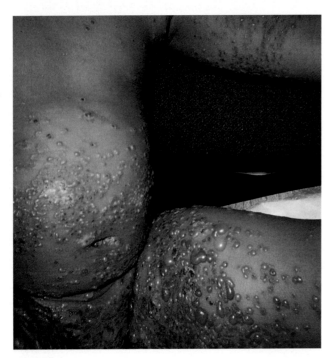

FIGURE 6–70. Linear IgA dermatosis in a 3-year-old child showing numerous tense bullae on the upper thigh, genitalia, abdomen, and arm.

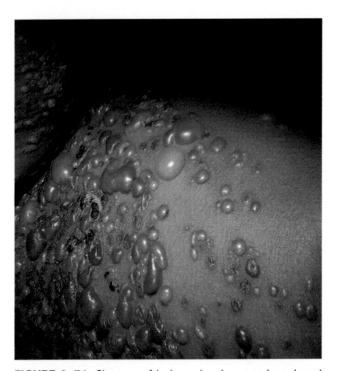

FIGURE 6–71. Close-up of lesions showing round, oval, and sausage-shaped bullae.

TABLE 6–27
Clinical Features of Linear IgA Disease of Childhood

Skin Lesions

Tense vesicles and bullae
Arranged in clusters or rosettes
Some are sausage-shaped
Common distribution
    Legs
    Buttocks
    Upper thighs
    Perineum
    Face
    Upper extremities

Other Features

Pruritus variable
Eruption may be recurrent

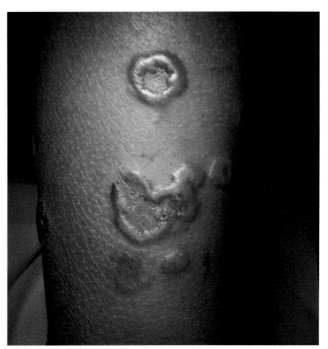

FIGURE 6–72. Sausage-shaped bullae in a ring configuration.

Pemphigus

DEFINITION

A chronic nonhereditary blistering disorder rarely seen in children

ETIOLOGY

1. The cause is unknown.
2. It is presumed to be an autoimmune disease.

EPIDEMIOLOGY

1. Rare in children
2. To date, fewer than 30 cases have been reported in the literature.

PATHOGENESIS

A circulating antiepithelial antibody binds with a pemphigus antigen in the membrane of the keratinocyte, resulting in acantholysis.

LABORATORY

A clinical diagnosis of pemphigus must be confirmed by the following three tests:

BOX 6–26   *Differential Diagnosis of Pemphigus*

Linear IgA disease of childhood
Dermatitis herpetiformis
Bullous pemphigoid
Erythema multiforme major
Herpetic gingivostomatitis
Bullous impetigo

---

1. Skin biopsy
   a. Pemphigus vulgaris: finding—a suprabasal acantholytic blister with eosinophils
   b. Pemphigus foliaceus: finding—a subcorneal blister with eosinophils
2. Direct immunofluorescence that shows intercellular (epidermal) deposits of IgG antibodies
3. Indirect immunofluorescence that demonstrates circulating antiepithelial antibody. Its titer correlates with disease activity.

COMPLICATION

Kaposi varicelliform eruption if patient is exposed to herpes simplex virus.

TREATMENT

1. Refer patient to a dermatologist.
2. Systemic corticosteroids
   a. Prednisone 2 to 4 mg/kg/day depending on severity of the disease
   b. The dose is continued until healing occurs (usually 2 to 5 months after start of therapy).
3. Immunosuppressive agents (e.g., methotrexate, azathioprine, or cyclophosphamide) or gold may be used if there is no response to high-dose corticosteroids.

KEY POINTS

Pemphigus

- The lesions of pemphigus consist of superficial blisters that leave eroded areas.
- The mucous membrane of the mouth is commonly involved.

TABLE 6–28
Clinical Features of Pemphigus

Skin Lesions

Flaccid blisters that leave eroded areas
Lesions localized or generalized
Lesions on mucous membranes (especially mouth) may precede
   skin eruption
Nikolsky sign positive
   Slightly rubbing the edge of a bulla enlarges the lesion
   This sign is *not* specific to pemphigus

Two Clinical Variants of Pemphigus in Children

Pemphigus vulgaris (as described above)
Pemphigus foliaceus (also called superficial pemphigus)
   Presents with diffuse crusting
   Bullae seldom remain intact

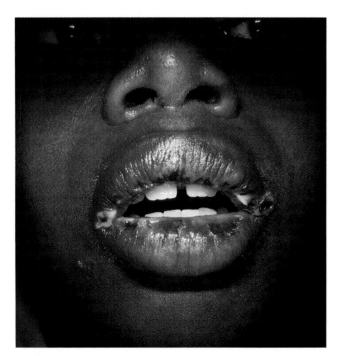

FIGURE 6–73. Pemphigus vulgaris presenting as recurrent oral lesions over 5 months in this 13-year-old boy.

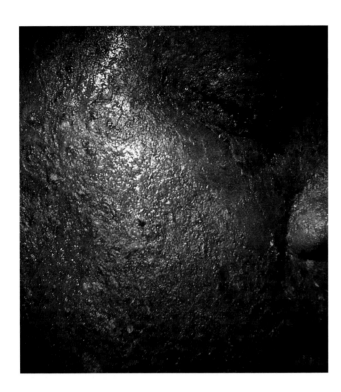

FIGURE 6-74. Pemphigus foliaceus showing crusting on the face of this 16-year-old.

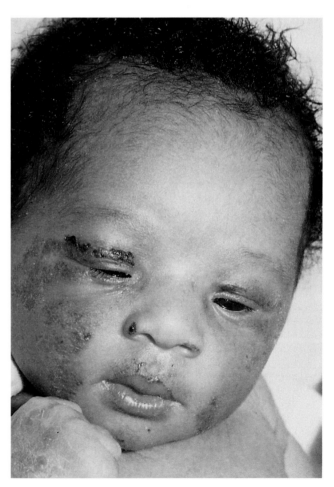

FIGURE 6-75. Neonatal pemphigus foliaceus in the newborn infant of patient shown in Figure 6-74. This benign condition is self-limiting and is caused by transplacentally acquired maternal pemphigus antibodies.

Dermatitis Herpetiformis

SYNONYM   Duhring's Disease

DEFINITION

A nonhereditary blistering disorder

ETIOLOGY

1. The cause is unknown.
2. It is presumed to be an autoimmune disease.

EPIDEMIOLOGY

Rare in children

LABORATORY

1. The clinical diagnosis of dermatitis herpetiformis must be confirmed by three tests:
   a. Skin biopsy, which shows a subepidermal blister with neutrophilic abscesses in the upper papillary dermis
   b. Direct immunofluorescence, which shows granular IgA deposits in the upper papillary dermis
   c. Indirect immunofluorescence, which shows circulating antibodies against reticulin, endomysium, and gliadin in some patients
2. Intestinal biopsy, if performed, demonstrates flattened intestinal villi in patients with associated gluten-sensitive enteropathy.

TREATMENT

1. Refer the patient to a dermatologist.
2. A course of dapsone or sulfapyridine
   a. The exact mechanism of action is unknown.
   b. Presumably they act because they are anti-inflammatory agents.
3. Gluten-free diet

KEY POINTS

Dermatitis Herpetiformis

- The skin lesions are pruritic papules end vesicles located symmetrically over the extensors of the extremities, shoulders, and buttocks.
- Dermatitis herpetiformis may be associated with a sprue-like enteropathy.

BOX 6-27 *Diagnosis of Dermatitis Herpetiformis*

Linear IgA disease of childhood
Vesicobullous lupus erythematosus
Herpes simplex virus infection
Widespread impetigo
Scabies

TABLE 6-29
Clinical Features of Dermatitis Herpetiformis

Skin Lesions

Minute
Pruritic
Papules and vesicles
Symmetrically distributed
    Knees
    Elbows (extensors)
    Buttocks
    Shoulders

Natural Course

Eruption is recurrent

Other Features

Mild intermittent diarrhea (in minority of cases)
Associated gluten-sensitive enteropathy (60% to 80% of cases)

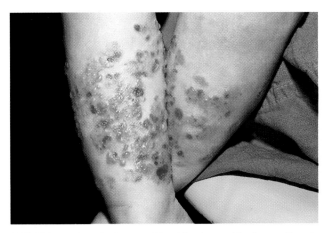

FIGURE 6-76. A 2-year-old with dermatitis herpetiformis showing lesions consisting of small vesicles on both legs.

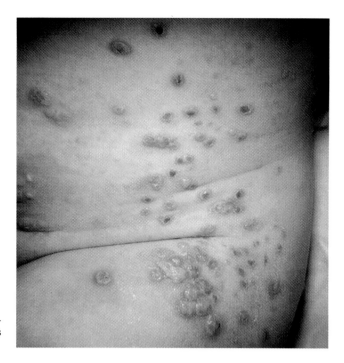

FIGURE 6–77. Pruritic papules and vesicles on the lower abdomen and upper thigh in an 18-month-old infant with dermatitis herpetiformis.

Bullous Pemphigoid

DEFINITION

A nonhereditary blistering disease of adults that may be seen in children

ETIOLOGY

1. Unknown
2. Presumably autoimmune

EPIDEMIOLOGY

1. Rare in children
2. May present in the first year of life

PATHOGENESIS

Autoantibodies to normal components of the dermoepidermal junction result in formation of a subepidermal blister.

LABORATORY

1. Skin biopsy shows a subepidermal blister with eosinophils in the blister cavity and the dermis.
2. Direct immunofluorescence shows IgG and C3 deposits in the dermoepidermal junction.
3. Indirect immunofluorescence shows circulating basement membrane zone antibodies (80% of cases)

COMPLICATION

Blindness in cicatricial pemphigoid of the eye

TREATMENT

1. Refer patient to a dermatologist.

BOX 6–28	*Differential Diagnosis of Bullous Pemphigoid*

Epidermolysis bullosa acquisita
Pemphigus vulgaris
Erythema multiforme
Linear IgA dermatosis of childhood
Vesicobullous lupus erythematosus
Dermatitis herpetiformis
Acute contact dermatitis

---

2. Treatment options include:
   a. Systemic corticosteroid
   b. Tetracycline and nicotinamide if the child is over 8 years of age
   c. Dapsone
3. Ophthalmology and oral surgery referrals are needed for patients with the cicatricial variant.

PROGNOSIS

1. Waxes and wanes
2. May be self-limiting in children

KEY POINTS

Bullous Pemphigoid

- Bullous pemphigoid is a rarer but more benign disease in children.
- Cicatricial pemphigoid of the eyes may lead to blindness.

TABLE 6–30
Clinical Features of Bullous Pemphigoid

Skin Lesions

Tense blisters
Appear on normal or erythematous skin
Distribution
    Mostly acral
    Face commonly involved in young children
    Mouth lesions may be present
    May be localized to vulvar area

Cicatricial Pemphigoid

Scarring variant localized to mouth and eyes

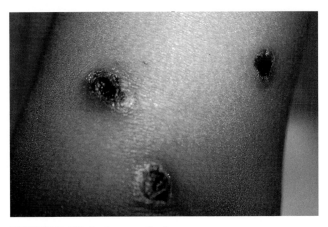

FIGURE 6–79. Lesions on the leg.

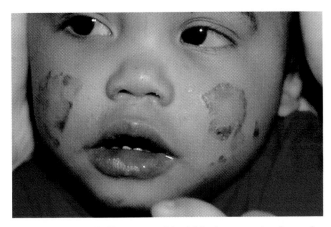

FIGURE 6–78. Bullous pemphigoid lesions on the face of a 1-year-old boy; onset occurred at 1 month of age.

Vitiligo

DEFINITION

An acquired disorder of pigmentation in which melanocytes are totally absent from the lesion.

ETIOLOGY

1. The exact cause is unknown.
2. An autoimmune theory implicates a process wherein circulating antibodies are responsible for melanocyte destruction.

EPIDEMIOLOGY

1. Common age at presentation
    a. Onset before 8 years of age in 25%
    b. Onset occurs before 20 years in 50%
    c. Uncommon during infancy
2. May be familial
3. More common in families with autoimmune diseases

LABORATORY

Thyroid function tests are indicated to rule out thyroid dysfunction.

BOX 6–29	*Differential Diagnosis of Vitiligo*

Postinflammatory hypopigmentation
Hypopigmented macule of tuberous sclerosis
Nevus depigmentosus
Piebaldism
Lichen sclerosus et atrophicus

COMPLICATIONS

1. Severe cosmetic disability may be experienced if the lesion is on the face of a dark-skinned individual.
2. Severe sunburn can occur on the vitiliginous lesions.

TREATMENT

1. Refer the patient to a dermatologist.
2. Mid to high-potency topical corticosteroids may be used.
3. If there is no response after 4 months of a topical corticosteroid, the next treatment of choice is

PUVA (topical or oral psoralen followed by ultraviolet A phototherapy).
4. Sunscreen to prevent sunburn of the affected areas
5. Camouflage make-up creams
6. Enroll the patient in the

National Vitiligo Foundation
Texas American Bank Building
P.O. Box 6337
Tyler, TX 75711

TABLE 6–31
Clinical Features of Vitiligo

Skin Lesion

If the lesion adjoins a hairy area, the hair is also depigmented. There may be islands of normal skin inside the white lesion.

Localized Vitiligo

One or few lesions of varying sizes
Ivory white in color surrounded by hyperpigmented convex border
Seen on any skin surface

Generalized Vitiligo

Depigmented symmetrical lesions
Distribution
    Periorificial areas: around eyes, nose, mouth, genitalia
    Hands, feet, wrists, knees

Segmental Vitiligo

Linear depigmented lesions
Unilateral distribution

PROGNOSIS

1. Lesions on the face respond better to treatment.
2. Generalized vitiligo has a poorer prognosis.

KEY POINTS

Vitiligo

- Vitiligo is an acquired loss of pigmentation.
- Treat children first with mid to high-potency topical steroids.

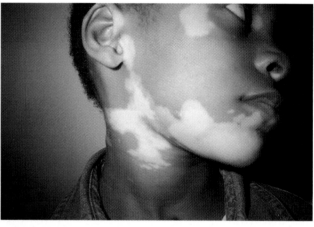

FIGURE 6–80. Vitiligo on the face of a 6-year-old boy.

Alopecia Areata

DEFINITION

A noninfectious localized nonscarring hair loss

ETIOLOGY

1. The cause is unknown.
2. It is presumed to be an autoimmune disorder.

EPIDEMIOLOGY

1. Common age at presentation
   a. Appears before 20 years of age in 50% of patients.
   b. Highest incidence: between 6 and 10 years of age
2. A positive family history for alopecia areata is present in 10% to 18% of patients.
3. More common in patients with
   a. Thyroid disease
   b. Vitiligo
   c. Other autoimmune disorders
   d. Down syndrome

BOX 6–30	*Differential Diagnosis of Alopecia Areata*

Tinea capitis
Trichotillomania
Traction alopecia
Anagen effluvium from chemotherapy

LABORATORY

Thyroid function test to rule out thyroid dysfunction

COMPLICATION

Severe alopecia may result in significant emotional and psychological stress.

TREATMENT

1. Refer the patient to a dermatologist.
2. Anthralin may be used topically for its contact irritant effect (stimulates hair regrowth).

3. Intralesional injection of triamcinolone solution in patchy lesions
4. Combination treatment with tretinoin solution twice a day and minoxidil solution once daily.
5. Oral corticosteroid pulse therapy, 5 mg/kg/dose of prednisone, once monthly until hair regrows
6. Use of a wig, especially for a girl, may be suggested.
7. Emotional support for the patient and family
8. Enroll the patient in the

> National Alopecia Areata Foundation
> P.O. Box 150760
> San Rafael, CA 94915-0760
> Telephone 415-456-4644
> Fax 415-456-4274

PROGNOSIS

1. Correlates positively with severity of disease
2. The following variants have poorer prognosis:
   a. Alopecia totalis
   b. Alopecia universalis
   c. Ophiasic alopecia

KEY POINTS

Alopecia Areata

- The well-circumscribed area devoid of hair has smooth skin.
- Alopecia totalis, alopecia universalis, and ophiasic alopecia have poorer prognoses.

TABLE 6–32
Clinical Features of Alopecia Areata

Sudden onset
One or more round circumscribed patches of hair loss
Scalp or any hair-bearing area may be involved
Skin where hair is lost is very smooth
Nail changes (pitting, longitudinal ridging) are seen in 50% of cases
Hair that regrows may have no pigment
Clinical variants (depending on extent of hair loss)
  Alopecia areata
  Alopecia totalis
  Alopecia universalis
  Ophiasic alopecia (headband distribution)

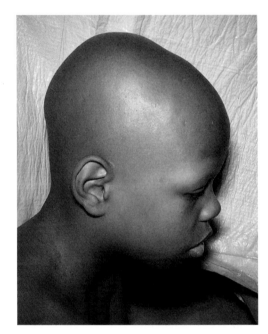

FIGURE 6–82. Alopecia universalis. The child had no scalp hair, eyebrows, or eyelashes.

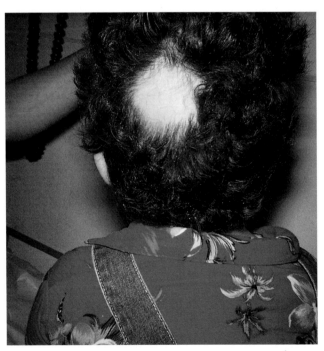

FIGURE 6–81. Alopecia areata in a 2-year-old child.

Hemangioma

DEFINITION

Hemangioma is a benign tumor consisting of proliferating immature capillaries.

ETIOLOGY

Hemangiomas are vascular hamartomas that occur sporadically.

EPIDEMIOLOGY

Female-male ratio is 4:1.

BOX 6-31 *Natural Course of Hemangioma*

Lesions increase in size in first 6 to 12 months.
Involution starts after first year.
  50% of hemangiomas are completely involuted by 5 years of age
  70% by 7 years of age
  90% by 9 years of age
Deep hemangiomas and hemangiomas in parotid region involute more slowly.

LABORATORY

1. MRI or CT scan of head
   a. Indicated in patients with hemangiomas covering a large area of the face and scalp
   b. Rules out structural brain abnormalities
   c. PHACE syndrome:
      (1) *P*osterior fossa malformation
      (2) *H*emangioma on the head
      (3) *A*rterial anomalies
      (4) *C*ardiac defects
      (5) *E*ye abnormalities
2. Early direct laryngoscopy
   a. In patients with hemangiomas located in the "beard area" (preauricular areas, chin, anterior neck, and lower lip)
   b. To rule out laryngeal involvement: if larynx is involved, intervention is indicated early.
3. Platelet count must be done in patients with very rapidly enlarging lesions as in Kasabach-Merritt syndrome.

TREATMENT

1. *Indications for treatment*
   a. Life- and function-threatening hemangiomas
      (1) Impairment of vision, hearing, urination, or defecation
      (2) Airway compromise
      (3) Congestive heart failure
      (4) Kasabach-Merritt syndrome

BOX 6-32 *Differential Diagnosis of Hemangiomas*

VASCULAR MALFORMATIONS

Types
  Capillary (e.g., port wine stain)
  Arteriovenous
  Venous
  Lymphatic (e.g., cystic hygroma)
All of these have the following characteristics:
  They are present at birth.
  Growth is commensurate with the child's growth.
  They do *not* involute.
  A bruit is heard when an arteriovenous malformation is auscultated.
  Female-male ratio is 1:1.

---

   b. Hemangiomas in certain anatomic locations that often leave permanent scars or deformities, especially of the nose and lip
   c. Large facial hemangiomas
   d. Ulcers
2. *Forms of treatment*
   a. Systemic corticosteroids: Prednisone 2 to 4 mg/kg/day, single dose in the morning for 4 weeks, then gradually tapering it to alternate days
   b. Intralesional injection of triamcinolone acetonide solution (40 mg/mL) 1 to 3 mg/kg every 2 weeks times 3
   c. Interferon alpha 2a: 1 million U/m^2/day subcutaneously; may be increased to 3 million U/m^2/day if tolerated. Caution: A 10% incidence of spastic diplegia with the use of interferon alpha 2a has been reported.
   d. Tunable pulse dye laser has been used on very early lesions with inconsistent results.
   e. Systemic antibiotics and local wound care are indicated for ulcerated lesions.
3. Patients with a complicated hemangioma should be referred to a dermatologist.

KEY POINTS

Hemangioma

- Hemangiomas involute spontaneously.
- Treatment is indicated in a few cases (see list under *Treatment*).
- They must be differentiated from vascular malformations.

TABLE 6–33
Clinical Features of Hemangioma

Three Types of Hemangioma

1. Superficial ("strawberry") hemangioma
   Most common type of hemangioma
   Lesion appears between 2nd and 4th weeks of life
   Asymptomatic
   Enlarging
   Blanching
   Compressible
   Red plaque or tumor
2. Deep (cavernous) hemangioma
   Lesion present at birth
   Overlying skin may be normal or slightly bluish
3. Mixed superficial and deep

Location

Hemangiomas are more common on the face and upper part of the body

TABLE 6–34
Complications of Hemangioma

Ulceration (with lesion in an area of friction)
Secondary infection (if hemangioma is ulcerated)
Compromise of a vital function (lesion by its location causing obstruction). Example: periorbital hemangioma obstructs vision, leading to amblyopia
Kasabach-Merrit syndrome
  A rapidly enlarging deep hemangioma
  Trapping of circulating platelets and coagulation factors leads to disseminated intravascular coagulation, which in turn leads to life-threatening hemorrhages
Multiple cutaneous hemangiomas (hemangiomatosis)
  May be associated with visceral hemangiomas (GI, liver, lung, CNS)

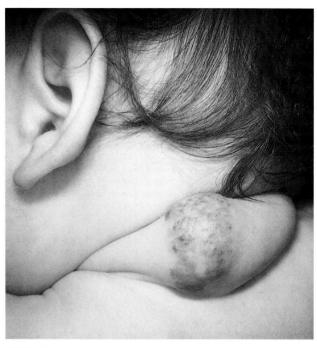

FIGURE 6–84. A 5-month-old girl with a mixed deep and superficial hemangioma on the posterior neck.

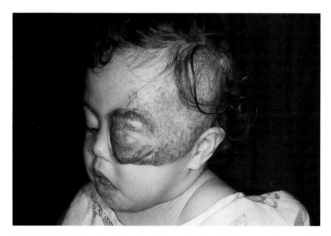

FIGURE 6–85. An infant with a big facial hemangioma that obstructed her vision. Head MRI was part of the work-up.

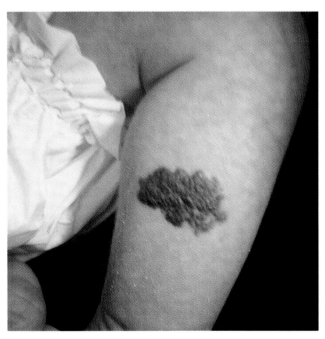

FIGURE 6–83. A 1-month-old infant with a superficial hemangioma on the leg.

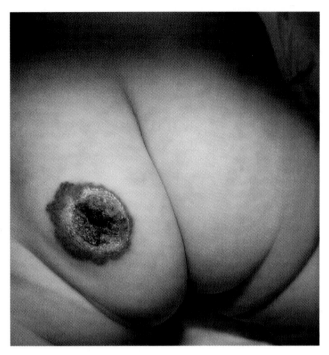

FIGURE 6–86. Ulcerated hemangioma.

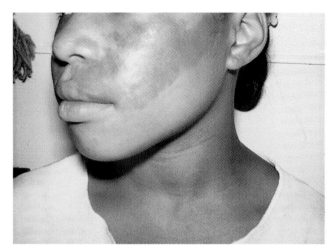

FIGURE 6–88. Port wine stain (capillary vascular malformation).

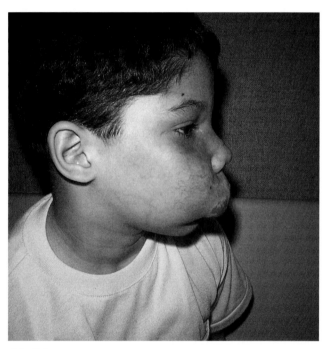

FIGURE 6–89. Vascular malformation on the right side of the face. A bruit was present.

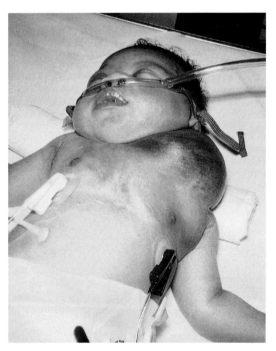

FIGURE 6–87. Kasabach-Merritt syndrome.

Klippel-Trenaunay Syndrome

SYNONYM   Angio-osteohypertrophy
                      Syndrome

DEFINITION

A sporadic disorder consisting of a vascular malformation and hypertrophy of the underlying structures.

ETIOLOGY

Unknown

EPIDEMIOLOGY

1. Equal sex distribution
2. The most common vascular malformation syndrome

LABORATORY

1. Radiographs of extremities to detect bone hypertrophy
2. Doppler studies of venous and lymphatic malformations

TREATMENT

1. Refer patient to the following specialists
   a. Vascular surgeon
   b. Orthopedist (to correct leg length discrepancy)
   c. Laser surgeon (for the pulse dye laser treatment of port wine stain)
2. Compression stockings
3. Sequential compression pump treatment

PROGNOSIS

1. Progressive limb hypertrophy
2. If arteriovenous fistula is present, the patient may develop high-output cardiac failure.

KEY POINTS

Klippel-Trenaunay Syndrome

- Klippel-Trenaunay syndrome is a sporadic (nonhereditary) disorder.
- Gradual limb hypertrophy occurs.

BOX 6–33	*Differential Diagnosis of Klippel-Trenaunay Syndrome*

Proteus syndrome
Phakomatosis pigmentovascularis

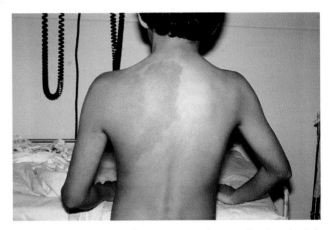

FIGURE 6–90. Klippel-Trenaunay syndrome affecting the left upper limb. There is hypertrophy of the left side of the body.

TABLE 6–35
Clinical Features of Klippel-Trenaunay Syndrome

Vascular Malformations

Capillary malformations (port wine stain)
    Unilateral
    On lower extremity (95%)
    On upper extremity (5%)
    Combined (85%)
    Swelling and increased redness of involved limb during
       febrile episodes can be mistakenly diagnosed as cellulitis
Venous malformations
    Phlebectasis
    Varicose veins
    Arteriovenous fistula presenting as a bruit (Klippel-Trenaunay-
       Parkes-Weber variant)
Lymphatic malformations—lymphedema

Hypertrophy of Affected Limb

Hypertrophy of muscle and bones
Affected limb is longer

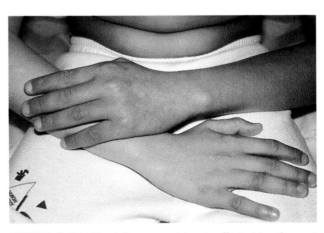

FIGURE 6–91. The left arm and hand, affected by the port wine stain, are bigger than the right arm and hand.

Congenital Pigmented Nevus (CPN)

DEFINITION

A pigmented hamartomatous lesion that is present at birth.

ETIOLOGY

CPN is a sporadically occurring hamartoma.

EPIDEMIOLOGY

One percent of newborns have CPN; 0.06% have giant CPN.

LABORATORY

1. MRI of head
   a. Indicated for large lesions anywhere on the body
   b. To exclude intracranial melanosis and Dandy-Walker malformation
2. Spinal MRI
   a. Indicated for CPN of any size that overlies midline or paraspinal area of the back
   b. To exclude underlying spinal or spinal cord defect
3. Skin biopsy
   a. May be performed if there is doubt about the true nature of a pigmented lesion
   b. CPN shows nests of nevus cells around skin appendages, in single file between collagen bundles, and deep in the subcutis and fascia.

BOX 6–34 *Congenital Pigmented Nevus and Risk of Transformation into Malignant Melanoma*

LIFETIME RISK FOR A CHILD

With giant CPN: 6% to 10%
With small CPN: <1%
With intermediate CPN: probably between these figures

GIANT CPN

Malignant melanoma starts in deeper subcutaneous tissues
By the time surface changes appear, it's too late
Some studies show a negative correlation between giant CPN on the extremities and malignant transformation

SMALL CPN

Changes of melanoma appear on the surface of small lesions
Patients may be observed except in some cases (see under *Treatment*)

COMPLICATIONS

1. Transformation into malignant melanoma (see Box 6–34)
2. Cosmetic concerns are a major problem with giant CPN, especially if it is located on exposed areas.

BOX 6–35 *Differential Diagnosis of Congenital Pigmented Nevus*

CAFÉ-AU-LAIT SPOTS
Normal skin texture
Absence of coarse hair
Absence of increased skin markings

TREATMENT

1. Refer the patient to a dermatologist and a plastic surgeon.
2. Surgical excision
   a. Recommended for giant CPN, especially those on the torso.
   b. The optimal time for surgery is the first decade of life.
3. Intermediate CPN may be observed or excised.
4. Small CPN may be observed for changes unless
   a. There is a family history of melanoma
   b. The lesion is in an area that is difficult to observe (e.g., scalp, genitalia)

KEY POINT

Congenital Pigmented Nevus

■ Congenital pigmented nevus can potentially transform into malignant melanoma.

TABLE 6-36
Clinical Features of Congenital Pigmented Nevus

Skin Lesion
Present at birth
Varies in size and shape
Varies in color from dark brown to deep black
Surface rough with prominent skin markings
Coarse terminal hair may be present
Distribution: any body surface
Arbitrarily classified as:
   Small: <2 cm
   Intermediate: 2-20 cm
   Giant: >20 cm or involving one whole anatomic area

Giant CPN (Garment Nevus)
Usually accompanied by multiple satellite lesions
Giant lesions on head and torso may have associated CNS
   involvement

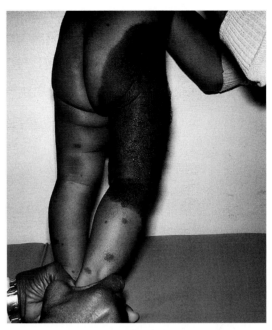

FIGURE 6-93. Giant congenital pigmented nevus involving the right buttock, thigh, and knee.

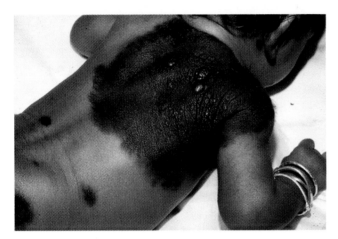

FIGURE 6-92. A 2-month-old infant with a giant congenital pigmented nevus on the shoulder with many satellite lesions. Coarse terminal hairs and neuroid tumors were present on the surface of the lesion.

Nevus of Ota, Nevus of Ito

SYNONYMS   Nevus Fuscoceruleus
               Ophthalmomaxillaris
               Nevus Fuscoceruleus
               Acromiodeltoidalis
               Dermal Melanocytosis

DEFINITION

A pigmentary disorder affecting specific anatomic locations

ETIOLOGY

Sporadic

EPIDEMIOLOGY

1. More common in Asians and African-Americans, although it is seen in all races
2. Female-male ratio is 3:1.

PATHOGENESIS

1. Failure of melanocytes to migrate completely from the neural crest to the epidermis during embryonic life
2. These melanocytes become arrested in the dermis, an abnormal location for them.

BOX 6-36	*Differential Diagnosis of Nevus of Ota and Nevus of Ito*
Mongolian spot (disappears) Postinflammatory hyperpigmentation Congenital pigmented nevus Café-au-lait spots	

LABORATORY

Skin biopsy shows melanocytes in the mid and upper dermis.

COMPLICATIONS

1. Cosmetic
2. A total of 37 cases of melanoma arising from nevus of Ota has been reported; all of them occurred in white patients.

TREATMENT

1. Camouflage make-up
2. Refer patient to an ophthalmologist.
3. Refer patient to a dermatologist for removal of lesion with a Q-switched ruby laser.

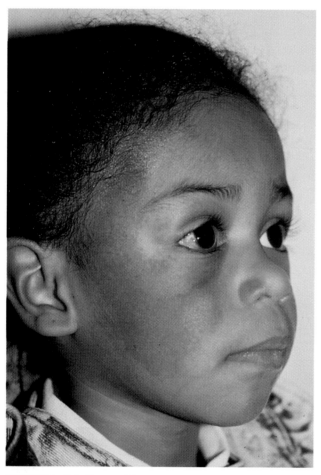

FIGURE 6–94. Nevus of Ota.

KEY POINTS

Nevus of Ota, Nevus of Ito

- Nevus of Ota and nevus of Ito are permanent lesions.
- They can be removed using a Q-switched ruby laser.

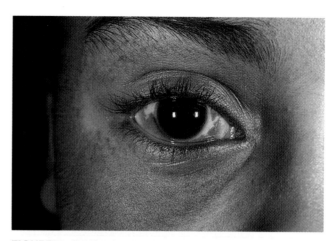

FIGURE 6–95. Eye involvement.

TABLE 6–37
Clinical Features of Nevus of Ota and Nevus of Ito

Skin Lesions

Present at birth in 60% of cases; remainder appear at puberty
Lesions are permanent

Nevus of Ota

Bluish-gray to brown macule on forehead and zygomatic
 region
Unilateral in most instances; rarely bilateral
Lesions may involve eye on the same side
Eye involvement may include
 Sclera
 Conjunctiva
 Iris
 Optic nerve
Other mucous membrane involvement is rare but may include
 Ear canal
 Pharynx
 Hard palate
 Nasal mucosa

Nevus of Ito

Bluish-gray macule on the shoulder and upper arm

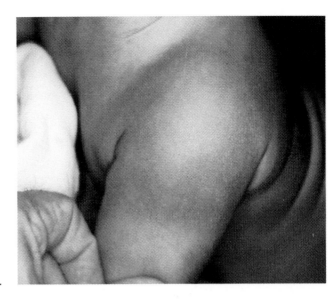

FIGURE 6–96. Nevus of Ito.

Nevus Sebaceus of Jadassohn

DEFINITION

A hamartomatous disorder consisting of immature sebaceous glands with a potential for transformation

ETIOLOGY

It is a sporadic hamartoma.

EPIDEMIOLOGY

1. It is seen in less than 0.5% of newborns.
2. Multiple nevus sebaceus lesions together with other structural anomalies (e.g., CNS or ocular defects) may be a component of the epidermal nevus syndrome.

LABORATORY

Skin biopsy

COMPLICATIONS

During adolescence, 15% of lesions may undergo hyperplasia and transformation into any of the following:

1. Basal cell epithelioma
2. Syringocystadenoma papilliferum
3. Squamous cell carcinoma
4. Keratoacanthoma
5. Malignant eccrine poroma
6. Apocrine carcinoma
7. Leiomyoma
8. Piloleiomyoma
9. Hidradenoma
10. Apocrine cystadenoma

TREATMENT

1. Refer patient to a dermatologist or pediatric surgeon.
2. Excise lesion before puberty.

KEY POINTS

Nevus Sebaceus of Jadassohn

- The lesion of nevus sebaceus is a hairless, yellowish-orange, velvety plaque that is commonly seen on the scalp.
- Malignant transformation into a nonmelanoma skin malignancy occurs after puberty in 15% of cases.

BOX 6–37	*Differential Diagnosis of Nevus Sebaceus of Jadassohn*
	Aplasia cutis congenita
	Juvenile xanthogranuloma
	Epidermal nevus (nevus verrucosus)

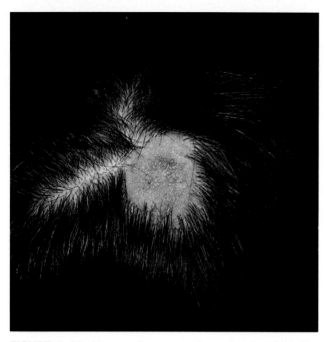

FIGURE 6–97. Nevus sebaceus on the scalp of a child. The lesion was a yellow plaque.

TABLE 6–38
Clinical Features of Nevus Sebaceus of Jadassohn

Skin Lesion
Solitary
Round or oval
Hairless plaque
Present at birth
Velvety surface
Yellowish to orange hue
Location
   Scalp is the most common location
   Face (lesions may appear as a string of yellowish papules)

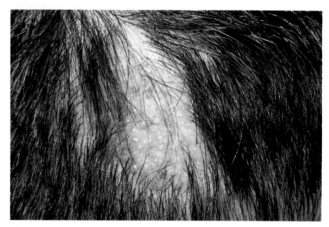

FIGURE 6–99. Nevus sebaceus that has undergone hyperplasia in an adult.

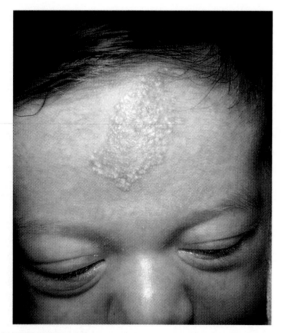

FIGURE 6–98. Nevus sebaceus on the forehead of a 1-month-old infant.

Epidermal Nevus (EN)

SYNONYMS   Nevus Unius Lateris
Nevus Verrucosus
Ichthyosis Hystrix

DEFINITION

A congenital malformation consisting of single or multiple scaling and wart-like overgrowths of the epidermis arranged in a linear and unilateral or bilateral and sometimes extensive distribution

ETIOLOGY

Believed to be the result of a genetic mosaicism that starts during embryogenesis

EPIDEMIOLOGY

1. Sexes are affected equally.
2. No racial predilection
3. No notable familial incidence

LABORATORY

1. Skin biopsy
   a. Determines if the epidermal nevus is epidermolytic
   b. If so, the patient's offspring may be at risk for epidermolytic hyperkeratosis, a chronic disease characterized by generalized thick scaling.
2. In patients with the EN syndrome, the work-up must be guided by the associated abnormal physical signs and symptoms.

TREATMENT

1. There is no satisfactory form of treatment to remove the lesions that does not result in recurrence or scarring.
2. In the EN syndrome, treatment depends on the systems involved.

TABLE 6–39
Clinical Features of Epidermal Nevus

Skin Lesions
Rough
Hyperpigmented, flesh-colored or slightly pink
Verrucous papules
Distribution
    Linear
    Segmental
    Whorled
    If generalized, lesions are patterned (systematized) and follow the lines of Blaschko
Lesions may be present at birth or shortly thereafter or may appear as late as puberty (tardive epidermal nevus)

BOX 6–38	*Epidermal Nevus Syndrome*

Epidermal nevus in association with two extracutaneous systemic abnormalities
    Neurologic: Seizures, mental retardation
    Skeletal: Hemihypertrophy, kyphoscoliosis, ankle and foot deformities, macrodactyly
    Ocular: Extension of nevus to lid and bulbar conjunctiva, colobomas, corneal opacity
May be associated with malignancies such as
Wilms' tumor
Rhabdomyosarcoma
Astrocytoma
Adenocarcinoma of salivary glands

KEY POINTS

Epidermal Nevus

- Epidermal nevus consists of permanent dark, verrucous lesions in different shapes and patterns.
- Epidermal nevus syndrome is the association of epidermal nevus with abnormalities in the CNS, skeletal and ocular systems.

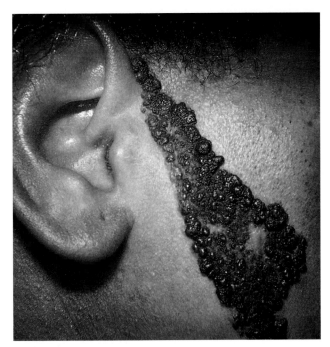

FIGURE 6–100. Localized epidermal nevus on the face. The lesion consists of a hyperpigmented verrucous plaque.

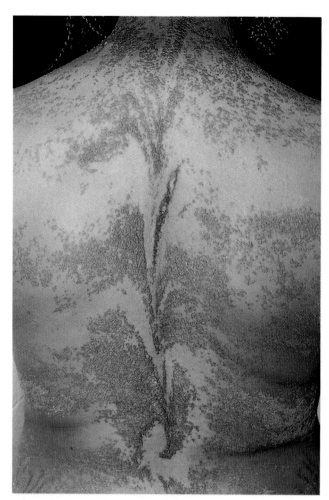

FIGURE 6-101. Generalized epidermal nevus. Lesions are whorled and systematized following Blaschko's line. The child had no extracutaneous abnormalities.

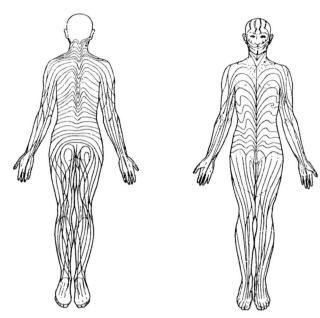

FIGURE 6-102. Lines of Blaschko.

Mastocytosis

SYNONYMS   Mast Cell Disease
                       Urticaria Pigmentosa

DEFINITION

A disorder of unknown etiology characterized by infiltration of the dermis and other tissues with mast cells.

ETIOLOGY

Unknown

EPIDEMIOLOGY

1. Ninety percent of cases are seen in children less than 3 years of age.
2. Equal sex distribution
3. More common in whites
4. Rarely, may be familial

5. The adult form (systemic mastocytosis with involvement of the liver, spleen, and bone marrow), telangiectasis macularis eruptiva perstans (TMEP), and mast cell leukemia are rare in children.

LABORATORY

Skin biopsy with Giemsa or methylene blue stain of the tissue demonstrates infiltration of the dermis with mast cells and their characteristic granules.

COMPLICATIONS

From massive release of histamines from the mast cells:

1. Diffuse urtication
2. Rarely, wheezing and anaphylaxis

DIFFERENTIAL DIAGNOSIS

Postinflammatory hyperpigmentation, nodular scabies, café-au-lait spots, urticaria, arthropod bite reaction

TREATMENT

1. Avoid vigorous toweling after baths.
2. Avoid histamine releasers such as hot spicy food, aspirin, codeine, radiologic contrast materials
3. Antihistamines (hydroxyzine, cyproheptadine, ketotifen) if patient is symptomatic
4. Topical corticosteroids during periods of acute urtication

PROGNOSIS

1. The course is benign in children.
2. The disorder remits permanently after several years.

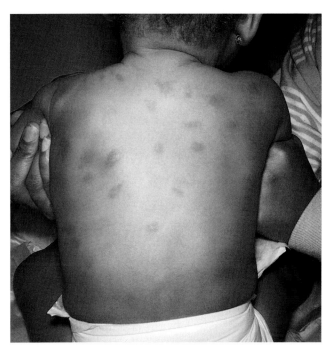

FIGURE 6–103. An 11-month-old infant who had had urticaria pigmentosa since the age of 2 months. She had multiple hyperpigmented flat lesions on the back.

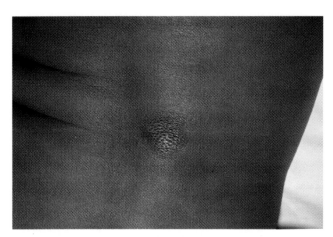

FIGURE 6–104. Positive Darier sign in an infant with solitary mastocytoma. Stroking the lesion caused urtication owing to histamine release by the mast cell.

BOX 6–39	*Positive Darier Sign in Mastocytosis*

Stroking results in urtication of the lesion due to release of histamine and other inflammatory mediators when mast cells are injured.

KEY POINTS

Mastocytosis

- Childhood-onset mastocytosis has a good prognosis.
- Positive Darier sign can be demonstrated in 95% of cases.

TABLE 6–40
Clinical Features of Mastocytosis

Three Clinical Forms in Children

Solitary mastocytoma
    Plaque measuring 1–3 cm
    Flesh-colored or yellowish, with a peau d'orange surface
    Present at birth or shortly thereafter
Urticaria pigmentosa
    Multiple lesions
    Pigmented macules, papules, or nodules
    Most common location: on trunk
    Onset: few weeks or months after birth
Diffuse cutaneous or erythrodermic mastocytosis
    Skin hard
    Scotch grain appearance and consistency
    May be present at birth

Other Features

Lesions may become bullous in young infant
Pruritus is variable
Positive Darier sign

Langerhans' Cell Histiocytosis

SYNONYMS   Histiocytosis X
Letterer-Siwe Disease

DEFINITION

A disease of unknown cause characterized by proliferation of histiocytes of the Langerhans' type.

ETIOLOGY

The exact cause is not known.

EPIDEMIOLOGY

1. The disseminated form is almost exclusively seen in children younger than 3 years.
2. The localized forms are more common in older children.

LABORATORY

1. Complete blood count, liver chemistries
2. Skeletal survey
3. Skin biopsy with light and electron microscopy. The latter demonstrates Langerhans' cells containing Birbeck granules.

BOX 6–40	*Differential Diagnosis of Langerhans' Cell Histiocytosis*

Seborrheic dermatitis
Leukemia
Candidal diaper dermatitis
Human immunodeficiency virus (HIV) infection
Streptococcal perianal dermatitis

COMPLICATION

Death if untreated.

TREATMENT

1. Hospitalization
2. Dermatology and hematology-oncology consultations
3. Chemotherapy: vinblastine either as monotherapy or in combination with vincristine, doxorubicin, and/or cyclophosphamide
4. Bone marrow transplant

PROGNOSIS

Guarded

KEY POINTS

Langerhans' Cell Histiocytosis

- Chronic erosive intertrigo in the diaper area, perianal erosions, and purpuric scalp lesions may be the first cutaneous signs of Langerhans' cell histiocytosis.
- Skin biopsy confirms the diagnosis.

TABLE 6–41
Clinical Forms of Langerhans' Cell Histiocytosis

Localized

Eosinophilic granuloma
  Consists of a solitary bone lesion
Hand-Schüller-Christian disease
  Bone lesions
  Diabetes insipidus
  Exophthalmos

Disseminated

Histiocytosis involving two or more organs

TABLE 6–42
Clinical Features of Langerhans' Cell Histiocytosis

Skin Lesions

Seen in 78% of patients
May comprise any combination or all of the following:
  Scaly, rose-yellow, translucent papules
    Location: scalp, especially above and behind ears, trunk, "seborrheic areas"
  Erosive intertrigo
    Location: groin and postauricular area
  Perianal erosions
  Purpuric lesions

Systemic Involvement

Hepatosplenomegaly
Lymphadenopathy
Diffuse pulmonary infiltrate
Bone lesions
Pancytopenia

Other Findings

Buccal and gingival ulcerations
Chronic recurrent otitis media

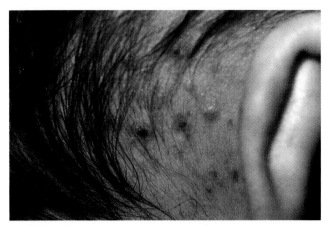

FIGURE 6–105. An 11-month-old child with Langerhans' cell histiocytosis. Skin lesions on the back of the ears were scaly purpuric papules.

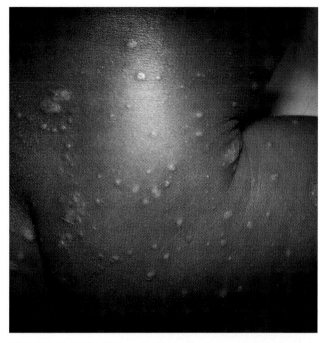

FIGURE 6–107. Diffuse infiltrated papular lesions in a 2-month-old child with Langerhans' cell histiocytosis.

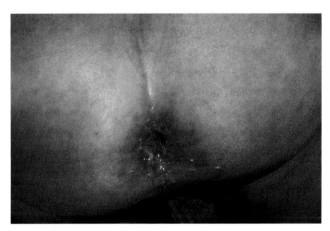

FIGURE 6–106. Perianal erosions in the same child.

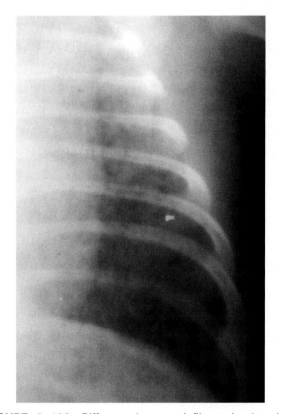

FIGURE 6–108. Diffuse pulmonary infiltrate in the child shown in Figure 6–107.

Ichthyosis

DEFINITION

A hereditary skin disorder characterized by dryness and excessive scaling

PATHOGENESIS

1. Increased epidermal cell turnover
2. Increased adhesiveness of the cells of the stratum corneum
3. Abnormal transepidermal water loss
4. Abnormalities of protein and lipid composition and metabolism affecting the cells and intercellular matrix of the stratum corneum

CLINICAL FEATURES

There are five major types of ichthyosis

1. Ichthyosis vulgaris (see Table 6–43)
2. X-linked ichthyosis (see Table 6–44)
3. Lamellar ichthyosis
   a. Inheritance: autosomal recessive
   b. Incidence: 1 in 300,000
   c. Cutaneous features
      (1) Collodion baby at birth
      (2) Plate-like scales
      (3) Palmar hyperkeratosis
   d. Associated findings
      (1) Premature birth
      (2) Ectropion
4. Nonbullous congenital ichthyosiform erythroderma
   a. Inheritance: autosomal recessive
   b. Incidence: 1 in 180,000
   c. Cutaneous features
      (1) Erythroderma at birth and thereafter
      (2) Fine white scales
5. Epidermolytic hyperkeratosis
   a. Synonym: bullous congenital ichthyosiform erythroderma
   b. Inheritance: autosomal dominant
   c. Incidence: rare; approximately 3000 Americans affected
   d. Cutaneous features
      (1) Bullae at birth and in early infancy
      (2) Verruciform or quill-like scales
      (3) Flexures involved
      (4) Keratoderma of palms and soles
   e. Associated finding: secondary bacterial infection

TREATMENT

1. Emollients (e.g., ammonium lactate cream, urea cream)
2. Keratolytics (e.g., salicylic acid in petrolatum)
3. Oral retinoids (e.g., acitretin)
4. Genetic counseling
5. Enroll patient in:

   Foundation for Ichthyosis and Related Skin Types (FIRST)
   P.O. Box 20921
   Raleigh, NC 27619-0921
   Telephone: 800-545-3286
            919-782-5728

PROGNOSIS

1. Chronic
2. Severe forms may be debilitating

BOX 6–41 *Syndromes Associated with Ichthyosis*

Netherton syndrome
Sjögren-Larsson syndrome
Rud syndrome
Congenital *h*emidysplasia *i*chthyosis *l*imb *d*efect (CHILD) syndrome
*K*eratitis, *i*chthyosis, *d*eafness (KID) syndrome
Refsum disease
Conradi-Hünermann syndrome
Trichothiodystrophy

KEY POINTS

Ichthyosis

- There are five major types of ichthyosis. Each is distinguished from the others by mode of inheritance, age of onset, and characteristics and distribution of scales.
- Ichthyosis may be a feature of a syndrome.

TABLE 6–43
Clinical Features of Ichthyosis Vulgaris

Inheritance: autosomal dominant
Incidence: 1 in 500 to 1 in 2000
Cutaneous features
  Onset—during childhood
  Diffuse fine scales over the extensors
  Sparing of the flexures
  Hyperlinear palms
Associated disorder: atopic dermatitis

TABLE 6–44
Clinical Features of X-linked Ichthyosis

Inheritance: X-linked recessive
Incidence: 1 in 2000 to 1 in 6000 males
Cutaneous features
  May be a collodion baby at birth
  Dirty-looking scales
  Sparing of palms, soles, flexures
Associated findings
  Corneal opacities
  Cryptorchidism
  Increased risk of testicular carcinoma
  Decreased skin steroid sulfatase

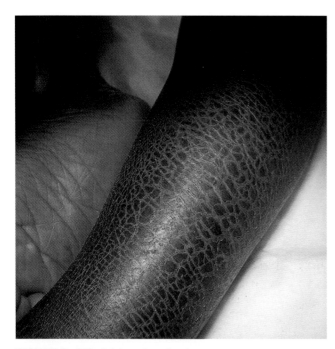

FIGURE 6-109. Ichthyosis vulgaris.

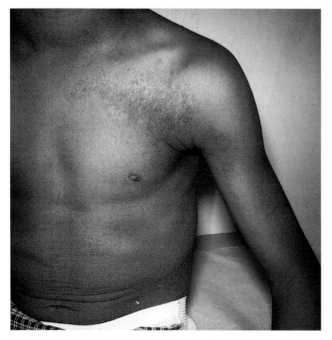

FIGURE 6-110. X-linked ichthyosis in a 10-year-old boy whose two brothers were also affected.

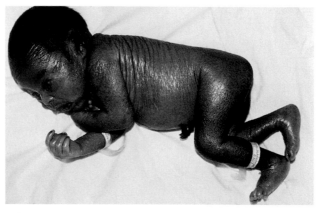

FIGURE 6-111. Collodion baby at birth. This child had lamellar ichthyosis.

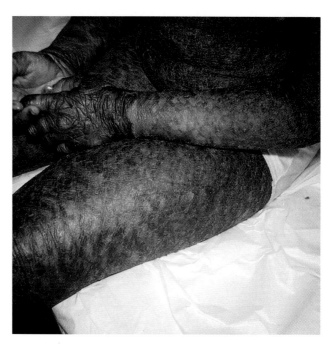

FIGURE 6-112. Lamellar ichthyosis. At age 6 years the same child had generalized thick scales.

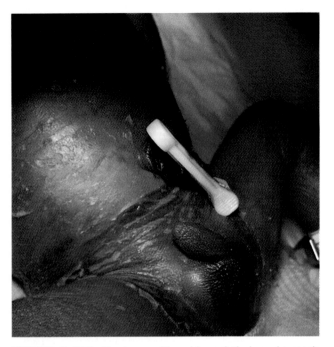

FIGURE 6–113. Newborn with epidermolytic hyperkeratosis showing eroded bullae.

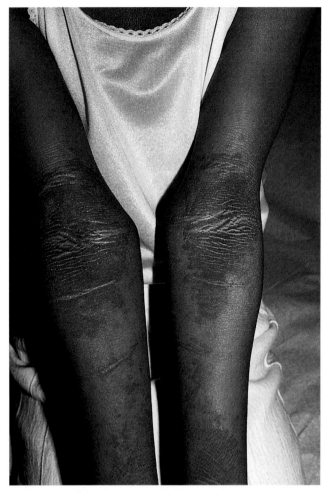

FIGURE 6–114. Sibling of newborn in Figure 6–113. She also has epidermolytic hyperkeratosis with quill-like lesions on the antecubital area.

Netherton Syndrome

SYNONYM   Ichthyosis Linearis Circumflexa

DEFINITION
A hereditary skin disorder characterized by a distinct eruption and abnormal hair shaft

ETIOLOGY
1. Autosomal recessive inheritance
2. Gene locus unknown

EPIDEMIOLOGY
1. Rare
2. Male-female ratio is 1:1.

LABORATORY
1. Light microscopy of a hair sample (from either the scalp or the eyebrow)
   a. Trichorrhexis invaginata (bamboo hair) is the most common finding
   b. Pili torti
2. Increased serum IgE level

DIFFERENTIAL DIAGNOSIS
Atopic dermatitis
Loose anagen syndrome
Conradi-Hünermann syndrome

TREATMENT
1. Monitor child at birth and during infancy for hypernatremia and failure to thrive.
2. Use emollients (skin moisturizers) liberally.
3. Treat atopic dermatitis (see p. 162)
4. Refer the patient to a dermatologist and an allergist.

PROGNOSIS
The condition may improve at puberty.

KEY POINTS
Netherton Syndrome
- Characteristic serpiginous migratory plaques with double-edged scales
- Hair shaft abnormalities (trichorrhexis invaginata)

TABLE 6–45
Clinical Features of Netherton Syndrome

At birth
  Generalized skin erythema and scaling (erythroderma)
  Secondary hypernatremia
  Failure to thrive
Infancy and later
  Atopic dermatitis
  Migratory, erythematous, serpiginous plaques with double-
    edged scales (ichthyosis linearis circumflexa)
  Poor hair growth
  Tendency toward food anaphylaxis

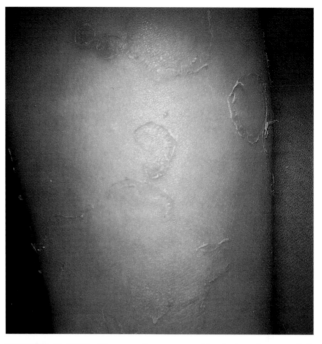

FIGURE 6–116. Close-up in same patient showing serpiginous lesions with double-edged scales.

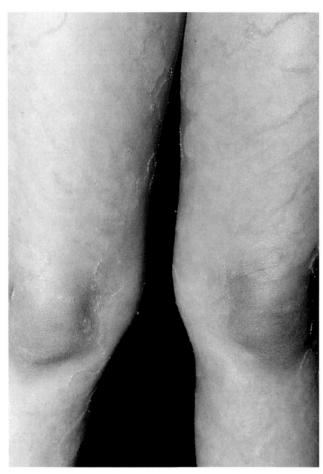

FIGURE 6–115. A 2-year-old girl with Netherton syndrome. Ichthyosis linearis circumflexa in a characteristic eruption.

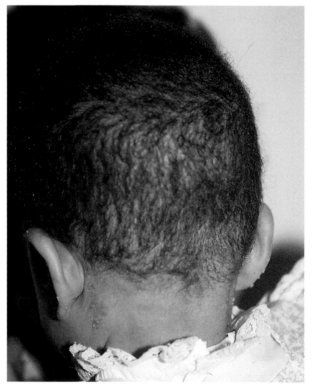

FIGURE 6–117. Poor hair growth in the same patient. She had trichorrhexis invaginata.

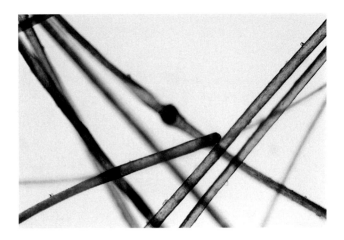

FIGURE 6-118. Trichorrhexis invaginata (bamboo hair) in Netherton syndrome.

Epidermolysis Bullosa (EB)

DEFINITION

A hereditary skin disorder characterized by bullae formed as a result of friction or minor mechanical trauma

ETIOLOGY

It is inherited in a manner that varies with the type of EB.

EPIDEMIOLOGY

It is a rare disorder.

CLINICAL FEATURES

1. There are three major groups
   a. Epidermolysis bullosa simplex (EBS)
   b. Junctional epidermolysis bullosa (JEB)
   c. Dystrophic epidermolysis bullosa (DEB)
2. Epidermolysis bullosa simplex (EBS)
   a. EBS of hands and feet
      (1) Synonyms: localized EBS, Weber-Cockayne variant of EBS
      (2) Inheritance: autosomal dominant
      (3) Cutaneous features
         (a) Onset in early infancy or childhood
         (b) Lesions consist of trauma-induced acral blisters.
         (c) It is worse in summer.
         (d) There is no scarring.
         (e) Condition improves with age.
   b. Generalized EBS
      (1) Synonym: EBS, Koebner variant
      (2) Inheritance: autosomal dominant
      (3) Cutaneous features
         (a) Onset at birth or in infancy or early childhood
         (b) Lesions consist of trauma-induced generalized tense blisters.
         (c) It is worse in summer.
         (d) There is no scarring.
         (e) Condition improves with age.
   c. EBS herpetiformis

   (1) Synonym: EBS, Dowling-Meara variant
   (2) Inheritance: autosomal dominant
   (3) Cutaneous features
      (a) Lesions consist of grouped herpetiform blisters with diffuse distribution.
      (b) There is no scarring.
      (c) There is palmar and plantar keratoderma.
      (d) Condition improves with age.
   d. EBS with neuromuscular involvement
      (1) Synonym: EBS lethalis
      (2) Inheritance: autosomal dominant
      (3) Cutaneous features
         (a) There are widespread erosions at birth.
         (b) These result in cutaneous scarring and atrophy.
      (4) Associated findings
         (a) Muscular dystrophy
         (b) Myasthenia gravis
3. Dystrophic epidermolysis bullosa (DEB)

BOX 6-42   *Junctional Epidermolysis Bullosa (JEB)*

Synonyms: JEB gravis (Herlitz type, JEB lethalis)
Inheritance: autosomal recessive
Cutaneous features
  Generalized blisters on trunk, extremities, and mucosae
  Hands and feet are spared
  Well-circumscribed exuberant granulation tissue on face
  Nails are involved
  Scarring is absent
Associated findings
  Blisters in gastrointestinal and respiratory tracts
  Pyloric atresia
  Growth retardation
Prognosis
  Mortality secondary to sepsis

a. DEB albopapuloid
  (1) Synonym: DEB of Pacini
  (2) Inheritance: autosomal dominant
  (3) Cutaneous features
      (a) There are generalized blisters at birth.
      (b) There is mucosal involvement.
      (c) Atrophic scarring results.
      (d) Papular scars (albopapuloid lesions) appear at puberty.
  (4) Associated findings
      (a) Squamous cell carcinoma
      (b) Growth retardation
b. DEB gravis
  (1) Synonym: DEB of Hallopeau-Siemens
  (2) Inheritance: autosomal recessive
  (3) Cutaneous features
      (a) There are generalized trauma-induced hemorrhagic blisters at birth.
      (b) There is resulting scarring and atrophy.
      (c) "Mitten hands" are caused by the digits fusing when healing occurs.
  (4) Associated findings
      (a) Mucosal lesions with scarring and stenosis of gastrointestinal and respiratory tracts
      (b) Squamous cell carcinoma
      (c) Dental and nail abnormalities
      (d) Eye abnormalities and scarring

      (e) Growth failure
      (f) Iron deficiency anemia
  (5) Prognosis
      Life span is shortened owing to complications.

LABORATORY

Clinical diagnosis is confirmed by the following tests:

1. Skin biopsy
2. Immunofluorescent mapping
3. Electron microscopy

TREATMENT

Treatment is mainly palliative. Refer the patient to a dermatologist.

1. Avoidance of trauma and heat
2. Low doses of systemic corticosteroids
3. Antisepsis of eroded areas
4. Plastic surgery on "mitten hands"
5. Esophageal dilatation
6. Enteral feeding including gastrostomy in selected patients
7. Genetic counseling
8. Enroll the patient in the

   Dystrophic Epidermolysis Bullosa Research Association of America, Inc. (DEBRA)
   141 Fifth Avenue, Suite 7-S
   New York, NY 10010
   Telephone (212) 995-2220

KEY POINTS

Epidermolysis Bullosa

- There are three major types of epidermolysis bullosa, all differing in mode of inheritance, clinical presentation, and findings on skin biopsy, direct immunofluorescence, and electron microscopy.
- Each and every patient must be registered with DEBRA, which is a major source of support and information for the patient, family, and physician.

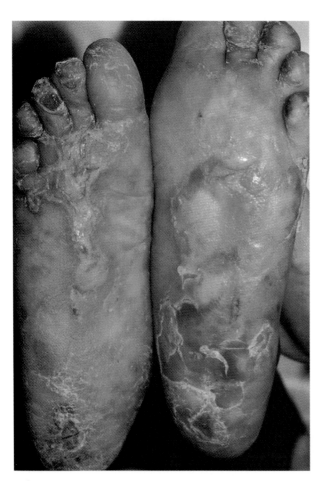

FIGURE 6–119. Epidermolysis bullosa simplex.

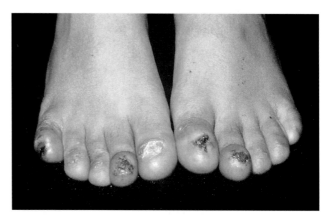

FIGURE 6–120. Junctional epidermolysis bullosa.

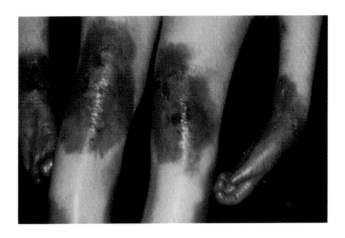

FIGURE 6-121. Dystrophic epidermolysis bullosa. Note hemorrhagic bullae, dystrophic scars, pseudosyndactyly, and claw-like (mitten hand) deformities of the hands. (Courtesy of Department of Dermatology, Yale University School of Medicine. From Hurwitz S: Clinical Pediatric Dermatology, 2nd ed. Philadelphia, WB Saunders, 1993.)

Incontinentia Pigmenti

SYNONYM   Bloch-Sulzberger Syndrome

DEFINITION

A rare, genetically transmitted disorder characterized by cutaneous and neuroectodermal malformations

ETIOLOGY

It is inherited as an X-linked dominant trait.

EPIDEMIOLOGY

1. The true incidence is unknown.
2. Majority of patients (97%) are females.
3. Males with XXY karyotype (Klinefelter syndrome) may be affected.
4. It is lethal to male fetuses.

BOX 6-43   *Associated Findings in Incontinentia Pigmenti*

Dental abnormalities (65%)
    Delayed dentition
    Pegged teeth
    Malocclusions
CNS abnormalities (50%)
    Seizures
    Psychomotor retardation
    Microcephaly
    Spasticity
Patchy alopecia (38%)
Eyes (35%)
    Cataract
    Strabismus
    Retinal atrophy
Dystrophic nail changes (7%)
Maternal history of spontaneous abortion of male fetuses

LABORATORY

1. Complete blood count shows associated peripheral eosinophilia.
2. Skin biopsy of a blister shows its intraepidermal location with numerous eosinophils.
3. Karyotyping of affected males

DIFFERENTIAL DIAGNOSIS

Herpes simplex neonatorum, epidermal nevus, nevoid hypermelanosis, hypomelanosis of Ito, postinflammatory hyperpigmentation

TREATMENT

1. Depends on the systems involved (e.g., anticonvulsants for seizures, dental surgery, ophthalmologic follow-up)
2. Genetic counseling
3. Enroll the patient in the

> National Incontinentia Pigmenti Foundation, Inc.
> 30 East 72nd St., 16th Floor
> New York, NY 10021
> Telephone 212-452-1231
> Fax 212-452-1406

PROGNOSIS

Normal life span

KEY POINTS

Incontinentia Pigmenti

■ There are four stages of the cutaneous lesions: vesicular, verrucous, whorled hyperpigmented macular, and atrophic.
■ The other systems most commonly involved are the CNS, dental, and ocular systems.
■ Majority of patients are females.
■ An affected male must undergo chromosome studies to rule out XXY karyotype.

TABLE 6–46
Clinical Features of Incontinentia Pigmenti

Skin Lesions

1st stage: linear vesicular lesions at birth
2nd stage: verrucous lesions replace the blisters
3rd stage: whorled hyperpigmented macular lesions that follow Blaschko's line appear de novo
4th stage: hypopigmented atrophic lesions appear after several years

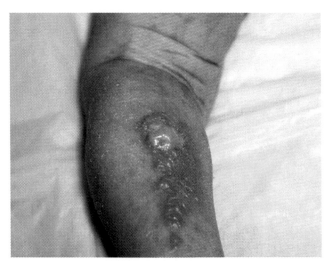

FIGURE 6–122. A child with incontinentia pigmenti. (Her mother was diagnosed with IP retrospectively.) At birth, linear vesicles are seen on the leg.

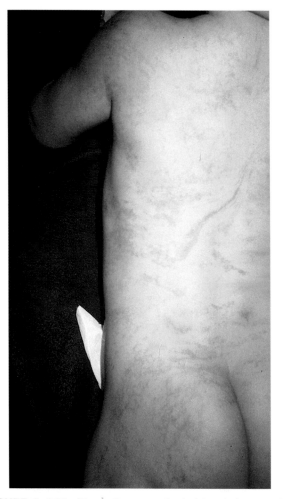

FIGURE 6–124. At age 2 years, whorled hyperpigmentation appears on the back following the lines of Blaschko.

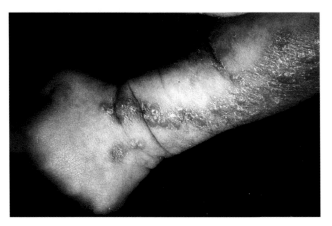

FIGURE 6–123. At age 6 months, verrucous lesions are visible on the arm.

Hypomelanosis of Ito

SYNONYM   Incontinentia Pigmenti Achromians

DEFINITION

A nonhereditary disorder characterized by a distinct hypopigmentation pattern and extracutaneous abnormalities in a small group of patients.

ETIOLOGY

Chromosomal or single gene mosaicism

EPIDEMIOLOGY

1. True incidence unknown
2. Equal sex distribution
3. No racial predilection

PATHOGENESIS

Mosaicism for chromosomal abnormality affects different pigmentary genes, producing the cutaneous phenotype.

LABORATORY

1. Radiographs of the limbs if there is leg length discrepancy
2. Head CT if there is CNS involvement

TREATMENT

Refer patient to subspecialists if he or she is symptomatic.

BOX 6–44	*Differential Diagnosis of Hypomelanosis of Ito*
Incontinentia pigmenti Nevus depigmentosus Tuberous sclerosis Vitiligo Postinflammatory hypopigmentation	

PROGNOSIS

1. Normal life span
2. Hypopigmentation may fade with time.

KEY POINTS

Hypomelanosis of Ito

- Hypomelanosis of Ito has a distinct skin finding: whorled and linear hypopigmentation that follows the lines of Blaschko.
- Associated abnormalities in other systems are seen in 23% of cases.

TABLE 6–47
Clinical Features of Hypomelanosis of Ito

Skin Lesions

Unilateral or bilateral involvement
Whorled, linear, "paintbrush" streaky hypopigmentation
Follow lines of Blaschko

Associated Findings (23% of cases)

CNS—microcephaly, psychomotor retardation, seizures
Musculoskeletal—limb length discrepancy, scoliosis
Ocular—strabismus, hypertelorism
Dental—malocclusion

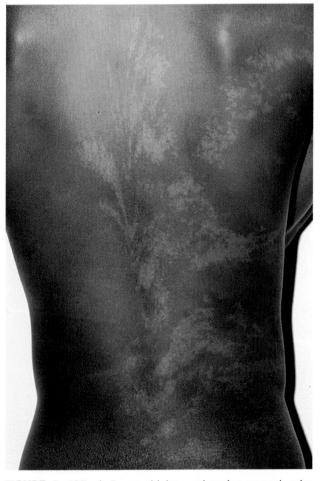

FIGURE 6–125. A 5-year-old boy, otherwise normal, who had hypomelanosis of Ito. The hypopigmentation had a paintbrush pattern following the lines of Blaschko.

Rothmund-Thomson Syndrome

SYNONYM   Poikiloderma Congenitale

ETIOLOGY

1. Autosomal recessive inheritance
2. Gene locus on chromosome 8

EPIDEMIOLOGY

Rare: only 200 reported cases

PATHOGENESIS

Possible abnormalities in DNA repair

LABORATORY

1. Radiographs of the bone to rule out abnormalities
2. Skin biopsy of suspected cutaneous malignancies

BOX 6–45	*Differential Diagnosis of Rothmund-Thomson Syndrome*

Dyskeratosis congenita
Ectodermal dysplasia
Bloom syndrome

COMPLICATIONS

Increased incidence of malignancies (14 in 200 cases)

1. Cutaneous: squamous cell carcinoma, Bowen disease, basal cell carcinoma
2. Noncutaneous: osteosarcoma

TREATMENT

1. Photoprotection (avoidance of sun exposure, use of sunscreen)
2. Refer to a dermatologist for surveillance for skin cancers
3. Refer to an ophthalmologist for yearly screening and cataract treatment
4. Refer to an orthopedist, dentist, or other specialist if the patient is symptomatic
5. Genetic counseling

PROGNOSIS

Normal life span if the patient does not develop malignancies.

KEY POINTS

Rothmund-Thomson Syndrome

■ Primarily a clinical diagnosis based on the combination of poikiloderma, alopecia, and juvenile cataract.
■ Affected individuals are prone to skin and skeletal malignancies.

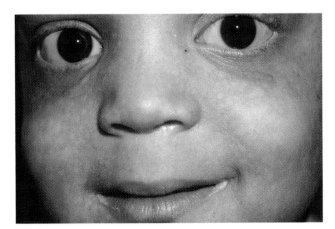

FIGURE 6–126. A 3-year-old boy with Rothmund-Thomson syndrome. Alopecia is seen here.

TABLE 6–48
Clinical Features of Rothmund-Thomson Syndrome

Common Features

Poikiloderma
  Reticulated
    Combination of hypopigmentation, hyperpigmentation, telangiectasia, and atrophy
Photosensitivity
Alopecia (scalp, eyebrows, eyelashes)
Keratotic skin lesions
Juvenile cataracts

Other Features

Short stature
Hypogonadism
Bony anomalies
Abnormal nails and teeth
Usually normal intelligence

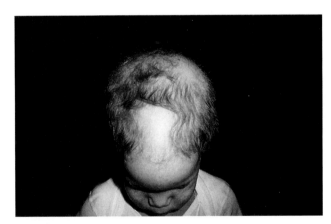

FIGURE 6–127. Poikiloderma of the face in the same child.

Anhidrotic Ectodermal Dysplasia (AED)

SYNONYMS   Hypohidrotic Ectodermal Dysplasia
                     Christ-Siemens-Touraine
                         Syndrome

DEFINITION

A hereditary disorder characterized by changes in the structures derived from the ectoderm: the skin and its appendages and the teeth

ETIOLOGY

It is inherited as an X-linked recessive trait.

EPIDEMIOLOGY

1. More than 90% of patients are boys.
2. The incidence is 1 in 100,000.

PATHOGENESIS

There is an embryologic ectodermal defect.

LABORATORY

1. Skin biopsy
   a. Best site: palm
   b. Shows diminished size and number of eccrine glands.

BOX 6–46   *Differential Diagnosis of Anhidrotic Ectodermal Dysplasia*

Hidrotic ectodermal dysplasia (Clouston syndrome) has the following features:
   Inherited as an autosomal dominant disorder
   Sparse hair
   Normal facies
   Keratoderma of palms and soles
   Dystrophic nails

---

2. Dental radiographs demonstrate whether tooth buds are present or not.

TREATMENT

1. Avoid overheating. The child must stay in an air conditioned or cool environment.
2. Refer the child to a dentist.
3. Treat sinopulmonary infections.
4. Genetic counseling
5. Enroll the patient in the

   National Foundation for Ectodermal Dysplasia
   219 East Main Street, P.O. Box 114
   Mascoutah, IL 62258-0114
   Telephone (618) 566-2020
   Fax (618) 566-4718

PROGNOSIS

Normal life span

KEY POINTS

Anhidrotic Ectodermal Dysplasia

- Affected individuals have characteristic facies.
- There is a tendency toward febrile episodes and sinopulmonary infections.

TABLE 6–49
Clinical Features of Anhidrotic Ectodermal Dysplasia

Decreased to absent sweating
Frequent febrile episodes during infancy
Sparse hair, eyebrows, and eyelashes
Absent to decreased number of teeth
Erupted teeth are peg-shaped
Increased susceptibility to sinopulmonary infections
Intelligence normal
Characteristic facies
    Saddle nose
    Frontal bossing
    Periorbital darkening
    Everted lips

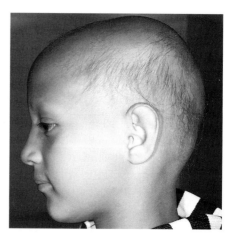

FIGURE 6–128. Anhidrotic ectodermal dysplasia, sparse hair.

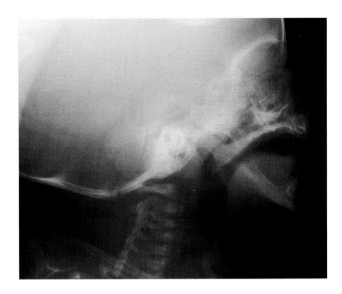

FIGURE 6–129. Anhidrotic ectodermal dysplasia in a 2-year-old; tooth buds are absent.

Keloids

DEFINITION

An overgrowth of scar tissues

ETIOLOGY

It is an exaggerated tissue response to injury.

EPIDEMIOLOGY

1. More common in dark-skinned individuals
2. More common between the ages of 10 and 30 years
3. Rare in infants

PATHOGENESIS

There is increased activity of the fibroblasts, leading to increased collagen synthesis; skin collagenase is inhibited, and collagen breakdown does not occur.

TABLE 6–50
Clinical Features of Keloids

Skin Lesions

Firm
Smooth
Hairless growth
Appears at a healed injury site
Claw-like prolongations may extend beyond edges of trauma site
May be pruritic
May be painful and tender
Most common sites
  Earlobes
  Anterior chest
  Upper back
  Shoulders

BOX 6–47	*Differential Diagnosis of Keloids*

Hypertrophic scar
  Limited to the edges of the trauma site

LABORATORY

None

TREATMENT

1. Refer the patient to a dermatologist.
2. Intralesional injections of triamcinolone 20 mg/mL
3. Excision followed by triamcinolone injections into the site
4. Silicone gel sheeting
5. Tretinoin liquid 0.05% applied twice daily over the lesion

KEY POINTS

Keloids

- Keloids are more common in dark-skinned people.
- The most common sites are the ear lobes, anterior chest, upper back, and shoulders.

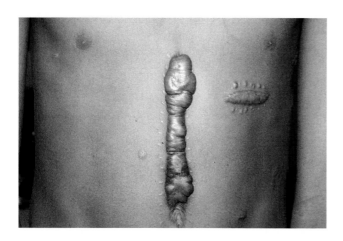

FIGURE 6–130. A keloid on the midline of the torso, and a hypertrophic scar on the left subcostal area.

Acanthosis Nigricans

DEFINITION

A disorder of unknown cause characterized by distinct skin findings. It may be associated with systemic disease.

BOX 6–48	*Acanthosis Nigricans and Associated Conditions*

Obesity
Hypertension
Lipid disorder
Hyperinsulinemia (insulin-resistant diabetes)
Polycystic ovary
Hyperandrogenic states
Endocrine disorders
Crouzon syndrome

ETIOLOGY

The exact cause is unknown.

EPIDEMIOLOGY

1. Acanthosis nigricans is seen in 7% of a selected pediatric population.
2. It is more common in obese African-American adolescents.
3. It may be familial.

PATHOGENESIS

Presumably there is a circulating keratinocyte growth factor.

LABORATORY

1. Fasting blood sugar, oral glucose tolerance test, HbA1C
2. Lipid profile
3. Other tests depending on other clinical associations

DIFFERENTIAL DIAGNOSIS

Confluent and reticulated papillomatosis of Gougerot and Carteaud, tinea versicolor, postinflammatory hyperpigmentation

TREATMENT

1. Treatment for the underlying disease
2. Weight reduction
3. Topical tretinoin solution

PROGNOSIS

Without weight reduction, the lesions do not respond well to topical treatment.

KEY POINTS

Acanthosis Nigricans

■ Acanthosis nigricans may be a marker for insulin-resistant diabetes mellitus.
■ The individual may be at risk for hypertension and hyperlipidemia.

TABLE 6–51
Clinical Features of Acanthosis Nigricans

Skin Lesions
Dark
Velvety
Dirty-looking
Thickened skin
Most common sites
  Posterior neck
  Axillae
  Intertriginous areas
  Interphalangeal areas

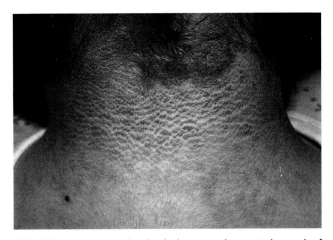

FIGURE 6–131. Acanthosis nigricans on the posterior neck of a child with Down syndrome. The lesions are dark and velvety in appearance.

Phytophotodermatitis

DEFINITION

An acute phototoxic skin eruption following contact with certain plants, fruits, or vegetables, and sun exposure.

ETIOLOGY

The plants, fruits, and vegetables that contain furocoumarin (psoralen), which is responsible for this reaction, include limes, lemons, bergamot, celery, parsnips, figs, and dill.

EPIDEMIOLOGY

1. It is common among handlers of the aforementioned produce.
2. Children may be exposed directly or indirectly.

PATHOGENESIS

1. It is a photoirritant contact dermatitis.
2. The furocoumarin reacts with the ultraviolet A spectrum of sunlight to produce the dermatitis.

BOX 6–49   *Differential Diagnosis of Phytophotodermatitis*

Ecchymoses from child abuse

LABORATORY

None

TREATMENT

None

PROGNOSIS

The hyperpigmentation resolves slowly over weeks to months.

KEY POINTS

Phytophotodermatitis

- The skin findings consist of hyperpigmented patches with a bizarre configuration.
- The most common produce containing the offending substance are limes and lemons, used in mixing drinks or in making lemonade.
- A history must be elicited because often it is thought by the parents to be irrelevant.
- May be mistaken for child abuse.

TABLE 6–52
Clinical Features of Phytophotodermatitis

Skin Lesions

Brown or erythematous patches
Puzzling, bizarre configuration (e.g., streaks, drip-marks, hand prints)
Occasionally, lesions may be bullous

Important Feature

Reaction occurs during hot and humid sunny days

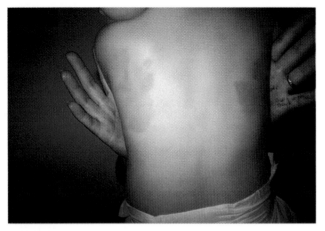

FIGURE 6–132. An infant with phytophotodermatitis of 3 weeks' duration. The mother, whose hands were wet with lime juice, picked her up while she was unclothed on a hot, humid sunny day. The hyperpigmentation corresponded to the mother's hands.

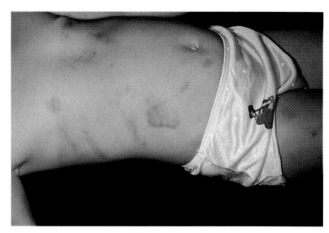

FIGURE 6–133. Phytophotodermatitis. Child presented with bizarre streaky hyperpigmentation on the torso. A history of mixing lemonade while at the beach was obtained.

Dermoid Cyst

DEFINITION

An epithelium-lined cyst that contains epidermal appendages, including hair, sebum, keratin, and apocrine glands

ETIOLOGY

1. Developmental
2. Arises as a consequence of displacement of dermal and epidermal cells into and along the embryonic lines of fusion.

EPIDEMIOLOGY

1. No racial predilection
2. Male-female ratio is 1:1.

PATHOGENESIS

It results from sequestration of skin at the lines of embryonic closure during skin development.

LABORATORY

CT scan or magnetic resonance imaging (MRI) of midline lesions to exclude sinus tract and intracranial extension

COMPLICATIONS

1. Secondary infection
2. Meningitis

BOX 6–50	*Differential Diagnosis of Dermoid Cyst*
Nasal glioma Encephalocele Meningocele Epidermoid cyst Hemangioma	

TREATMENT

Refer patient to a pediatric surgeon for surgical excision.

KEY POINT

Dermoid Cyst

- MRI must be performed on midline lesions to exclude intracranial extension, nasal glioma, or encephalocele.

TABLE 6-53
Clinical Features of Dermoid Cysts

Skin Lesions

Present at birth or early infancy
Firm
Skin-colored nodules
Asymptomatic unless infected
If in midline, there may be an associated sinus tract with
  intracranial extension

Location

Head or neck
Common around eyes, particularly the lateral eyebrow

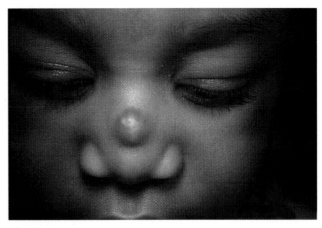

FIGURE 6-134. A 1-year-old child with dermoid cyst on the midline of the nose. CT scan was negative for intracranial extension. The cyst was surgically excised.

Hidradenitis Suppurativa

DEFINITION

A chronic suppurative, cicatricial disease of the apocrine sweat glands

ETIOLOGY/PATHOGENESIS

1. Primary keratinous occlusion of the apocrine duct is followed by secondary bacterial infection and then rupture of the apocrine gland, leading to extension of the infection or inflammation to adjacent areas and scarring.
2. Bacteria are *not* the underlying cause of hidradenitis; they participate in the process and thus represent a secondary infection.
3. Microbiology of early lesions
   a. Coagulase-positive staphylococci or streptococci
   b. Anaerobes
   c. Gram-negative pathogens including *Escherichia coli* or *Pseudomonas aeruginosa* are occasional contaminants.
4. Several factors that predispose to the occurrence of hidradenitis are
   a. Obesity
   b. Warm tropical climates
   c. Hormonal factors (low estrogens or presence of androgenic progestins)
   d. End-organ hypersensitivity to androgens
5. Use of antiperspirants or deodorants may exacerbate the condition.

EPIDEMIOLOGY

1. More common in African-Americans than in whites
2. More common in adults than in adolescents
3. Age at presentation (in pediatric population)
   a. Most commonly seen during puberty (with the development of the apocrine glands)
   b. Rarely seen in children before the onset of puberty.
4. Female-male ratio is 3 to 4:1.
5. Axillary lesions are more common in females; groin lesions are more common in males.
6. May be associated with endocrinopathies (e.g., diabetes, Cushing disease)

INHERITANCE

1. Most cases are sporadic.
2. Familial occurrence with autosomal dominant inheritance (with a tendency to follicular occlusion) has been seen.

BOX 6-51   *Follicular Occlusion Triad*

Hidradenitis suppurativa
Cystic acne vulgaris
Dissecting cellulitis of scalp

CLINICAL FEATURES

1. Involvement is often bilateral
2. Most common areas of involvement
   a. Axillae
   b. Anogenital areas
   c. Inguinal creases
   d. Buttocks
   e. Upper inner thighs
3. Less common areas of involvement
   a. Areolae, periareolar and submammary regions of the breasts
   b. Periumbilical region
   c. Scalp, face, posterior neck, shoulders

4. Characteristics of lesions
   a. They begin as deep-seated tender, inflammatory nodules that tend to coalesce, enlarge, and within few days become purulent.
   b. Malodorous discharge may be thin and serous or frankly purulent.
   c. Milder cases resolve spontaneously or after incision and drainage of the abscess.
   d. In severe cases, new lesions develop, leading to subsequent suppuration and rupture.
   e. During healing, deep fibrosis occurs, leaving sinus tracts and fistulas admixed with the new inflammatory lesions.
5. There is wide variation in the extent and severity of the disorder among patients.

LABORATORY

1. Culture and sensitivity of skin lesions may help in guiding the therapy.
2. Serum values of androgen may be elevated in some patients.

COMPLICATIONS

1. Painful, draining abscesses and accompanying odor often produce considerable physical and social debilitation.
2. Rare complications include:
   a. Urethral, bladder, or rectal fistulas
   b. Squamous cell carcinoma (in an area affected for more than 10 years)
   c. Pyoderma gangrenosum

TREATMENT

1. Early in the course
   a. Antibiotic therapy
      (1) Topical (e.g., clindamycin)
      (2) Long-term oral therapy (e.g., erythromycin, first-generation cephalosporin)
   b. Incision and drainage of abscesses
   c. Intralesional corticosteroids (e.g., triamcinolone acetonide) injected into inflamed areas may reverse the process.
   d. Systemic corticosteroids (e.g., prednisone) may be necessary in severe cases.
   e. Oral retinoids have been shown to be effective.
2. In recalcitrant cases
   a. Surgical extirpation of apocrine glands
   b. Total excision of the hair-bearing area, followed by split-thickness skin grafting may be the only curative option
3. General measures
   a. Weight reduction
   b. Loose-fitting clothes
   c. Improved local hygiene
   d. Antiseptic compresses (e.g., povidone-iodine or chlorhexidine) or Burow's solution soaks

PROGNOSIS

1. Recurrences are common.
2. The course is chronic; if severe, the disease leads to fistulas, dermal scarring, lymphedema, and even restriction of arm or leg movement.

KEY POINTS

Hidradenitis Suppurativa

- A chronic, recurrent inflammatory disease of the apocrine sweat glands
- Clinically seen as painful nodules or abscesses with chronically draining sinuses involving the axillae, groin, or perineum

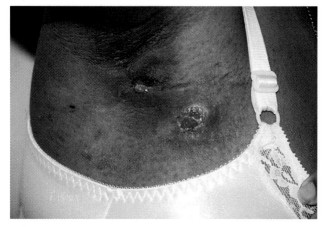

FIGURE 6–135. Hidradenitis suppurativa showing nodules, abscess, and draining sinus tract. Both axillae were involved in this 15-year-old African-American girl. This was the third recurrence of the lesion.

TABLE 6–54
Differential Diagnosis of Hidradenitis Suppurativa

Axillary Region	Anogenital Region
Suppurative lymphadenitis (from any cause)	Furunculosis
Furunculosis	Crohn's disease
Nodulocystic acne	Ulcerative colitis
Deep fungal infections (e.g., actinomycosis)	Granuloma inguinale
Cat-scratch disease	Lymphogranuloma venereum
Scrofuloderma	Bartholin gland abscesses

Spider Bites

SYNONYM   Arachnidism

DEFINITION

A reaction to the bites of two major species of spiders.

ETIOLOGY

1. Brown recluse spider (*Loxsoceles reclusa*)
   a. 1 to 5 cm long
   b. Violin-shaped mark on the cephalothorax
   c. It likes corners and warm dark places such as closets and storage boxes.
2. Black widow spider (*Latrodectus mactans*)
   a. Size of a quarter
   b. Red hourglass mark on the abdomen
   c. Seen in outhouses.

BOX 6-52   *Differential Diagnosis of Spider Bites*

Cellulitis
Erysipelas
Ecthyma gangrenosum
Purpura fulminans
Bacterial or rickettsial infections
Other arthropod bite reactions

EPIDEMIOLOGY

1. The brown recluse spider is found everywhere in the United States and is indigenous in the south-central states.
2. The black widow spider is found in the southwest and west coast states.

PATHOGENESIS

1. The brown recluse spider produces a toxic enzyme, sphingomyelinase, which is responsible for the local tissue necrosis.
2. The black widow spider produces a neurotoxin.

LABORATORY

1. Complete blood count
2. Electrolytes

TREATMENT

1. Clean the wound, rest and elevate the area.
2. Give a booster tetanus shot.
3. Cold compresses over the area slow the spread of the venom.
4. Local injection of steroid is given when severe swelling and inflammation are present.
5. In patients with extensive necrosis, debridement and skin grafting may be necessary.
6. Muscle relaxants help in patients with black widow spider envenomation.
7. Supportive treatment with fluids and analgesics.

PROGNOSIS

Guarded in patients with severe systemic reactions.

KEY POINTS

Spider Bites

- The best treatment is prevention: keep children away from places where there may be spiders.
- Spiders are indigenous to some areas of the United States but may be found anywhere.

TABLE 6-55
Clinical Features of Brown Recluse Spider Bite

Local Reactions

"Flag sign" (red, white, and blue): Wound has a pale center surrounded by a dusky purple area and then an area of erythema
Dark eschar in the center may be seen
With severe envenomation: Extensive necrosis of the area may develop

Systemic Reactions

Nausea, vomiting, malaise, fever, chills
Severe hemolysis and renal failure (in 1% of patients)

TABLE 6-56
Clinical Features of Black Widow Spider Bite

Local Reactions

Area is nondescript
Mild erythema

Systemic Reactions

Headache, nausea, vomiting
Pain, paralysis, profuse sweating
Cramping and rigidity of muscle groups
May be mistaken for appendicitis (with abdominal muscle involvement)

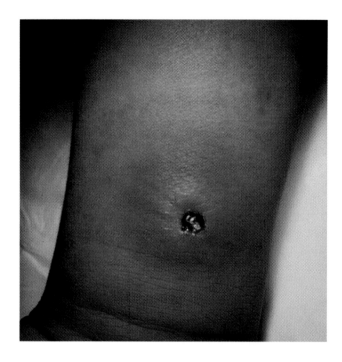

FIGURE 6–136. Local reaction to brown recluse spider bite.

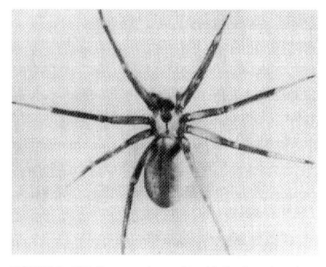

FIGURE 6–137. Brown recluse spider. Violin-shaped mark on the cephalothorax. (From Goddard J. Physician's guide to arthropods of medical importance. 2nd ed. Boca Raton, CRC Press, 1996.)

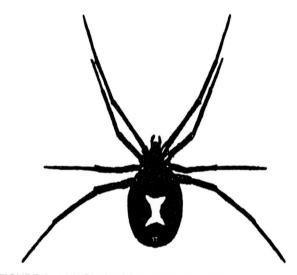

FIGURE 6–138. Black widow spider. Hourglass-shape mark is visible on the abdomen. (From Goddard J. Physician's guide to arthropods of medical importance. 2nd ed. Boca Raton, CRC Press, 1996.)

7

Hematology and Oncology

Binita R. Shah, M.D.

Iron Deficiency Anemia

DEFINITION

Insufficient amount of iron leading to a decrease in hemoglobin (Hgb) production and resulting in a hypochromic microcytic anemia.

ETIOLOGY (see also Table 7–1)

1. Consumption of a large quantity (a quart or more) of unsupplemented milk
2. Rapid growth spurt leading to expansion of red cell mass
   a. Early infancy
   b. Adolescence
3. Low-birth-weight premature infants
   a. Lower iron stores at birth (in utero transplacental transfer of iron occurs during 3rd trimester)
   b. Rapid growth rate postnatally
   c. These infants may deplete their iron stores as early as 2 months of age.
4. History of pica (eating of non-nutritious substances like plaster, dirt, clay)
5. Chronic diseases
   a. Juvenile rheumatoid arthritis
   b. Cystic fibrosis

BOX 7–1   *Iron Metabolism*

- Newborn's iron content = 0.3–0.5 g; adult's iron content = 5 g
- To make up the 4.5 g difference in the first 15 years of life 0.8 mg/day of iron must be absorbed
- Normal iron loss = 1 mg/day
- For a positive iron balance during childhood 0.8–1.5 mg/day of iron must be absorbed from the diet
- Normal iron absorption from the average mixed diet = 10%
- Thus, for optimum nutrition 8–15 mg/day of iron is necessary

---

EPIDEMIOLOGY

1. Anemia caused purely by inadequate dietary iron is unusual before 4 to 6 months of age
2. In term infants the common age for nutritional iron deficiency is between 9 and 24 months. Thereafter it is relatively infrequent until adolescence.

PATHOPHYSIOLOGY (see Box 7–1)

1. Availability of iron becomes rate limiting in Hgb production $\Rightarrow$ fall in red blood cell (RBC) production in the bone marrow.
2. RBCs produced are small and lack hemoglobin.

LABORATORY (see also Table 7–4)

1. Nutritional iron deficiency anemia can often be diagnosed by the dietary history.
2. Complete blood test
   a. Leukocyte count normal
   b. Hypochromic microcytic anemia (low mean corpuscular hemoglobin [MCH] and mean corpuscular volume [MCV]; RBCs have decreased hemoglobin content and are smaller than normal in size) (see Fig. 7–2).
   c. Reticulocyte percentage is normal or minimally elevated.
   d. Thrombocytosis ($>600,000/mm^3$) or thrombocytopenia (rare)
   e. Elevated red cell distribution width (an index of the variation in size of RBCs)
      (1) One of the earliest signs of iron deficiency
      (2) It is also more sensitive in screening for iron deficiency than serum values of iron or ferritin or transferrin saturation.
3. Decreased serum ferritin values (<10 ng/mL) reflect depletion of iron stores
4. Decreased serum iron and increased iron-binding capacity result in serum transferrin saturation (serum iron/iron-binding capacity) of $<15\%$.
5. Hemoccult test for blood in stool
6. Bone marrow (not routinely indicated)
   a. Hypercellular with erythroid hyperplasia
   b. Normoblasts with poor hemoglobinization

TREATMENT

1. Iron therapy (see also Table 7–3)
   a. Given *orally* as a ferrous sulfate
   b. Dosage: 3 to 6 mg/kg/day of elemental iron given in two or three divided doses
   c. Preferably given with food high in ascorbic acid, which increases iron absorption (e.g., orange juice)
   d. Iron therapy should be continued for at least 8 weeks after a normal Hgb value to replenish the stores. This should be followed by a daily maintenance requirement.
2. Parenteral iron therapy
   a. Painful
   b. Response is same as that obtained by oral therapy.
   c. *Not* indicated unless malabsorption or poor compliance is present
3. Red cell transfusion
   a. Rarely required unless signs and symptoms associated with anemia pose a serious threat
   b. When indicated, it should be done slowly in the presence of hypervolemia and cardiac dilation.
4. Nutritional counseling
   a. Iron-fortified infant formula or breastfeeding is recommended until the infant is 1 year old.
   b. Milk or formula intake should not exceed 1 L/day to encourage the intake of variety of iron-rich solid foods.

KEY POINTS

Iron Deficiency Anemia

- Most common nutritional deficiency causing anemia
- *Suspect* blood loss if iron deficiency anemia develops within the first 4 to 6 months of life in full-term infants or if anemia persists or recurs after iron therapy at any age.
- Full-term infants should be given elemental iron 1 mg/kg/day (maximum 15 mg/day) starting no later than 4 months of age and continuing until 3 years of age.
- Preterm or low-birth-weight infants should be given elemental iron 2 to 4 mg/kg/day (maximum 15 mg/day) starting at 1 month of age.
- For infants younger than 12 months, only iron-fortified formula should be used for weaning or supplementing breast milk.

TABLE 7–1
Etiology of Iron Deficiency Anemia

Blood loss (overt or occult) from GI tract ⇒ chronic iron deficiency
  Chronic intestinal blood loss induced by heat-labile protein in whole cow's milk
  Meckel diverticulum
  Polyp
  Hemangioma
  Peptic ulcer
Blood loss through heavy menstrual flow
Chronic blood loss into lung parenchyma
  Primary pulmonary hemosiderosis (chronic pulmonary disease with chronic blood loss [iron sequestered and not available for re-utilization])

TABLE 7–2
Clinical Features of Iron Deficiency Anemia

Mild to moderate anemia (Hgb 7–10 g/dL)	Other features
Nonspecific symptoms or asymptomatic	Splenomegaly (10% to 15% of cases)
Severe anemia	Systemic signs
Pallor	Blue sclera
Irritability or lethargy	Alteration in cognitive performance
Anorexia, poor weight gain	Koilonychia
High-output cardiac failure	
Tachycardia	
Gallop rhythm	
Systolic murmur	
Cardiac dilation	

TABLE 7–3
Response to Iron Therapy in Iron Deficiency Anemia

Time After Iron Therapy	Response
12–24 hours	Replacement of intracellular iron enzymes Decreased irritability; increased appetite
48–72 hours	Reticulocytosis, peak at 5–7 days
4–30 days	Increase in Hgb level (as much as 0.5 g/dL/day)
1–3 months	Repletion of stores

Modified from Schwartz E: Iron deficiency anemia. In Behrman RE et al (eds): Nelson Textbook of Pediatrics, 15th ed. Philadelphia; W.B. Saunders, 1995. An appropriate response can be used for both diagnostic and therapeutic purposes.

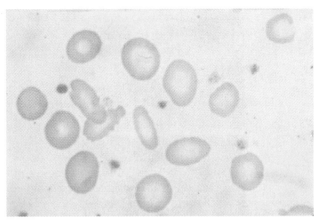

FIGURE 7–2. Iron deficiency anemia. Peripheral smear showing hypochromia, microcytosis, and variation in size (anisocytosis) and shape (poikilocytosis). (From Schwartz E: Iron Deficiency Anemia. In Behrman RE, Kliegman R, Arvin AM (eds): Nelson Textbook of Pediatrics, 15th ed. Philadelphia, WB Saunders, 1996.)

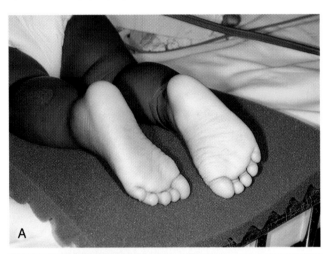

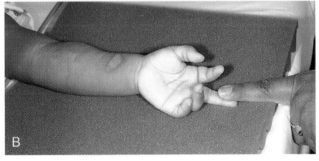

FIGURE 7–1. *A* and *B*, Extreme pallor on the foot and hand of an 18-month-old child with nutritional iron deficiency anemia (Hgb 3.0 g/dL, mean copuscular volume [MCV] 56, ferritin 2.1 ng/mL). He consumed about 48 oz of cow's milk daily and ate hardly any iron-fortified solid food.

TABLE 7–4
Differential Diagnosis of Hypochromic Microcytic Anemia

	Fe	TIBC	Ferritin	RDW	Hgb A$_2$	Lead	FEP
Iron deficiency	↓	↑	↓	↑	nl	nl	↑
Lead poisoning	nl	nl	nl	nl	nl	↑	↑
Beta thalassemia trait	nl	nl	nl	nl	↑	nl	nl
Alpha thalassemia trait	nl	nl	nl	nl	nl	nl	nl
Anemia of chronic disease	↓	↓	nl or ↑	nl	nl	nl	↑

Fe, iron; TIBC, total iron-binding capacity; RDW, red cell distribution width; Hgb A$_2$, hemoglobin A$_2$; FEP, free erythrocyte protoporphyrin.

Acute Hemolytic Anemia and Glucose-6-Phosphate Dehydrogenase (G6PD) Deficiency

INTRODUCTION/PATHOGENESIS

1. Reduced glutathione level in the red blood cells (RBCs) normally protects the sulfhydryl groups of hemoglobin and the RBC membrane from oxidation. On exposure to an oxidant stress (e.g., drug, toxin, infection), the amount of glucose that is metabolized via the hexose-monophosphate shunt is increased severalfold, leading to regeneration of reduced glutathione.
2. Individuals with an inherited defect in the hexose-monophosphate shunt (G6PD deficiency being most common) are unable to maintain an adequate level of reduced glutathione in their RBCs, making hemoglobin susceptible to oxidant insult. This leads to hemoglobin precipitation, membrane damage, and RBC destruction.
3. G6PD deficiency is the most common inherited shunt defect of RBCs.

ETIOLOGY (see also Table 7–5)

1. Degree of hemolysis varies with the drug (or oxidant stress), the amount ingested, and the severity of the enzyme deficiency in the patient.
2. Exposure to naphthalene products (e.g., moth balls)
   a. One of the most common offending oxidants, inducing moderate to severe life-threatening hemolysis in G6PD deficient African-American children (in our experience)
   b. Naphthalene is still commonly used as a moth repellent and is available in the form of balls, flakes, or cakes.
   c. It is a metabolite of naphthalene, alpha-naphthol, which is a potent hemolytic agent. Thus, hemolysis may be delayed by 1 to 3 days because naphthalene must be converted to alpha-naphthol by the liver.

EPIDEMIOLOGY

1. More than 100 distinct enzyme variants of G6PD have been documented.
2. Normal G6PD enzyme found in most whites is designated G6PD B or B$^+$.
3. Incidence of G6PD deficiency varies among different ethnic groups (e.g., Chinese 5%; Kurdish Jews as high as 75%)
4. The World Health Organization (WHO) classifies G6PD variants by degree of enzyme deficiency and tendency to hemolysis. There are at least four major G6PD deficiency variants associated with either acute drug or infection-induced hemolytic anemia.
   a. G6PD A$^-$ (most common variant in the United States; present in 13% of African-Americans males and 2% of females)
   b. G6PD Mediterranean (Israelis, Greeks)
   c. G6PD Canton (Chinese)

   d. G6PD Chicago (Americans of North European descent)

INHERITANCE

1. Synthesis of red cell G6PD is determined by a gene on the X chromosome. Thus, the deficiency is an X-linked trait and is caused by inheritance of any of the abnormal alleles of the gene responsible for synthesis of the G6PD molecule.
2. Affected males (hemizygotes) inherit the abnormal gene from their mothers, who are usually asymptomatic carriers (heterozygotes).
3. According to the Lyon hypothesis (inactivation of one of the two X chromosomes), the heterozygote female has two populations of RBCs; on average, half are normal and half are deficient in G6PD. Female carriers with a high proportion of deficient cells resemble the male hemizygote.
4. Absolute deficiency of G6PD is not compatible with life.

CLINICAL FEATURES (see also Table 7–6)

1. The majority of G6PD-deficient people are clinically and hematologically normal (minimal or no hemolysis) in the steady state.
2. The most classic manifestation of a G6PD-deficient child is acute hemolytic anemia secondary to an oxidant stress (see Table 7–5).
3. Clues in the history include ethnicity of patient and family, history of similar episodes in the past, and a family history of hemoglobinopathies or anemia.

LABORATORY (see also Table 7–7)

1. Normally, G6PD enzyme activity decreases as RBCs age. Thus, during acute hemolytic crises the oldest RBCs with the least G6PD activity are the first to hemolyze, followed by younger RBCs.
2. Heinz bodies:
   a. Are seen by supravital staining with crystal violet
   b. Are rapidly removed by the spleen and may not be seen after the first day or two
   c. Their removal (by "pinching off" the peripheral portion of the RBCs) leads to "bite cells" and fragmentation (from multiple bites).
3. Quantitative assay of G6PD enzyme activity
   a. Following an acute hemolytic episode, reticulocytes and young RBCs (which have a significantly higher G6PD enzyme activity than older RBCs) predominate in the circulation.
   b. Diagnosis of G6PD may be obscured at the time of acute hemolysis (because of "false" normal levels).
   c. After recovery, patient requires a repeat G6PD enzyme assay to confirm the diagnosis.
   d. G6PD assays of patient's mother (for a male child) or both parents (for a female child) may reveal evidence of heterozygosity or hemizygosity.

TREATMENT

1. Hospitalization
2. Oxygen therapy and close monitoring of vital signs including cardiac and pulse oxymetry
3. Removal of oxidant stressor (e.g., discontinue suspected drug) and/or treat infection
4. Packed red blood cell transfusion is usually indicated for
   a. Hemodynamically unstable or symptomatic patients
   b. Patients with hemoglobin value of ≤6 g/dL
   c. Patients with Hgb value of between 6 and 9 g/dL with ongoing hemolysis (ongoing hemoglobinuria)
5. Parenteral hydration to maintain adequate urine output (to prevent renal damage from hemoglobinuria) with urinary alkalinization if necessary

PREVENTION

1. Counseling of family to prevent acute hemolytic episodes related to known oxidants
   a. Removal of the offending agent (e.g., naphthalene products) from the child's environment
   b. Avoidance of medications known to induce hemolysis (see Table 7–5).
   c. Avoidance of fava beans in the diet
2. Education of family about signs/symptoms of hemolysis (to promote early detection and treatment)

3. Males belonging to ethnic group with a significant incidence of G6PD deficiency should be tested for the defect *before* drugs that are potent oxidants are prescribed.

KEY POINTS

Acute Hemolytic Anemia and G6PD Deficiency

- The majority of G6PD deficient people are normal with minimal or no hemolysis in the steady state.
- Acute hemolytic anemia develops when G6PD-deficient RBCs are exposed to oxidant stress.
- Sudden onset of dark urine, pallor, and jaundice in a male child with a history of exposure to an oxidant suggests intravascular hemolysis with G6PD deficiency.
- A G6PD level in low to "normal" range in the presence of reticulocytosis *actually* suggests G6PD deficiency.

TABLE 7–5
Oxidant Stressors for Acute Hemolysis in G6PD Deficiency

Infections	Drugs
Bacterial	Antimalarials
Viral	Primaquine
	Chloroquine
Chemicals	Sulfonamides and sulfones
Exposure to naphthalene	Sulfafurazole
products	Sulfapyridine
Ingestion	Dapsone
Inhalation of vapors*	Nitrofurans
Absorption through skin*†	Nitrofurantoin
Transplacental exposure in	Analgesics
newborn (from mother)	Acetylsalicylic acid
	Acetophenetidin
Miscellaneous	
Ingestion of fava beans	

* For example, playing in room where mothballs are stored.
† For example, wearing diapers stored in moth products.

TABLE 7–6
Clinical Features of Acute Hemolytic Anemia with G6PD Deficiency

Pallor ⇒ fatigue, malaise
Tachycardia
Splenomegaly (moderately enlarged, tender)
Hepatomegaly
Hypovolemic shock or heart failure (severe, rapid drop in Hgb/Hct)
Dark urine (often described as brown, red, tea-colored, or cola-colored)
Acute hemolytic episodes
  Usually self-limited
  Hemolysis occurs 24–48 hours after an oxidant stress
  Spontaneous recovery is heralded by reticulocytosis
  Hgb concentration increases starting 4–5 days after acute hemolysis

---

TABLE 7–7
Laboratory Findings in Acute Hemolytic Anemia

Anemia (usually normochromic normocytic)
Reticulocytosis (evidence of bone marrow response to anemia)
Hemolysis on peripheral smear (fragmented RBCs, blister cells, anisocytosis, poikilocytosis)
Heinz bodies (precipitates of denatured Hgb within the RBCs)
Jaundice
  Indirect hyperbilirubinemia
  Direct bilirubin and liver chemistries normal
Elevated serum lactate dehydrogenase
Transient elevation of urea nitrogen (renal failure uncommon)
Decreased or undetectable serum haptoglobin
Hemoglobinemia (free hemoglobin in the plasma; seen as pink-red supernatant)
Methemoglobinemia
Hemoglobinuria (from intravascular hemolysis)
  Strongly positive result on dipstick for blood
  After centrifugation, supernatant is as dark as before
  RBCs absent or normal (0–5 RBCs/HPF) on microscopic examination

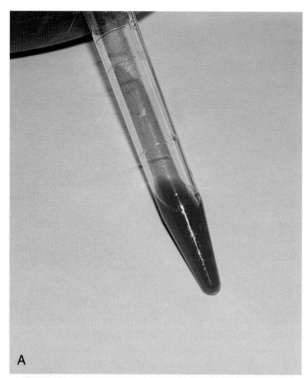

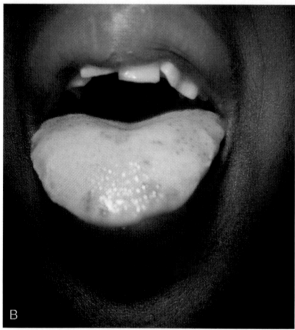

FIGURE 7–3. *A,* Reddish urine (hemoglobinuria) and extreme pallor (*B*) in a 3-year-old African-American male child who presented with lethargy and a hemoglobin value of 3.2 g/dL.

TABLE 7–8
Differential Diagnosis of "Red Urine"*

Hematuria (see Box 15–6)
Hemoglobinuria
  Acute transfusion reaction
  G6PD deficiency
  Paroxysmal cold
    hemoglobinuria
  Blackwater fever (malaria)
  Physical trauma (e.g., march
    hemoglobinuria)
Food ingestion
  Beets
  Blackberries
  Azo dyes
  Red food color

Drugs
  Nitrofurantoin
  Pyridium
  Phenolphthalein
  Deferoxamine mesylate
  Rifampin
Urates

* Red, tea-colored, cola-colored, pink, burgundy, or dark brown urine.

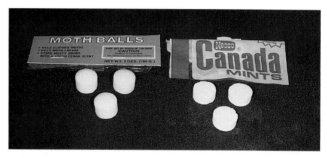

FIGURE 7–4. Naphthalene moth balls (which look like candy as shown here) were ingested by the same child (mentioned in Fig. 7–3) 2 days prior to the onset of above symptoms. Mothballs were used by this family in the bedroom closets as moth repellents.

Acute Immune Thrombocytopenic Purpura

SYNONYM   Acute Idiopathic
               Thrombocytopenic Purpura

DEFINITION

1. Immune thrombocytopenic purpura (ITP) in children is an *acquired* hemorrhagic disorder that results from excessive destruction of circulating platelets.

2. It is classified as
   a. Acute ITP
   b. Chronic ITP (thrombocytopenia persisting >6 months)

ETIOLOGY

1. About 70% of patients have an antecedent viral infection.
2. Both the usual childhood illnesses (e.g., varicella, rubella, rubeola, mumps, upper respiratory tract infection, infectious mononucleosis) and immunizations have been associated with ITP.

EPIDEMIOLOGY

1. Immune thrombocytopenic purpura is the most common cause of acquired thrombocytopenia in childhood with a frequency of 4 to 8 in 100,000 children per year.
   a. Acute ITP: seen in about 85% to 90% of cases
   b. Chronic ITP: seen in about 10% to 15% of cases
2. Common age at presentation (two peaks)
   a. Acute ITP: 1 to 4 years
   b. Chronic ITP: adolescence
3. Gender predilection
   a. Acute ITP: Male and female ratio equal
   b. Chronic ITP: Female-male ratio is $3:1$.

PATHOGENESIS

1. An immune mechanism is the basis for thrombocytopenia.
2. Sensitization by viral antigens leads to production of antibodies that cross-react with glycoprotein on the platelet membrane, causing subsequent premature destruction of the antibody-coated platelets in the spleen.

LABORATORY

1. Complete blood count (CBC)
   a. White blood cell count, differential and morphology, and hemoglobin level are normal
   b. Smear is normal except for thrombocytopenia:
      (1) Severity of thrombocytopenia is variable.
      (2) Platelet count is usually less than 50,000/mm^3 (a count of $<150,000$ indicates thrombocytopenia; normal platelet count ranges from $150,000-400,000$/mm^3).
      (3) Platelets seen on the smear are large (megathrombocytes), reflecting active thrombopoiesis and increased turnover of platelets.
   c. Anemia may develop after significant bleeding.
2. Prothrombin time, partial thromboplastin time, fibrinogen, and fibrin split product are normal.
3. Bleeding time and clot retraction (tests that depend on platelets) are abnormal.
4. Bone marrow aspiration (see also Box 7–2)
   a. Normal erythrocytic and granulocytic series
   b. Megakaryocytes are normal or increased.
5. Antinuclear antibody and human immunodeficiency virus (HIV) tests, especially in an adolescent or as indicated

---

| BOX 7–2 | *Bone Marrow Aspiration and ITP* |

Not routinely indicated
Usually indicated in patients presenting with features *atypical* of acute ITP; examples include
   Anemia
   Neutropenia
   Reticulocytopenia
   Hepatosplenomegaly

DIFFERENTIAL DIAGNOSIS (see also Tables 7–10 and 7–11)

1. Acute ITP is a clinical diagnosis reached by exclusion of other causes of thrombocytopenia.
2. Immune thrombocytopenia can be a presenting sign of systemic lupus erythematosus or acquired immunodeficiency syndrome (AIDS), especially in adolescents.

COMPLICATIONS

1. Intracranial bleeding
   a. Seen usually with a platelet count of less than 10,000 to 20,000/mm^3 and when signs of significant hemorrhage are present (e.g., oral mucosal bleeding, hematuria, or hematochezia).
   b. It occurs in less than 0.5% of patients.
   c. Accounts for virtually all the mortality seen in this disease
2. Gastrointestinal hemorrhage (rare)
3. Hematuria (rare)

TREATMENT

1. Mild ITP (platelet count between 30,000 and 50,000/mm^3)
   a. In the absence of mucosal or retinal hemorrhage, patients can be observed with no specific therapy.
   b. Usually the patient can be followed on an outpatient basis with CBC performed once or twice weekly.
2. Hospitalization and hematology consultation, especially for
   a. Patients with mucosal or retinal hemorrhages
   b. Patients at high risk for bleeding (platelet count $<30,000$/mm^3)
3. Treatment alternatives (any of the following may be used for patients with a platelet count of $<30,000$/mm^3 and/or mucosal bleeding):
   a. Intravenous immune globulin (IVIG)
      (1) Advantages include rapid onset of action and high effectiveness ($>90\%$)
      (2) It can be given *without* prior bone marrow examination
      (3) Usual dose is 1 g/kg for 1 to 2 days
   b. Intravenous methylprednisolone (30 mg/kg/day for 3 days)
   c. Prednisone

(1) Advantages include low cost, oral administration, and effectiveness in 75% to 80% of patients.

(2) A bone marrow examination is required prior to starting the therapy.

(3) Usual dose is 2 mg/kg/day for 2 to 4 weeks followed by a tapering dose.

d. Intravenous anti-D immunoglobulin

(1) Immune globulin against D antigen of Rh blood group system; when given to Rh+ children with ITP, it produces a rise in platelet count

(2) Useful adjunct as outpatient therapy

4. Platelet transfusions

a. Antiplatelet antibodies continue to be produced in patients with acute ITP, and transfused platelets are consumed rapidly.

b. Platelet transfusions are *not* effective in increasing and sustaining platelet counts for a long time. However, this may be a life-saving measure in life-threatening situations.

5. Life-threatening hemorrhages (e.g., intracranial bleeding or retroperitoneal bleeding)

a. IVIG 1 g/kg/day for 2 days *and*

b. Methylprednisolone IV 30 mg/kg/day for 3 days

c. Platelet transfusions every 6 to 8 hours

d. Splenectomy (usually reserved for the rare child with severe acute ITP and intracranial bleeding)

6. Education of family and patient

a. Activities that increase the risk of head injury, falls, or trauma should be restricted (e.g., rollerskating, ice-skating, contact sports).

b. Laws on use of helmets and seat belts should be strictly enforced.

c. Avoid rectal temperature taking and intramuscular injections.

d. Avoid platelet-inhibiting drugs (e.g., aspirin, antihistamines).

e. Avoid direct exposure to sunlight for prolonged periods. This produces petechiae and purpura in a child with thrombocytopenia.

f. Educate patient about signs and symptoms of increased intracranial pressure.

g. A rule of thumb for children with a low platelet count: "avoid any activity in which one foot is not on the ground at all times."

PROGNOSIS

1. This is a self-limited disorder in 90% of children.

2. Complete recovery occurs in 75% of patients within 12 weeks and in 90% by 9 to 12 months after onset. Most recover in 8 weeks.

3. Acute phase with mucocutaneous hemorrhage lasts approximately 1 to 2 weeks. Thrombocytopenia may persist after this, but hemorrhage subside.

4. Relapses may be seen during the first several months to years after diagnosis.

5. Chronic ITP develops in 10% of children. It is usually not possible at diagnosis to predict which patients have acute ITP and which ones will go on to develop chronic ITP.

KEY POINTS

Acute Immune Thrombocytopenic Purpura

- Most common thrombocytopenia of childhood
- Acute onset of petechiae, purpura, and epistaxis in a well-appearing child with otherwise normal findings on physical examination suggests acute ITP.
- Prednisone therapy is usually not given without a bone marrow examination because of the risk of temporarily masking acute leukemia.

BOX 7–3   *Purpura*

- Purpura = blood in the skin or mucous membranes
- Purpuric lesions *do not* blanch
- Purpura is subdivided into:

  Petechiae: small (pinpoint) reddish macular lesions

  Ecchymoses: larger lesions that may be tender and, when severe, may be raised above the skin surface

---

TABLE 7–9
Clinical Features of Acute ITP

Antecedent viral infection
  About 70% of cases
  Interval between infection and onset of purpura: 1–4 weeks
    (average 2 weeks)
Onset of ITP is usually acute
Patient appears clinically well
  Absence of symptoms/signs suggestive of malignancy or
    collagen disease
  Absence of anorexia, fever, or weight loss
  Absence of bone pain, hepatosplenomegaly,
    lymphadenopathy, or joint swelling; mild splenomegaly
    may be present (5% to 10%)
Mucocutaneous bleeding
  Occurs spontaneously or after minor trauma
  Sites of hemorrhage (any of the following)
    Skin: pinpoint petechiae to large areas of ecchymosis
    Head, eyes, ears, nose, throat: petechiae in buccal
      mucosa, epistaxis, gum bleeding, retinal hemorrhage
    Gastrointestinal: melena
    Genitourinary: menorrhagia, hematuria
  Mucous membrane hemorrhages ("wet purpura")
    May suggest an increased tendency toward serious
      bleeding
    Usually occur in patients with platelet count <20,000/mm³

TABLE 7–10
Differential Diagnosis of Thrombocytopenia

Decreased Platelet Production (Megakaryocytes Decreased or Abnormal Function)

Infection-induced thrombocytopenia (with or without leukopenia and/or anemia)
  Viral (e.g., rubella, varicella, Epstein-Barr virus, human immunodeficiency virus [HIV])
  Bacterial (e.g., syphilis, septicemia)
  Parasitic (e.g., malaria, toxoplasmosis)
Leukemia
Aplastic anemia
TAR (*T*hrombocytopenia, *A*bsent *R*adius) syndrome
Familial thrombocytopenia
  Wiskott-Aldrich syndrome
  May-Hegglin anomaly
  Chediak-Higashi anomaly
Drug-induced thrombocytopenia
  Anticonvulsants
  Antibiotics (e.g., sulfonamides, chloramphenicol)

Increased Platelet Consumption or Destruction

Antibody mediated (acute or chronic ITP)
Disseminated intravascular coagulopathy
Hypersplenism
Kasabach-Merrit syndrome
Hemolytic uremic syndrome

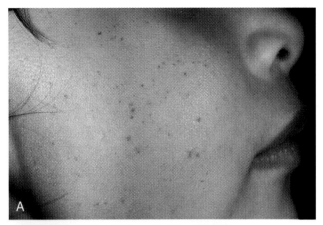

FIGURE 7–5. *A,* Petechiae over face. *B,* Petechiae and ecchymoses over lower extremity in this 2-year-old girl, who had normal values of WBC, differential, and Hgb. Her platelet count was 13,000/mm^3. Interestingly, she had received chickenpox vaccine 3 weeks prior to the onset of purpura. Purpura is most prominent over the legs and typically is *asymmetric* in acute ITP. In Henoch-Schönlein purpura, purpuric lesions are *symmetrically* distributed over the lower extremities (see pp. 186–188).

TABLE 7–11
Differential Diagnosis of Purpura

Trauma
  Accidental
  Child abuse
Henoch-Schönlein purpura
Scurvy
Letterer-Siwe disease
Ehlers-Danlos syndrome
Factor deficiencies (e.g., hemophilia)
	Infection
	  Bacterial (e.g., meningococcemia, endocarditis)
	  Viral (e.g, EBV, measles)
	  Rickettsial (e.g., Rocky mountain spotted fever)
	Drugs (e.g., sulfonamides, penicillins)

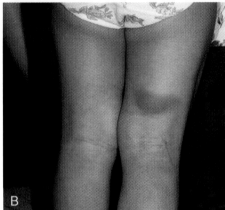

Sickle Cell Anemia

DEFINITION

Homozygous hemoglobin sickle cell disease (Hb SS) is characterized by chronic hemolytic anemia, recurrent painful vaso-occlusive episodes (crisis), and an increased tendency toward frequent infection with encapsulated bacteria.

ETIOLOGY/PATHOGENESIS

1. Substitution of valine for glutamic acid at the 6th position of the B-globin chain results in production of sickle hemoglobin (Hb S).

2. Consequences of this mutation include
    a. Polymerization of Hb S within the RBCs when they are deoxygenated, distorting their shape
    b. Sludging and stasis in the microvasculature secondary to obstruction of blood flow by tangled masses of abnormally shaped (sickled) cells, leading to distal ischemia and tissue infarction
    c. Acute and chronic organ dysfunction
    d. Shortened RBC lifespan of 10 to 20 days (normal RBC survival: 120 days)

EPIDEMIOLOGY

1. Sickle cell disease has a significant prevalence worldwide; it is found in equatorial Africa, the United States, the Caribbean, northern Europe, Australia, throughout the Mediterranean basin (Turkey, Italy, and Greece), Middle East, and India.
2. Incidence of Hb SS: 1 in 600 African-American newborns
3. About 8% of African-Americans carry the Hb S gene.
4. Male-female ratio is equal (no gender predominance).
5. People with sickle cell trait (carrier state) are asymptomatic.

BOX 7-4 *Sickle Cell Trait*

About 8% of African-Americans have sickle cell trait

Individuals with the trait have one normal and one abnormal gene

RBCs in sickle trait contain 30% to 40% Hb S

Individuals with trait are protected from falciparum malaria (unlike patients with sickle cell disease)

Benign, asymptomatic clinical course

Anemia or hemolysis should *not* be attributed to sickle trait

Sickling is absent under normal physiologic conditions

Sickling may occur if patient flies at high altitudes in unpressurized aircraft or during general anesthesia

Spontaneous gross hematuria (usually from left kidney)

Hyposthenuria (older children and adults)

Complications of traumatic hyphema (e.g., rebleeding) occur more commonly

---

INHERITANCE

1. Autosomal recessive
2. Inheritance of Hb S gene from both parents results in homozygous sickle cell anemia (Hb SS)

ANTENATAL DIAGNOSIS

1. Antenatal complete blood count (CBC) and hemoglobin electrophoresis for both parents in groups at risk
2. Chorionic villous sampling at 8 to 11 weeks of gestation
3. Amniocentesis

CLINICAL FEATURES (see also Table 7–12)

1. Hand-foot syndrome or acute sickle dactylitis
    a. Seen in about 33% of patients with sickle cell anemia
    b. Most common age: 6 months to 3 years (range 3 months to 5 years)
    c. Often the first clinical manifestation of sickle cell anemia during infancy
    d. Symmetrical infarction of metacarpals, metatarsals, or phalanges
    e. Seen clinically as symmetrical painful swelling of the hands and feet
    f. Patient refuses to bear weight.
    g. Episodes of dactylitis may recur.
2. Vaso-occlusive crisis of bones and joints
    a. Typically seen in children after the age of 3 or 4 years
    b. Infarction of the cortical bone, bone marrow, or periarticular tissue
    c. Swelling, tenderness, erythema, and limitation of movement

LABORATORY

1. CBC (evidence of hemolytic anemia and compensatory responses evoked by hemolytic anemia)
    a. Moderate to severe normochromic, normocytic anemia: average Hgb 7.5 g/dL (range 5.5 to 9.5 g/dL)
    b. Reticulocytosis: range 5% to 15%
    c. Increased nucleated RBCs
    d. Increased white blood cell count: range 10 to 25/mm^3
    e. Hyperbilirubinemia
        (1) Usually indirect hyperbilirubinemia (secondary to hemolysis)
        (2) Direct hyperbilirubinemia secondary to cholestasis (cholelithiasis)
2. Peripheral smear (see Fig. 7–6): irreversibly sickled RBCs (secondary to spontaneous sickling seen in vivo in sickle cell anemia)
3. "Sickle cell prep"
    a. RBCs are suspended in a 2% solution of a reducing agent (e.g., sodium metabisulfite).
    b. RBCs containing reduced Hb S assume a sickled shape.
    c. A positive sickle prep does not differentiate between sickle cell anemia and sickle cell trait or other hemoglobinopathies with Hb S.
4. Hemoglobin electrophoresis (after infancy)
    a. *Absence* of Hb A
    b. Hb S of more than 90%
    c. Normal amount of Hb A$_2$ (<3.5%)
    d. Variable amount of Hb F (2% to 20%)

e. Patients with sickle cell trait have Hb A (Hb A/ Hb S ratio is 60:40)
5. Radiographs (as indicated)
   a. Hand-foot syndrome
      (1) Initially soft tissue swelling only
      (2) Evidence of osteolysis, periostitis, bone reabsorption, and subperiosteal new bone formation after 1 to 2 weeks
   b. Chest radiograph for suspected acute chest syndrome or cardiomegaly
6. Abdominal ultrasound for suspected gallstones or cholecystitis
7. Bone scan and bone marrow scan to differentiate bone infarction from osteomyelitis

DIFFERENTIAL DIAGNOSIS

1. Other sickle cell syndromes (e.g., Hb SB thalassemia, Hb SC disease)
2. For bone infarction (swelling, tenderness of bone or joint)
   a. Trauma
   b. Osteomyelitis
   c. Acute rheumatic fever
   d. Systemic juvenile rheumatoid arthritis
   e. Leukemia

TREATMENT

1. Principles of management
   a. Management of vaso-occlusive episodes
   b. Prevention of serious complications
   c. Blood transfusions as indicated (see Tables 7–13 and 7–14)
   d. Folic acid supplementation
2. Vaso-occlusive crisis
   a. Hydration (oral or parenteral)
   b. Analgesics (therapy should be individualized as indicated)
      (1) Non-narcotic oral analgesics (e.g., acetaminophen)
      (2) Narcotic analgesics (e.g., acetaminophen with codeine, morphine, meperidine, ketorolac)
3. Antisickling agents
   a. Examples: hydroxyurea and butyrate
   b. Stimulates fetal hemoglobin synthesis
4. Allogeneic bone marrow transplantation from an identical sibling donor offers a hematologic cure for sickle cell disease, especially when performed in young children who have not suffered chronic organ damage.

5. Education of parents and patient about the need to seek immediate medical care for
   a. Fever
   b. Enlarging splenic size
   c. Vaso-occlusive episodes that fail to respond to analgesic therapy
   d. Increasing pallor and/or jaundice
   e. Significant headache or any neurologic signs or symptoms

PREVENTION

1. Universal newborn screening for hemoglobinopathy
2. Infants identified with Hb SS are seen at 4 months of age for confirmation of diagnosis, parent education, and beginning penicillin prophylaxis.
3. Prevention of infections
   a. Administration of a 23-polyvalent pneumococcal vaccine
      (1) Given at ages 2 and 5 years
      (2) Consider continued booster dose every 3 to 5 years
   b. Administration of *Haemophilus influenzae* vaccine: same schedule as normal children
   c. Administration of hepatitis B vaccine: same schedule as normal children
   d. Prophylactic penicillin G therapy
      (1) Penicillin VK 125 mg given orally twice a day starting at 4 months of age
      (2) Dose of penicillin VK is increased to 250 mg given orally twice a day at 3 years of age
      (3) Penicillin is usually discontinued in most patients after age 5 (after administration of pneumococcal vaccine).
      (4) Erythromycin is given to patients who are allergic to penicillin.

KEY POINTS

Sickle Cell Anemia

- Sickle hemoglobin is the most common hemoglobin variant in the world.
- Manifestations of sickle cell anemia do not usually appear until the second 6 months of life, which coincides with the postnatal decrease in fetal hemoglobin and an increase in Hb S.
- Vaso-occlusive crises are the most frequent clinical symptom.
- Hand-foot syndrome is often the first clinical manifestation during infancy.

TABLE 7–12
Clinical Features of Sickle Cell Anemia

Vaso-occlusion

Vaso-occlusive crisis
   Musculoskeletal, hand-foot syndrome
   Abdominal
Splenic sequestration (see p. 259)
   Splenomegaly
   Extreme pallor
   Hypovolemic shock
Acute chest syndrome (see p. 261)
Priapism (see p. 266)
Stroke (see p. 263)
Leg ulcers
Proliferative retinopathy
Renal
   Isosthenuria, natriuresis, enuresis
   Papillary necrosis, hematuria
   Chronic renal failure, nephropathy

Other features

Psychological problems
Narcotic addiction
Effects of chronic illness

Hemolysis

Chronic anemia
   Pallor
   Flow murmur, cardiomegaly
Hyperbilirubinemia, scleral icterus
Reticulocytosis
Hemolytic crisis (with G6PD deficiency)
Aplastic crisis
Cholelithiasis, cholecystitis
Growth failure, delayed puberty

Functional Asplenia

Septicemia
Meningitis
Bacterial pathogens
   Streptococcus pneumoniae
   Haemophilus influenzae
   Salmonella (osteomyelitis)

Pregnancy

Increased fetal loss
Small babies

TABLE 7–13
Current Indications for Blood Transfusion in Sickle Cell Anemia

Acute exacerbation of anemia
   Aplastic crisis
   Hemolytic crisis (with G6PD deficiency)
Life-threatening or organ-threatening vaso-occlusive crisis
   Acute chest syndrome
   Stroke or transient ischemic attack
   Priapism
   Acute multiorgan failure

Sequestration crisis
   Splenic
   Hepatic
High-risk procedures
   Prior to general anesthesia
   Prior to angiography

TABLE 7–14
Current Indications for Chronic Blood Transfusion in Sickle Cell Anemia

Stroke	Chronic organ failure
Recurrent splenic sequestration	Intractable leg ulcers
Recurrent acute chest syndrome	Severe debilitating pain

TABLE 7–15
Complications Related to Blood Transfusion

Transfusion reactions
Transmission of viral infections (HIV, hepatitis B, C, D, or E, cytomegalovirus (CMV), EBV)
Hemosiderosis (parenchymal damage to liver, heart, and pancreas)
Hyperviscosity (worsening vaso-occlusion and organ injury)
Alloimmunization to minor RBC antigens

TABLE 7–16
Common Causes of Mortality in Sickle Cell Anemia

Overwhelming bacterial infections due to *Streptococcus pneumoniae*
   Most common cause of death in children <3 years old
   Peak mortality: around age 2 years
Acute splenic sequestration
   Typical age at sequestration crisis: infants (6 months to 3 years old)
Stroke
   Typical age at stroke: childhood
   Median age: 6 years (about 80% of cases occur in children <15 years old)

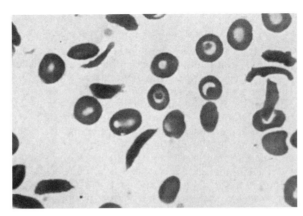

FIGURE 7–6. Sickle cell anemia. Peripheral smear showing target cells and fixed (irreversibly sickled) cells. (From Honig GR: Hemoglobin Disorders. In Behrman RE, Kliegman R, Arvin AM (eds): Nelson Textbook of Pediatrics, 15th ed. Philadelphia, WB Saunders, 1996.)

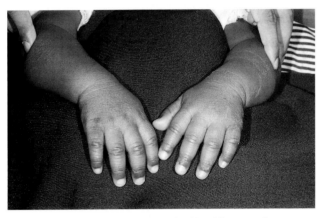

FIGURE 7–7. Vaso-occlusive crisis. Hand-foot syndrome was the first manifestation of Hb SS in this 7-month-old infant, who presented with bilateral symmetrical, cylindrical swelling of the soft tissues of both hands and feet.

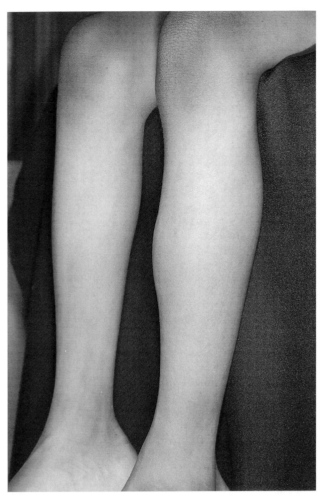

FIGURE 7–8. Vaso-occlusive crisis. Swelling and tenderness of the left lower extremity in sickle cell anemia.

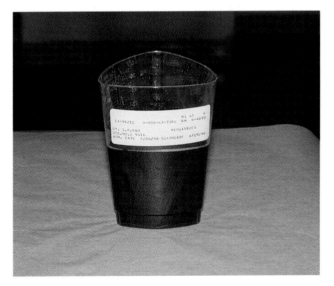

FIGURE 7–9. Gross hematuria secondary to papillary necrosis in an 8-year-old patient with Hb SS. (Courtesy of S.P. Rao, M.D., State University of New York, Brooklyn, NY.)

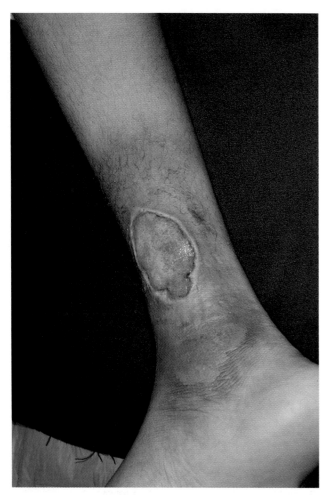

FIGURE 7–10. Leg ulcer in a 15-year-old patient with Hb SS. Chronic leg ulcers are common in adolescents and young adults. The most common location of such ulcers is over the lower tibia.

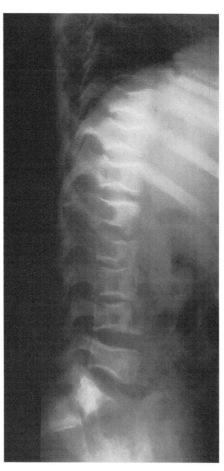

FIGURE 7–11. Lateral view of the thoracolumbar spine. There is uniform biconcavity of the vertebral bodies. The thoracic spine has a characteristic "fish-mouth" appearance. In the lumber spine, note destruction of the intervertebral space with areas of vertebral angulation.

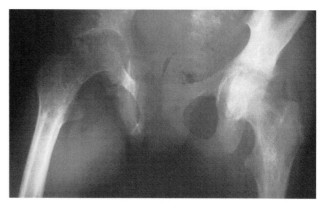

FIGURE 7–12. Bilateral avascular necrosis of the femoral head. Infarction and necrosis of the right femoral head with secondary acetabular deformity are evident. Left femoral head is sclerotic and flattened with narrowing of the hip joint. Note coarsening of the trabecular pattern.

Sickle Cell Anemia and Acute Sequestration Crisis

SYNONYM   Splenic Sequestration

DEFINITION

Rapid enlargement of the spleen due to acute trapping of blood resulting in a fall in Hgb level of more than 2 g/dL despite a persistently elevated reticulocyte count

ETIOLOGY/PATHOGENESIS

1. Triggering factors are unclear.
   a. It may occur during a viral illness.
   b. It may occur with other manifestations of sickle cell disease (e.g., acute chest syndrome, aplastic crisis).
2. A large amount of blood is trapped in the abdominal organs.
   a. Probably because egress of blood from spleen (or liver) is blocked while arterial inflow continues
   b. Most commonly involved organ: spleen
   c. Rarely, sequestration may also occur in the liver (liver is not as distensible as the spleen; thus, trapping of RBCs is rarely significant enough to cause cardiovascular collapse).
3. Splenic sequestration occurs in children with previously palpable spleens, prior to the development of splenic fibrosis and autosplenectomy.

EPIDEMIOLOGY

1. Incidence of splenic sequestration
   a. Occurs in about 10% to 30% of children with sickle cell anemia (Hb SS)
   b. Seen also in other hemoglobinopathies (e.g., Hb SC, sickle B+ thalassemia)
2. Sequestration crisis in children with Hb SS
   a. Typically occurs in infants and young children
   b. Most common age: 6 months to 3 years
   c. Rarely seen in infants under 6 months or in older children and adolescents
3. Sequestration crisis with other hemoglobinopathies may occur in older children and adults (owing to delayed development of splenic fibrosis and autosplenectomy)

TREATMENT

1. Hospitalization and hematology consultation
2. Frequent serial monitoring of splenic size and vital signs (cardiac and pulse oxymetry)
3. Frequent serial monitoring of hemoglobin levels
4. Prompt restoration of intravascular volume and oxygen-carrying capacity
   a. Plasma expanders (crystalloid therapy while awaiting blood products)
   b. Packed red cell or whole blood transfusions

PROGNOSIS

1. An important cause of morbidity and mortality in children
2. If shock can be reversed, much of the sequestered blood is remobilized, and dramatic regression of splenomegaly occurs within a few days. Thrombocytopenia also resolves.
3. Rarely, splenomegaly may persist following acute sequestration episode, and patient may develop hypersplenism.

PREVENTION

1. Parents *must* be taught to recognize early signs and symptoms of splenic sequestration.
2. Parents *must* be taught about abdominal (splenic) palpation and instructed to seek immediate medical help if splenic enlargement occurs.
3. In a patient who has more than one severe (life-threatening) episode, therapeutic options include:
   a. Splenectomy (carries a risk of overwhelming bacterial infection in splenectomized young children), preferably after pneumococcal immunization.
   b. Chronic transfusion therapy

KEY POINTS

Sickle Cell Anemia and Transient Aplastic Crisis

- May be a first clinical manifestation of sickle cell disease
- May progress rapidly to cardiovascular collapse and death
- Predilection for recurrence is high; up to 50% of patients with a first episode have a second episode within 2 years.

TABLE 7–17

Clinical and Laboratory Features of Sequestration Crisis

Signs/symptoms depend on severity of blood pooling
Mild episodes may escape detection
Sudden, rapid, massive enlargement of spleen
Abdominal fullness (massive splenomegaly)
Left upper quadrant pain ($\pm$)
Sudden onset of lethargy, weakness
Pallor
Signs of circulatory collapse
    Poor tissue perfusion, cold, clammy extremities
    Tachycardia $\Rightarrow$ hypotension $\Rightarrow$ shock $\Rightarrow$ death
Rapid drop in Hgb
Mild to moderate thrombocytopenia (sequestering of platelets in spleen)
Elevated reticulocyte count
Increased nucleated RBCs

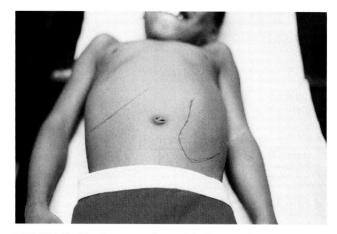

FIGURE 7–13. Sequestration crisis in a patient with sickle cell disease who presented with a rapidly enlarging spleen, extreme pallor, and tachycardia. (Courtesy of Drs. S. P. Rao and N. Desai, State University of New York, Brooklyn, NY.)

Sickle Cell Anemia and Transient Aplastic Crises (TAC)

DEFINITION

A state of severe anemia combined with profound reticulocytopenia

ETIOLOGY

Human parvovirus B19 (about 70% to 100% of cases of TAC)

CLINICAL FEATURES

1. A prodromal illness with fever, malaise, and myalgia may be present.
2. Typical rash seen with parvovirus B19 infection in normal children is uncommon (erythema infectiosum: a "slapped cheek" appearance with circumoral pallor and a lace-like maculopapular rash symmetrically distributed on the arms, thighs, trunk, and buttocks.)
3. Patient may have a concurrent vaso-occlusive crisis.
4. Signs and symptoms of severe anemia
    a. Weakness, listlessness, dizziness
    b. Extreme pallor
    c. Tachycardia
    d. Signs of congestive heart failure (tachypnea, tachycardia, pulmonary congestion)

TREATMENT

1. Hospitalization
    a. Patients with symptoms
    b. Patients with a severe degree of anemia

2. Isolation of hospitalized patients with TAC
    a. Respiratory droplet precautions for those caring for such patients
    b. Such precautions should be maintained for 7 days.
    c. Patient with TAC should be isolated from other patients with hemoglobinopathies.
    d. Pregnant health care workers should be informed about the risk to the fetus from parvovirus infections and preferably should not be involved in the care of such patients.
3. Oxygen therapy, continuous cardiac and pulse oxymetry monitoring
4. Packed RBC transfusion (to improve oxygen-carrying capacity)
    a. If degree of anemia is severe enough to cause or threaten cardiovascular instability
    b. If patient is symptomatic

KEY POINTS

Sickle Cell Anemia and Transient Aplastic Crisis

- Parvovirus infection leads to production of protective levels of antibodies; thus, an aplastic crisis due to parvovirus does not recur in the same patient.
- Parvovirus probably causes a transient aplasia in most individuals, but patients with shortened RBC survival (e.g., those with Hb SS) are unable to compensate for RBC destruction and manifest an abrupt decrease in hematocrit level.

TABLE 7–18
Diagnosis of Transient Aplastic Crisis

Worsening of degree of anemia
Profound reticulocytopenia (<5%)
Decrease in jaundice
Absence of erythrocyte precursors in bone marrow
Erythropoiesis increases 6–8 days after hematocrit reaches its
   nadir
Serum for parvovirus antibodies assays
   Serum B19-specific IgM antibody (confirms infection within
      past several months)
   Serum IgG antibody (indicates previous infection and
      immunity)

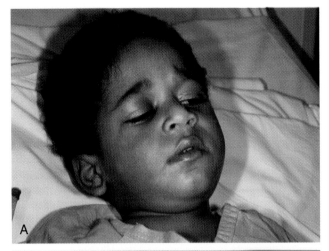

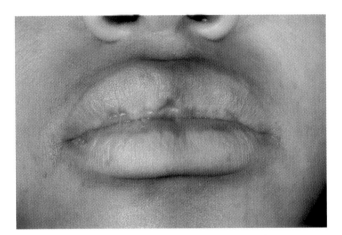

FIGURE 7–14. Transient aplastic crisis presented as extreme pallor and easy fatigability in this 10-year-old patient with Hb SS. The Hgb was 3.4 g/dL, and the reticulocyte count was 1%.

FIGURE 7–15. *A*, Human parvovirus B19 infection with "slapped cheek" appearance and circumoral pallor. *B*, Close-up showing erythematous cheek in a child with Hb SS who was admitted with TAC. Serum parvovirus B19 specific IgM antibody was positive. (Courtesy of Dr. S.P. Rao, State University of New York, Brooklyn, NY.)

Sickle Cell Anemia and Acute Chest Syndrome (ACS)

DEFINITION

An acute illness with a new pulmonary infiltrate on chest radiographs in patients with sickle hemoglobinopathies.

ETIOLOGY (see Table 7–19)

1. Etiology is often unclear; in many cases it is multifactorial.
2. Infectious causes include bacterial, viral, and atypical pathogens; however, in many cases an infectious cause is not proved.
3. Acute chest syndrome may develop on the 2nd or 3rd day of hospitalization in patients hospitalized with vaso-occlusive crisis (especially patients receiving therapies that are not closely monitored such as intravenous hydration [fluid overload] and parenteral analgesic therapy [respiratory depression]).

EPIDEMIOLOGY

1. ACS occurs in more than 50% of pediatric patients with sickle cell anemia (Hb SS).
2. Leading cause of mortality in sickle cell disease

CLINICAL FEATURES

1. Presenting symptoms include varying degrees of fever, cough, and chest and/or back pain.
2. Presenting signs include varying degrees of tachypnea, evidence of respiratory distress (increased respiratory rate and effort, flaring, grunting), and hypoxemia.

LABORATORY

1. Complete blood count: usually shows a significant drop in Hgb value from baseline, a decrease in

platelet count, and an elevated number of nucleated RBCs
2. Arterial blood gases
3. Type and cross-match for blood transfusion
4. Baseline values of serum electrolytes, urea nitrogen, and lactic dehydrogenase, and liver function tests.
5. Chest radiograph
   a. Pulmonary infiltrates are seen unilaterally or bilaterally.
   b. They are either confined to a single lobe or diffusely spread.
   c. Pleural effusions may be present.
   d. Radiologic findings may lag behind clinical findings; a repeat chest radiograph may be required to confirm the diagnosis.

TREATMENT

1. Hospitalization (preferably in an intensive care unit) and hematologist consultation
2. Oxygen therapy, continuous cardiac and pulse oxymetry monitoring
3. Aggressive but closely monitored analgesic therapy to prevent hypoventilation (leading to subsequent atelectasis and hypoxemia) secondary to splinting
4. Hydration: Give 1½ times maintenance fluids with close monitoring of intake and output to avoid pulmonary edema and worsening of acute chest syndrome.
5. Antibiotic therapy
   a. Cefuroxime or ceftriaxone to cover common bacterial pathogens such as *Streptococcus pneumoniae* and *Haemophilus influenzae* and
   b. Erythromycin to cover *Mycoplasma pneumoniae* and *Chlamydia pneumoniae*
6. Blood transfusion
   a. Simple transfusion with packed RBCs is usually given for moderately severe episode, especially when associated with a drop in Hgb concentration.
   b. Exchange transfusion is usually reserved for:
      (1) Patients who do not respond to simple transfusion
      (2) Patients with severe hypoxemia
      (3) Patients with severe bilateral disease
      (4) Patients with rapidly progressive disease
7. Incentive spirometry

PREVENTION

1. Incentive spirometry is given to reduce the risk of ACS (e.g., for patients with thoracic bone pain or those requiring narcotic analgesia).
2. For patients with recurrent episodes of ACS, chronic blood transfusion therapy may prevent subsequent episodes.

PROGNOSIS

Repeated episodes of ACS predispose adolescents and adults to the development of chronic restrictive lung disease, pulmonary hypertension, and cor pulmonale.

KEY POINTS

Sickle Cell Anemia and Acute Chest Syndrome

- Diagnosis of ACS mandates hospitalization.
- Maintain a high index of suspicion for ACS in any patient with Hb SS who presents with fever, chest pain, back pain, or any respiratory symptoms.
- Chest radiograph may be negative despite clinical findings suggestive of ACS during early course; repeat radiographs 12 to 24 hours later may show evidence of pulmonary infiltrates.
- Pulse oxymetry can be used to screen for hypoxemia in patients presenting with signs and symptoms suggestive of ACS.

TABLE 7–19
Etiologies of Acute Chest Syndrome

Infectious	Noninfectious
Common	Pulmonary infarction
Mycoplasma pneumoniae	Sickling, thrombosis in
Chlamydia pneumoniae	pulmonary circulation
Uncommon	Pulmonary fat embolism
Streptococcus pneumoniae	Bone marrow necrosis
Haemophilus influenzae	(vaso-occlusive crisis
Staphylococcus aureus	in bones)
Klebsiella sp.	Hypoventilation
Parvovirus	Splinting due to thoracic
Other respiratory viruses	bones infarction (ribs,
(e.g., respiratory	sternum)
syncytial virus)	Respiratory depression
	due to narcotic
	analgesia
	Postoperative

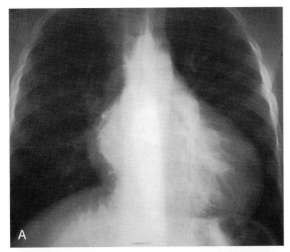

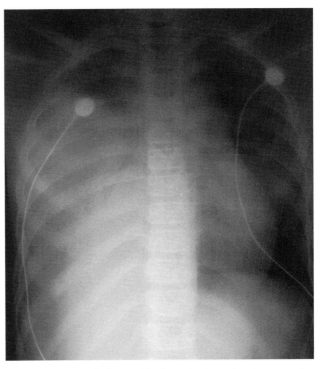

FIGURE 7–17. Radiographic frontal view showing massive consolidation of the right lower lobe, right middle lobe, and portions of the right upper lobe in a 10-year-old patient with Hb SS who presented with respiratory distress and hypoxemia.

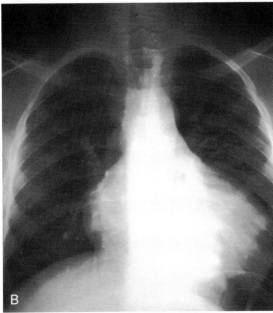

FIGURE 7–16. Acute chest syndrome. *A,* Frontal view in a 9-year-old patient with Hb SS shows cardiomegaly and a mild patchy retrocardiac infiltrate. *B,* Six hours later, a significant consolidation is apparent in the retrocardiac region.

Sickle Cell Anemia and Stroke

DEFINITION

An acute, clinically evident neurologic event in patients with sickle hemoglobinopathies.

EPIDEMIOLOGY

1. Incidence of stroke: 7% to 8% of patients with Hb SS
2. Stroke can occur any time after the first year of life.
3. Risk of stroke is higher in young patients
   a. Median age at diagnosis: 6 years
   b. About 80% of patients are under 15 years old.

PATHOGENESIS

1. Two types of strokes
   a. Ischemic stroke: cerebral infarction caused by thrombosis with complete occlusion or severe narrowing of large cerebral vessels
   b. Hemorrhagic stroke: accompanied by subarachnoid or intracerebral hemorrhage
2. Cerebral infarction secondary to vasculopathy
   a. Most common type of stroke in pediatric patients (about 70% to 90% of cases)
   b. Most commonly involved vessels are arteries near the circle of Willis
      (1) Internal carotid artery
      (2) Middle cerebral artery
      (3) Anterior cerebral artery

c. The exact mechanism by which sickle cell disease causes endothelial damage and intimal hyperplasia in these vessels is unclear.
3. Hemorrhagic stroke is more common in older patients.

LABORATORY

1. Complete blood count
2. Computed tomography
   a. Is performed to exclude hemorrhage
   b. May miss a new stroke
3. Magnetic resonance imaging (MRI) or magnetic resonance angiography (MRA)
   a. More sensitive for ischemia or infarction
   b. MRI: may be abnormal in patients without stroke (about 15% of patients)
   c. MRA: abnormal with stroke
4. Lumbar puncture, if indicated (especially in febrile patients)

TREATMENT

1. Stroke, either diagnosed or suspected clinically, mandates hospitalization.
2. Hematologist and neurologist consultations
3. Blood transfusion therapy prevents progression of neurologic injury and maximizes the chances for full recovery. Therapy options vary in different centers and include:
   a. Exchange transfusion to lower Hb S to less than 30%
   b. Simple transfusion in a stable patient without progressive neurologic symptoms
4. Chronic transfusion program is started and continues indefinitely:
   a. To suppress erythropoiesis sufficiently, to provide enough normal RBCs (with Hg A), and to maintain patient's Hg S concentration at less than 30%
   b. Iron chelation therapy
   c. Frequency of chronic transfusions may be reduced to maintain Hb S at less than 60% after 4 years
5. Bone marrow transplant may be considered if a histocompatible donor is available.

PROGNOSIS

1. With aggressive treatment including prompt blood transfusion: complete or nearly complete neurologic recovery occurs in about 50% of patients.
2. Frequent consequences include intellectual impairment and serious neurologic sequelae.
3. Mortality (up to 50%)
4. Rate of recurrence
   a. Without transfusion therapy, the risk of a second stroke within 3 years is about 60% to 90%.
   b. With chronic transfusion program aiming to maintain Hb S at less than 30%, the risk of recurrence is reduced to about 10%.

PREVENTION

1. Transcranial Doppler ultrasonography identifies patients with Hb SS who have abnormally increased blood velocity, which reflects narrowed cerebral vessels.
2. Currently, trials are under way to evaluate the effect of prophylactic chronic transfusion therapy in reducing the risk of stroke in such children.

KEY POINTS

Sickle Cell Anemia and Stroke

- Most common cause of stroke in children is cerebral infarction.
- Painless limp or weakness (hemiparesis) is the most common presentation.
- Most events occur as a result of large cerebral vessel occlusion.
- All patients with Hb SS presenting with a seizure or neurologic symptoms or signs must be emergently evaluated for possible stroke.

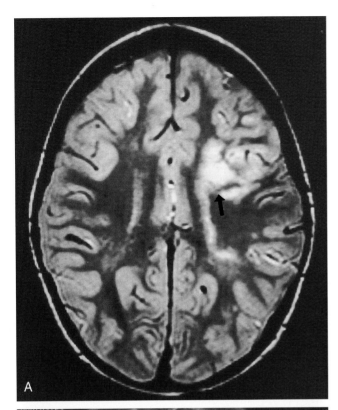

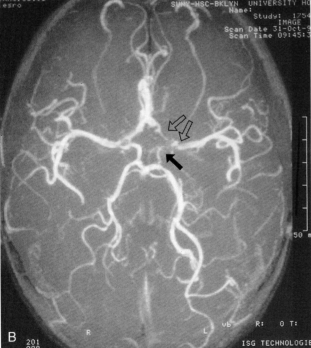

FIGURE 7-18. *A*, Sickle cell anemia and stroke. T2-weighted image in MRI scan of the brain shows areas of increased signal intensity involving the gray and white matter of the left parietal lobe that are consistent with an acute infarct (*arrow*). *B*, MRI angiography of the circle of Willis in the same patient shows areas of stenosis in the left anterior cerebral artery and proximal middle cerebral artery (*two open arrows*). The left posterior communicating artery shows less signal intensity (*closed arrow*), compared with the right, a finding that is consistent with decreased flow. (Courtesy of Scott Miller, M.D., State University of New York, Brooklyn, NY.)

TABLE 7-20
Clinical Features of Sickle Cell Anemia and Stroke

Most common presenting signs and symptoms
   Hemiparesis or monoparesis
   Gait disturbances
   Aphasia or dysphagia
   Focal or generalized seizures
Alterations of sensorium (coma, semicoma)
Transient ischemic attack with subsequent complete resolution of neurologic findings
Usually stroke develops as an isolated event
May occur during other types of crisis (e.g., aplastic crisis, vaso-occlusive crisis, or splenic sequestration)

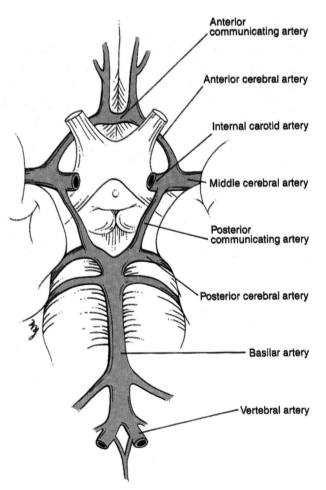

FIGURE 7-19. The circle of Willis. (From Swartz MH: Textbook of Physical Diagnosis, 2nd ed. Philadelphia, WB Saunders, 1994.)

Sickle Cell Anemia and Priapism

DEFINITION

Priapism is defined as a state of persistent, painful penile erection unaccompanied by sexual stimulation. The word priapism is derived from Priapus, the Greek god of fertility, who was depicted in statues as having an erect phallus of exaggerated proportions.

PATHOGENESIS (see Fig. 7–21)

1. Nocturnal erections, mild acidosis related to hypoventilation, and relative dehydration may be triggering events.
2. Obstruction of communication between the corpora cavernosa and corpora spongiosa
3. Sickling of RBCs produces sludging and stasis in the erectile tissues of the corporal bodies.
4. Stagnant blood within the corpora cavernosa leads to further hypoxia, acidosis, and more sickling.
5. Engorgement of the corpora cavernosa with sparing of the corpus spongiosum and the glans penis results.
6. Pain results from ischemia.
7. Prolonged erection results in edema, inflammation leading to thrombosis, fibrosis, and impotence.

EPIDEMIOLOGY

1. Sickle cell disease accounts for 75% of all pediatric cases of priapism.
2. Age at presentation: bimodal peaks:
   a. First peak: between the ages of 5 and 13 years
   b. Second peak: between the ages of 21 and 29 years
3. Types of priapism
   a. "Low-flow" or ischemic type
      (1) Requires a more aggressive approach
      (2) More common in postpubertal males
      (3) Permanent impotence common after priapism lasting more than 24 hours
   b. "High-flow" or nonischemic type
      (1) Usually responds to conservative treatment (hydration, analgesia)
      (2) Usually better prognosis

BOX 7-5   *Differential Diagnosis: Priapism*

Leukemia
Idiopathic priapism
Excessive sexual stimulation
Anticoagulation therapy
Paraphimosis
Phimosis with erection
Urethral foreign body
Diabetes mellitus
Trauma
    Cervical or thoracic spinal cord injury (lack of sympathetic output)
    Local trauma (straddle injury)

LABORATORY

1. A clinical diagnosis in a patient with a history of a sickle cell disease
2. Noninvasive methods used to assess penile perfusion
   a. Radionuclide penile scan
   b. Doppler ultrasonography

COMPLICATIONS

1. Complications related to priapism:
   a. Acute complication: urinary retention
      (1) Mechanical obstruction secondary to engorged corpora cavernosa impedes flow through the urethra.
      (2) Patient hesitates to void because of pain.
   b. Recurrence of priapism
   c. Long-term complication: impotence (about 20% to 25%)
      (1) The risk of impotence increases with number of recurrent episodes and increased duration of episodes.
      (2) The prognosis is better in young patients.
2. Complications related to surgery
   a. Necrosis, cellulitis, sloughing of the penile skin and penile gangrene
   b. Urethral fistula

TREATMENT

1. Hospitalization for any patient with priapism lasting more than 2 to 3 hours
2. Hematologist and urologist consultations
3. Principles of therapy
   a. Relieving pain (analgesics) and acute complications (catheterization for urinary retention)
   b. Achieving detumescence
   c. Preservation of sexual potency
4. Intravenous hydration at 1½ to 2 times maintenance level
5. Oxygen therapy
6. For priapism lasting more than 24 hours, treatment options include:
   a. Transfusion (simple packed RBCs or exchange transfusion to reduce the percentage of Hb S to about 30%)
   b. Cavernosal aspiration
   c. Cavernosal injection or irrigation with solutions containing an alpha-adrenergic agent (e.g., epinephrine, pseudoephedrine, hydralazine)

BOX 7-6   *Priapism*

- In priapism, unlike in normal erection, only the dorsal paired corpora cavernosa are involved; the glans and ventral surface (corpus spongiosum) remain flaccid.
- Although priapism may occur as a result of sexual stimulation, tumescence is neither associated with continued sexual pleasure nor is relieved by ejaculation.

---

d. Winter shunt procedure (glans-cavernosal procedure)
7. For frequently recurrent (stuttering) episodes therapeutic options include:
    a. Chronic transfusion program
    b. Self-administered injection of alpha-adrenergic agents

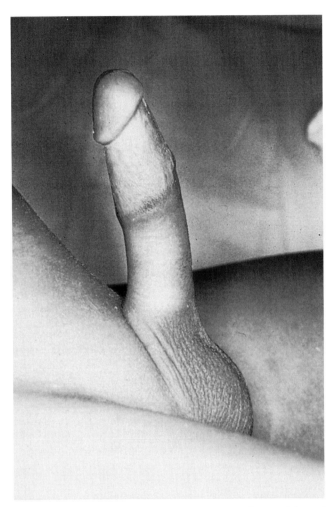

FIGURE 7–20. Priapism. Prolonged erection of several hours' duration in a prepubertal 6-year-old child with sickle cell disease. Examination reveals an erect penis, but the glans and corpus spongiosum may remain flaccid, unlike those of a normal erection. (Courtesy of A.I. Hashmat, M.D., The Brooklyn Hospital Center, Brooklyn, NY.)

KEY POINTS

Sickle Cell Anemia and Priapism

- Sickle cell disease is the most common cause of priapism in children and adolescents.
- Long-standing priapism can lead to impotence.

TABLE 7–21
Clinical Features of Priapism and Sickle Cell Anemia

Penis swollen, edematous, and very tender (pain prominent)
Urinary retention or difficult urination
Duration (severity) of priapism
   May be prolonged lasting >24 hours
   Isolated or infrequent recurrent episodes of <3 hours duration
   "Stuttering" priapism (multiple, brief [<3 hour] episodes several times a week for 4 weeks or more)
Characteristics of priapism (see also Box 7–6)
   Onset most often at night or in early morning
   Frequently an isolated finding (without vaso-occlusive crisis at other sites)

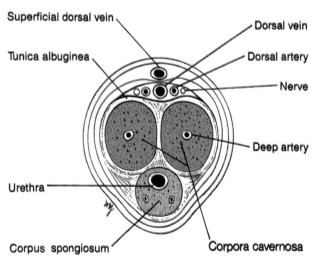

FIGURE 7–21. Cross-sectional view through the penis. (From Swartz MH: Textbook of Physical Diagnosis, 2nd ed. Philadelphia, WB Saunders, 1994.)

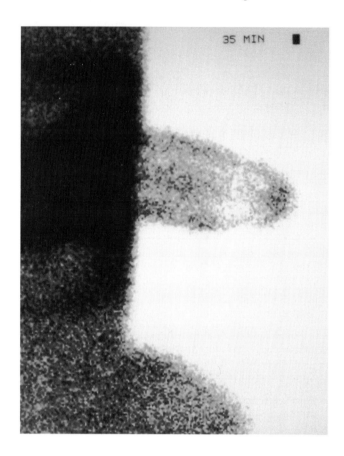

FIGURE 7–22. Radionuclide penile scan showing low-flow (persistent stagnant) priapism. Following intravenous administration of ^{99m}Tc pertechnetate, continuous computer data are acquired for one-half hour starting at the time of injection. Five-minute grouped frames are generated from the computer recording. In this 8-year-old Hb SS patient with priapism (>24-hour duration), there was a persistent lack of activity in the corpora cavernosa throughout the entire examination. One of the frames is shown here.

Hemophilia A

SYNONYMS   Classic Hemophilia
            Factor VIII Deficiency
            Antihemophilic Factor Deficiency

DEFINITION

Hemophilias are genetically determined quantitative deficiencies or qualitative defects of coagulation factors that lead to frequent and excessive bleeding.

1. Hemophilia A: deficiency of or abnormal function of factor VIII
2. Hemophilia B (Christmas disease): deficiency of or abnormal function of factor IX
3. Hemophilia C: deficiency of or abnormal function of factor XI

ETIOLOGY/PATHOGENESIS

1. Factors VIII and IX are involved in the activation of factor X in the intrinsic pathway of coagulation.
2. Factor VIII molecule
   a. Hemophilia A = a defect in factor VIII procoagulant activity *and normal* platelet function
   b. Von Willebrand disease = a variable abnormality of factor VIII procoagulant activity *and defective* platelet function (due to defective or decreased von Willebrand factor [a substance necessary for platelet adhesion to blood vessel walls and for maintenance of a normal bleeding time])

EPIDEMIOLOGY/INHERITANCE

1. Hemophilia A is the most common type of hemophilia (occurs in about 80% of hemophilia cases).
2. Incidence: 1 in 7500 to 10,000 live male births
3. The defective gene is carried on X chromosome.
4. Inherited as sex-linked recessive disorder; thus, males are affected while females are carriers
5. Each male infant born to a woman who is a carrier has a 50% risk of having the disease.
6. Family history is positive in 80% of cases.
7. Sporadic cases represent new mutations and therefore there is a negative family history (about 33% of cases).
8. Following the Lyon hypothesis (random inactivation of the X chromosome), if by chance the normal X chromosome is affected, a mutant X chromosome is expressed in most cells. Some carrier females are symptomatic; they represent the lower end of the predicted bell-shaped distribution of factor levels for carrier females.

ANTENATAL DIAGNOSIS

1. Chorionic villus biopsy sample for chromosome 22 inversion (at 8 to 11 weeks' gestation)
2. Direct assay of factor VIII activity on fetal periumbilical cord blood sampling (after 18 weeks' gestation)

**BOX
7-7**   *Hemarthrosis: Hallmark of Hemophilia*

May occur spontaneously or following trauma
Seen at beginning of toddler stage
Most commonly involved joints
  Elbows
  Knees
  Ankles
Less frequently involved joints
  Shoulders
  Wrist
  Hips
Clinically
  Acute joint swelling
  Pain
  Warmth
  Limitation of movement
  Sometimes accompanied by erythema or discoloration

DIFFERENTIAL DIAGNOSIS

1. Von Willebrand disease
2. Hemophilia B
3. Hemophilia C

TREATMENT

1. Hematology consultation
2. Replacement therapy with factor VIII is the mainstay of therapy.
   a. Types of products available
      (1) Recombinant non–plasma-derived factor VIII concentrate

---

**BOX
7-8**   *Intracranial Hemorrhage in Hemophiliacs*

Most common cause of death (25%)
Only 50% of patients have a history of trauma (thus "treat first and confirm later")
Suspect with any of the following:
  Unusual headache
  Neurologic deficits
  Sensorium changes (lethargy, coma)
  Seizures
Diagnosis made by either CT scan or MRI of head
About 50% of survivors have serious neurologic deficits
Rebleeding within 1 year is common

KEY POINTS

CT scan or MRI of head must be done if there is any suggestion of head trauma, even if symptoms are minimal.
All head injuries should be treated very aggressively with factor infusion even if there are no signs of intracranial bleeding.

---

(2) Monoclonal purified plasma derived factor VIII concentrate
   (3) Cryoprecipitate (rarely used)
   b. Dosage of factor VIII prescribed depends on plasma level needed to treat specific bleeding episode
   c. Each unit of factor VIII per kilogram of body weight increases plasma level by 2% (half-life of 8 to 12 hours)
   d. Desired therapeutic factor VIII levels (some examples)
      (1) Life-threatening hemorrhage or major surgery: 80% to 100% (40 to 50 U/kg)
      (2) Hemarthrosis: at least 50% (25 U/kg)
      (3) Soft tissue bleeding: 40% (20 U/kg)
3. Desmopressin acetate (DDAVP) therapy
   a. For mild hemophilia
   b. Mechanism of action
      (1) Stimulates endogenous release of factor VIII (causes a three- to fivefold rise in baseline factor VIII)
      (2) Stimulates endogenous release of von Willebrand factor
   c. Mode of administration: intranasal spray or intravenous
4. Fibrinolytic inhibitors (e.g., aminocaproic acid)
   a. As adjunctive therapy
   b. For mucous membrane bleeding involving the gums, tongue, or teeth
5. Adjuvant therapy for hemarthrosis
   a. During acute phase
      (1) Immobilization as required by bed rest
      (2) Ice
      (3) Compression
      (4) Elevation
   b. Physical therapy, splints, crutches as required for abnormalities in gait or joint function after resolution of acute hemorrhage
   c. Prednisone therapy
      (1) For patients with evidence of inflammation or synovitis after resolution of hemarthrosis
      (2) Dose: 1 to 2 mg/kg/day for 3 to 5 days

PREVENTION

1. Protection from trauma
   a. Padded cribs and playpens during infancy
   b. Avoidance of contact sports
   c. Avoidance of football, ice hockey
4. Immunizations given intramuscularly should be given after factor VIII replacement by the smallest-bore needle or given by subcutaneous route.
5. Immunizations against hepatitis B and hepatitis A
6. Medications to avoid: aspirin
7. Bleeding complications have rarely occurred in female carriers (especially during surgery); thus, factor XIII levels should be measured in all carriers.

PROGNOSIS

1. Repeated hemarthrosis in the same joint
   a. Combination of soft tissue, cartilage and bony abnormalities ⇒ anatomically abnormal joint ⇒ patient prone to successive bleeds

b. Development of bony cysts
2. Development of antibodies to transfused factor VIII ("factor VIII inhibitors"), making management of subsequent bleeds increasingly difficult

KEY POINTS

Hemophilia A

- Most common congenital coagulation disorder
- Transmitted as X-linked trait; thus, males are affected, and females are carriers

- Lifelong tendency toward serious and often life-threatening hemorrhage
- Hemarthrosis and deep soft tissue bleeding are the cardinal signs.
- Factor VIII does not cross the placenta; excessive bleeding from either the circumcision site or the umbilical cord may be an initial presentation.

TABLE 7–22
Clinical Features of Hemophilia

During Neonatal Period

Bleeding from circumcision site (about 33% to 50% of affected cases)
Hematoma after injections
May not exhibit any clinical signs (about 50% escape detection)

During Infancy and Childhood

Bleeding either spontaneously (in severe hemophiliacs) or following trauma (in mild to moderate hemophiliacs)
Infancy (typically during second 6 months after birth)
 Excessive bruising (associated with ambulation)
 Mucous membrane bleeding during primary teeth eruption
 Hematomas over common areas of trauma (forehead, arms pretibial areas)
Excessive bleeding after torn frenulum
Hemarthrosis (see Box 7–7)
Petechiae/purpura uncommon (unlike von Willebrand disease)
Intramuscular hematomas
Deep soft tissue bleeding
Prolonged bleeding (hours to days)
Hematuria

TABLE 7–23
Laboratory Tests for Hemophilia A

Platelet count: normal
Tests for platelet function: usually normal
Bleeding time: normal in 90% of cases
Bleeding time: prolonged in 10% of cases (severe hemophiliacs)
Thrombin time: normal
Prothrombin time: normal
Partial thromboplastin time (PTT): usually prolonged; may be normal in mild hemophiliacs
Fibrinogen concentration: normal
Level of factor VIII in plasma: reduced; determines clinical severity
 Mild cases: 6% to 30% (6–30 units/dL) of normal factor activity
 Moderate cases: 1% to 5% (1–5 units/dL) of normal factor activity
 Severe cases: <1% (1 unit/dL) of normal factor activity
Von Willebrand factor assay: normal
Carrier detection (factor VIII levels of <50%)
 Ratio of factor VIII coagulant activity to von Willebrand factor antigen: <0.8 (normal ratio is 1:1)
 Genetic determination using restriction fragment length polymorphism
 Inversion affecting chromosome 22

TABLE 7–24
Complications of Hemophilia

Complications Related to Disease	Complications Related to Therapy
Life-threatening hemorrhages	Transmission of viruses (transfusion-related)
Intracranial	HIV
Neck or pharynx (airway compromise)	Hepatitis B
Retroperitoneal	Hepatitis C
Gastrointestinal tract	Hepatitis A
Compartment syndrome (intramuscular bleeding)	Parvovirus
Hemophilic arthropathy	Development of inhibitor
Synovial damage and hypertrophy	Inhibitors against factor VIII
Muscular atrophy, contraction of ligaments	Seen in 15% to 20% of cases
Joint contracture, fixed unstable joint	Inactivates infused factor
Degenerative changes (osteoporosis)	
Limited range of motion, chronic pain	
Poor wound healing (factors VIII and IX required for wound healing)	

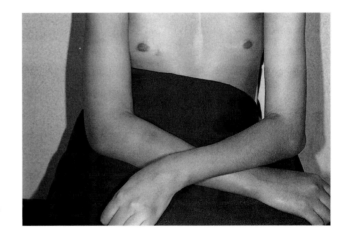

FIGURE 7–23. Hemarthrosis of the right elbow in a 14-year-old patient with hemophilia A.

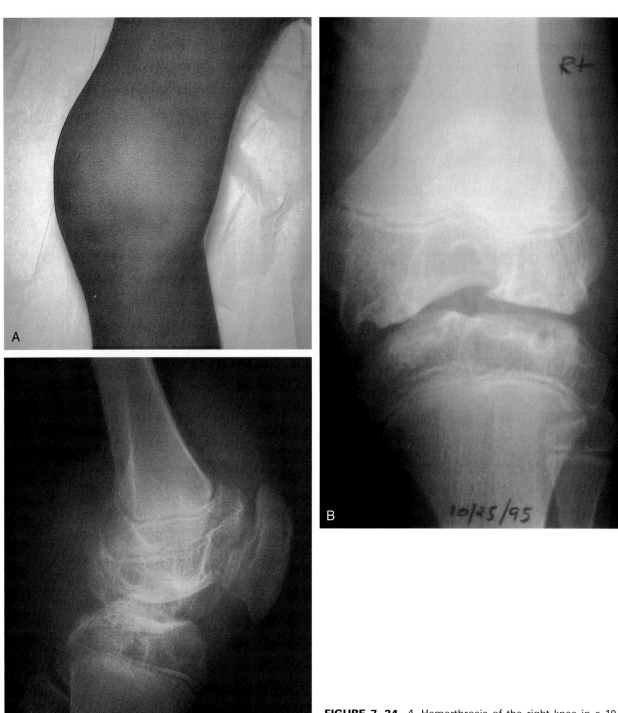

FIGURE 7–24. *A,* Hemarthrosis of the right knee in a 10-year-old with hemophilia A. *B* and *C,* Frontal and lateral views of the right knee show diffuse osteopenia, widening of the intercondylar notch, cortical irregularity, and a suprapatellar effusion. There is a subcortical cyst, and increased synovial density secondary to hemosiderin deposition.

Acute Lymphoblastic Leukemia (ALL)

DEFINITION

Acute lymphoblastic (or lymphocytic) leukemia (ALL) is a malignant disorder of the lymphoblast that results from clonal proliferation of a single lymphoblast that has undergone malignant transformation.

ETIOLOGY/PATHOGENESIS

1. Cause of ALL remains unknown; random mutations are believed to cause most cases.
2. Genetic, host, and environmental factors may play a role (see Box. 7–9).
   a. Siblings of a child with ALL have a two- to fourfold increased risk of developing ALL.
   b. Concordant ALL occurs in monozygotic twins
   c. Viral infections: human T-cell lymphotropic virus (HTLV)-I associated with adult T-cell leukemia and HTLV-II with adult hairy cell leukemia, Ebstein-Barr virus (EBV)
   d. Exposure to ionizing radiation or hydrocarbons

EPIDEMIOLOGY

1. Among all acute leukemias:
   a. ALL: 80% of cases
   b. Acute myeloid (or nonlymphoblastic) leukemia: 20% of cases
2. ALL in the United States:
   a. Incidence: 40 cases/1 million children under 15 years of age
   b. About 2500 new cases are diagnosed annually in children under 15 years of age
   c. Peak age at diagnosis: 2 to 4 years
   d. Higher incidence in whites than in African-Americans (ratio 1.8:1)
   e. Higher incidence in boys than in girls (ratio 1.2:1)

LABORATORY (see also Table 7–26)

1. Complete blood count with differential
2. Serum concentrations of electrolytes, urea nitrogen, creatinine, calcium, phosphorus, uric acid, lactate dehydrogenase, liver enzymes
3. Bone marrow aspirate (leukemic lymphoblast >25% required for diagnosis)
4. Cerebrospinal fluid examination (to look for central nervous system [CNS] involvement [found in <5% of patients at diagnosis])
5. Coagulation profile (prothrombin time, partial thromboplastin time, fibrinogen)
6. Radiographs (changes may be seen in 50% to 100% of patients)
   a. Chest: anterior mediastinal mass (found in 66% of patients with T-cell ALL) or hilar adenopathy
   b. Long bones: multiple punctate osteolytic lesions (most common), diffuse demineralization, metaphyseal lucent bands, and periosteal reaction
7. Karyotyping and immunophenotyping of blasts

PATHOLOGY/CLASSIFICATION

1. There is no staging system for ALL because most patients have disseminated disease (bone marrow, spleen, liver, lymph nodes, and blast cells in peripheral circulation) at diagnosis.
2. ALL is subclassified for diagnostic, prognostic, and therapeutic purposes based on morphologic, immunologic, and genetic features of the leukemic blast cells.
   a. French-American-British classification (L_1, L_2, L_3) is based on the morphology of the lymphoblast (size, character, and amount of cytoplasm, and so on.)
   b. Immunologic classification: B-cell lineage, T-cell lineage, immunologic markers
   c. Cytogenetics: karyotype of leukemic blast cells (translocations, Philadelphia chromosome, hyperdiploidy [>50 chromosomes] or hypodiploidy [<46 chromosomes])

DIFFERENTIAL DIAGNOSIS (see also Table 7–27)

1. Infectious mononucleosis
   a. EBV infection can present with lymphocytosis, thrombocytopenia, hemolytic anemia with hepatosplenomegaly and lymphadenopathy
   b. Atypical lymphocytes may resemble leukemic lymphoblasts
2. Systemic-onset juvenile rheumatoid arthritis
   a. Signs/symptoms of fever, anemia, leukocytosis, arthralgia or arthritis, lymphadenopathy, and hepatosplenomegaly resemble ALL
   b. ALL *must* be excluded by a bone marrow exam-

BOX 7–9	*Conditions Associated With Increased Risk for Leukemia*
Down syndrome (10- to 15-fold increased risk)	Ataxia telangiectasia
Bloom syndrome	X-linked agammaglobulinemia
Fanconi anemia	Severe combined immune deficiency
Aplastic anemia	Wiskott-Aldrich syndrome
Shwachman-Diamond syndrome	IgA deficiency
Neurofibromatosis	

ination, especially prior to starting corticosteroid therapy

TREATMENT

1. Hospitalization
2. Pediatric hematology-oncology consultation for confirmation and management (as per ongoing clinical therapeutic trial protocols)
3. Combination chemotherapy is the principal modality.
   a. Induction and consolidation therapy: Commonly used drugs include vincristine, prednisone, L-asparaginase with or without doxorubicin or daunorubicin
   b. CNS therapy: commonly used regimens include intrathecal methotrexate and cranial irradiation or intrathecal methotrexate, hydrocortisone, and ara-C.
4. Management of complications of the leukemic burden (tumor lysis syndrome)

PROGNOSIS

1. Second cancer

   a. Brain tumor (patients who have received cranial irradiation at ≤5 years of age)
   b. Acute myeloid leukemia (patients treated with epipodophyllotoxins)
2. Late sequelae secondary to cranial irradiation
   a. Neuropsychological deficits
   b. Endocrine dysfunction (short stature, obesity, precocious puberty, osteoporosis)

KEY POINTS

Acute Lymphoblastic Leukemia

- Most common malignancy diagnosed in children
- Most common presenting symptoms are fever, pallor, purpura, and bone pain.
- The diagnosis of leukemia cannot be made from peripheral smear alone; bone marrow examination is required to make the diagnosis.
- Untreated ALL leads to pancytopenia and organ failure (bone marrow and organ infiltration), resulting in death (infection, bleeding) in 100% of cases.

TABLE 7–25
Clinical Features of Acute Lymphoblastic Leukemia

Symptoms	Signs
Fatigue, anorexia, lethargy	Splenomegaly
Bone pain (arthralgia, limp)	Lymphadenopathy (generalized)
Fever	Hepatomegaly
Pallor	Bone tenderness
Bleeding (skin, mucosal, epistaxis)	Ecchymosis or petechiae
Headache, vomiting (↑ intracranial pressure; rare)	Testicular enlargement (rare)

TABLE 7–26
Presenting Laboratory Findings of Acute Lymphoblastic Leukemia

Leukocyte Count/mm³		Platelet Count/mm³		Hemoglobin (g/dL)	
<10,000	50%	<20,000	20%	<7.5	46%
10,000–50,000	34%	20,000–100,000	51%	7.5–10	30%
>50,000	22%	>100,000	29%	>10	24%

Modified from Acute lymphoblastic leukemia in childhood. *In* Johnson KB, Oski FA (eds): Oski's Essential Pediatrics. Philadelphia, Lippincott-Raven, 1997, p. 365.

TABLE 7–27
Differential Diagnosis of Acute Lymphoblastic Leukemia

Nonmalignant Conditions	Malignancies
Idiopathic thrombocytopenic purpura	Acute myeloid leukemia
Leukemoid reaction (e.g., pertussis, bacterial sepsis)	Metastasis to bone marrow
Aplastic anemia	Neuroblastoma
Myelofibrosis	Retinoblastoma
Infectious mononucleosis	Rhabdomyosarcoma
Systemic-onset juvenile rheumatoid arthritis	Lymphoma
Acute infectious lymphocytosis	Ewing sarcoma

TABLE 7–28
Complications of Acute Lymphoblastic Leukemia

Hyperleukocytosis (WBC >100,000/mm³)
   Infarction (CNS hemorrhage, pulmonary)
Hemorrhage (platelet count <20,000/mm³)
   Mucous membranes, CNS, GI tract
Infections due to granulocytopenia
   Bacterial (gram-negative enteric bacilli, gram-positive cocci)
Infections due to lymphopenia
   Viral (e.g., varicella, herpes simplex virus, cytomegalovirus)
   Fungal (e.g., *Candida, Aspergillus*)
   Opportunistic (e.g., *Pneumocystis*)
Relapse
   Bone marrow (most common site)
   Other sites (CNS, testes)

Metabolic complications (tumor lysis)
   Hyperuricemia
   Hyperkalemia
   Hyperphosphatemia
   Hypocalcemia
   Hypercalcemia
   Hyponatremia
   SIADH
   Lactic acidosis

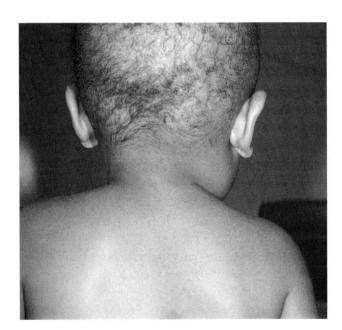

FIGURE 7–25. Acute lymphoblastic leukemia in a patient who presented with a prominent cervical adenopathy. The patient also had generalized lymphadenopathy and hepatosplenomegaly. Her WBC count was 45,000/mm³, the platelet count was 28,000/mm³, and Hgb was 6.0 g/dL.

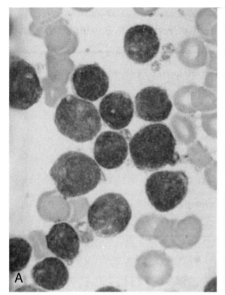
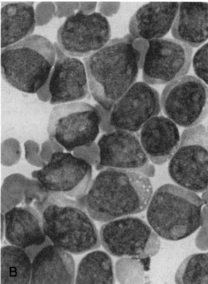
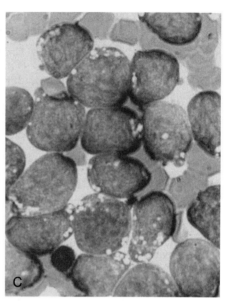

FIGURE 7–26. Morphologic appearance of ALL cells classified according to the French-American-British (FAB) system. *A,* L1 morphology (seen in about 85% of cases). L1 blasts are small and have scanty cytoplasm. *B,* L2 morphology (seen in fewer than 15% of cases). L2 blasts are larger and have more cytoplasm. *C,* L3 morphology (seen in about 1% of cases). L3 blasts have basophilic cytoplasm with vacuolization. (From Crist WM, Pui Ching-Hon: The leukemias. *In* Behrman RE, Kliegman R, Arvin AM (eds): Nelson Textbook of Pediatrics, 15th ed. Philadelphia, WB Saunders, 1996.)

Neuroblastoma

DEFINITION

A malignant tumor arising from the neural crest cells, which normally give rise to the adrenal medulla and the sympathetic ganglia

EPIDEMIOLOGY

1. Incidence: 1 in every 7,000 to 10,000 live births
2. Most common extracranial solid tumor in children
3. Most frequently diagnosed tumor in infants
4. The fourth most common of all pediatric neoplasms, exceeded only by leukemia, lymphoma, and brain tumors. It accounts for 8% to 10% of all childhood cancers.
5. Age at presentation
   a. Median age at diagnosis: 22 months
   b. About 50% of patients are diagnosed during the first 2 years.
   c. About 90% of patients are diagnosed before the age of 5 years.
   d. Diagnosis is rare after the age of 10 years.
6. Other associated conditions
   a. Hirschsprung disease
   b. Fetal hydantoin syndrome
   c. Neurofibromatosis
   d. Nesidioblastosis
   e. Beckwith-Wiedemann syndrome

BOX 7–10   *Neuroblastoma and Paraneoplastic Syndromes*

Seen in <5% of patients
Signs and symptoms unrelated to local mass effect
Secretion of vasoactive intestinal polypeptide (VIP syndrome)
    Intractable secretory diarrhea
    Abdominal distention
    Electrolyte disturbances (hypokalemia)
    Symptoms resolve after surgical removal of tumor
Opsomyoclonus syndrome ("dancing eyes/dancing feet" syndrome)
    Acute myoclonic encephalopathy
    Sustained irregular multidirectional conjugate eye movements
    Myoclonic jerks
    Acute cerebellar and truncal ataxia
    Symptoms may *not* resolve after therapy

<table>
<tr><td>

BOX 7-11   *Anatomic Locations of Neuroblastoma**

Abdominal (70%)
  Adrenal medulla (50%)
  Paraspinal ganglia (20% to 25%)
Mediastinal paraspinal ganglia (15%)
Pelvic paraspinal ganglia (5%)
Cervical sympathetic ganglia (3%)
No identifiable primary sites (1%)

*About 75% to 80% of tumors occur below the diaphragm

</td></tr>
</table>

INHERITANCE

Familial occurrence has been reported but is rare.

PATHOLOGY

1. Neuroblastoma can arise in sympathetic nervous tissue from the brain to the pelvis.
2. Neuroblastomas are classified into three histologic subgroups
   a. Neuroblastomas
   b. Ganglioneuroblastoma
   c. Ganglioneuroma
3. Metastasis occurs through hematogenous and lymphatic routes and involves the liver, bone marrow, skin, lymph nodes, skeleton, brain, and lungs.

LABORATORY (see also Table 7–31)

1. Radiographs
   a. Chest (anteroposterior and lateral): to exclude posterior mediastinal mass, lung metastasis
   b. Abdominal (flat plate): finely stippled calcifications may be seen in 25% to 50% of patients with abdominal neuroblastoma.
   c. Skeletal survey: skeletal metastases are usually osteolytic and may show a periosteal reaction.
2. Computed tomography and/or magnetic resonance imaging of chest, abdomen, and head
3. Bone scan (technetium-99m diphosphonate scan) or meta-iodobenzylguinidine (MIBG) scan to detect metastasis
4. Bone marrow aspirate and bone marrow biopsy from each of the posterior iliac crests

TREATMENT

1. Hospitalization
2. Hematology-oncology and surgery consultations for confirmation of diagnosis and management
   a. Pathologic diagnosis from tumor tissue
   b. Accurate staging (e.g., International Neuroblastoma Staging) is essential because treatment is based on age of patient and extent of disease.
   c. Various treatment protocols include surgery, radiation, chemotherapy, and bone marrow transplantation.

KEY POINTS

Neuroblastoma

- Most common tumor in infants under 1 year of age in the United States
- Most common extracranial solid tumor of childhood
- Most common tumor to metastasize to the orbit in childhood
- Metastatic disease is present in 75% of patients at the time of diagnosis.
- Up to 90% to 95% of patients have elevation of either VMA or HVA at the time of diagnosis.

| BOX 7-12 | *Catecholamine Synthesis and Metabolism* |

Phenylalanine

↓

    (by phenylalanine hydroxylase)

↓

Tyrosine

↓

    (by tyrosine hydroxylase)

↓

DOPA ——————— ⇒ urinary metabolite ⇒ homovanillic acid (HVA)

↓

    (by DOPA decarboxylase)

↓

Dopamine ——————— ⇒ urinary metabolite ⇒ HVA

↓

    (by dopamine B-hydroxylase)

↓

Norepinephrine ——————— ⇒ urinary metabolite ⇒ vanillylmandelic acid
                                                  (VMA)

↓

    (by phenylethanolamine-*N*-methyltransferase)

↓

Epinephrine ——————— ⇒ urinary metabolite ⇒ VMA

- About 90% to 95% of neuroblastomas secrete catecholamines.
- About 5% to 10% of neuroblastomas do not secrete catecholamines but may secrete acetylcholine.
- Production and release of dopamine and norepinephrine occur at the axonal terminals of neurons.
- Epinephrine (along with norepinephrine) is released by the adrenal medulla.
- More differentiated tumors produce norepinephrine (and thus elevated levels of VMA).
- Serial urinary catecholamine determinations are valuable in following the response to treatment.

TABLE 7–29
Clinical Features of Neuroblastoma

Signs/Symptoms (depending on anatomic location)
Abdominal neuroblastoma
   Abdominal or flank mass (firm, fixed, frequently crosses
      midline)
   Asymptomatic
   Abdominal pain (hemorrhage in necrotic center of the
      tumor)
   Signs of bowel obstruction (mass effect)
   Genital or lower extremity edema (mass effect)
   Hypertension (renin-mediated due to compromised renal
      vasculature)
Paravertebral tumor extending into extradural space
   ("dumbbell" tumor)
   Paralysis or paresis, bladder or bowel dysfunction (spinal
      cord compression)
Lower cervical or upper thoracic paravertebral mass
   Horner syndrome (unilateral ptosis, miosis, anhidrosis,
      enophthalmos)
   Respiratory distress or stridor
Constitutional symptoms
   Fever
   Failure to thrive

TABLE 7–30
Clinical Features of Metastatic Neuroblastoma

Hutchinson Syndrome (widespread bone/bone marrow
   disease)
Bone disease
   Bone pain/irritability in infants
   Limping
   Refusal to walk
   Pathologic fractures
Bone marrow failure
   Anemia
   Bleeding
   Increased risk of infection
   Fever

Orbit ("raccoon eyes")

Orbital proptosis; unilateral or bilateral
Ecchymosis (upper or lower eyelids, surrounding tissues)

Pepper Syndrome

Massive involvement of liver
Respiratory compromise (hepatomegaly)

Skin/Subcutaneous Tissue ("blueberry muffin" nodules)

Most frequently seen in newborns
Firm, nontender, bluish subcutaneous nodules

TABLE 7–31
Laboratory Findings of Neuroblastoma

Anemia	Thrombocytopenia or Thrombocytosis
Elevated serum values of	Elevated urinary values of
Lactate dehydrogenase (LDH)	Catecholamines
Urea nitrogen	Epinephrine
Creatinine	Dopamine
Calcium (uncommon)	Catecholamine metabolites
Ferritin	VMA
Vasoactive intestinal peptide	HVA
Neuron-specific enolase (NSE)	
Catecholamines	

TABLE 7–32
Prognosis of Neuroblastoma

Clinical findings with adverse prognosis	Biochemical markers with adverse prognosis
Age >1–2 years	Serum ferritin >142 ng/mL
Bone metastasis	Serum NSE >100 ng/mL
Extensive bone marrow involvement	Serum LDH >1500 U/L
Tumor cell features with adverse prognosis	Urine VMA/HVA ratio <1.0
N-myc proto-oncogene >3–10 copies	

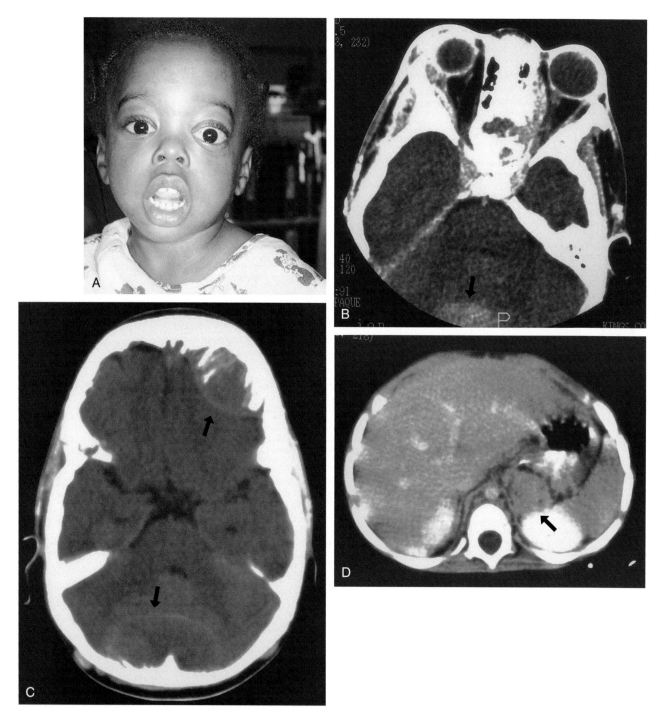

FIGURE 7–27. *A,* Metastatic neuroblastomas in a 22-month-old child presenting with proptosis of the left eye and ecchymosis of the right eye. The primary site of the neuroblastoma was in the left adrenal medulla. Orbital proptosis results from retrobulbar and orbital infiltration with tumor. In this patient proptosis was misdiagnosed as orbital cellulitis and treated with antibiotics for 2 weeks with no improvement. (Courtesy of Dr. S.P. Rao, State University of New York, Brooklyn, N.Y.) *B,* CT scan of the orbits shows a large mixed lytic and blastic bony lesion involving the ethmoid and sphenoid sinuses. An adjacent left orbital subperiosteal lesion with lateral deviation of the optic nerve and proptosis is also visible, as is a small right subperiosteal lesion. A portion of a large lesion in the occipital region is also visualized (*arrow*). *C,* CT scan with bone windows demonstrates the sclerotic occipital skull lesion (*arrow*) as well as a large frontal sclerotic lesion (*arrow*). *D,* CT scan of the abdomen at the level of the adrenals demonstrates a left heterogeneous adrenal mass (*arrow*). The mass contained small flecks of calcium.

TABLE 7–33
Differential Diagnosis of Neuroblastoma

Other Catecholamine-Secreting Tumors

Ganglioneuroma
Ganglioneuroblastoma
Pheochromocytoma

Neuroblastoma/Disseminated Bone Disease

Osteomyelitis
Juvenile rheumatoid arthritis

Neuroblastoma/VIP Syndrome

Infectious diarrhea
Inflammatory bowel disease

Neuroblastoma/Opsomyoclonus Syndrome

Primary neurologic disease

Neuroblastoma/Abdominal Mass

Wilms tumor
Teratomas
Primative neuroectodermal tumors

Neuroblastoma/Metastatic Bone Marrow Disease

Rhabdomyosarcoma
Ewing sarcoma
Lymphoma
Leukemia

Osteosarcoma

SYNONYM   Osteogenic Sarcoma

DEFINITION

A malignant pleomorphic spindle cell tumor of the bone in which the proliferating tumor cells produce new bone

EPIDEMIOLOGY

1. Primary malignant tumors of the bone are the second most common group of solid malignant tumors in adolescents and young adults.
2. Most common age at diagnosis
   a. During adolescence
   b. Median age: 15 years
   c. More than 75% of patients present between 10 and 20 years of age.
3. Rarely seen in prepubertal children
4. Most commonly involved bones
   a. Distal femur, proximal tibia or fibula (about 50% to 80% of patients)
   b. Proximal humerus (about 9% to 15% of patients)
5. Uncommon sites of involvement
   a. Central axis lesions are involved in less than 10% of patients.
   b. Involvement of axial skeleton (pelvis, spine) is uncommon in children.
   c. Flat bones of the trunk or skull are not common sites of involvement.

PATHOGENESIS

1. This is a malignant tumor of mesenchymal origin. It is composed of large osteoid-producing spindle cells.

2. Typically, it arises in the metaphyseal end of a long bone but may extend into the diaphysis or epiphysis.

LABORATORY

1. Complete blood count (usually normal)
2. Serum alkaline phosphatase value (Alk. phosphatase) may be elevated, reflecting increased osteoblastic activity.
3. Serum lactate dehydrogenase value (LDH) may also be elevated.
4. Radiographs of the involved extremity show
   a. An eccentric metaphyseal lytic lesion or a mixed lytic lesion with calcification or evidence of new bone formation
   b. A characteristic "sunburst" appearance produced by horizontal bone spicules that traverse the eroded cortex into the surrounding soft tissue.
   c. Extensive periosteal reaction (Codman triangle) may be present.
5. Computed tomography of chest to exclude pulmonary metastasis
6. Magnetic resonance imaging of the involved extremity provides information about tumor extent in the medullary cavity and in the soft tissues.
7. Tissue biopsy (for confirmation and differentiation from Ewing sarcoma)

TREATMENT

1. Hospitalization for confirmation of the diagnosis and management
2. Multidisciplinary approach with pediatric hematology-oncology and surgery consultations

---

BOX 7-13 *Differential Diagnosis of Bone Tumors*

INFECTION

Osteomyelitis

BENIGN TUMORS

Eosinophilic granuloma
Unicameral bone cyst
Osteoblastoma
Osteochondroma
Aneurysmal bone cyst
Giant cell tumor

MALIGNANT TUMORS

Osteosarcoma
Ewing's sarcoma
Fibrosarcoma

BONE METASTASIS

Lymphoma
Neuroblastoma
Rhabdomyosarcoma

---

3. Goals of therapy
   a. To achieve local control of the tumor
   b. To eradicate micrometastasis
   c. To prevent new systemic spread of disease
4. Treatment modalities include
   a. Neoadjuvant chemotherapy preoperatively
      (1) To decrease tumor viability
      (2) To treat micrometastatic disease, if present at the time of diagnosis

---

TABLE 7-34
Etiologies/Predisposing Conditions for Osteosarcoma

Primary Osteosarcoma

Without pre-existing bone lesion
Without prior treatment of bone (e.g., radiation therapy)
Accounts for >95% of osteosarcomas in children and young adults

Secondary Osteosarcoma Arises

With preexisting bone condition
  Fibrous dysplasia
  Osteocartilaginous exostosis
  Osteochondroma
  Paget disease
As second malignancy within field of radiation exposure (after radiation therapy for other childhood malignancies)
In children with familial form of retinoblastoma (with or without prior exposure to radiation)
Li-Fraumeni syndrome

---

   b. Surgery: removal of tumor with wide margins either:
      (1) By amputation *or*
      (2) By resection, leaving uninvolved distal parts (limb salvage surgery)
5. Osteosarcoma is unresponsive to radiation therapy.

PROGNOSIS

Unfavorable

1. Involvement of axial skeleton
2. Involvement of proximal primary site (e.g., proximal femur)
3. Elevated serum LDH value
4. Elevated serum Alk. phosphatase value
5. Clinically detectable metastasis at diagnosis
6. Tumor response after initial chemotherapy
   a. Viable tumor—unfavorable
   b. Necrotic tumor—favorable

KEY POINTS

Osteosarcoma

- Most common primary malignant bone tumor in children
- About 50% to 80% of osteosarcomas involve the area around the knee (metaphyseal ends of either the distal femur or the proximal tibia or fibula).

TABLE 7-35
Clinical Features of Osteosarcoma

Symptoms
  Localized pain and swelling of affected area
  Patient often relates pain to recent trauma (usually an incidental history)
Signs
  Most common sites: most rapidly growing ends of long bones (distal femur, proximal tibia)
  Palpable mass that is usually tender and warm
  Limited range of movement (especially when tumor is adjacent to joint)
  Pathologic fracture of involved bone
  Metastasis at presentation (about 15% of patients)
  Most common site of metastasis: lungs

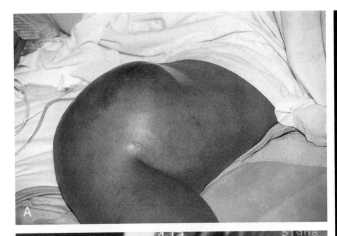

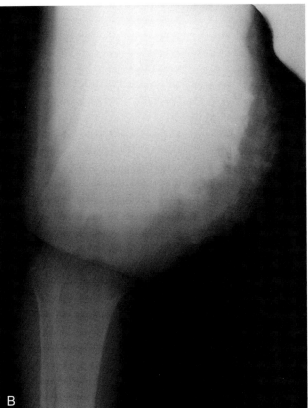

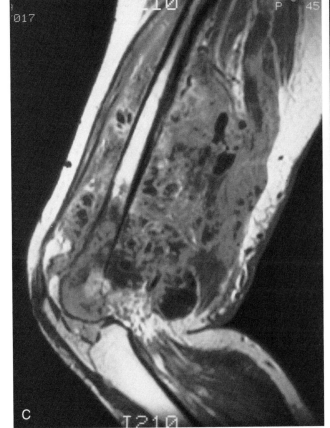

FIGURE 7–28. *A,* Osteosarcoma of distal femur in a 14-year-old girl with an enlarging right leg mass of 8 months duration. *B,* Frontal radiograph demonstrates a large lesion along the medial metaphysis. There is abundant calcification with an ill-defined cortex and significant soft tissue swelling. *C,* Sagittal gadolinium-enhanced T1-weighted image shows tumor involvement of the epiphysis and metadiaphysis. There is marked soft tissue involvement with heterogeneous enhancing signal representing areas of calcification, necrosis, and peri-tumoral edema.

TABLE 7–36
Differential Diagnosis: Osteosarcoma versus Ewing Sarcoma

Osteosarcoma

Epidemiology
   Most common malignant bone tumor
   Most common age: second decade
   All races
Sites
   Typically involves appendicular skeleton
   Uncommon: axial skeleton (pelvis, spine)
   Typically metaphysis of a long bone
   Most common site of metastasis: lungs
Radiography
   "Sunburst" pattern
   Sclerotic destruction (less commonly lytic)
Therapy
   Unresponsive to radiation therapy.

Ewing Sarcoma

Epidemiology
   Second most common bone tumor
   Most common age: second decade
   Primarily whites
Sites
   Common: axial skeleton
   Typically diaphysis of a long bone
   Metastasis: lungs, bone, bone marrow
Radiography
   "Onionskin" pattern
   Primarily lytic
Therapy
   Sensitive to radiation therapy

Modified from Meyer W: Neoplasms of bone. *In* Nelson Textbook of Pediatrics, 15th ed. Philadelphia, W.B. Saunders, 1996, p. 1467.

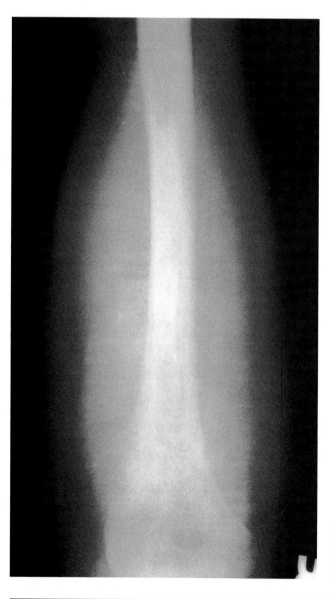

FIGURE 7–29. Osteosarcoma of the distal humerus in 15-year-old girl. Frontal view demonstrates a combined sclerotic and lytic lesion originating in the metaphysis and spreading to the diaphysis. Note significant cortical destruction with classic malignant "sunburst" periosteal reaction.

Mature Cystic Ovarian Teratoma

SYNONYMS   Mature Cystic Teratoma
                Benign Cystic Teratoma
                Dermoids

DEFINITION

Teratoma is an embryonal neoplasm that may be benign or malignant and contains tissue derived from the ectoderm, mesoderm, and endoderm.

EPIDEMIOLOGY

1. Most common pelvic neoplasm in patients under 20 years of age is of ovarian origin.
2. Most common ovarian neoplasm in an adolescent is teratoma.
3. Mature cystic teratoma
   a. Is the most common germ cell tumor
   b. Accounts for 10% to 20% of all ovarian neoplasms
   c. Occurrence rate for bilateral mature cystic teratomas is 10% to 15%.

PATHOLOGY

1. Ovarian teratomas
   a. Benign (90% to 95%)
   b. Malignant (5% to 10%)
2. Two forms
   a. Mature (99%)
   b. Immature (1%)
3. Mature teratomas are further classified as
   a. Cystic or solid: Teratoma consisting of well-differentiated tissues derived from the three germ cell layers (ectoderm, mesoderm, and endoderm)
   b. Monodermal lesions containing neuroectodermal tumors, carcinoid, thyroid tissue, or a combination of thyroid tissue and carcinoid.
      (1) Thyroid tissue is a relatively frequent constituent of mature cystic teratoma and has been demonstrated in 5% to 20% of cases.
      (2) Struma ovarii implies a tumor composed entirely or predominantly of thyroid tissue that may produce thyrotoxicosis.
4. Cystic ovarian teratomas are more common than solid ovarian teratomas.
5. Solid tumors are more likely to be malignant than cystic tumors.

LABORATORY

1. To exclude malignancy and organ damage from mass effect
   a. Complete blood count
   b. Serum values of electrolytes, urea nitrogen, creatinine, uric acid, lactate dehydrogenase, and liver enzymes
2. Tumor markers used to exclude malignant tumors (specific tests)
   a. Serum values of alpha-fetoprotein (e.g., elevated in most patients with yolk sac tumor)
   b. Serum values of beta-human chorionic gonadotropin (e.g., usually elevated in patients with pure embryonal carcinoma)
   c. Mature cystic ovarian teratomas are not associated with tumor markers.
3. Serum beta-human chorionic gonadotropin (to exclude pregnancy)
4. Pelvic ultrasonography
   a. To delineate the size, location, and characteristics of the tumor
   b. To exclude pregnancy
5. Plain abdominal radiographs
   a. Calcium deposits may be seen in the tumor.
   b. Teeth without root canals may be seen in the tumor.
6. Computed tomography of pelvis
   a. To evaluate the extent or size, location, and characteristics of the tumor
   b. To exclude malignancy and local or distant metastasis

TREATMENT

1. Hospitalization
2. Pediatric hematology-oncology and surgery consultations
3. Surgery is the mainstay of therapy.
   a. An ovary-sparing technique such as cystectomy is the preferred approach whenever possible to preserve the reproductive and hormonal functions. However, oophorectomy may be performed when cystectomy is technically impossible.
   b. Attempts are usually made to remove the cyst completely to avoid recurrence.
   c. In patients with torsion and necrosis, a necrotic ovarian tumor as well as a necrotic fallopian tube are removed.
   d. The opposite ovary should also be evaluated (by careful inspection and palpation) during surgery, and a biopsy specimen should be obtained if any pathology is suspected. A suspicious cyst can be aspirated; if the fluid is oily and immiscible with saline, the cyst should be removed.

PROGNOSIS

1. Excellent with ovarian preservation
2. Full surgical excision is curative for mature cystic ovarian teratoma.
3. Malignancy associated with mature cystic teratoma is rare and complicates only 1% to 2% of cases.
   a. Most common cancer is invasive squamous cell carcinoma.
   b. Other cancers include sarcomas, carcinoids, and adenocarcinoma.

KEY POINTS

Mature Cystic Ovarian Teratoma

- Most common type of ovarian teratoma
- Most common ovarian tumor in patients under 20 years old
- Presence of calcification on the abdominal radiograph is often a hallmark of a benign teratoma.

TABLE 7–37
Clinical Features of Cystic Ovarian Teratoma

Most common age at presentation: adolescents
Most common presentation: suprapubic mass
Completely asymptomatic patients: 60% of cases
Tumor incidentally discovered: 19% of cases
Laterality: unilateral (85% to 90%); bilateral (10% to 15%)
Other presentations
  Local compression on surrounding organs (mass effect)
    Abdominal pain
    Constipation
    Urinary tract symptoms
    Backache
  Volvulus of ovarian pedicle/adjacent fallopian tube
    Acute abdominal pain, nausea, vomiting

TABLE 7–38
Complications of Cystic Ovarian Teratoma

Spontaneous rupture of cystic teratoma (uncommon)
  Intraperitoneal rupture
    Sudden rupture of tumor contents ⇒ ⇒ acute peritonitis
    Ruptured cyst may leak chronically ⇒ ⇒ inflammatory
      response
      Granulomatous peritonitis (multiple small white peritoneal
        implants/ dense adhesions)
      Mass effect involving omentum or bowel and pelvic
        lymphadenopathy
  Spontaneous rupture into bladder, small bowel, rectum,
    sigmoid colon, or vagina
Ovarian torsion (3.5% of cases): torsion seen more frequently
  in larger tumors than in smaller ones
Local compression on surrounding organs from mass effect

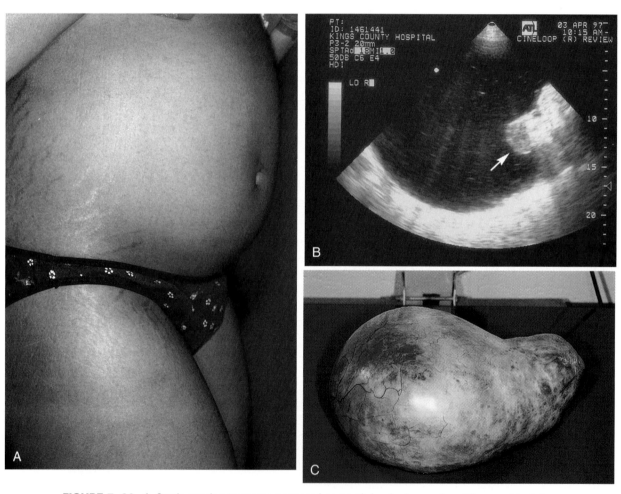

FIGURE 7–30. *A,* Cystic ovarian teratoma appeared as an abdominal mass in a 12-year-old adolescent female. She had "fullness" of the abdomen and a history of chronic constipation for the past 6 months. The abdominal contour resembled that of pregnancy (on three separate occasions a pregnancy test had been ordered by pediatricians to exclude pregnancy). *B,* Ultrasound examination of the right adnexa demonstrates a complex cystic mass containing a peripheral echogenic component with posterior shadowing representing calcification (*arrow*). CT scan of the abdomen and pelvis showed a large complex cystic and solid mass containing fat, fluid, soft tissue, and calcifications. *C,* Close-up of the cystic teratoma weighing 10 lb that was removed from this patient. Grossly, a mature cystic teratoma is usually a globular or cystic tumor as seen here. A smooth glistening capsule that is milky-white in color is also very characteristic (if fat or hair has accumulated beneath the capsule, the tumor may appear yellow or gray). This large tumor usually destroys any adjacent functional ovarian tissue.

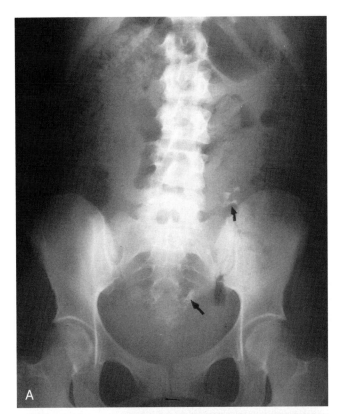

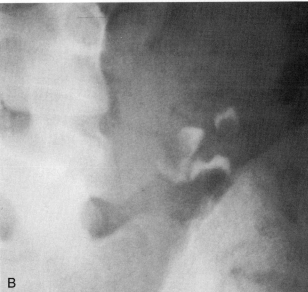

TABLE 7–39
Differential Diagnosis of Cystic Ovarian Teratoma

Abdominal mass in an adolescent
  Pregnancy
    Hematocolpos or hematometrocolopos (imperforate hymen)
    Lymphoma
    Sarcoma
Ovarian torsion presenting as acute abdomen
    Acute appendicitis
    Ectopic pregnancy
Other benign ovarian tumors
    Mature solid teratomas
    Cystic adenoma
    Granulosa cell tumor
Malignant ovarian tumors
    Immature teratoma
    Endodermal sinus tumor (yolk sac tumor)
    Embryonal carcinoma
    Malignant teratoma
    Dysgerminoma

FIGURE 7–31. *A,* Bilateral ovarian teratoma in a 17-year-old girl presenting with pelvic pain. Supine kidney-ureter-bladder (KUB) film of the abdomen shows two clusters of calcifications (*arrows*), which represented bilateral masses with intrinsic dental structures. The larger right mass displaced the left mass above the iliac bone. *B,* Close-up of the left mass demonstrates the cluster of teeth.

Hodgkin Lymphoma

DEFINITION

A lymphoid malignancy arising in a single lymph node or lymphoid region. Initially it spreads to contiguous lymph node areas. If untreated, it disseminates and may involve any organ in the body including the spleen, liver, lungs, bone, and bone marrow.

BOX 7–14   *Lymphadenopathy and Hodgkin Disease*

Almost always presents as lymphadenopathy
Primary site: above the diaphragm in two thirds of patients
Primary site: below the diaphragm in one third of patients
Most common first presenting sites
  Lower cervical (60% to 90%) or supraclavicular
Infrequent first presenting sites
  Axillary or inguinal
Mediastinal adenopathy
  Present in 75% of patients
  Almost always seen with low cervical or supraclavicular involvement
Characteristics of lymph nodes
  Painless
  Rubbery
  Firmer than inflammatory nodes
  Discrete or matted together
  Enlarged nodes slowly progress in size
  Occasionally the size may wax and wane
  Lymph nodes may be sensitive to palpation if they have grown rapidly

---

EPIDEMIOLOGY

1. Lymphomas represent the third largest group of malignancies in children (after acute leukemias and brain tumors).
2. Age: bimodal distribution
   a. United States and other industrialized countries
      (1) First peak: mid to late 20s
      (2) Second peak: after age 50
   b. Developing countries: first peak before adolescence
   c. Rare: under 5 years of age
3. Three distinct forms
   a. Childhood form: patients under 14 years old
   b. Young adult form: patients between 15 and 34 years old
   c. Adult form: patients 55 to 74 years old
4. Gender predeliction
   a. Male-female ratio is equal during adolescence.
   b. Slight male predominance in patients under 10 years of age
5. Genetic predisposition: clustering of Hodgkin disease occurs in families.

BOX 7–15   *Conditions Associated with Increased Frequency of Hodgkin Disease*

AIDS
Epstein-Barr viral infection
Lupus erythematosus
Rheumatoid arthritis
Congenital agammaglobulinemia
Ataxia telangiectasia

LABORATORY

1. Measurement of enlarged lymph nodes and careful assessment of all node-bearing areas including Waldeyer ring (nasopharynx, tonsils, and base of tongue)
2. Complete blood count: nonspecific
   a. Neutrophilic leukocytosis, lymphopenia, eosinophilia, and monocytosis
   b. Anemia may be seen in advanced disease and results from impaired mobilization of iron stores.
3. Erythrocyte sedimentation rate (important for monitoring clinical course of disease and for detecting recurrences)
4. Renal and hepatic function tests (unreliable indicators of hepatic disease)
5. Uric acid and lactate dehydrogenase levels (more frequently elevated in patients with non-Hodgkin lymphoma)
6. Chest radiographs (anteroposterior and lateral views)
7. Computed tomographic (CT) scan or magnetic resonance imaging (MRI) of thorax to detect involvement of lungs (best evaluated by CT), pleura, pericardium, and chest wall that may not be apparent on chest radiographs
8. Abdominal and pelvic CT scan or MRI
9. Lymphangiography
10. Lymph node biopsy to establish a histologic diagnosis
11. Staging laparotomy (in selected cases only)
12. Bone marrow biopsy (in clinical stage IIB or higher)
13. Bone scan with corresponding plain radiographs of abnormal areas to exclude skeletal metastasis (indicated in patients with bone pain, increased alkaline phosphatase level, or extranodal disease)

PATHOLOGY

1. Histologic subtypes
   a. Nodular sclerosis (most common in children and adolescents)
   b. Lymphocytic predominance
   c. Mixed cellularity
   d. Lymphocytic depletion
2. Hallmark of Hodgkin disease is the presence of Reed-Sternberg cells.

DIFFERENTIAL DIAGNOSIS

1. Lymphadenopathy (due to other causes)
   a. Bacterial (e.g., cat-scratch disease)
   b. Tuberculous
   c. Viral (e.g., Epstein-Barr virus)
2. Non-Hodgkin lymphoma characterized by
   a. Rapid growth
   b. Peak age: 7 to 10 years
   c. Primary extranodal or nodal
   d. Metabolic abnormalities

TREATMENT

1. Hospitalization for diagnostic work-up, confirmation of diagnosis, and treatment.
2. Therapy planning involves multidisciplinary approach with pediatric, pediatric hematology-oncology, surgery, radiology, pathology, and radiation-oncology consultations.
3. The anatomically based Ann Arbor staging system is used (see Table 7-41).
4. Pediatric protocols include multiagent chemotherapy used alone or in combination with low-dose involved-field radiation, or high-dose extended-field radiation therapy used alone.

PROGNOSIS

1. Untreated Hodgkin disease: fatal in 80% of patients within 6 to 24 months; in virtually all by 5 years.
2. With appropriate staging and therapy: cure in up to 90% of children and adolescents.

KEY POINTS

Hodgkin Lymphoma

- Most common presentation in children is painless, progressive cervical or supraclavicular lymphadenopathy (which may fluctuate over time).
- Masses located completely anterior to the sternocleidomastoid muscle are benign (exception: thyroid tumor)
- About 50% of masses in the posterior triangle or multiple masses extending across both anterior and posterior triangles represent malignancies, the majority of which are of lymphoid origin.
- Suspect malignancy with large, painless, firm, and rubbery lymph nodes in the posterior triangle.

TABLE 7-40
Clinical Features of Hodgkin Disease

Fever*	Lymphadenopathy (see Box 7-14)
Night sweats*	Hepatosplenomegaly (uncommon)
Weight loss*	Pruritus
Tracheal, bronchial, or esophageal compression	Superior vena cava syndrome
Nonproductive cough	Facial edema
Dysphagia	Distended neck veins
Dyspnea	Pleural effusion

* Fever, night sweats, and weight loss together are seen in 25% to 30% of children.

TABLE 7-41
Ann Arbor Clinical Staging Classification for Hodgkin Lymphoma

Stage	Definition
I	Involvement of a single lymph node region (I) or of a single extralymphatic organ or site (I$_E$)
II	Involvement of two or more lymph node regions on the same side of the diaphragm (II) *or* localized involvement of one extralymphatic organ or site and one or more lymph node regions on the same side of the diaphragm (II$_E$)
III	Involvement of lymph node regions on both sides of the diaphragm (III), which may also include: involvement of spleen (III$_S$) or localized extralymphatic involvement (III$_E$) or both (III$_{SE}$)
IV	Diffuse or disseminated involvement of one or more extralymphatic sites with or without lymph node involvement

All stages are subclassified as A or B to indicate absence or presence of unexplained fever, night sweats, or unexplained loss of 10% or more weight in the preceding 6 months.

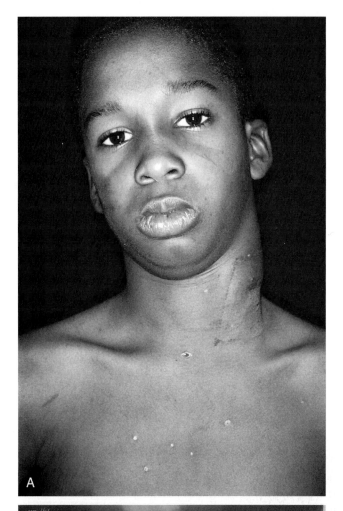

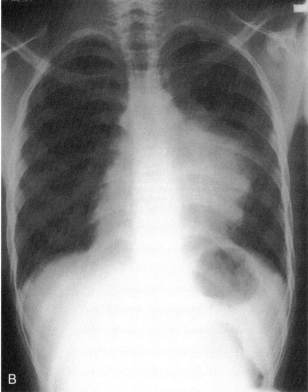

FIGURE 7–32. *A,* Hodgkin lymphoma. A 12-year-old adolescent male presented with a painless, rubbery, firm cervical lymphadenopathy (a group of lymph nodes matted together) of 6 months' duration. Enlarged lymph nodes extended over both posterior and anterior triangles of the neck. Lymph node biopsy (note scar on the neck) confirmed the diagnosis. There was a dramatic decrease in the size of the lymph nodes within 1 week after chemotherapy. (Courtesy of S.P. Rao, M.D., State University of New York, Brooklyn, NY.) *B,* Frontal view of the chest demonstrating a large left hilar mass. This mass also showed significant improvement within a week following therapy.

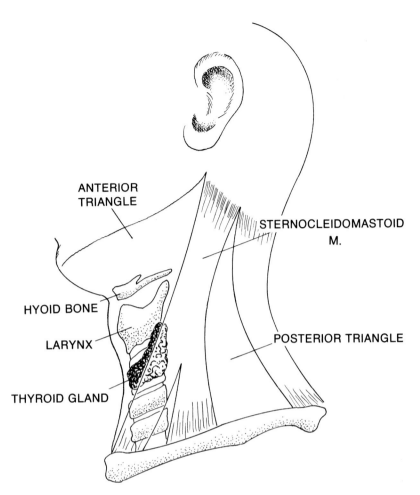

ANTERIOR
TRIANGLE

STERNOCLEIDOMASTOID
M.

HYOID BONE

LARYNX

POSTERIOR TRIANGLE

THYROID GLAND

FIGURE 7–33. Surface anatomy of the neck. The neck is bounded superiorly by the lower margin of the mandible and inferiorly by the clavicles and a line through the spinous process of the 7th cervical vertebra. Two cervical triangles are formed by the sternocleidomastoid (SCM) muscle. Anterior to the SCM is the anterior triangle (bounded by the clavicle inferiorly and the midline anteriorly). Posterior to the SCM is the posterior triangle (bounded by the trapezius muscle posteriorly and the clavicle inferiorly). (From Zitelli BJ: Neck masses in children: Adenopathy and malignant disease. Pediatr Clin North Am 28(4):813, 1981.)

Endocrinology

Binita R. Shah, M.D.

Adolescent Gynecomastia

DEFINITION

Gynecomastia is defined as any palpable mammary gland development in the male. The Greek word *gyne* means woman and *mastos* means breast (gynecomastia = "womanlike breast").

ETIOLOGY/PATHOGENESIS (see also Tables 8–1 to 8–3)

1. Estrogen stimulates, whereas androgens inhibit, mammary growth; thus, gynecomastia is almost always a sign of an altered ratio of estrogen to androgen.
2. Increase in free estrogens
   a. Increased secretion of estrogens or estrogen precursors (testes, adrenal)
   b. Extraglandular (muscle, fat, skin) conversion (aromatization) of androstenedione and testosterone to estrone and estradiol, respectively
   c. Exogenous administration
3. Decrease in endogenous free androgens
   a. Decreased secretion
   b. Increased metabolism

EPIDEMIOLOGY

1. Gynecomastia is frequently seen at three distinct periods during life:
   a. Neonatal (gynecomastia occurs in 60% to 90% of newborn males owing to the transplacental passage of estrogens). It resolves spontaneously. (See also Fig. 1–23, p. 20)
   b. Pubertal
   c. Senescent
2. Transient pubertal gynecomastia
   a. Seen in about 40% of boys between 10 and 16 years of age
   b. Peak prevalence (about 65% to 75%) at 14 years (midpuberty, sexual maturity ratings [SMR] 2–4).
3. There are no racial differences in the prevalence of gynecomastia.

CLINICAL FEATURES

1. A healthy adolescent boy with signs of male sexual development

   a. Testicular enlargement (>3 cm in length or 8 mL in volume), pubic hair development, pigmentation of scrotal skin *preceding* the onset of breast enlargement
   b. Note that testicular enlargement is the first sign of puberty in adolescent males; thus, breast enlargement should *not* precede testicular enlargement.
2. Breast enlargement
   a. Most often bilateral (75%); unilateral (25%)
   b. Both breasts may enlarge at disproportionate rates or at different times
   c. Enlarged tissue may be tender and is nonadherent to the skin or underlying tissue.
   d. Mild gynecomastia
      (1) Usually measures up to 3 cm (enlargement is usually not visible until it reaches a diameter of 1.5 to 2 cm or more)
      (2) Seen in majority of boys
   e. Pubertal macrogynecomastia
      (1) Refers to breast enlargement extending 5 cm or more in diameter
      (2) Often areola and nipple form a secondary mound above the dome-shaped breast (resembling female breast development; SMR 4–5).
      (3) Seen in 5% to 15% of pubertal males

BOX 8–1 *Evaluate Patients with Gynecomastia IF*

Onset before puberty
Onset after completion of physical maturity
Associated with hypogonadism
Macrogynecomastia
Persistent (duration more than 2 years)
Abnormal history or physical examination

LABORATORY

1. Gynecomastia is easily diagnosed by clinical examination.
2. A physician must determine whether gynecomastia is physiologic or pathologic by taking a thorough

history (duration, timing, pain, progression) and performing a physical examination (height, weight, size of breasts, any discharge, tenderness, careful palpation and measurement of the testes, SMR of the genitalia).

3. Majority of patients require no laboratory tests.
4. Serum values of follicle-stimulating hormone (FSH), luteinizing hormone (LH), estradiol, testosterone, dehydroepiandrosterone sulfate (DHEAS), human chorionic gonadotropin (hCG), and prolactin
   a. Values are the same in healthy pubertal boys with or without gynecomastia.
   b. However, if correlated with the stage of puberty, a decreased ratio of testosterone to estradiol is found in patients with gynecomastia.
5. Serum chemistry profiles to assess hepatic, renal, and thyroid functions, if indicated
6. Karyotype, especially if the testes are less than 3 cm in length or 8 mL in volume

DIFFERENTIAL DIAGNOSIS (see Tables 8–1 to 8–3)

Pseudogynecomastia/lipomastia

1. Soft subcutaneous fat deposition (without glandular proliferation) in obese boys that simulates the appearance of gynecomastia
2. No disk of firm and tender subareolar glandular tissue is palpated in such patients.

TREATMENT/PROGNOSIS

1. Pubertal gynecomastia less than 4 cm in diameter (similar to early breast budding in female):
   a. Requires no therapy other than education about the transient and physiologic nature of this phenomenon and reassurance
   b. Gynecomastia of this size resolves *spontaneously* without treatment in about 75% of patients within 2 years and in about 90% of patients within 3 years.
2. If enlargement is striking (macrogynecomastia) or persistently produces anxiety, embarrassment, or serious emotional problems and interference with patient's daily life, medical or surgical therapy may be considered.
3. Medical therapy with consultation with an endocrinologist
   a. Principles of therapy: alteration of estrogen-androgen ratio either by reducing estrogens or by increasing androgens
   b. A placebo-controlled, double-blind, randomized study in a large number of patients with pubertal gynecomastia is lacking.

   c. Drugs (rarely used because of poor success rate and significant side effects)
      (1) With antiestrogenic effects: tamoxifen (not approved in the United States), clomiphene citrate
      (2) Aromatase inhibitor (prevents conversion of androgen to estrogen): testolactone
      (3) Increase androgens: administration of testosterone (aggravates gynecomastia), dihydrotestosterone
3. Surgical therapy for definitive resolution
   a. Common procedure is transareolar reduction mammoplasty and liposuction
   b. Surgery should not be done in early puberty because after insufficient surgical removal of tissue, regrowth may occur as puberty progresses.
   c. Indications
      (1) For persistent macrogynecomastia of 4 years or longer duration (after 4 years, breast tissue shows fibrosis and hyalinization, which is frequently irreversible)
      (2) For cosmetic and psychological reasons
4. Correction of any contributory causes, especially those due to medications or substance abuse, and treatment of any underlying disorders
5. Encourage weight loss and physical activity to increase pectoralis muscle development.
6. Pubertal gynecomastia is *not* associated with an increased risk of breast cancer.

KEY POINT

Adolescent Gynecomastia

- Adolescent boy with gynecomastia must be educated about the physiologic and transient nature of this entity and reassured that he is not "becoming a female."

TABLE 8–1
Etiologies of Gynecomastia

Pubertal (25%)	Testicular tumors (3%)
Idiopathic (25%)	Secondary hypogonadism (2%)
Drugs (10–20%)	
Primary hypogonadism (8%)	Hyperthyroidism (1.5%)
Cirrhosis or malnutrition (8%)	Renal disease (1%)

TABLE 8–2
Pathologic Causes of Gynecomastia

Endocrine

Hypogonadism
    Primary hypogonadism (hypergonadotropic hypogonadism, e.g., Klinefelter syndrome)
    Secondary hypogonadism (hypogonadotropic hypogonadism)
Congenital virilizing adrenal hyperplasia

Tumors

Testicular (Leydig cell, Sertoli cell, germ cell)
Adrenal (feminizing tumors)
Pituitary (prolactinoma [gynecomastia with galactorrhea])
Ectopic production of human chorionic gonadotropin by cancer (lung, liver, kidney)

Systemic Disorders

Liver disease
Renal failure
Malnutrition (recovery phase)
Acquired immune deficiency syndrome (AIDS)

TABLE 8–3
Drug-Induced Gynecomastia

Hormones	Estrogens, androgens, anabolic steroids, human chorionic gonadotropin
Cardiovascular	Digitalis, calcium-channel blockers, captopril
Testosterone antagonist	Ketoconazole, spironolactone, cimetidine
Chemotherapeutic agents	Cyclophosphamide, chlorambucil, methotrexate
Substance abuse	Marijuana, amphetamines, alcohol, heroin, methadone
Psychoactive drugs	Diazepam, tricyclic antidepressants, haloperidol, phenothiazines

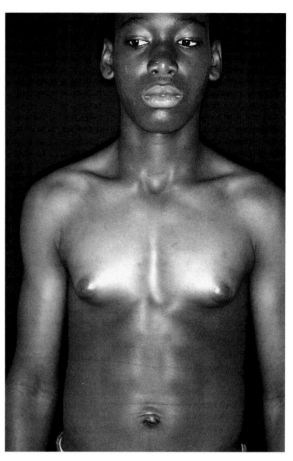

FIGURE 8–2. Mild gynecomastia (Tanner 2) in a 13-year-old adolescent male. With the patient in the supine position, the breast tissue is pinched between the thumb and forefinger. When the two digits are gently moved while squeezing the breast tissue toward the nipple, a firm or rubbery freely movable disk of glandular tissue arising concentrically from beneath the nipple and areolar region is felt in gynecomastia.

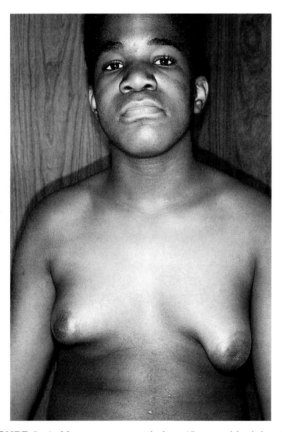

FIGURE 8–1. Macrogynecomastia in a 15-year-old adolescent male. Breast enlargement may be striking and may mimic female breast development (up to SMR 3–5). (Courtesy of Amy Suss, M.D., State University of New York, Brooklyn, NY.)

Premature Thelarche

SYNONYM   Incomplete (Partial) Precocious
                     Puberty

DEFINITION

Isolated, transient breast tissue development in prepubertal girls (prior to age 8 years) without other signs of puberty

ETIOLOGY/PATHOGENESIS

1. Unclear in the majority of patients
2. Possible causes include:
   a. Persistent neonatal mammary hyperplasia: some girls with premature thelarche have a prior history of physiologic breast enlargement (in neonatal period) that has persisted.
   b. Increased sensitivity of breast tissue to estradiol stimulation

c. Transient elevation of plasma estradiol in some girls

d. Transient episodic formation of ovarian cyst (graafian follicles that have become cystic and luteinized, secreting estrogens). Regression and recurrence of thelarche suggest functioning follicular cysts.

EPIDEMIOLOGY

1. Puberty in normal girls occurs after 8 years of age, and the first sign of puberty is usually the appearance of the "breast buds."
2. Most common age for premature thelarche:
   a. Girls less than 3 years of age (range, infancy to 8 years)
   b. 60% of patients are between 6 months and 2 years of age
3. Epidemics of premature thelarche have been reported secondary to consumption of foods contaminated with estrogen (e.g., chicken breasts)

INHERITANCE

1. Most cases occur sporadically.
2. Rarely familial (family history of early puberty)

LABORATORY

1. Serum values of gonadotropins (luteinizing hormone [LH], follicle-stimulating hormone): prepubertal
2. Serum value of estradiol: prepubertal or early pubertal
3. LH response to gonadotropin-releasing hormone (GnRH): prepubertal
4. Serum value of dehydroepiandrosterone sulfate (DHEAS): normal or minimally increased for age
5. Bone age (BA): consistent with chronologic age
6. Pelvic ultrasound: normal prepubertal size of ovaries; however, a few small follicular cysts are not uncommon

TREATMENT

1. Reassurance about the benign nature of this entity
2. Regular follow-up to note the progression or regression of breast enlargement and to watch for any other signs of puberty
3. Endocrinology consultation for any patient who shows any of the following signs during follow-up:
   a. Progressive continued enlargement of the breast
   b. Signs of secondary sex characteristics (development of pubic or axillary hair)
   c. Growth spurt

d. Advancement of skeletal age (BA) in relation to chronologic age

e. Vaginal bleeding

PROGNOSIS

1. Breast development may regress and completely disappear after several months to 2 years, or it may persist for 3 to 5 years; it is rarely progressive.
2. Normal puberty (onset, appearance of secondary sexual maturation, and menarche) occurs at an appropriate age.

KEY POINTS

Premature Thelarche

- Premature thelarche is a benign and self-limited condition.
- Since breast enlargement is a first sign of true puberty, patients with premature thelarche should be followed closely to exclude the possibility of true precocious puberty.
- Premature thelarche is a diagnosis of exclusion; the diagnosis should not be made in the presence or progression of other signs of puberty.
- Breast enlargement in girls over 3 years of age usually suggests a cause other than benign premature thelarche.

TABLE 8–4
Clinical Features of Premature Thelarche

Breast enlargement
  Bilateral; very rarely only unilateral
  Unilateral breast enlargement may proceed to contralateral breast enlargement
  Asymmetry in size between two breasts ($\pm$)
  Breast tenderness ($\pm$)
  No further significant increase in size of breasts until puberty
Nipples and areola
  Infantile appearance (not prominent)
  Absence of pigmentary changes
  Absence of galactorrhea
External genitalia
  Appearance of vulva, labia minora, vagina: infantile
  Evidence of estrogenization of vaginal epithelium ($\pm$)
Absence of other signs of puberty
  Absence of growth spurt (growth velocity curve appropriate for chronologic age)
  Absence of axillary or pubic hair
  Absence of menses
  Body habitus childlike (does not show mature contours)
Absence of café-au-lait spots suggestive of McCune-Albright syndrome

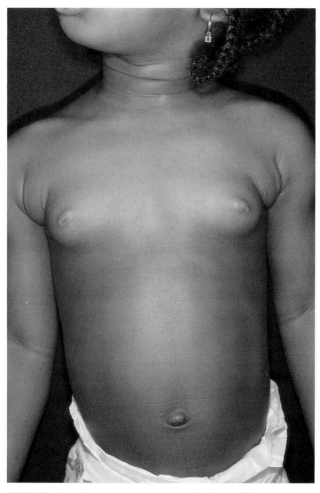

FIGURE 8–3. Premature thelarche. Isolated bilateral breast enlargement in a 2-year-old girl that began at the age of 8 months. There may be asymmetry in size between the two breasts (as in the early stages of normal puberty, during which asymmetric breast development is quite common).

TABLE 8–5
Differential Diagnosis of Premature Thelarche

Neonatal physiologic enlargement of the breast
True precocious puberty
Obesity with adipose tissue giving appearance of breast tissue
Environmental exposure to exogenous estrogens
   Ingestion or cutaneous absorption of medicinal forms (birth control pills, estrogen creams)
   Ingestion of foods contaminated with estrogen
Tumors of mammary gland (exceedingly rare in children)

Juvenile Graves Disease

DEFINITION

1. A multisystem disease characterized by three distinctive features:
   a. Hyperthyroidism with diffuse goiter
   b. Ophthalmopathy
   c. Dermopathy
2. These three features appear in varying combinations and frequencies and may run courses that are independent of each another.

EPIDEMIOLOGY

1. Common age at presentation
   a. Peak incidence occurs during adolescence
   b. More than two-thirds of cases are seen in patients between 10 and 15 years of age.
   c. Onset occurs from birth to 5 years of age in about 15% of children.
2. Female-male ratio is 5 to 8:1.

PATHOGENESIS

1. Graves disease is an immunogenetic disorder associated with thyroid-stimulating immunoglobulins, most notably:
   a. Antithyroglobulin antibodies
   b. Antimicrosomal antibodies (antithyroid peroxidase)
   c. Thyroid-stimulating hormone (TSH) receptor antibody.
2. TSH receptor-stimulating antibodies
   a. Are detected in 93% of children with untreated active disease
   b. Bind to the TSH receptor and stimulate thyroid follicular cell function, leading to increased synthesis and secretion of T_4 and T_3
   c. This process is independent of the pituitary-thyroid axis of feedback control
3. A family history of autoimmune thyroid disease is present in up to 60% of patients.

Graves Disease and Other Associated Autoimmune Diseases

Hashimoto thyroiditis
Addison disease
Myasthenia gravis
Systemic lupus erythematosus
Insulin-dependent diabetes mellitus
Vitiligo
Pernicious anemia

4. Thyrotoxicosis results from excessive circulating levels of unbound thyroid hormones (free T_4 and/or free T_3).

CLINICAL FEATURES (see also Table 8-6)

1. Clinical course is variable with signs and symptoms developing insidiously over several months; the usual interval between onset of symptoms and diagnosis is 6 to 12 months.
2. Thyroid "storm"
   a. Results from a sudden release of thyroid hormone into the circulation
   b. A life-threatening presentation
   c. Seen less commonly in children than in adults
   d. Patients present acutely with the following signs:
      (1) Hyperthermia
      (2) Severe tachycardia progressing to cardiogenic shock
      (3) CNS manifestations of restlessness, agitation, psychosis, delirium, or coma
3. Graves dermopathy (pretibial myxedema)
   a. Rare in children
   b. A raised, thickened, well-demarcated area over the dorsum of the legs or feet with a peau d'orange appearance

LABORATORY

1. Elevated values of T_4, free T_4, and T_3 in association with a suppressed value of TSH in the serum, and the presence of TSH receptor-stimulating antibodies establishes the diagnosis of Graves disease.
2. A serum TSH value above 1.0 mU/mL suggests TSH-dependent hyperthyroidism, whereas suppression of TSH indicates that hyperthyroidism is not pituitary in origin.
3. Antithyroglobulin antibodies
4. Antimicrosomal antibodies

TREATMENT

1. Referral to a pediatric endocrinologist for management once the diagnosis is made
2. Treatment options include
   a. Medical management (most frequently used)
      (1) Antithyroid drugs (propylthiouracil or methimazole)
      (2) Beta-adrenergic blocking agent (propranolol) for cardiac symptoms, if indicated
   b. Surgical (subtotal thyroidectomy)
   c. Radioiodine ablation

PROGNOSIS

Ophthalmopathy resolves gradually and usually independently of the hyperthyroidism.

KEY POINTS

Juvenile Graves Disease

- Graves disease accounts for 95% of cases of thyrotoxicosis in children
- Behavioral abnormalities including emotional lability and declining academic performance are frequently early signs
- Goiter is *almost always* present in Graves disease; its absence should raise serious doubt about the diagnosis, and other causes of hyperthyroidism must be considered

TABLE 8-6
Clinical Features of Graves Disease

Goiter	Voracious appetite with weight loss or poor weight gain
Ophthalmopathy	Emotional disturbances
Seen in >50% of patients	Hyperdefecation
Lid lag, stare	Heat intolerance
Exophthalmos	Menstrual irregularities
Cardiac	Restless, nervous, fidgety
Tachyarrhythmias	Skin (smooth, flushed, excessive sweating)
Systolic hypertension	
Increased pulse pressure	Fine tremors (fingers, tongue)
Myopathy	
Fatigue	
Muscle weakness	
Periodic paralysis	

TABLE 8-7
Differential Diagnosis of Graves Diseases

Surreptitious exogenous T_4 or T_3
  Thyrotoxicosis *without* goiter and low thyroglobulin value
Autonomously functioning thyroid nodule
TSH-induced hyperthyroidism
  TSH-secreting pituitary adenoma
  Pituitary unresponsiveness to thyroid hormone
McCune-Albright syndrome
  Precocious puberty
  Polyostotic fibrous dysplasia
  Café-au-lait spots
  Hyperfunction of endocrine glands including hyperthyroidism

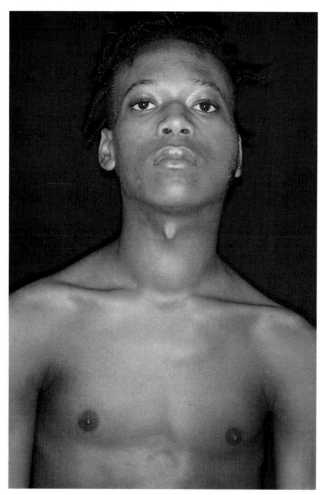

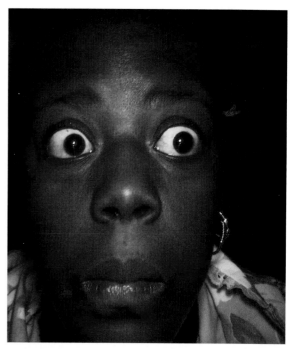

FIGURE 8–5. Exophthalmos (due to infiltration of lymphocytes, mucopolysaccharides, and edema fluid in the orbit) causing the appearance of a stare in a 14-year-old female with Graves disease. The stare results from retraction of the upper lid and wide palpebral apertures due to sympathetic hyperactivity.

FIGURE 8–4. Graves disease with goiter in a 13-year-old patient with a diffuse, soft, nontender, symmetrically enlarged thyroid gland that moved with swallowing. A bruit was heard over the enlarged gland.

Autoimmune Thyroiditis

SYNONYMS   Hashimoto Thyroiditis
            Chronic Lymphocytic Thyroiditis
            Lymphadenoid Goiter

DEFINITION

An autoimmune disease of the thyroid gland

ETIOLOGY/PATHOGENESIS

1. Organ-specific autoimmune disease
2. Hyperplasia of the thyroid gland, followed by lymphocytic and plasma cell infiltration between the follicles, and subsequently atrophy of the follicles

EPIDEMIOLOGY

1. Most common cause of acquired hypothyroidism
2. Incidence: about 1% among high school children
3. Female-male ratio is 4 to 7:1
4. Age at presentation
   a. Peak during adolescence
   b. Uncommon before 6 years of age
5. Autoimmune thyroiditis is more frequently seen with other conditions (see Table 8–8).

INHERITANCE

1. Occurs in genetically predisposed persons
2. People with tissue types HLA-DR4 and DR5, and HLA-DQW-7 are prone to develop autoimmune thyroiditis.
3. Family history of thyroid disease is positive in 30% to 40% of patients.
4. Autosomal dominant inheritance (with decreased penetrance in males) among family members for autoantibodies to thyroglobulin and thyroid peroxidase

DIFFERENTIAL DIAGNOSIS

1. Acquired hypothyroidism due to other causes
   a. TSH deficiency hypothyroidism (secondary hypothyroidism)
      (1) Tumors (craniopharyngioma)
      (2) Granulomatous disease
      (3) Infections (meningitis)
      (4) Head trauma
      (5) Cranial irradiation
   b. Iatrogenic (radioactive iodine, postsurgery [e.g., removal of thyroglossal duct cyst])
   c. Exposure to goitrogenic agents (e.g., iodine in large amounts, drugs)
2. Other rare causes of thyroiditis
   a. Acute bacterial suppurative thyroiditis
   b. Viral causes (e.g., mumps)
   c. Granulomatous conditions (e.g., tuberculosis, sarcoidosis)
   d. Cat-scratch disease

TREATMENT

1. Patients with evidence of hypothyroidism
   a. Replacement therapy with a single daily dose of levo-thyroxine (L-thyroxine)
   b. L-thyroxine is the most effective thyroid preparation for the treatment of hypothyroidism.
   c. Monitor thyroid function tests while adjusting the dose of L-thyroxine
   d. Serum TSH is the most useful test to monitor; with optimal replacement therapy, TSH level should be maintained in the normal range. Serum T_4 (or free T_4) helps to determine whether patient is receiving excessive L-thyroxine.
   e. Schedule follow-up thyroid function tests every 3 to 6 months until growth ceases, and then yearly thereafter.
   f. Because of the possibility of spontaneous remission, therapy may be discontinued (after completion of growth) for 6 to 8 weeks; a repeat TSH test is then performed. If TSH rises, therapy should be restarted, and patient needs lifelong replacement therapy.

2. Patients who are euthyroid initially become hypothyroid gradually within months to years. Thus, untreated patients need periodic thyroid function test monitoring.
3. Treatment of children during the euthyroid phase of the disease is controversial. Treatment of euthyroid goiter has not been shown either to reduce the size of the thyroid gland or to prevent the development of hypothyroidism.
4. Goiter may decrease somewhat in size or may persist for years. However, a nodule that persists despite therapy should undergo histologic examination to exclude thyroid cancer.

PROGNOSIS

1. Spontaneous remission is seen in about 30% of adolescent patients.
2. Yearly incidence of hypothyroidism in adult patients with Hashimoto thyroiditis is 5% to 7%.
3. Antibody levels fluctuate in both treated and untreated patients and may persist for years.

KEY POINTS

Autoimmune Thyroiditis

- The most common cause of thyroid disease in children and adolescents
- The most common cause of acquired hypothyroidism and goiter in children over 6 years of age in North America
- Most common presenting signs are growth failure and goiter
- Thyroid deficiency *must* be excluded in any child who demonstrates growth failure.

TABLE 8–8
Autoimmune Thyroiditis and Other Associated Conditions

Autoimmune Disorders

Diabetes mellitus
Pernicious anemia
Alopecia
Vitiligo
Chronic active hepatitis
Systemic lupus erythematosus
Rheumatoid arthritis
Sjögren syndrome

Polyglandular Autoimmune Syndrome, Type I

Autoimmune thyroiditis
Hypoparathyroidism
Addison disease
Mucocutaneous candidiasis

Polyglandular Autoimmune Syndrome, Type II (Schmidt Syndrome)

Autoimmune thyroiditis
Insulin-dependent diabetes mellitus
Addison disease

Abnormal Chromosome Karyotype

Down syndrome
Turner syndrome
Klinefelter syndrome
Noonan syndrome

Other Diseases

Congenital rubella

TABLE 8–9
Clinical Features of Autoimmune Thyroiditis

Growth retardation (short stature, decreased growth velocity)
Goiter (variable course with any of the following)
　Seen in 33% to 50% of patients
　Insidious onset
　Small or large (feeling of local pressure, swallowing difficulty)
　Diffusely enlarged or lobular/nodular
　Rubbery or firm consistency, with or without mild tenderness
　May disappear spontaneously or persist for years
Thyroid function (variable course with any of the following)
　Euthyroid (about 70%)
　Clinical signs of hypothyroidism (about 20%; see Table 8–10)
　Only biochemical evidence of hypothyroidism
　Evidence of hyperthyroidism (about 5% to 10%)
　Concurrent signs of Graves disease (see Table 8–6); "hashitoxicosis")

TABLE 8–10
Clinical Symptoms and Signs of Acquired Hypothyroidism

Fatigue
Lethargy
Puffy eyes
Deteriorating school performance
Constipation
Cold intolerance
Skin dry, cool, coarse, or carotenemia
Hair loss or thinning of hair
Weight gain (weight for age > height for age)
Menstrual irregularities
Sexual precocity (rare)
　Girls: Breast development, galactorrhea, vaginal bleeding
　Boys: Testicular and penile enlargement

Short stature, increased upper-lower body ratio
Goiter
Dull facial expression
Bradycardia
Muscle weakness
Hyporeflexia
Nonpitting edema
Paresthesias
Delayed puberty
Delayed bone age
Delayed dentition

TABLE 8–11
Laboratory Features of Autoimmune Thyroiditis

Serum thyroid function tests at presentation
　Thyroid-stimulating hormone (TSH): usually normal or may be elevated
　Thyroxine (T_4): usually normal
　Triiodothyronine (T_3): usually normal
Serum thyroid function tests with progressive thyroid failure
　TSH: elevated
　T_4: decreased; free thyroxine: decreased
　T_3: decreased
Thyroid antiperoxidase antibodies (antimicrosomal antibodies): positive (90% to 95%)
Antithyroglobulin antibodies: positive (<50%)
Thyrotropin receptor-blocking antibodies: positive (in patients with hypothyroidism)
Evidence of antithyroid antibodies in siblings or parents (in absence of thyroid disease)
Tests indicated rarely (only if nodular thyroid disease is suspected)
　Thyroid ultrasound: scattered hypoechogenicity
　Thyroid scan: irregular, patchy distribution of radioisotope
　Biopsy of thyroid gland

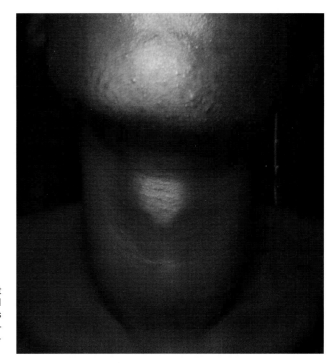

FIGURE 8–6. A goiter was seen in this 14-year-old adolescent female, who presented with excessive menstrual bleeding and "fullness in her neck." A diagnosis of autoimmune thyroiditis with hypothyroidism was confirmed by elevated antithyroglobulin and antiperoxidase antibody titers, elevated TSH, and decreased T_4 and T_3 levels.

Addison Disease

SYNONYM   Primary Adrenocortical Deficiency

DEFINITION

1. Adrenal insufficiency can result from a primary adrenal disorder or may be secondary to hypopituitarism (resultant adrenocorticotropic hormone [ACTH] deficiency)
2. Addison disease is a primary adrenal insufficiency.

ETIOLOGY

1. Autoimmune destruction (most common cause—over 80% of cases)
   a. Autoimmune adrenalitis (isolated)
   b. As part of autoimmune polyglandular syndromes, types 1 and 2 (see Table 8–8)
   c. About 45% of patients with autoimmune Addison disease develop one or more other autoimmune endocrinopathies (most often thyroid disease)
2. Infection
   a. Tuberculosis (most common cause in past)
   b. Acquired immune deficiency syndrome (AIDS)
   c. Other: histoplasmosis, coccidioidomycosis, cryptococcosis
3. Other causes
   a. Hemorrhage (Waterhouse-Friderichsen syndrome)
   b. Congenital adrenal hypoplasia
   c. Abdominal irradiation
   d. Sarcoidosis
   e. Neoplastic infiltration
   f. Medications

(1) Decreased steroid synthesis (e.g., ketoconazole)
(2) Increased steroid metabolism (e.g., phenobarbital, rifampin)

EPIDEMIOLOGY

1. Incidence in children: unknown
2. Incidence in adults: 1 in 25,000
3. Age at presentation
   a. Rare in children
   b. Most patients present between 20 and 50 years of age
4. Females are affected more often than males.

PATHOGENESIS

1. Bilateral destruction of adrenal cortices leads to decreased production of all three groups of steroid hormones:
   a. Cortisol
   b. Aldosterone
   c. Adrenal androgens
2. Destruction must involve more than 90% of the gland before adrenal insufficiency appears.
3. Decreased production of cortisol leads to compensatory increased production of ACTH and beta-melanocyte-stimulating hormone (β-MSH) by the pituitary gland.

DIFFERENTIAL DIAGNOSIS

1. Physiologic pigmentation
   a. Seen normally in African-Americans
   b. May be difficult to differentiate at times from Addison disease; however, a *recent* and *progres-*

sive increase in pigmentation is highly suggestive of gradual adrenal destruction.

   c. Physiologic pigmentation remains indefinitely; the hyperpigmentation seen with Addison disease improves with steroid therapy.

2. Familial glucocorticoid deficiency (ACTH unresponsiveness; see p. 304)
3. Adrenoleukodystrophy
   a. Glucocorticoid deficiency
   b. Neurologic involvement
   c. Elevated levels of very long chain fatty acids
4. Other conditions with similar electrolyte abnormalities
   a. Renal disorders (e.g., obstructive uropathy)
   b. Isolated aldosterone deficiency

BOX 8-3   *Hyperpigmentation and Addison Disease*

PRESENCE OF HYPERPIGMENTATION

One of the most prominent features

Seen in 92% of cases

Diffuse brown, tan, or bronze darkening of skin or certain areas of skin

May be equally intense over entire body or accentuated in sun-exposed areas

Most common sites

   Oral mucosa, tongue, gingiva, hard palate

   Pressure or friction points (elbows), creases of palms and soles

   Genitalia, nipples, areola

   Umbilicus, axilla, sun-exposed skin

Hyperpigmentation improves with steroid therapy (unlike physiologic pigmentation in African-Americans that remains indefinitely)

ABSENCE OF HYPERPIGMENTATION

Does not exclude the diagnosis

Usually absent when adrenal destruction is rapid (e.g., in bilateral adrenal hemorrhage)

TREATMENT

1. "Physiologic replacement" therapy with glucocorticoids and mineralocorticoids
   a. Hydrocortisone (cortisol)
      (1) This is the mainstay of therapy.
      (2) Usual dose: 10 to 15 mg/m^2/day given orally in divided doses
      (3) To simulate normal diurnal rhythm: two thirds of the dose is taken in the morning; one third is taken in the late afternoon.
   b. Florinef: 0.1 mg given orally once a day

2. Adequate intake of salt (3 to 4 g/day)
3. "Stress dose"
   a. For major stress (e.g., surgery, serious infection)
      (1) Intravenous hydrocortisone 100 mg/m^2 followed by 50 to 100 mg/m^2/24 hours in six divided doses
      (2) Taper to physiologic doses over a few days once the patient's condition improves
   b. For minor stress (e.g., infection)
      (1) Usually the physiologic dose of hydrocortisone is doubled or tripled and given orally.
      (2) Usually given for 24 hours, after which the usual dose is resumed
   c. Increase the dose of fludrocortisone and add salt to the normal diet during extremely hot weather, strenuous exercise with excessive sweating, and gastrointestinal illness.
4. For adrenal crisis, see Table 8–15

PROGNOSIS

1. Long-term prognosis for Addison disease is good provided adrenal crisis is prevented and patient gets appropriate therapy during periods of stress.
2. Hyperpigmentation regresses with adequate treatment.

PREVENTION AND FOLLOW-UP

1. Education of family and patient for signs and symptoms of adrenal crisis
2. Medic Alert bracelet must be worn all the time so that patient receives appropriate immediate treatment for adrenal crisis.
3. Patients should be regularly followed and screened for signs of other autoimmune diseases.

KEY POINTS

Addison Disease

- Adrenal insufficiency should always be considered in a patient with increased pigmentation of the skin.
- Failure of a suntan to disappear may be the first clue.
- Long-term survival of patients with adrenocortical insufficiency depends largely on prevention and treatment of adrenal crisis.
- Glucocorticoid dosage *must* be increased during periods of stress.

TABLE 8-12
Clinical Features of Addison Disease

Most Frequent Signs and Symptoms

Weakness (asthenia)
  A cardinal symptom
  First noted during periods of stress
  Becomes progressively worse (as adrenal function
    deteriorates)
  Eventually patient becomes continuously fatigued
Hyperpigmentation of skin (see Box 8-3)
Pigmentation of mucous membranes
Weight loss or poor weight gain
Anorexia, nausea, vomiting
Dehydration, postural hypotension
Diarrhea or constipation

Less Frequent Signs and Symptoms

Syncope
Salt craving
Abdominal pain
Vitiligo (may present concomitantly with hyperpigmentation)
Decreased pubic and axillary hair
Decreased libido

TABLE 8-13
Common Laboratory Findings of Addison Disease

Normocytic anemia
Eosinophilia
Lymphocytosis
Chest x-ray: small heart
  (hypovolemia)
Electrocardiography
  Peak T waves, absent P waves
    widened QRS complex
  Arrhythmias (hyperkalemia)

Hyponatremia
Hypochloremia
Hyperkalemia
Hypoglycemia
Acidosis
Azotemia (hypovolemia)
Hypercalcemia (10% to
  20%)

TABLE 8-14
Specific Laboratory Tests of Addison Disease

Serum cortisol level
  Levels may vary from zero to low normal range
  Cortisol level alone is of little diagnostic value
  Diagnosis should *never* be excluded based on a normal
    cortisol level
Serum aldosterone level: usually decreased
Plasma renin levels: elevated
Serum levels of androgens: decreased in adolescents
Plasma levels of ACTH, β-MSH: elevated
Antiadrenal antibodies ($\pm$)
Antibodies to other endocrine glands ($\pm$)
ACTH stimulation tests
  Most important tests for confirmation of the diagnosis
  Help to assess adrenal reserve capacity for steroid
    production
  In severe adrenal insufficiency
    Basal cortisol levels subnormal
    Serum levels of cortisol and aldosterone fail to increase
      after ACTH administration
    24-hour urine cortisol excretion: low to absent

TABLE 8-15
Acute Adrenal Crisis (Addisonian Crisis)

Precipitating Events

Infections, surgery, trauma

Clinical

Fever, apathy, or weakness
Abdominal pain, nausea, vomiting
Hypoglycemic seizures
Hypovolemia $\Rightarrow$ tachycardia
Hypotension $\Rightarrow$ shock $\Rightarrow$ cardiovascular collapse $\Rightarrow$ death

Laboratory

Hyponatremia
Hypochloremia
Hyperkalemia
Acidosis
Hypoglycemia (or normal glucose)

Treatment

Volume repletion (lactated Ringer's or 0.9 normal saline)
Correction of hypoglycemia (D25 or D10)
Stress dose of hydrocortisone (100 mg/m^2)
Followed by hydrocortisone 100 mg/m^2/24 hours in divided
  doses at 6-hour intervals
With satisfactory oral intake
  Daily oral cortisol replacement therapy
  Daily oral mineralocorticoid replacement therapy

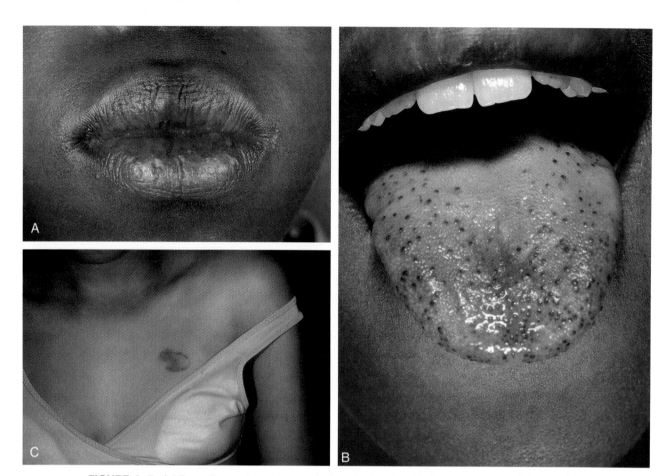

FIGURE 8–7. Addison disease in a 14-year-old female showing black pigmentation of the lips (*A*), spotty pigmentation of the tongue (*B*), and pigmentation of the scar (patient had been bitten by a classmate 2 months earlier) (*C*). She presented with weight loss, anorexia, and progressive weakness of a few months' duration.

Familial Glucocorticoid Deficiency (FGD)

SYNONYMS   Familial Glucocorticoid
                         Insufficiency
                     Adrenocorticotropic Hormone
                         (ACTH) Unresponsiveness
                     Hereditary or Congenital
                         Adrenocortical Unresponsiveness
                         to ACTH
                     Triple A Syndrome
                     Allgrove Syndrome

DEFINITION

A multisystem disorder characterized by glucocorticoid deficiency with normal mineralocorticoid activity, achalasia of the cardia, and alacrima

ETIOLOGY/PATHOGENESIS

1. Preservation of mineralocorticoid function with simultaneous loss of glucocorticoid production may be attributable to different stimuli:
   a. Only stimulus for glucocorticoid secretion: ACTH

BOX 8–4	*Triple A Syndrome*

ACTH unresponsiveness
Alacrima
Achalasia of cardia

---

   b. Stimuli for aldosterone secretion: angiotensin, potassium, ACTH
2. Most commonly cited explanations for adrenal failure in patients with FGD include:
   a. Primary adrenocortical unresponsiveness to ACTH
      (1) Abnormality at adrenal ACTH receptor or postreceptor site
      (2) A number of mutations in the gene for ACTH receptor have been described.
      (3) Both endogenous and exogenously administered ACTH fail to stimulate cortisol production, making a defect in the endogenous ACTH molecule unlikely.

(4) Aldosterone secretion is not affected because its secretion is controlled by factors other than ACTH.
b. Progressive degeneration of adrenal cortex leading to atrophy with:
  (1) *Involvement* of only glucocorticoid-producing zones (zona fasciculata and zona reticularis)
  (2) *Sparing* of aldosterone-producing zone (zona glomerulosa)
c. Persistence of a fetal-like adrenal gland
d. Autonomic dysfunction manifested by (relationship of this to adrenal disorder is unclear)
  (1) Alacrima
  (2) Achalasia of cardia

EPIDEMIOLOGY

1. Rare entity
2. Usual age at presentation
   a. Most patients present after first year of life and almost always by 5 years of age
   b. Some patients are symptomatic with hyperpigmentation at birth or shortly thereafter
3. Males and females are equally affected

INHERITANCE

1. Inherited defect in the ACTH receptor
2. Most common mode of inheritance: autosomal recessive
3. Rarely X-linked recessive mode of inheritance is suggested.
4. Adrenal function may be impaired in asymptomatic family members.

DIFFERENTIAL DIAGNOSIS

1. Addison disease (see p. 301)
2. Adrenoleukodystrophy
   a. Adrenal insufficiency (glucocorticoid deficiency)
   b. Neurologic findings (behavioral changes, dysarthria, poor memory to severe dementia)
   c. Elevated levels of very long chain fatty acids

TREATMENT

1. Glucocorticoid deficiency
   a. Physiologic replacement of glucocorticoid (see page 302)
   b. Stress dose of glucocorticoid during periods of stress (e.g., infection, operative procedures; see page 302)
2. Artificial tears for alacrima
3. Achalasia cardia
   a. Gastroenterology and surgical consultations
   b. Modified Heller esophageal myotomy

KEY POINTS

Familial Glucocorticoid Deficiency

- Preservation of mineralocorticoid function with simultaneous loss of glucocorticoid production
- Salt-losing manifestations *do not* occur
- Most common presenting signs and symptoms are hyperpigmentation and hypoglycemic seizures.
- Many affected children receive other treatment for seizures before the hypoglycemic origin is recognized.

TABLE 8-16
Clinical Features of Familial Glucocorticoid Deficiency

Usually presents with features of chronic adrenal insufficiency during childhood
Hyperpigmentation
  Involvement of skin and mucous membranes (see Box 8–3)
  Pigmentation may be seen at birth or shortly thereafter
Hypoglycemia presenting as
  Seizures
  Lethargy or coma
Failure to thrive
Mental retardation
Alacrima
  Deficient tear production
  Dryness of conjunctiva
Achalasia of cardia
  Nocturnal cough
  Inspiratory stridor
  Vomitus containing undigested food particles
  Weight loss

TABLE 8-17
Laboratory Features of Familial Glucocorticoid Deficiency

Isolated glucocorticoid deficiency
  Serum cortisol (AM and PM): decreased
  Plasma ACTH: increased
  Plasma β-MSH: increased
  Urinary 17-hydroxycorticosteroid (17-OHCS) excretion: decreased
Normal mineralocorticoid function
  Serum electrolytes: normal
  Serum aldosterone: normal
ACTH stimulation test
  Failure of serum cortisol (AM and PM) values to rise
  Failure of urinary 17-OHCS values to increase
Achalasia of cardia
  Chest radiograph
  Barium swallow

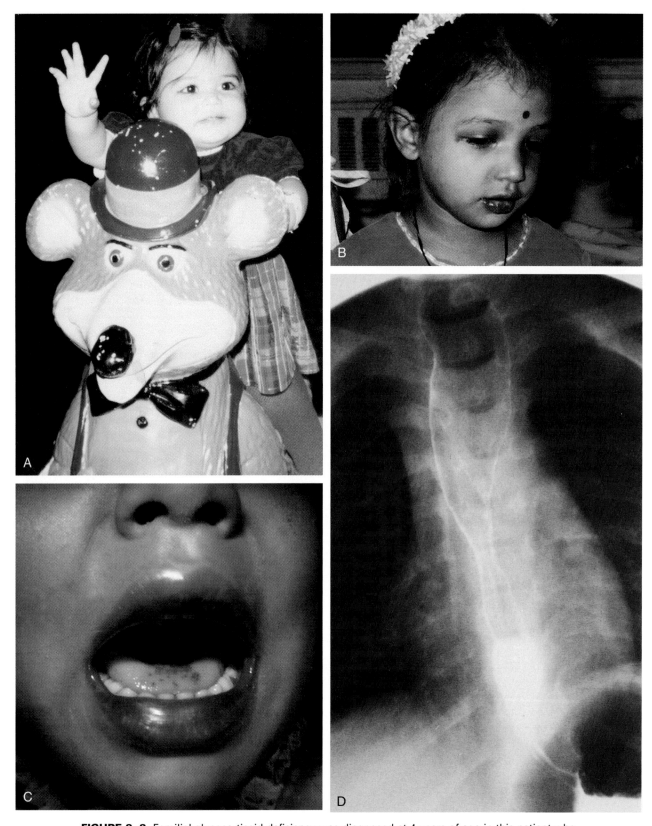

FIGURE 8–8. Familial glucocorticoid deficiency was diagnosed at 4 years of age in this patient who had suffered a hypoglycemic seizure at 3½ years leading to severe hypoxic encephalopathy. *A,* Fair complexion during infancy. *B,* Uniformly pigmented skin of the same patient with hyperpigmentation of the lips at 3 years of age. *C,* Hyperpigmentation of lips and tongue. This hyperpigmentation disappeared after therapy with glucocorticoids. Hyperpigmentation in patients with FGD (or Addison disease) improves with steroid therapy; physiologic pigmentation remains indefinitely. *D,* Achalasia of the cardia was diagnosed in this patient at 4½ years of age. Frontal view of the chest during a barium swallow study. Note marked tapering of the esophagus at the gastroesophageal junction and secondary distention of the proximal esophagus.

Cushing Syndrome (CS)

DEFINITION

Hypercortisolism is excessive secretion of cortisol by the adrenal cortex.

1. Cushing syndrome is a state of hypercortisolism with a characteristic pattern of obesity, hypertension, and other clinical features.
2. Cushing disease is a state of hypercortisolism secondary to an adrenocorticotropic hormone (ACTH)-producing pituitary adenoma (macro or microadenoma).
3. Cushingoid syndrome refers to a characteristic pattern of obesity and other clinical features of CS resulting from prolonged exogenous administration of ACTH or cortisol or its analogs.

ETIOLOGY/PATHOGENESIS

1. Cushing syndrome may be endogenous or exogenous and may be ACTH-dependent or ACTH-independent (see Table 8–18).
2. Adrenal adenomas usually secrete cortisol with minimal amounts of mineralocorticoids or androgens.
3. Adrenocortical carcinoma usually secretes both cortisol and androgens.

EPIDEMIOLOGY

1. Incidence of CS: 2 to 4 new cases per million population per year
2. Female predominance
3. Many patients first seen as adults with CS actually experience onset of symptoms in childhood or adolescence.
4. Congenital hemihypertrophy may be associated with adrenal adenoma or carcinoma.
5. Adrenocortical carcinoma accounts for more than 50% of CS in children under 7 years of age.
6. ACTH-dependent CS accounts for about 80% of cases of hypercortisolism in children over 7 years of age and in adults.

TREATMENT

1. Hospitalization for definitive treatment
2. Pediatric endocrinology, surgery, and neurosurgery consultations
3. Surgery is the therapeutic approach
   a. For ACTH-independent CS
      (1) Unilateral adrenalectomy for benign cortical adenoma
      (2) Subtotal adrenalectomy for bilateral adenomas
      (3) Total adrenalectomy for bilateral adrenocortical carcinoma
   b. For ACTH-dependent CS
      (1) Transsphenoidal surgery for pituitary adenoma (treatment of choice)
      (2) Pituitary radiation is an alternative treatment for patients unsuitable for surgery or in whom surgery has failed

KEY POINTS

Cushing Syndrome

- Growth retardation is often the first manifestation of hypercortisolism.
- Any obese child who stops growing should be evaluated for CS.
- Most common cushingoid features include truncal or generalized obesity, round, plethoric "moon" face, and increased dorsal fat pad ("buffalo hump").
- Most common cause of CS is iatrogenic administration of pharmacologic doses of glucocorticoids as anti-inflammatory or immunosuppressive agents.
- CS associated with virilization suggests adrenal carcinoma.

TABLE 8–18
Etiology of Cushing Syndrome

Endogenous/ACTH-Independent CS

Adrenocortical tumors (infants)
  Carcinoma
  Adenoma
  Nodular hyperplasia
Bilateral hyperplasia (older children)
McCune-Albright syndrome
  Adenoma
  Nodular hyperplasia
Primary pigmented nodular adrenocortical disease

Exogenous/ACTH-Independent CS

Glucocorticoid therapy
  Most common cause of CS
  High-dose and/or long duration of therapy
  Oral, intradermal, or topical (occlusive dressing)

Endogenous/ACTH-Dependent CS

Pituitary ACTH-producing tumor
  Adenoma
Ectopic ACTH-producing tumor
  Islet cell carcinoma of pancreas
  Neuroblastoma
  Ganglioneuroblastoma
Ectopic corticotropin-releasing factor (CRF)-producing tumor
Hypothalamic CRF-producing tumor

Exogenous/ACTH-Dependent CS

ACTH therapy

TABLE 8–19
Clinical Features of Cushing Syndrome

Weight gain with growth retardation	Signs of virilization (androgen excess)
Most consistent feature	Hypertrichosis (face, trunk)
Rapid weight gain, deceleration of linear growth	Acne
Hypertension	Deepening of voice
Heart failure	Premature pubic or axillary hair
Fatigue, weakness	Enlargement of clitoris
Menstrual irregularities	Precocious puberty
Pubertal delay	Violaceous skin striae (flanks, thighs)
Amenorrhea	Facial plethora
Muscle weakness	Hyperpigmentation (excess ACTH)
Radiographic abnormalities	Acanthosis nigricans
Osteoporosis (most evident on spine)	Easy bruisability
Pathologic fractures	Increased infections
Slipped capital femoral epiphysis	Poor wound healing

TABLE 8–20
Laboratory Findings of Cushing Syndrome

Common Laboratory Findings

Polycythemia, lymphopenia, eosinopenia
Alkalosis, hypokalemia, hypochloremia (serum sodium normal)
Hypercalcemia, hypercalciuria (renal stones)
Glucose tolerance test abnormal, glycosuria

Specific Tests (As Indicated)

Serum cortisol value
   Loss of diurnal rhythm* of cortisol
   Elevated cortisol level at 8 PM
Plasma ACTH value
   High ACTH value with hypercortisolism: Cushing disease
   Low ACTH value with hypercortisolism: Adrenal tumor
Serum androgen value
   High: adrenocortical carcinoma
   Low: benign cortisol-secreting adenoma
24-hour urinary excretion
   Free cortisol: *always* increased *(best screeing test)*
   17-hydroxy corticosteroids: usually increased
Overnight dexamethasone-suppression test†
Abdominal CT (adrenal carcinoma, adenoma, bilateral
   hyperplasia)
Pituitary MRI with gadolinium (pituitary adenoma)

---

* Normal diurnal rhythm (children >3 years): Serum cortisol level is normally elevated at 8 AM, and cortisol level is <50% (of AM value) at 8 PM.

† Overnight dexamethasone suppression test: give 0.3 mg/m² of dexamethasone at 11 PM. Measure serum cortisol next morning (cortisol value >5 mg/mL suggests hypercortisolism [normal cortisol value after dexamethasone: <5 mg/mL])

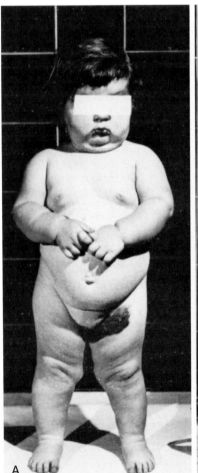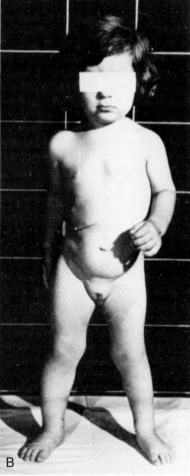

A   B

FIGURE 8–9. Patient with Cushing syndrome caused by adrenocortical carcinoma prior to (*A*) and following (*B*) surgical removal of the tumor. The time interval between *A* and *B* was 3 months. (From Kaplan SA: Disorders of adrenal cortex I. Pediatr Clin North Am 26(1):66, 1979.)

TABLE 8–21
Differential Diagnosis of Cushing Syndrome Versus Exogenous Obesity

	Cushing Syndrome	**Exogenous Obesity**
Clinical	Striae	Striae
	Hypertension	Hypertension
	Rapid weight gain	Weight gain
	Decelerating linear growth	*Growth rate rapid or normal*
	Short stature	*Tall for age (early years)*
Urinary Corticosteroids	Elevated	Elevated
	Not suppressed by dexamethasone	*Suppressed by dexamethasone*

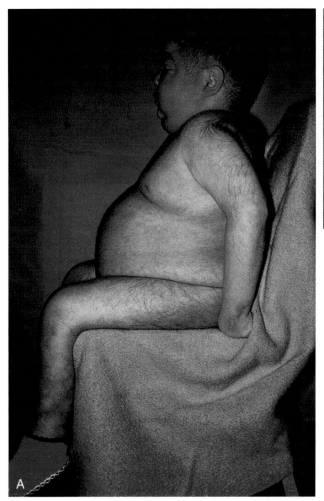

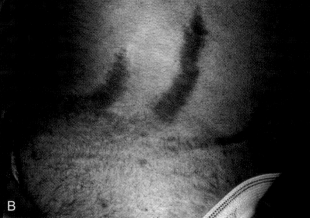

FIGURE 8–10. *A,* Cushing syndrome in a 6-year-old child. Note marked obesity and generalized hypertrichosis. *B,* Violaceous skin striae over flank and thighs of the same patient. (Courtesy of Max Salas, M.D., St. Peter's University Hospital, New Brunswick, NJ.)

Pheochromocytoma

DEFINITION

Catecholamine-secreting adrenomedullary tumors are termed pheochromocytomas. Pheochromocytomas arising from chromaffin cells in or about the sympathetic chain ganglia are termed either extra-adrenal pheochromocytoma or functioning paraganglioma.

EPIDEMIOLOGY

1. Uncommon tumor of childhood; nevertheless, 20% of all pheochromocytomas are diagnosed in children.
2. About 0.5% to 1% of cases of childhood hypertension are due to pheochromocytoma.
3. Typical age at presentation
   a. Between 8 and 14 years of age (average age at onset of signs or symptoms: 9.5 years)
   b. Peak incidence: between third and fourth decades of life
4. Children have a higher incidence of bilateral, multiple, or extra-adrenal tumors and a lower incidence of malignancy than adults with pheochromocytoma (see Table 8–24)
5. Pheochromocytoma is benign in more than 90% of pediatric patients.
6. Right adrenal involvement is more common than left adrenal involvement (by about 2:1).

BOX 8–5	*Sites of Pheochromocytoma in Children*

Adrenal medulla
   Most common site in children (about 70%)
   Bilateral involvement (about 25%)
   May involve multiple sites (both adrenal and extra-adrenal)
Extra-adrenal sites (about 25% to 30%)
   Most common site is *within* the abdominal cavity in the organ of Zuckerkandl (near aortic bifurcation close to the origin of the inferior mesenteric artery)
   Urinary bladder (about 1%)
   Thoracic cavity (about 1%)
   Cervical region (<1%)

PATHOGENESIS (see Box 7–12, p. 278)

1. Pheochromocytoma arises from the chromaffin cells. It can arise from the chromaffin cells anywhere from the neck to the base pelvis in or about the sympathetic ganglia.
2. Chromaffin cells synthesize, store, and release catecholamines.
3. Chromaffin cells of the adrenal medulla convert 75% of norepinephrine to epinephrine, whereas extra-adrenal chromaffin cells (of the sympathetic ganglia and nerves) do not have this ability.

4. Catecholamines released by pheochromocytoma
   a. Tumors arising in the adrenal medulla produce both epinephrine and norepinephrine.
   b. Most extra-adrenal tumors produce only norepinephrine.
   c. Relative proportions of norepinephrine and epinephrine may influence the signs/symptoms produced by pheochromocytoma.
   d. Majority of childhood pheochromocytoma contain (but do not secrete) substantial quantities of dopamine. Increased dopamine production is uncommon in patients with benign lesions but may occur in those with malignant pheochromocytoma.
   e. Norepinephrine activates predominantly alpha-adrenergic receptors, resulting in effects such as increased peripheral vasoconstriction, diastolic hypertension, and sweating.
   f. Epinephrine activates alpha- and beta-adrenergic receptors, resulting in systolic hypertension, tachycardia, and arrythmias.

BOX 8–6	*Differential Diagnosis of Catecholamine-Secreting Tumors*

Pheochromocytoma
Ganglioneuroma
Neuroblastoma
Ganglioneuroblastoma
Chemodectoma (derived from carotid body)

---

5. Bone, liver, lymph node, and lung are the most common distant metastatic sites in patients with malignant pheochromocytomas.

INHERITANCE

1. About 90% of pheochromocytomas occur sporadically.
2. About 10% of pheochromocytomas are familial and are inherited as an autosomal dominant trait either alone or in association with multiple endocrine neoplasia syndromes (see Table 8–25).
3. Bilateral adrenal pheochromocytomas are present in more than 50% of familial cases.

LABORATORY

1. Complete blood count
2. Urinalysis, serum electrolytes, urea nitrogen, and creatinine (to exclude renal causes of hypertension)
3. Plasma catecholamine measurements
4. A 24-hour urine collection for catecholamines or their metabolites (see Box 7–12, p. 278)
   a. Vanillylmandelic acid (VMA)—end product of epinephrine and norepinephrine
   b. Free catecholamines
   c. Metanephrine
   d. Homovanillic acid (HVA)—end product of dopamine

5. For localization of pheochromocytoma (first in the adrenal region and abdomen, then as indicated)
   a. Abdominal ultrasonography
   b. Computed tomography with contrast enhancement
   c. Magnetic resonance imaging
   d. ^{131}I-metaiodobenzylguanidine (MIBG) scan
      (1) Detects presence of functional chromaffin tissue
      (2) This guanidine analog has a molecular structure similar to that of norepinephrine and is concentrated in catecholamine storage vesicles.
      (3) Permits the entire patient to be screened for tumor deposits (including extra-adrenal sites) in a simple, safe, and noninvasive manner
      (4) If available, whole body MIBG scan is the initial test of choice for tumor localization.

TREATMENT

1. Hospitalization for confirmation, localization, and surgical excision of pheochromocytoma
2. Consultations with pediatric nephrology, surgery, anesthesia, and radiology services

3. Treatment is surgical excision.
   a. This requires extensive, well-planned medical therapy aimed at preoperative and perioperative management of hypertension, tachyarrhythmias, and maintenance of intravascular blood volume.
   b. Alpha-adrenergic blocking drugs (to lower blood pressure, increase intravascular volume, and prevent paroxysmal hypertension) and beta-adrenergic blocking drugs (to control arrythmias) are usually required.

FOLLOW-UP

1. After successful surgery, catecholamine excretion returns to normal in about 1 week; this confirms complete resection of the tumor.
2. Following surgical resection, patients need regular follow-up including monitoring of blood pressure and urinary catecholamines every year for several years or when symptoms reappear. Recurrence of pheochromocytoma has been described (30% of children in one series).
3. Siblings and parents of patient with pheochromocytoma also require periodic evaluations because of increased familial incidence.

KEY POINTS

Pheochromocytoma

- Catecholamine-secreting tumor
- Hypertension is a cardinal sign, although it is present in only 70% to 80% of patients.
- It is a curable cause of hypertension in about 75% of patients if properly diagnosed and treated, but may be fatal if undiagnosed or mistreated.
- Elevated urinary norepinephrine values indicate an extra-adrenal site, whereas elevated urinary epinephrine values indicate an adrenal lesion.
- Hypertensive paroxysms are an important diagnostic clue.

TABLE 8–22
Clinical Features of Pheochromocytoma: "The Great Mimic"*

Hypertension

Cardinal sign
Sustained (about 60%)
Paroxysmal (about 40%)
Hypertensive paroxysms or "crises" (seen in >50%)
  Sudden onset
  May last from a few minutes to hours
  Throbbing headaches (misdiagnosed as migraine)
  Palpitations, tachycardia, arrhythmias
  Apprehension, feeling of "impending doom"
  Nausea, vomiting
  Excessive sweating
  Visual disturbances
  Chest or abdominal pain
  Pallor (followed by flushing)
  Symptom-free intervals between crisis
Hypertensive encephalopathy (convulsions, coma)
Orthostatic hypotension (decreased plasma volume, blunted sympathetic reflexes)
Cardiomegaly
Eye findings (papilledema, hemorrhages, exudates)

Other Signs/Symptoms

Hyperglycemia, glycosuria
Polyuria, polydipsia
Weight loss (increased metabolism)
Voracious appetite
Abdominal mass
Emotional lability
Constipation

* Clinical manifestations of pheochromocytoma are protean, ranging from life-threatening to asymptomatic; hence, it has been labeled "the great mimic."

TABLE 8–23
Differential Diagnosis of Hypertension in Children

Renal (e.g., pyelonephritis, glomerulonephritis)	Familial dysautonomia
	Essential hypertension
Renovascular (e.g., renal artery stenosis)	Pheochromocytoma
	Cushing syndrome
Coarctation of the aorta	Neuroblastoma
Increased intracranial pressure	Congenital adrenal hyperplasia
	Hyperparathyroidism
Neurofibromatosis	Hyperthyroidism
Drugs (e.g., steroids, sympathomimetics)	Primary aldosteronism
	Adrenal cortical tumors

TABLE 8-24
Comparison of Pheochromocytomas: Children versus Adults (Approximate Percentages)

Characteristics	Children (%)	"Rule of 10" for Adults (%)
Multiple sites	30	10
Bilateral	25	10
Extra-adrenal	25–30	10
Familial	10–30	10
Malignant	Rare	10
Recurrence	30	<10

TABLE 8-25
Pheochromocytomas and Other Associated Conditions

Neurocutaneous syndrome
  Neurofibromatosis
  Tuberous sclerosis
  Sturge-Weber syndrome
Von Hippel-Lindau disease
Multiple endocrine neoplasia, type IIa (Sipple syndrome)
  Pheochromocytoma
  Hyperparathyroidism
  Medullary carcinoma of thyroid
Multiple endocrine neoplasia, type IIb (mucosal neuroma syndrome)
  Pheochromocytoma
  Ganglioneuromatosis
  Submucosal neuromas (lips, tongue, eyelids)
  Medullary carcinoma of thyroid

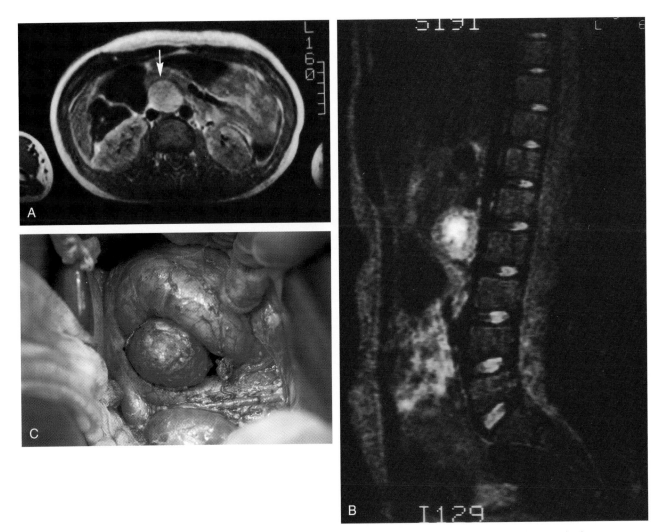

FIGURE 8-11. *A,* Pheochromocytoma was suspected in a 12-year-old boy whose headaches had been misdiagnosed as migraine since the age of 10 years. His headaches were associated with profuse sweating and "heart beating very fast." He also had a history of being admitted for seizures associated with high blood pressure. His urinary catecholamine levels were markedly elevated. *A,* Axial T1-weighted MRI showing a high signal mass arising in the sympathetic chain at the organ of Zuckerkandl *(arrow). B,* On the sagittal T2-weighted image, the mass has a characteristic very high signal intensity. *C,* A golf-ball sized tumor, seen in the center of this intraoperative field, was resected, and the diagnosis of pheochromocytoma was confirmed. The patient has remained completely symptom free after surgery.

McCune-Albright Syndrome

SYNONYM   Albright Syndrome

DEFINITION

A syndrome of polyostotic fibrous dysplasia, café-au-lait spots, and endocrine dysfunction with precocious puberty, especially in girls

EPIDEMIOLOGY

1. Sporadic occurrence; rarely seen
2. Seen more commonly in females than in males (10:1)

PATHOGENESIS

1. Somatic mutation in the gene encoding the subunit G_s (G protein) that controls the regulation of cyclic AMP-dependent hormone receptors
2. Thus, the receptors (TSH, ACTH, FSH, and LH receptors) are activated even though the target organs are not exposed to high levels of hormones or other stimuli (which would normally be required for activation), leading to a hyper-responsive state.
3. Somatic mutation is expressed in variable amounts in affected tissues, resulting in variable clinical expression in affected patients.

CLINICAL FEATURES

1. Clinical course is variable with age at presentation ranging from birth to first few months of life
2. Bone disease (see Table 8–26)
3. Endocrine dysfunction (see Table 8–27)
4. Café-au-lait spots (see Box 8–7)

BOX 8–7   *Café-au-lait Spots*

IN McCUNE-ALBRIGHT SYNDROME

Present in about 50% of patients
Clinical appearance
  Evenly pigmented macules with light brown to medium brown color
  Large
  Unilateral with an irregular border ("coast of Maine")
  Usually stop abruptly at midline
  May follow a dermatomal distribution on same side as skeletal lesions
  May actually overlie skeletal lesions
  As a rule, there are fewer than six lesions
  Size ranges from 1 cm to lesions covering very large areas (back or buttocks)

IN NEUROFIBROMATOSIS

Numerous
More widely distributed than in fibrous dysplasia
Smooth border ("coast of California")
Multiple axillary freckles are pathognomonic of neurofibromatosis

---

LABORATORY

1. Serum alkaline phosphatase values are elevated in approximately one third of patients.
2. Serum values of calcium and phosphorus are normal (unless rickets is present).
3. Tests for endocrine gland dysfunction (thyroid, adrenal, and pituitary) as clinically indicated
4. With sexual precocity (gonadotropin-independent precocious puberty)
   a. Serum estradiol levels are high.
   b. LH and FSH levels are very low.
5. Radiographs
   a. Of bone (corresponding to the site of café-au-lait spot)
   b. Skeletal age is advanced, especially in patients with sexual precocity.
6. Ultrasound examination of ovaries may show bilateral multiple large ovarian cysts

DIFFERENTIAL DIAGNOSIS

1. Neurofibromatosis with café-au-lait spots (see Box 8–7)
2. Brown tumors of hyperparathyroidism with lytic skeletal lesions
   a. Absence of cutaneous pigmentation
   b. Abnormal calcium and phosphorus values

TREATMENT

1. Refer patient to pediatric endocrinologist
   a. For evaluation and management of endocrine gland dysfunctions
   b. Sexual precocity
      (1) May be treated with variable success by blocking estrogen synthesis with the aromatase inhibitor testolactone
      (2) Functioning ovarian cysts leading to sexual precocity often disappear spontaneously and rarely require surgical intervention.
2. Refer patient to orthopedist.
   a. Fibrous dysplasia is not curable.
   b. Orthopedic intervention may be necessary for bony deformities and fractures.

PROGNOSIS

Normal lifespan with disabilities related to bony deformities and repeated fractures

KEY POINTS

McCune-Albright Syndrome

- A syndrome of polyostotic fibrous dysplasia, café-au-lait spots, and endocrine dysfunction with precocious puberty, especially in girls
- Menstrual bleeding in girls under 2 years of age has been the first symptom of McCune-Albright syndrome in 85% of patients.

TABLE 8–26
Clinical Features of McCune-Albright Syndrome

Bone Disease

Skeletal lesions may occur in absence of other features
Long bones and craniofacial bones are commonly involved
Pain, recurrent fractures or deformities (bowing, limb length
   discrepancies)
Hearing loss and obliteration of external ear canal (if temporal
   bones involved)
Facial asymmetry, proptosis, and optic nerve compression (if
   orbital bones involved)
Short stature related to premature closure of epiphyses

TABLE 8–27
Endocrine Features of McCune-Albright Syndrome

Endocrine Dysfunction

Peripheral sexual precocity (gonadotropin-releasing hormone
   independent)
   Occurs more frequently in females than in males
   Not due to pituitary or hypothalamic dysfunction; thus
      production of estradiol is stimulated without increased
      gonadotropins
   May be a presenting sign (occasionally appears before
      skeletal symptoms)
   Girls: premature development of breasts, axillary or pubic
      hair, and vaginal bleeding
   Boys: testicular and phallic enlargement

Other Endocrine Abnormalities

Autonomous hyperfunction of glands ⇒ excessive hormone
      production
   Hyperthyroidism (about 50% of patients)
   Cushing syndrome
   Gigantism or acromegaly
Hypophosphatemia leading to rickets or osteomalacia

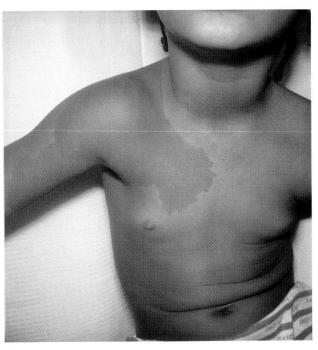

FIGURE 8–12. Café-au-lait spot and breast enlargement in a 4-year-old girl with McCune-Albright syndrome. The café-au-lait spot is large and unilateral, has an irregular border, and does not cross the midline.

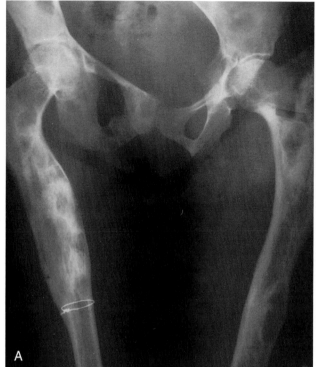

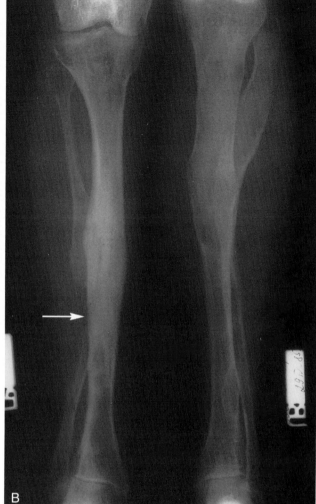

FIGURE 8–13. McCune-Albright Syndrome. *A* and *B,* Frontal views of the lower extremities show multiple areas of mixed fibrotic and cystic involvement, giving the bones a characteristic "ground glass" amorphous appearance with areas of sclerosis. Pseudarthrosis of the right (*arrow*) and left fibulas is apparent, as well as a "shepherd's crook" deformity of the left femoral head.

Ambiguous Genitalia

DEFINITION
Sexual ambiguity in a neonate

ETIOLOGY
Four major conditions result in sexual ambiguity (see Tables 8–28 to 8–31).

1. Female pseudohermaphroditism (FPH; virilized genotypic female)
2. Male pseudohermaphroditism (MPH; undervirilized genotypic male)
3. True hermaphroditism
4. Mixed gonadal dysgenesis

PATHOGENESIS

1. External genitalia of male and female fetuses are identical until 8 weeks of gestation.
2. Circulating testosterone secreted by the fetal testis masculinizes the external genitalia of a male fetus.
3. In absence of androgenic stimulation, female phenotype develops.
4. Incomplete masculinization of male fetus results when testosterone production is inadequate or when there is partial nonresponsiveness to testosterone.
5. Virilization of female fetus occurs between 8 and 12 weeks of gestation in the presence of testosterone or androgen from any source.
6. Sources of androgens
   a. Exogenous androgens (e.g., anabolic steroids) used in the treatment of endometriosis
   b. Excess endogenous androgen production (e.g., congenital adrenal hyperplasia)

CLINICAL FEATURES (see Tables 8–28 to 8–32)

1. Mobile, oval palpable masses below the inguinal ligament are testes until proved otherwise (even if they are within the labia majora).
2. Gonadal symmetry

a. Gonadal symmetry refers to the position of one gonad relative to the other, above or below the external inguinal ring.
b. Both gonads are symmetrically placed, either above or below the inguinal ring, if the etiologic influence leading to the abnormality is applied equally to both sides.
c. Gonadal symmetry may be seen in FPH and in MPH.
d. Gonadal asymmetry is seen in mixed gonadal dysgenesis or true hermaphroditism because one gonad has differentiated predominantly as a testis (and descends on one side), and the other has as a differentiated ovary (which does not descend).

LABORATORY

1. The following issues must be urgently addressed:
   a. Determine whether the genital abnormality is an isolated problem or is part of a multiple congenital malformation syndrome.
   b. Determine the chromosomal sex.
   c. Determine the gonadal sex.
   d. Determine the phenotypic sex.
2. Chromosomal analysis
   a. Rapid karyotype on lymphocyte (result within 2 to 5 days)
   b. Bone marrow chromosomes (result within 6 to 12 hours)
3. Buccal smear for Barr chromatin bodies: inaccurate, unreliable method
4. Tests for congenital adrenal hyperplasia (see Table 8–32)
5. Imaging studies
   a. Pelvic ultrasound to assess uterus, ovaries, fallopian tubes, undescended testes
   b. Renal ultrasound to assess urinary tract
   c. Genitogram with retrograde injection of contrast media via the urogenital orifice
      (1) To detect the presence of müllerian structures
      (2) To outline anatomy of urethra

TREATMENT/MANAGEMENT

1. Important points while sharing the news with the family
   a. The first question parents ask is "Is it a boy or a girl?" Telling them that the baby is partly male and partly female is inappropriate.
   b. Share the examination of the external genitalia with the parents and describe the observed findings.
   c. Explain that further testing is necessary that will help in determining "the sex the baby is meant to be."
2. Transfer to a secondary or tertiary level nursery may be required to accomplish a prompt and expert evaluation of the baby.
3. Multidisciplinary team approach involving consultations with pediatric urologists or surgeons, an endocrinologist, geneticist, radiologist, and social worker is used. Management of these patients begins in the neonatal period and often extends throughout adolescence.
4. General principles of management
   a. Female pseudohermaphrodite is usually raised as a female even when highly virilized.
   b. Gender assignment is based on the infant's anatomy (e.g., size of the phallus) and not on the karyotype.

KEY POINTS

Ambiguous Genitalia

- A newborn with ambiguous genitalia is a medical and "social" emergency.
- Most frequent cause of ambiguous genitalia is congenital adrenal hyperplasia due to 21-hydroxylase deficiency.
- Females with classic 21-hydroxylase deficiency (salt-losing type) tend to show a greater degree of virilization than those with the nonsalt-losing type.

TABLE 8–28
Female Pseudohermaphroditism

Incidence	About 33% to 50% of patients with ambiguous genitalia
Karyotype	46,XX
Commonest cause	Congenital adrenal hyperplasia (see Table 8–32)
Clinically	Ambiguity limited to external genitalia only; External genitalia virilized (masculinized); Clitoral hypertrophy; Labioscrotal fusion
Gonads	Both gonads are ovaries; testes are absent
Present	Müllerian duct structures (uterus, fallopian tubes, upper vagina)
Absent	Wolffian duct structures (seminal vesicles, epididymidis, vasa deferens)

TABLE 8–29
Male Pseudohermaphroditism

Karyotype	46,XY
Clinically	External genitalia ambiguous or completely female or incompletely virilized; Genital appearance ranges from completely feminized to milder forms
Gonads	Both gonads are testes; testes are either rudimentary or fully developed
Absent	Müllerian duct structures (uterus, fallopian tubes, upper vagina); Exception: Persistent Müllerian duct syndrome
Absent or hypoplastic	Wolffian duct structures (seminal vesicles, epididymidis, vasa deferens)

TABLE 8-30
True Hermaphroditism

Definition	Presence of both ovarian follicles and seminiferous tubules in same patient
Karyotype	46,XX (most common type; seen in about two thirds of patients)
Clinically	External genitalia usually ambiguous but may be male or female
Gonalds	Bilateral ovotestis (most frequent) *or* ovary or testis on one side and ovotestis on other side *or* ovary on one side and testis on other side
	Ovarian tissue is usually normal; testicular tissue is dyskinetic
Present	Uterus almost always present
	Müllerian structures usually present on the same side as ovary or ovotestis
	Wolffian structures on the side of testis
Tumors	Increased incidence of gonadal tumors

TABLE 8-31
Mixed Gonadal Dysgenesis

Definition	Presence of a testis and a streak gonad in the same patient
Incidence	Second most common type of intersexuality
Karyotype	45,X/46,XY (most common karyotype) or 46,XY
Clinically	External genitalia ambiguous
	Asymmetry of external genitalia (descent of testicular tissue on one side, while the streak gonad does not descend)
Gonads	Ovotestis on one side, streak ovary on other side *or* one dysgenetic testis and no ovarian tissue
Present	Müllerian structures (uterus, fallopian tubes, upper vagina) on the side of a streak gonad
	Wolffian structures (seminal vesicles, epididymidis, vasa deferens) on side of ovotestis
Tumors	Increased incidence of gonadal tumors

TABLE 8-32
Congenital Adrenal Hyperplasia Due to 21-Hydroxylase Deficiency

Congenital adrenal hyperplasia (CAH)	Most common cause of ambiguous genitalia
Most common defect in CAH	21-hydroxylase deficiency (classic form)
Key features (classic form)	Ambiguous genitalia in females (masculinization)
	Most common cause of FPH (see Table 8-28)
	Enlargement of clitoris, varying degrees of labial fusion
	Urogenital sinus (common opening of vagina and urethra)
	Genital hyperpigmentation
	Males have normal genitalia at birth, but develop premature isosexual development
Karyotype in affected patients	46,XX in females, 46,XY in males
Salt losers	About two thirds of patients
Adrenal crisis	Hypovolemic shock, death
Laboratory findings	Hyponatremia, hypochloremia, hyperkalemia
	Hypoglycemia, elevated urea nitrogen
	Serum 17-OH-progesterone (markedly elevated)
	Serum androstenedione (elevated)
	Serum testosterone (elevated)
	Serum cortisol (usually low)
	Urinary 17-ketosteroids (elevated)
	Urinary pregnanetriol (elevated)

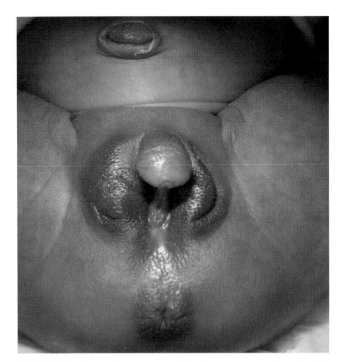

FIGURE 8-14. Ambiguous genitalia in a newborn female (46, XX) infant with virilizing congenital adrenal hyperplasia. An enlarged clitoris (phallic-like structure), genital hyperpigmentation, empty labioscrotal folds, and a single perineal opening into a urogenital sinus were present.

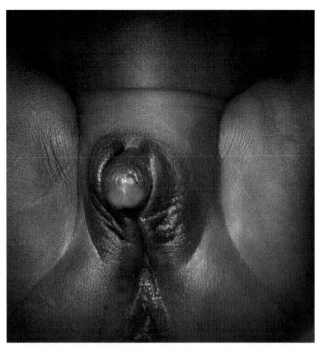

FIGURE 8-15. Ambiguous genitalia of newborn who was found to be a 46,XX true hermaphrodite. Note labioscrotal folds and phallus. This infant had an ovary on one side and a contralateral ovotestis. The ovotestis was removed and this patient was raised as female.

Urology and Surgery

Binita R. Shah, M.D.

Hydrometrocolpos with Imperforate Hymen

DEFINITION/ETIOLOGY

Congenital vaginal obstruction with a patent cervix and a uterus leads to hydrocolpos or one of its variants.

1. Hydrocolpos or mucocolpos
   a. Vaginal distention with mucous secretions
   b. Caused by excessive intrauterine stimulation of the infant's cervical mucus glands by maternal estrogens
2. Hydrometrocolpos
   a. Distention of the uterus and vagina with mucous secretions
   b. Caused by excessive intrauterine stimulation of the infant's mucus glands by maternal estrogens
3. Hematocolpos
   a. Vaginal distention with menstrual products
   b. Seen at the time of menarche
4. Hematometrocolpos
   a. Distention of the uterus and vagina with menstrual products
   b. Seen at the time of menarche

ETIOLOGY/EPIDEMIOLOGY

1. Two most common anomalies causing congenital vaginal obstruction are
   a. Imperforate hymen
   b. Vaginal atresia (transverse vaginal septum)
2. Imperforate hymen is usually an isolated anomaly.
3. Transverse vaginal septum is often associated with major genitourinary or gastrointestinal anomalies. Examples include
   a. Imperforate anus
   b. Bicornuate uterus
   c. Renal hypoplasia

LABORATORY

1. Imperforate hymen is a clinical diagnosis.
2. Ultrasonography
   a. Pelvic: to detect the extent of vaginal/uterine distention and any other associated anomalies

b. Renal: to detect secondary obstructive effects (e.g., hydronephrosis)
3. Renal function tests

BOX 9–1 *Normal Anatomy*

- A normal perforate hymen can be seen on a careful examination of the newborn.
- Vaginal length can be determined by inserting a moistened cotton-tipped applicator into the vagina.
- A normal vagina in the full-term infant is approximately 4 cm long.

COMPLICATIONS

1. Acute urinary retention
2. Hydronephrosis or hydroureter secondary to chronic extrinsic pressure

DIFFERENTIAL DIAGNOSIS

Labial agglutination

TREATMENT

Hymenotomy with decompression

KEY POINTS

Hydrometrocolpos with Imperforate Hymen

- An abdominal mass with a visible bulging mass or membrane at the introitus
- Inspect the hymen in any pubescent girl who has never menstruated and who presents with an abdominal mass.
- Imperforate hymen is usually an isolated anomaly.

TABLE 9–1
Clinical Features of Imperforate Hymen in Infancy

Asymptomatic
Difficulty in micturition
Hydrocolpos or hydrometrocolpos presenting as
    Palpable lower midline abdominal mass
    Mass extending superiorly to umbilicus
    A visible bulging mass/membrane at introitus

TABLE 9–2
Clinical Features of Imperforate Hymen in Adolescents

Abdominal pain (which may be cyclic)
Normal pubertal changes with "primary amenorrhea"
Urinary retention or symptoms of urgency, dysuria, or frequency
Hematocolpos or hematometrocolpos presenting as
    Lower abdominal mass
    A visible bulging mass at introitus (mass may appear blue from hematocolpos)
    Persistent low back pain (sacral plexus or nerve root irritation secondary to a large hematocolpos)

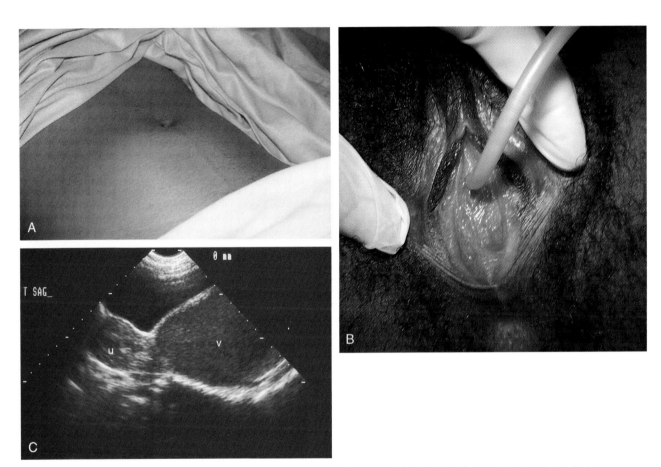

FIGURE 9–1. *A,* Abdominal pain was a presenting complaint in this 13-year-girl. An abdominal mass was palpable in the mid to lower abdomen. She also had difficulty in voiding. About 5 weeks prior to this, she had been treated with antacids at another institution when she presented with similar abdominal pain. She denied having prior menstruation. *B,* A bulging mass is visualized at the introitus, and urinary catheter is visible. *C,* Longitudinal view of the pelvis shows a large hypoechoic mass in a distended vagina (V) and fluid and debris in the distended uterus (U).

Labial Adhesions

SYNONYMS   Labial Agglutination
            Vulvar Agglutination
            Labial Fusion
            Labial Synechiae

DEFINITION

Fusion of the labia minora usually extends from an area immediately inferior to the clitoris to the fourchette. The extent of the adhesions is variable, they are thickest posteriorly and stop below the clitoris.

ETIOLOGY

1. An *acquired* condition
2. Fusion of the medial surfaces of the labia minora to each other secondary to local inflammation (e.g., vulvovaginitis) *in the presence of* a hypoestrogenic state in a preadolescent child (inflamed or injured epithelium is more likely to agglutinate in a low-estrogen environment)
3. Nonspecific vulvovaginitis and poor perineal hygiene are the most common factors contributing to labial adhesions.

BOX 9-2   *Differential Diagnosis of Labial Adhesions*

Imperforate hymen
Congenital absence of the vagina

EPIDEMIOLOGY

1. Most common age
   a. Between 3 months and 5 years
   b. Median age at diagnosis: 2 years
2. Labial adhesions are rare in
   a. Newborns (owing to exposure to high levels of maternal estrogens)
   b. Postpubertal premenopausal women

LABORATORY

Diagnosis of a labial adhesion is made clinically.

COMPLICATIONS

1. Urinary tract infection related to pooling of urine in the vagina and recurrent vulvovaginitis
2. Recurrent labial adhesions

TREATMENT/PROGNOSIS

1. Education of caretaker about good perineal hygiene

   a. Regular changing of diapers
   b. Thorough wiping after each bowel movement; wiping from anterior to posterior
   c. Loose-fitting cotton underwear
   d. Sitz baths (with either tap water or Burow solution)
2. No specific treatment may be indicated for patients with asymptomatic adhesions. Spontaneous resolution with no therapy does occur.
3. At puberty, with endogenous estrogen production, this condition resolves spontaneously.
4. Agglutinated tissue should *not* be manually forced apart; it is very painful, and the resulting raw surfaces have a greater tendency to re-agglutinate.
5. Estrogen cream (e.g., Premarin)
   a. This treatment may be used if parents are worried.
   b. A small quantity is applied topically at bedtime for 2 to 8 weeks.
   c. Very effective in majority of patients
   d. Prolonged use of topical estrogen cream should be discouraged; side effects (reversible) include
      (1) Breast enlargement and/or tenderness
      (2) Vulvar pigmentation
      (3) Vulvar erythema
   e. An additional few weeks' application of an inert ointment (e.g., Vaseline) keeps the labia apart while healing is completed.

KEY POINTS

Labial Adhesions

- A thin vertical raphe in the midline over the site of the vaginal orifice (where the labia are adherent) is pathognomonic of labial adhesions.
- Labial adhesions should not be separated manually with force; this leads to adhesion of the raw surfaces and is painful.
- Labial adhesions (including recurrent episodes) resolve completely with puberty.

TABLE 9-3
Clinical Features of Labial Adhesions

Majority of patients are asymptomatic
Usually noted incidentally by parent or physician
Absence of "apparent vaginal opening"
Thin vertical raphe in the midline over the site of the vaginal orifice (where labia are adherent)
Normal female genitalia
With complete adhesions
   Urethra is usually not visualized
   Urine may be seen dribbling at anterior end (just posterior to clitoris)
   Urinary symptoms of dysuria, frequency, or urinary retention may be present
With partial adhesions
   Central line of fusion is seen at posterior fourchette (extending to varying lengths anteriorly)

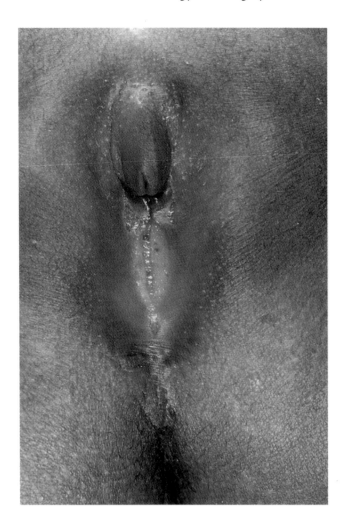

FIGURE 9–2. Labial agglutination incidentally noted by a parent in a 3-year-old girl. She was rushed to a pediatrician because the parent feared "absence of the vagina." A thin vertical raphe is seen in the midline over the site of the vaginal orifice, where the labia are adherent.

Urethral Prolapse

DEFINITION

An eversion of the distal urethral mucosa that protrudes through the urethral meatus

ETIOLOGY/PREDISPOSING FACTORS

1. Hypoestrogenism in the premenarcheal and postmenopausal age groups
2. Poor cleavage plane attachments between the inner longitudinal and outer circular-oblique smooth muscle layers of the urethra combined with episodes of increased intra-abdominal pressure (e.g., violent coughing, constipation).
3. Preceding trauma (e.g., straddle injury, sexual abuse)

EPIDEMIOLOGY

1. Exclusively seen in two age groups:
   a. Premenarcheal girls
   b. Postmenopausal women
2. Premenarcheal age: peak incidence 4 to 10 years
3. Racial predilection

a. Premenarcheal girls: African-Americans (95%)
b. Postmenopausal women: none

PATHOGENESIS

1. Constriction of prolapsed mucosa at the urethral meatus leads to impairment of venous blood flow, resulting in edema and erythema or purplish appearance of the mucosa
2. Thrombosis and necrosis of the mucosa result if the process is not corrected.

LABORATORY

1. Urethral prolapse is a clinical diagnosis.
   a. Prolapse may be a large enough circle to conceal the introitus.
   b. Careful examination reveals the vaginal introitus as a separate structure *posterior* to the prolapsed urethra.
   c. Urethral prolapse is the only lesion that has a circular mass of tissue surrounding the urethral meatus.
   d. If in doubt, catheterization of the bladder through the central dimple of the mass or ob-

BOX 9–3	*Differential Diagnosis of Urethral Prolapse*
Prolapsed ectopic ureterocele	Condylomata acuminata
Prolapse of urethral polyp	Hydrometrocolpos
Prolapsed bladder	Sexual abuse
Periurethral abscess	Sarcoma botryoides

servation of the child during voiding will aid in the diagnosis.

2. Urinalysis: red blood cells may be present because of the external irritation of the urethral meatus.
3. Urine culture: usually negative
4. Ultrasonography (for atypical presentation)
   a. Pelvic: to exclude tumor
   b. Renal: to exclude hydronephrosis caused by ureterocele

TREATMENT

1. Conservative therapy is used for mild cases with no necrotic mucosa.
   a. Warm sitz baths
   b. Emollient cream or, if indicated, topical antibacterial therapy
   c. Topical estrogen therapy for 10 to 14 days
   d. Usually resolves spontaneously or with above therapy in 2 to 3 weeks
2. Indications for surgery
   a. Prolapse with necrotic mucosa at time of presentation

b. Persistent prolapse
c. Recurrence of prolapse following medical therapy

PROGNOSIS

1. Mild prolapse resolves in a few weeks in majority of cases.
2. Recurrences may occur weeks to months after the initial resolution following medical therapy.
3. Recurrence is uncommon after surgical excision and reapproximation of the mucosal edges.

KEY POINTS

Urethral Prolapse

- Most common cause of "apparent vaginal bleeding" in premenarcheal girls
- Urethral prolapse is the only lesion that has a circular mass of tissue surrounding the urethral meatus.
- Clinical findings of urethral prolapse can be mistakenly attributed to sexual abuse.

TABLE 9–4
Clinical Symptoms of Urethral Prolapse

Painless bleeding or spotting on underwear
  Most common symptom (90% of patients)
  Bleeding most often mistaken for "vaginal bleeding"
  Bleeding occasionally mistaken for hematuria or rectal
    bleeding
Urinary symptoms
  Dysuria and/or frequency (urethral inflammation)
  Difficulty in voiding
  Urinary retention (depending on size of mass and whether
    or not it precludes urethral meatus)
Patient asymptomatic; prolapse noted during routine
  examination

TABLE 9–5
Clinical Signs of Urethral Prolapse

"Cherry-red doughnut" or "prolapsed cervix"–like mass at
  introitus
Center of the "doughnut" is the urethral orifice
Usually not tender
May be a friable rosette of red or hemorrhagic tissue
May be ulcerated, gangrenous, or necrotic or infected
Prolapse may be partial or complete

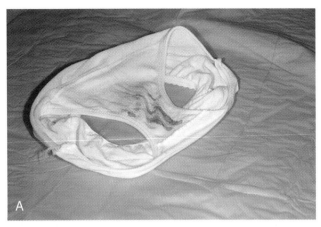

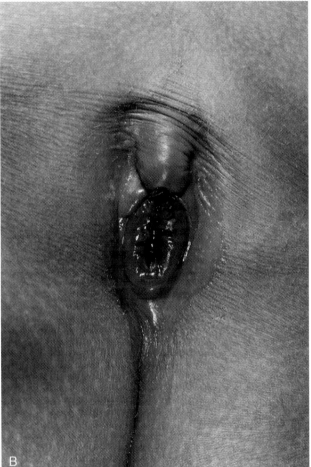

FIGURE 9–3. *A,* Blood-stained underwear from a 4-year-old girl who was brought to the emergency room with a complaint of "vaginal bleeding." *B,* A doughnut-shaped, hyperemic, edematous mass with a hemorrhagic center that obscures the vaginal introitus is seen here. Mucosal prolapse, as seen here, usually appears as a complete circle forming a doughnut with a small dimple in the center indicating the urethral meatus.

Testicular Torsion

DEFINITION

Twisting of the testis leading to venous engorgement, edema, progressive arterial compromise, and subsequent infarction

ETIOLOGY/PATHOGENESIS

1. The testes enter the scrotum by the 32nd week of gestation, projecting into the distal end of the processus vaginalis.
2. At birth, the processus is usually obliterated, leav-

ing the tunica vaginalis, a serosal membrane of the peritoneal sac.

3. Normally the testis is attached in the intrascrotal subcutaneous tissue by the tunica vaginalis except posteriorly at the upper pole, where the epididymis and the spermatic cord are attached (see Fig. 9–4).

4. Intravaginal torsion
   a. Most common form of testicular torsion
   b. Occurs secondary to a "bell-clapper" deformity (see Fig. 9–4)
      (1) This anomaly is almost always bilateral.
      (2) When the tunica vaginalis covers the testis, epididymis, and distal part of the spermatic cord, the testis can rotate freely within this serosal sac like a clapper in a bell.
      (3) Twisting of the testis and of the spermatic cord on a vertical axis leads to venous engorgement, obstruction, and secondary edema of the spermatic cord with progressive arterial compromise and subsequent infarction.

5. Extravaginal torsion
   a. Testis not fixed in the scrotum; entire cord, tunica vaginalis, and testis rotate within the lax subcutaneous tissue of the scrotum, producing torsion
   b. Seen in neonates or in infants with cryptorchidism

EPIDEMIOLOGY

1. Age at presentation
   a. Common between 10 and 20 years of age; however, it can occur at any age
   b. Peak incidence: around 13 years of age (coincides with onset of puberty)
   c. About 66% of cases: between 12 and 18 years of age
   d. Second most frequent time: neonatal period

2. Torsion affects the left testis twice as often as the right (most likely due to the longer length of the left spermatic cord).

3. Although unilateral testicular torsion is more common, bilateral torsion has been reported in the newborn period.

CLINICAL FEATURES (see also Tables 9–6 and 9–7)

1. A thickened cord and an anterior location of the epididymis may be palpated early in the course of the torsion. With intense swelling and edema, the testis and epididymis are indistinguishable by palpation as separate structures.

2. Clinical distinction between testicular torsion and epididymo-orchitis is often difficult.

3. Henoch-Schönlein purpura
   a. Pain and swelling of spermatic cord and testicle occur in 2% to 38% of patients.
   b. Purpura usually precedes scrotal swelling by a few days; however, acute scrotal swelling may be an initial presentation *before* the onset of purpura.

LABORATORY

1. Testicular torsion is a clinical diagnosis.
2. Urinalysis: negative (usually absence of pyuria or bacteriuria)
3. When diagnosis cannot be made on clinical grounds alone, imaging study may be considered.
4. Most commonly used imaging studies include
   a. Testicular real-time color-flow Doppler ultrasonography
      (1) Diagnostic study of choice
      (2) May be helpful for differentiating between torsion and epididymo-orchitis
      (3) Decreased or absent blood flow is seen with torsion.

BOX 9–4   *Differential Diagnosis of Acute Pediatric Scrotum*

PAINFUL AND SWOLLEN

Testicular torsion
Epididymo-orchitis
Mumps orchitis
Torsion of appendix testis
Torsion of appendix epididymis
Trauma
   Fracture/rupture of testis
   Testicular hematoma
Testicular tumor (hemorrhage within tumor)
Incarcerated inguinal hernia
Acute hydrocele
Vasculitis
   Henoch-Schönlein purpura
   Kawasaki disease
   Familial Mediterranean fever

NOT PAINFUL AND SWOLLEN

Acute idiopathic scrotal edema
Hydrocele
Reducible inguinal hernia
Varicocele
Testicular tumor

(4) Blood flow is increased in epididymo-orchitis.
  b. Testicular scintigraphy
    (1) Analyzes testicular perfusion
    (2) Testicular torsion: produces "cold spot" (decreased or absent blood flow)
    (3) Epididymo-orchitis: increased blood flow

TREATMENT

1. Surgical (or urologic consultation) must be obtained emergently.

BOX 9-5 *Testicular Torsion*

- Imaging study should be performed *only* after surgical consultation and *only* when the clinical impression is *against* testicular torsion.
- Scrotal exploration should *not* be inappropriately delayed to await a diagnostic study or attempt at manual detorsion.
- *No* radiologic tests are either 100% accurate or pathognomonic for testicular torsion.

---

2. Surgical exploration for
  a. Detorsion
  b. Evaluation for testicular viability
    (1) Viable testis: scrotal orchiopexy (fixing the testis to the scrotal wall)
    (2) Infarcted testis: removal
  c. Fixation orchiopexy of contralateral testis (contralateral testis is malfixed [bell-clapper deformity] in >50% of cases)
3. Manual detorsion (if timely surgical intervention is not available)
  a. May be attempted if symptoms are less than 4 to 6 hours old
  b. Sedation prior to detorsion
  c. Usually torsion occurs in a medial direction. Detorsion can be tried by lifting the scrotum and rotating the testis (on its vascular pedicle) outward toward the thigh.
  d. Successful detorsion is indicated by
    (1) Relief of pain
    (2) Attainment of a lower testicular position (from a prior high-riding position)
  e. Surgical fixation *must* be performed following successful detorsion to prevent recurrence.

PROGNOSIS

1. Time is a critical factor for testicular salvage. Damage to the gonad varies with the degree of torsion (one turn = 360 degrees), its tightness, and its duration (see Table 9-8).
2. If the blood supply has been obstructed totally for more than 6 hours, surgical detorsion is unlikely to salvage the testis.

KEY POINTS

Testicular Torsion

- Most common cause of acute painful scrotal swelling
- A true surgical emergency; for testicular salvage prompt diagnosis and treatment are required.
- Boys with acute scrotal pain should be presumed to have testicular torsion until proved otherwise.
- Any male child presenting with abdominal pain *must* have a testicular examination to exclude torsion.
- Preceding history of testicular trauma is often misleading.

TABLE 9-7
Clinical Signs of Testicular Torsion

Scrotal/Testicular Examination

Red, swollen, and tender hemiscrotum
Testis swollen, exquisitely tender
Testis riding high in scrotum; horizontal lie
Epididymis may be difficult to palpate owing to intense edema (normal position of epididymis is posterolateral to testis; with torsion it is in abnormal position and axis)
Absent cremasteric reflex on affected side
Negative Prehn's sign
  Elevation of affected testis above pubic symphysis does not relieve pain and may even cause a sharp increase in pain

---

TABLE 9-6
Clinical Symptoms of Testicular Torsion

Scrotol or Testicular Pain

Most common symptom (>80% of patients)
Usually sudden onset or may be gradual onset increasing in severity (excruciating character)
Pain may awaken patient from sleep
Pain may radiate to ipsilateral inner thigh or to abdomen
Previous history of short-lived episodes of testicular pain with spontaneous resolution (30% to 50% of patients)
Associated abdominal pain, nausea, vomiting (*often mimics acute appendicitis*)
Preceding history of trauma (20% of patients)
Absence of urinary symptoms such as dysuria, frequency, urgency

---

TABLE 9-8
Duration of Torsion and Testicular Salvage

Duration of Torsion (Hours)	Testicular Salvage (%)
Less than 6	85–97
6–12	55–85
12–24	20–80
Greater than 24	Less than 10

Modified from Smith-Harrison LI, Knoontz WW Jr: Torsion of the testis. Changing concepts. *In* Ball TP Jr, et al (eds): American Urological Association Update Series, Vol. IX, Lesson 32. Houston, AUA Office of Education, 1990.

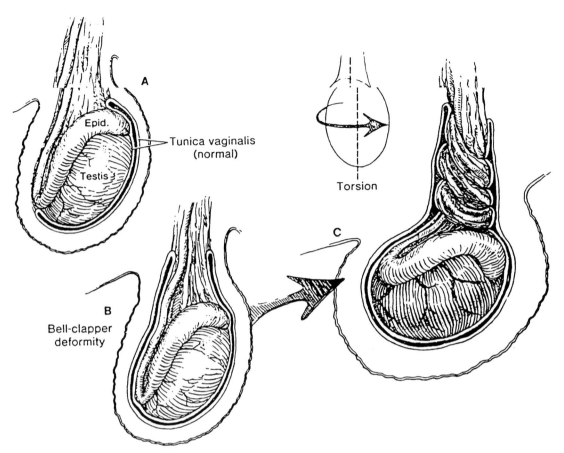

FIGURE 9–4. *A–C,* Mechanism of testicular torsion associated with the "bell-clapper" deformity (an abnormally high investment of tunica on the spermatic cord). (From Fleisher GR, Ludwig S: *In Textbook of Pediatric Emergency Medicine, 3rd ed. Baltimore, Williams & Wilkins, 1993.)

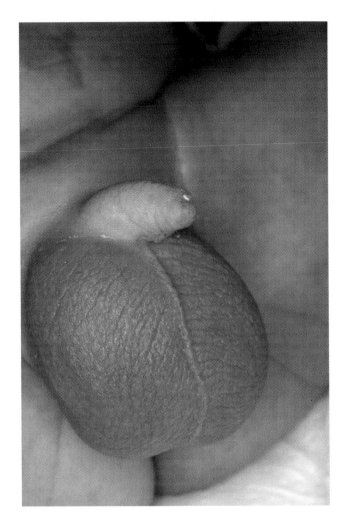

FIGURE 9–5. Erythematous scrotal swelling with right-sided testicular torsion was noted in this neonate shortly after birth. An infarcted testis was found.

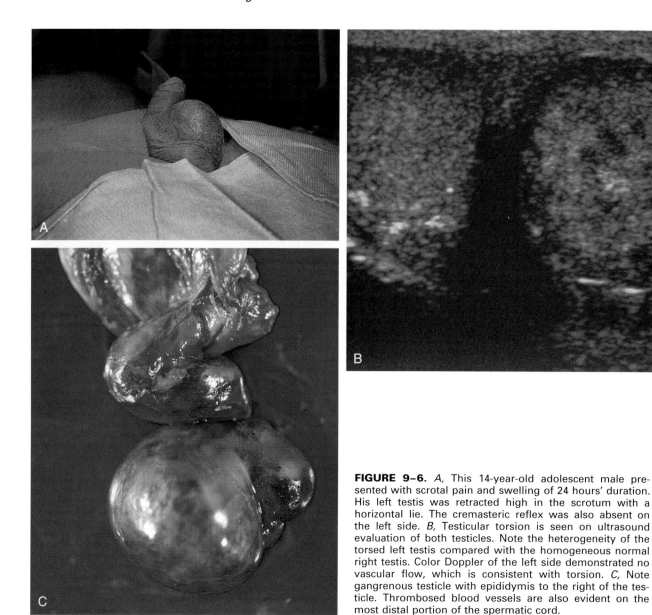

FIGURE 9–6. *A,* This 14-year-old adolescent male presented with scrotal pain and swelling of 24 hours' duration. His left testis was retracted high in the scrotum with a horizontal lie. The cremasteric reflex was also absent on the left side. *B,* Testicular torsion is seen on ultrasound evaluation of both testicles. Note the heterogeneity of the torsed left testis compared with the homogeneous normal right testis. Color Doppler of the left side demonstrated no vascular flow, which is consistent with torsion. *C,* Note gangrenous testicle with epididymis to the right of the testicle. Thrombosed blood vessels are also evident on the most distal portion of the spermatic cord.

Torsion of the Appendix Testis

DEFINITION

Torsion of the appendix testis (testicular appendage or hydatid of Morgagni)

ETIOLOGY/PATHOGENESIS

1. Appendix of the testis
   a. A vestigial embryonic remnant representing the degenerated müllerian (mesonephric) duct
   b. Among all embryonic remnants (see Fig. 9–7), it is the appendage most commonly involved in torsion.
   c. It is located on the superior pole of the testis or between the testis and the epididymis.
   d. At the onset of puberty, it enlarges under the influence of human chorionic gonadotropin.
   e. When pedunculated, it may twist around its base, producing venous engorgement, edema, and subsequent infarction.

EPIDEMIOLOGY

1. Common age at presentation
   a. Between 7 and 12 years
   b. Average age: 10 years
   c. Rare in adolescents
2. Right and left testes are equally affected (unlike testicular torsion, in which the left testis is affected more often than the right testis).

LABORATORY

1. Torsion of the appendix testis is a clinical diagnosis.
2. If the likely diagnosis is torsion of the appendix testis and additional confirmation is desired, testicular real-time color-flow Doppler ultrasonography can be done.
   a. It may be helpful to differentiate between torsion, epididymo-orchitis, and torsion of the appendix testis.
   b. Decreased or absent blood flow is seen with testicular torsion.
   c. Blood flow is increased in epididymo-orchitis.
   d. Blood flow to the testis is increased with torsion of the appendix testis.

DIFFERENTIAL DIAGNOSIS

1. Testicular torsion
2. Epididymo-orchitis

TREATMENT

1. Surgical (or urology) consultation.

2. Surgical exploration
   a. *Not required:* if a diagnosis of torsion of the appendix is entertained *and* the examiner is confident about the diagnosis.
   b. *Required:* if diagnosis of testicular torsion cannot be excluded because of the intensity of the pain and edema.
3. Supportive therapy includes bed rest and nonsteroidal anti-inflammatory medication.
4. Patient can be discharged home to be followed in 48 to 72 hours.

KEY POINTS

Torsion of the Appendix Testis

- Torsion of the appendage is very likely if tenderness is present at the upper pole of the testis and the remainder of the testis is nontender.
- "Blue dot" sign, a pathognomonic sign of an infarcted appendage, is often not seen because of the overlying scrotal wall edema

---

TABLE 9–9
Clinical Features of Torsion of Appendix Testis

Symptoms

Most frequently seen in prepubertal boys
Gradual onset of scrotal pain and swelling
Nausea/vomiting rare
Fever rare
Urinary symptoms (dysuria, pyuria) rare

Genitourinary Examination

Tenderness and swelling localized to superior lateral aspect of
 testis (where appendage is located)
Firm swelling distinct from epididymis
Testis normal or enlarged
Erythema and edema of scrotal wall
Cremasteric reflex present
"Blue dot" sign
 A localized area of bluish discoloration (secondary to
 infarction of appendage)
 Rarely seen because of overlying scrotal edema

Natural Course

Inflammation resolves gradually following infarction
Usually resolves completely within 7–10 days from the onset
 of symptoms

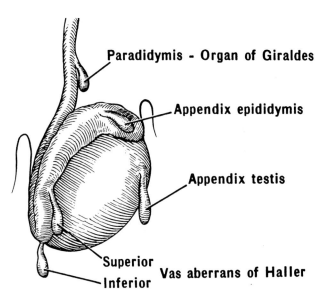

FIGURE 9–7. Lateral view of the testis showing posterior location of the epididymis and testicular appendages. The appendix testis is present in almost all boys, the appendix epididymis is present in approximately 50% of boys, and the other appendages are rarely present. (From Kelalis PP, King LR, Belman AB [eds]: Clinical Pediatric Urology, 2nd ed. Philadelphia, WB Saunders, 1985.)

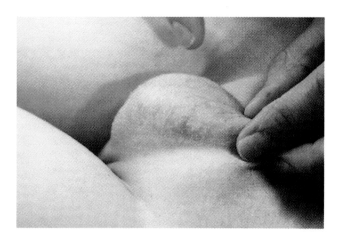

FIGURE 9–8. Blue dot sign in torsion of the appendix testis. This sign is best seen by holding the skin taut over the testicular appendix. (Courtesy of Javier A. Gonzalez del Rey, M.D. From Bondesson JD: Testicular torsion. *In* Knoop KJ, Stack LB, and Storrow AB [eds]: Atlas of Emergency Medicine. New York, McGraw-Hill, 1997.)

Epididymitis (Epididymo-Orchitis)

DEFINITION

1. Epididymitis is an inflammatory process involving the epididymis. If the inflammatory process also involves the testis, it is referred to as epididymo-orchitis.
2. Orchitis is an inflammatory process involving the testis. Orchitis as an isolated infection is uncommon.

EPIDEMIOLOGY

1. Most common age
   a. Postpubertal, sexually active adolescents
   b. Rare: younger preadolescent children
2. Predisposing conditions in younger children
   a. Anatomic abnormality of genitourinary tract
      (1) Congenital anomaly of the wolffian duct (e.g., ectopic ureter entering the vas, ectopic vas deferens)
      (2) Neurogenic bladder
      (3) Hypospadias
      (4) Urethral stricture
   b. Recent urinary tract infection
   c. Recent urinary surgery or instrumentation (e.g., catheterization)
   d. Anatomic abnormality of the gastrointestinal tract (e.g., imperforate anus, rectourethral fistula)
3. Mumps epididymo-orchitis
   a. Seen in adolescents and adults (most common age)
   b. Testis is often affected with or without epididymis.
   c. Epididymitis may occur alone.
   d. Bilateral orchitis is uncommon (seen in about 2% of patients).
   e. Unilateral testicular involvement occurs in about 30% of patients.
   f. Usually follows parotitis; however, it may precede parotitis or occur as an isolated manifestation of mumps.

PATHOGENESIS

1. Epididymitis results from a urethral infection that passes in a retrograde fashion through the vas deferens to the epididymis.
2. If it is diagnosed and treated promptly, the testis may not be involved.

LABORATORY

1. In patients with sexually transmitted epididymitis
   a. Urinalysis may suggest urethritis with any of the following:
      (1) Positive leukocyte esterase test on first-void urine
      (2) Microscopic examination of first-void urine showing 10 or more white blood cells (WBCs) per high-power field (HPF)
      (3) Presence of bacteriuria (Gram-stained smear of uncentrifuged urine)
   b. Urethral discharge or intraurethral swab specimen
      (1) Gram-stained smear demonstrating WBCs containing intracellular gram-negative diplococci suggests gonococcal infection.
      (2) Gram-stained smear of urethral secretions showing 5 or more WBCs per oil immersion field may suggest urethritis.
      (3) Culture and sensitivity or nucleic acid amplification test for *Neisseria gonorrhoeae* and *Chlamydia trachomatis*
   c. Syphilis serology
   d. Human immunodeficiency virus (HIV) testing
2. Not all prepubertal boys with epididymitis have an abnormal urinalysis.
3. Urine culture and sensitivity
4. To differentiate between testicular torsion and epididymo-orchitis (if diagnosis is in doubt), the following studies may be helpful:
   a. Testicular real-time color-flow Doppler ultrasonography
      (1) Diagnostic study of choice
      (2) Decreased or absent blood flow is seen with torsion.

(3) Increased blood flow is seen in epididymo-orchitis.
  b. Testicular scintigraphy
    (1) Analyzes testicular perfusion
    (2) Testicular torsion: produces "cold spot" (decreased or absent blood flow)
    (3) Epididymo-orchitis: increased blood flow

DIFFERENTIAL DIAGNOSIS (see Box 9–6)

1. Testicular torsion versus epididymitis
  a. In epididymitis:
    (1) An enlarged epididymis can be distinguished from the testis by palpation early in the course. However, with time, edema spreads to the testis as well as to the scrotal wall, and it may become difficult to differentiate torsion from epididymo-orchitis.
    (2) The testis is in the normal position, and the long axis is usually in the axis of the body.
2. Torsion of the appendix testis

BOX 9–6 *Acute Pediatric Scrotum*

THREE MOST COMMON CAUSES

Testicular torsion
Epididymo-orchitis
Torsion of appendix testis

TREATMENT

1. Supportive measures until fever and local inflammation subside.
  a. Bed rest
  b. Scrotal support
  c. Ice pack
  d. Nonsteroidal anti-inflammatory medications for pain

2. Antibiotic therapy pending culture results in adolescents for sexually transmitted epididymitis (1998 Centers for Disease Control and Prevention (CDC) recommendations):
  a. For epididymitis most likely caused by *N. gonorrhoeae* or *C. trachomatis:*
    (1) Ceftriaxone 250 mg IM in a single dose *and*
    (2) Doxycycline 100 mg orally twice a day for 10 days
  b. For epididymitis most likely caused by enteric organisms or for patients allergic to cephalosporins and/or tetracyclines: ofloxacin given orally for 10 days
3. For nonsexually transmitted epididymitis associated with urinary tract infection in prepubertal children
  a. Trimethoprim-sulfamethoxazole
  b. Urology consultation

PREVENTION

1. Sex partners should be evaluated and treated when sexually transmitted epididymitis is either suspected or confirmed.
2. Counseling is needed about refraining from sexual intercourse until patient and his sexual partners have been treated and cured (completion of therapy and absence of symptoms).

KEY POINTS

Epididymitis (Epididymo-Orchitis)

■ Epididymitis is the most common cause of acute painful scrotal swelling in young adults older than 18 years.
■ Epididymitis in a younger child signals an underlying urinary tract anomaly.
■ Sexually transmitted epididymitis is usually associated with urethritis (which often is asymptomatic).

TABLE 9–10
Etiology of Epididymitis

Sexually Transmitted Epididymitis	Nonsexually Transmitted Epididymitis (associated with UTI)
Occurs in sexually active adolescents	Occurs in younger children
Causative organisms	Causative organisms
Chlamydia trachomatis	*Escherichia coli*
Neisseria gonorrhoeae	Other gram-negative uropathogens
Mycoplasma	
Escherichia coli (homosexual men)	

TABLE 9–11
Clinical Features of Epididymitis

Symptoms

Pain and swelling typically more gradual than in testicular
    torsion
Adolescents: urethral discharge, urinary frequency, urgency,
    dysuria
Preadolescent boys: urinary symptoms (dysuria or pyuria)
Fever

Genitourinary Examination

Tenderness and firm swelling initially localized to epididymis
May involve testis after a few hours
Scrotal erythema may be present
Cremasteric reflex present
Tender boggy prostate
Prehn's sign
    Not very reliable
    Elevation of scrotum (above pubic symphysis) may relieve
        pain in epididymo-orchitis (unlike torsion, in which pain
        may get worse)

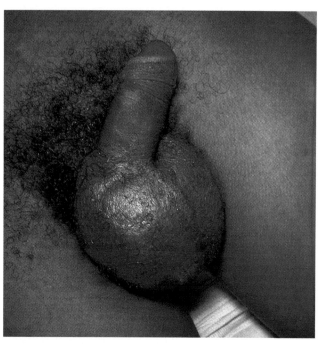

FIGURE 9–10. Erythematous right-sided scrotal swelling and pain of 4 days' duration occurred in this 15-year-old sexually active adolescent whose urethral discharge was positive for *Neisseria gonorrhoeae*. The swelling and erythema shown here are nonspecific; however, this patient's pain was localized to the epididymis. Cremasteric reflexes were present bilaterally.

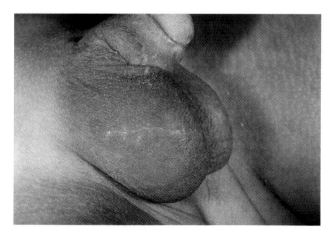

FIGURE 9–9. An erythematous right-sided scrotal swelling of about 12 hours' duration occurred in this 3-year-old child. He had previously undergone two surgical procedures (hypospadias repair and scrotal exploration for a similar episode of scrotal swelling when he was found to have epididymo-orchitis; note the scar on the scrotum). During this episode, the testis was in the normal position with the long axis in the axis of the body. Doppler studies also showed increased flow.

Balanoposthitis

DEFINITION

1. Posthitis refers to an inflammation and cellulitis of the foreskin (prepuce) only.
2. Balanitis refers to an infection/inflammation of the glans penis.
3. Balanoposthitis refers to an infection/inflammation of the glans penis and prepuce. Both of the aforementioned entities usually occur in conjunction.

ANATOMY (see Fig. 9–11)

1. The foreskin is the free fold of skin that covers the glans penis in the flaccid condition.
2. The preputial space is a potential space between the foreskin and the glans penis.
3. The preputial ring is the opening from the preputial space to the outside of the foreskin.
4. Normally the preputial ring stretches easily to allow retraction of the foreskin.

BOX 9-7   *Balanoposthitis*

Balanitis: Inflammation or infection of glans
Posthitis: Inflammation or infection of prepuce (foreskin)

ETIOLOGY/PATHOGENESIS

1. Sloughed epithelial debris and secretions (smegma) trapped beneath the foreskin in uncircumcised boys may be a contributory factor.
2. Bacteria, yeasts, and fusospirillary organisms are abundant in the preputial sac, and although they are normally saprophytic, under conditions of lowered local or general resistance, they may become pathogens.
3. In infants and children
   a. *Candida*
   b. Overgrowth of normal bacterial flora
   c. Chronic irritation (e.g., poor hygiene, wet diapers, smegma collection, soap, laundry detergents, alkalis, friction, and trauma)
4. Trauma (e.g., zipper injuries)
5. In adolescents and adults
   a. Sexually transmitted diseases (STDs)
      (1) *Chlamydia*
      (2) *Trichomonas*
      (3) *Mycoplasma*
      (4) Syphilis (rare)
   b. Candidal infections
      (1) Immunocompromised states (e.g., diabetes mellitus, AIDS)
      (2) Elderly

EPIDEMIOLOGY

These infections are more common in uncircumcised boys.

LABORATORY

1. Balanoposthitis is a clinical diagnosis.
2. Microscopy and culture for *Candida*
3. Cultures of exudates usually show mixed organisms.
4. Investigation for STD in adolescents (as indicated)
   a. Urethral discharge or intraurethral swab specimen for Gram-stained smear and culture and sensitivity
   b. Nucleic acid amplification test either on intraurethral swab or first-voided urine for *C. trachomatis*
   c. Wet mount examination and culture of intraurethral swab specimen for *Trichomonas*

COMPLICATIONS

1. Phimosis may occur when chronic infection due to poor hygiene causes fibrosis and contracture of the preputial ring (especially with recurrent episodes of balanoposthitis).
2. Gangrenous balanoposthitis from anaerobic infection may lead to erosion and ulceration

DIFFERENTIAL DIAGNOSIS

1. Contact dermatitis
2. Lichen sclerosus et atrophicus

TREATMENT

1. Education
   a. Proper cleansing of prepuce
   b. Improvement of hygiene
   c. Lukewarm baths may help if condition is associated with difficult micturition
2. Treatment is directed at suspected cause
   a. Warm soaks
   b. Topical antibacterial agent for bacterial infections (e.g., bacitracin)
   c. Oral antibiotic therapy may be required if condition is associated with cellulitis.
   d. Topical antifungal agent for candidal infections (e.g., nystatin [Mycostatin])
   e. Treatment of suspected STD in adolescents (including treatment of sexual partners)
      (1) Metronidazole for trichomonal balanitis
      (2) Doxycycline or Azithromycin for *Chlamydia* balanitis
3. Surgery (or urology) consultation for the rare patient who may require a dorsal slit because of edema causing severe phimosis
4. Circumcision may be considered as an option for further management.

KEY POINT

Balanoposthitis

- Candidal balanoposthitis may be a presenting sign of undiagnosed immunocompromised state.

TABLE 9–12
Clinical Features of Balanoposthitis

Foreskin and/or glans
  Pain
  Erythema
  Edema
  Malodorous discharge (may be purulent)
  Extension of erythema and edema may result in phimosis
  Erosion and ulceration (rare; invasion by gram-negative
    bacteria)
Urinary symptoms
  Dysuria
  Urinary retention (meatal obstruction secondary to edema)
Signs related to specific etiology
  Candida (beefy red color, involvement of scrotum/
    intertriginous areas, satellite lesions, scaling)
  Chlamydia (nongonococcal urethritis)
  Trichomonas (urethritis)

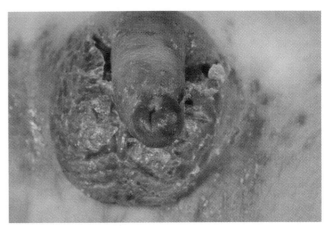

FIGURE 9–12. Candida balanoposthitis in an uncircumcised toddler. Note erythema, scaling, severe edema, and constricted preputial orifice. This patient also had urinary retention.

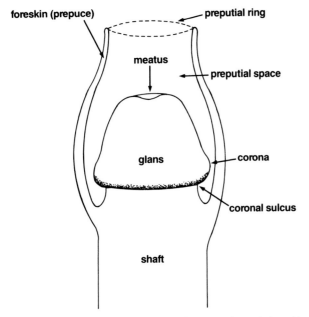

FIGURE 9–11. Normal anatomy of the penis and foreskin. (From Ashcraft KW, Holder TM [eds]: Pediatric Surgery, 2nd ed. Philadelphia, WB Saunders, 1985.)

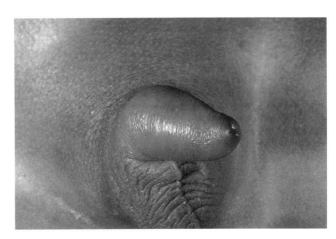

FIGURE 9–13. Posthitis with erythema and edema of the foreskin in an uncircumcised toddler.

Paraphimosis

DEFINITION

1. Phimosis is a stenosis of the preputial ring, such that the foreskin cannot be retracted back over the glans penis.
2. Paraphimosis is a retracted foreskin that cannot be brought forward over the glans penis.

ANATOMY/PATHOGENESIS (see Fig. 9–11)

1. The foreskin cannot be retracted in newborns without disrupting the natural adhesions, which attach the epithelial layers of the inner prepuce and the glans.
2. After birth, sloughed epithelial debris and secretions (smegma) accumulate beneath the foreskin, elevating it from the glans penis and eventually facilitating separation.
3. The foreskin is retractable in infants as follows:
  a. Neonates: in 4%
  b. By 1 year: in 50%
  c. By 2 years: in 80%
  d. By 3 years: in 90%
3. Paraphimosis is more likely to result from the

tight, partially retractable foreskin of infants and young children. A partially stenotic preputial ring that is retained at the coronal sulcus proximal to the corona creates a tourniquet effect and results in tension greater than lymphatic pressure, leading to subsequent edema of the prepuce and glans distal to the ring.

4. Paraphimosis can rarely develop in boys with a fully retractable foreskin, which becomes entrapped, or in a circumcised boy who has some residual foreskin.
5. Physicians may forcibly retract a tight foreskin during cleansing prior to bladder catheterization and may produce paraphimosis if the prepuce is not reduced afterward.
6. A tight foreskin retracted behind the glans and left in that position forms a constricting ring that results in the impairment of lymphatic and venous return from the glans. This leads to edema of the prepuce, penile shaft, and glans distal to the incarcerated foreskin. If this is not reduced promptly, arterial insufficiency, ischemia, and gangrene of the glans may develop.
7. Once the constriction is relieved, normal blood flow into and out of the foreskin and glans penis will return.

LABORATORY

Paraphimosis is a clinical diagnosis.

COMPLICATIONS

1. Necrosis of the glans penis if the condition is not reduced promptly.
2. Complications related to treatment:
   a. Injury to the glans and foreskin with overly zealous attempts at manual reduction
   b. Cold injury related to application of ice

DIFFERENTIAL DIAGNOSIS

Penile strangulation by a hair tourniquet: a constricting band of hair just proximal to the glans in a circumcised male

TREATMENT

1. Nonsurgical reduction techniques
   a. Conscious sedation or a local anesthetic block on the dorsal nerve of the penis
   b. Gentle manual reduction:
      (1) Hold one gauze sponge in each hand, and place the index and third fingers of each hand proximal to the foreskin (with the gauze under the fingers to allow traction) and both thumbs on the end of the glans penis.
      (2) Use thumb pressure to push the glans back through the paraphimotic ring between the

four fingers, which are behind this ring and are supporting it (see Fig. 9–15).
      c. If this is unsuccessful, try to reduce the swelling by using
         (1) Either gentle, continuous compression by the clinician's hand (for 3 to 5 minutes), *or*
         (2) A mixture of ice and water sealed in a rubber glove for brief periods (3 minutes at a time)
         (3) Patient requires close monitoring to prevent pressure injury or cold injury.
         (4) With reduction of the swelling, manual reduction is attempted.
      d. Postreduction bleeding, if it occurs, is slight and generally responds to pressure.
      e. Reduction using noncrushing (Babcock) clamps.
      f. Successful reduction using hyaluronidase (disperses extracellular edema) has been reported in adults
2. Patient can be discharged home after successful reduction with follow-up recommended with a pediatric surgeon (or urologist).
3. Surgical reduction:
   a. Urologic/surgical consultation
   b. Puncture of the edematous prepuce with a 25-gauge needle. Gentle compression is applied to express the fluid and relieve the edema; manual reduction then follows.
   c. Dorsal slit
   d. An emergency circumcision, if all other measures fail

PREVENTION

1. Counseling parents that no special care is required for the uncircumcised penis. The external surface of the foreskin requires gentle cleaning like other parts of the body, and the foreskin should not be forcibly retracted for cleaning.
2. Uncircumcised older boys with a retractable foreskin should be taught to return the foreskin to its unretracted (normal) position after cleaning.

KEY POINTS

Paraphimosis

- A surgical emergency that requires prompt reduction to prevent ischemia to the glans penis
- Prompt reduction obviates a later difficult reduction of an extremely swollen foreskin and glans penis.
- Prolonged and painful attempts at manual reduction must be avoided.
- Inability to retract the foreskin completely is normal in young children (up to 4 to 5 years); attempting to retract it may cause paraphimosis.

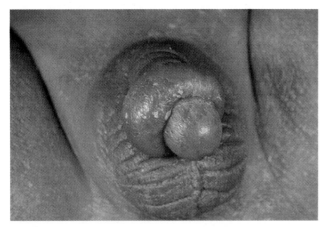

FIGURE 9-14. Paraphimosis in an 18-month-old infant who presented with pain (i.e., inconsolable crying) and swelling of 2 days' duration. The edematous foreskin trapped proximal to the glans penis is seen.

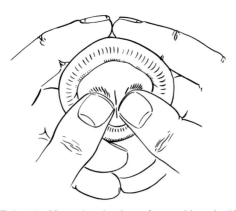

FIGURE 9-15. Manual reduction of paraphimosis. With the thumbs on the glans penis and the fingertips on the tight band of foreskin, the glans is pushed as the foreskin is pulled over the glans penis. The foreskin can be reduced by applying pressure on the glans as if one were "turning a sock inside out." (From Kelalis PP, King LR, Belman AB: Clinical Pediatric Urology, 2nd ed. Philadelphia, WB Saunders, 1985.)

TABLE 9-13
Clinical Features of Paraphimosis

Most common age
  Uncircumcised young infants and children
Most common presentation
  Pain and swelling of glans penis
Young infants
  Swelling usually pricked by a caretaker during a diaper change
  May present with inconsolable crying because of pain
Older children
  Severe pain as swelling increases leading to ischemia of glans penis

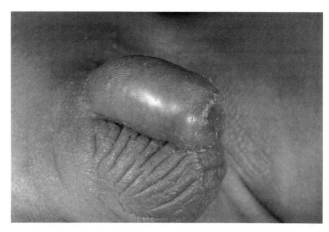

FIGURE 9-16. Penis after manual reduction of paraphimosis. Residual edema may take hours to days to fully resolve.

Intussusception

DEFINITION

Intussusception occurs when one part of the intestine invaginates into the lumen of the distal adjoining bowel.

EPIDEMIOLOGY

1. Incidence: 1 to 4 in 1000 live births
2. Male-female ratio is 2:1 to 4:1
3. Age at presentation
   a. Peak incidence: 5 to 12 months
   b. Range: between 2 months and 5 years
   c. About 66% to 80% of patients are less than 2 years of age.

PATHOGENESIS

1. Most common sites: ileocolic (90% of cases) and ileo-ileocolic
2. Less common sites: cecocolic, rarely just ileoileal
3. Usually starts with a lead point just proximal to the ileocecal valve, which leads to an ileocolic invagination. The intussusceptum continues through the colon a variable distance, occasionally as far as the rectum, where it can be palpated on rectal examination.
4. During telescoping, the mesentery is dragged along with the *intussusceptum* (proximal invaginating portion of the bowel) into the *intussuscipiens* (adjacent distal recipient portion of the bowel).
5. The mesentery of the intussusceptum becomes compressed, leading to venous engorgement,

edema, and bleeding from the mucosa (clinically evident by bloody stools mixed with mucus). Further pressure from entrapment may lead to obstruction of the mesenteric arteries, causing gangrene, perforation of the bowel, and peritonitis.

COMPLICATIONS

1. Intestinal hemorrhage
2. Necrosis secondary to local ischemia
3. Bowel perforation
4. Peritonitis, sepsis
5. Shock

BOX 9–8   *Clinical Features of Intussusception*

CLASSIC TRIAD

- Intermittent colicky abdominal pain (85% of patients)
- Bilious vomiting (75% of patients)
- Currant jelly stools (60% of patients)

Classic triad is seen in only 21% of patients
Two symptoms are seen in 70% of patients

BOX 9–9   *"Neurologic" Signs of Intussusception*

"Neurologic" signs (often misdiagnosed as sepsis or a postictal state)
    Lack of interaction
    Extreme lethargy
    Coma or shock-like state (because of intense visceral pain)
    Apnea
    Seizures
    Seizure-like activity
    Opisthotonic posturing
    Weak cry
    Hypotonia
    Pinpoint pupils

DIFFERENTIAL DIAGNOSIS

1. In infants: gastroenteritis, trauma, incarcerated inguinal hernia
2. In older children: appendicitis

DIAGNOSIS AND TREATMENT

1. Prompt surgical consultation, insertion of nasogastric tube, and fluid resuscitation
2. Complete blood count, serum electrolytes, glucose, type and cross-match.
3. Antibiotic coverage for both gram-positive and gram-negative pathogens (e.g., ampicillin and gentamicin)

4. Plain radiographs and sonography
  a. Acute abdomen series
  b. Sonogram to make a diagnosis and color Doppler sonogram to determine whether intussusception is likley to be reducible
  c. Negative radiographs or sonograms should *not* deter one from performing a barium enema in an infant in whom intussusception is strongly suspected.
5. Hydrostatic reduction using barium (use for both diagnosis and therapy, see Box 9–10)
6. Reduction of intussusception by air insufflation is an alternative to barium. Air contrast obviates the risk of barium peritonitis if perforation is present.
7. Intraoperative manual reduction is done in patients in whom hydrostatic reduction has been unsuccessful. If indicated, resection of gangrenous bowel or a recognizable lead point can be performed.
8. Hospitalization after reduction for observation for possible recurrence.

BOX 9–10   *Intussusception and Barium Enema*

A high index of suspicion for intussusception mandates either hydrostatic reduction or pneumatic reduction
Hydrostatic reduction using barium, a procedure for both diagnosis and therapy
Contraindications for barium enema
    Evidence of peritonitis
    Intestinal perforation
    Shock
Sedation is often helpful for relaxing the infant during study
Follow "rule of 3" to avoid perforation:
    Weight of barium column should be not more than 3 feet above abdomen
    Maximum three attempts
    Each attempt should not exceed 3 minutes
Successful reduction occurs in 50% to 75% of cases
Success rate is directly related to timing of diagnosis; the later the referral, the lower the success rate
Reduction is confirmed *only* with an adequate reflux of barium into the ileum

---

PROGNOSIS

1. Recurrence rate after barium enema reduction ranges from 3% to 5%. It occurs relatively soon after the reduction. The rate of recurrence after surgical reduction is about 1% to 5%.
2. Recurrence is more common in older children. An anatomic lead point must be suspected.

KEY POINTS

Intussusception

- Most common cause of acute intestinal obstruction between 3 months and 2 years of age
- Intussusception rarely reduces spontaneously; if left untreated it would result in death in most cases.

- Currant jelly stool is a late finding, and its absence does *not* exclude the diagnosis
- Infants with "neurologic" or "painless" intussusception present with lethargy or unresponsiveness without striking gastrointestinal symptoms

---

TABLE 9-14
Etiology of Intussusception

Infants

Idiopathic (90% to 95% of cases)
Lead point: hypertrophied Peyer patches and lymph nodes
    following a viral infection (e.g., adenovirus)

Older Children

Recognizable anatomic lead point is the rule (75% of cases)
Few examples:
    Meckel diverticulum (most common)
    Polyp
    Tumors (lymphoma, hemangioma)
    Duplication cysts
    Appendix
    Henoch-Schönlein purpura with intramural hematoma
    Cystic fibrosis with meconium ileus equivalent
    Intestinal parasites
    Hemophilia with intramural hematoma
    Hemangioma proximal to ileocecal valve

TABLE 9-15
Clinical Features of Intussusception
(see also Box 9-8)

Abdominal pain (85%)
    Pattern of pain fairly characteristic
    Episodic severe colicky pain, often leading to episodic bouts
      of crying
    Guarded position with knees pulled up onto abdomen
    Infant may sleep or may appear listless, lethargic, or playful
      between episodes of pain
Abdominal mass (65% of cases)
    Ill-defined, variably tender sausage-shaped mass
    Mass palpable in right upper quadrant or midabdomen *with*
      absence of bowel in the right lower quadrant (Dance
      sign)
Bilious vomiting (75%)
Stool (currant jelly stools in 60% of cases)
    Diarrheal stool with gross blood or mucus (either passed
      spontaneously or following rectal examination) *or*
    Normal appearing stool positive for occult blood
Rectal examination
    Presence of blood mixed with stool
    Occasionally intussusception can be felt on rectal
      examination
Signs of systemic toxicity (due to gangrenous bowel or
    peritonitis)
    Fever
    Marked abdominal distention
    Leukocytosis

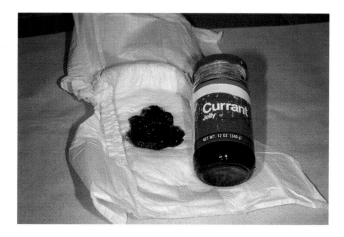

FIGURE 9-17. Commercially available "currant jelly."

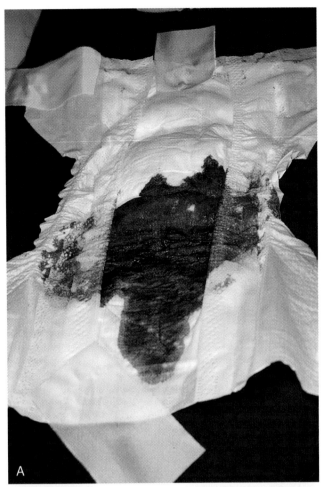

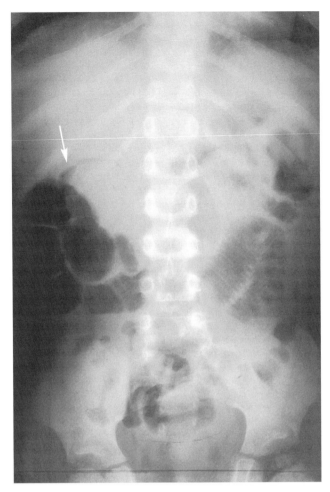

FIGURE 9–19. Supine view of the abdomen demonstrates a soft tissue mass with a surrounding crescent of air in the right midabdomen *(arrow).*

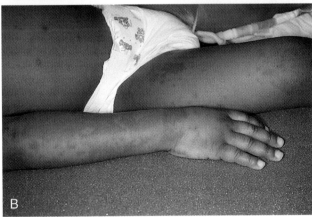

FIGURE 9–18. *A,* Dark maroon blood mixed with mucus in the stool (currant jelly stool) was passed by a 3-year-old child with Henoch-Schönlein purpura. *B,* This child was admitted with a purpuric eruption, angioedema of hands, severe vasculitis of the ear (see Fig. 2–32), abdominal distention, and bilious vomiting.

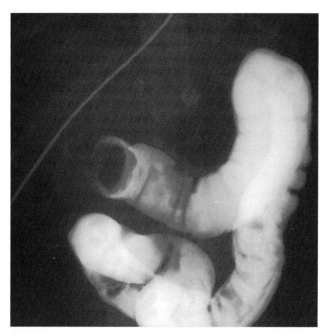

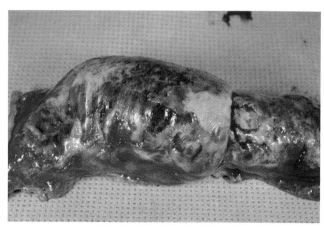

FIGURE 9-21. Magnified view of ileo-ileo colic intussusception after bowel resection. On the right side, the proximal portion of the ileum (intussusceptum) telescopes into the more distal ileum and cecum (intussuscipiens). This picture illustrates necrosis of both the intussusceptum and the intussuscipiens.

FIGURE 9-20. Frontal abdominal radiograph after a barium enema in the same patient. A large filling defect in the hepatic flexure is seen. Intussusception could not be reduced, and surgical intervention was required. During surgery, attempts at manual reduction failed, and resection of the gangrenous bowel was required.

Hirschsprung Disease

SYNONYM   Congenital Aganglionic Megacolon

DEFINITION

Hirschsprung disease results from an absence of ganglionic cells in the bowel wall extending proximally from the anus for a variable distance

ETIOLOGY/PATHOGENESIS

1. Bowel histology in Hirschsprung disease
   a. Absence of intramural ganglionic cells at the submucosal plexus and myenteric plexus of the intestine results in failure of normal bowel relaxation and peristalsis
   b. High concentration of acetylcholine esterase between muscular layers and in submucosa
2. Absence of neural innervation results from an arrest of neuroblast migration from the proximal to distal bowel.
3. The abnormally innervated bowel becomes hypertonic and functions as a stenotic bowel.
4. The normal bowel proximal to the aganglionic segment becomes dilated.

EPIDEMIOLOGY

1. Incidence: 1 in 5000 to 8000 live births
2. Male-female ratio is 4:1
3. Family history is positive in 3% to 7% of affected children.

BOX 9-11	*Aganglionic Bowel Involvement in Hirschsprung Disease*

Starts at the anus and extends proximally to a variable extent
Aganglionic segment is limited to
  Rectosigmoid (75%)
  Entire colon (10%)
  Entire intestine (rare)

4. Other associated syndromes
   a. Down syndrome
   b. Waardenburg syndrome
   c. Laurence-Moon-Biedl syndrome
   d. Multiple endocrine neoplasia

CLINICAL FEATURES

1. Newborns
   a. Delayed passage of meconium (see Box 9-12)
   b. Enterocolitis
      (1) Most commonly seen between 2 and 4 weeks of life
      (2) Abdominal distention
      (3) Vomiting
      (4) Explosive diarrhea (following digital rectal examination) that rapidly becomes bloody
      (5) High fever

Hirschsprung Disease

DELAYED PASSAGE OF MECONIUM

- About 94% of patients with Hirschsprung disease fail to pass meconium within the first 24 hours.
- About 90% of normal full-term neonates pass meconium within 24 hours after birth; 99% pass it within 48 hours.

(6) Lethargy
(7) Colonic perforation
(8) Peritonitis and shock
  c. Complete intestinal obstruction associated with bilious vomiting, abdominal distention, and obstipation
2. Infants
  a. Chronic constipation that frequently requires enemas, suppositories, or rectal stimulation
  b. Rectal examination
    (1) An empty vault that is not dilated
    (2) Explosive release of feces may result with withdrawal of the examining finger.
  c. Hydroureter secondary to ureteral compression from dilated colon

LABORATORY

1. Abdominal radiographs
2. Barium enema
  a. Barium enema should be done *without* prior rigorous colonic emptying.
  b. Key to the diagnosis is the presence of a transition zone; however, a transition zone is not usually present before 1 to 2 weeks of age.
3. Rectal suction mucosal biopsy
  a. Absence of ganglion cells
  b. Large number of hypertrophied nerve bundles that show increased acetylcholinesterase staining
4. Anal manometry: difficult to perform in young infants

TREATMENT

1. Surgical consultation
2. Operative options include a temporary colostomy initially followed by definitive repair when infant is 6 to 12 months old.
3. Full-thickness biopsy is done at the time of surgery for confirmation and to determine the level of involvement.

PROGNOSIS

1. Most patients achieve fecal continence after surgery.
2. Long-term postoperative problems include
  a. Stricture formation
  b. Fecal soiling
  c. Recurrent enterocolitis
  d. Perianal abscess

KEY POINTS

Hirschsprung Disease

- Most common cause of lower intestinal obstruction in the neonate
- Suspect Hirschsprung disease in any full-term neonate who does not pass meconium within 48 hours.
- Most ominous presentation and most common cause of death is enterocolitis.

TABLE 9–16
Differential Diagnosis of Constipation

Common Causes

Diet (lack of fiber)
Anal fissure
Hypothyroidism
Functional constipation
Hirschsprung disease

Uncommon Causes

Anal atresia
Anal stenosis
Cerebral palsy
Hypercalcemia
Disorders of spinal cord
Hypotonia
Diabetes insipidus
Renal acidosis

Medications

Antacids (aluminum containing)
Cough medications (codeine containing)
Elevated Mg^{++} in neonate (mother given Mg^{++} during labor)

TABLE 9–17
Differential Diagnosis: Functional Constipation Versus Hirschsprung Disease

	Functional Constipation	Hirschsprung Disease
Onset of constipation	After 2 years	Birth
Encopresis	Common	Very Rare
Abdominal distention	Rare	Common
Enterocolitis	None	Possible
Poor weight gain	Rare	Common
Rectal exam	Feces-packed ampulla	Ampulla empty
Anal tone	Normal	Normal
Barium enema	No transition zone	Transition zone
	Dilated rectum	Delayed evacuation (>24 hours)
	Massive amount of stools	
Anorectal manometry	Distention of rectum causes relaxation of internal sphincter	No sphincter or paradoxical relaxation or increase in pressure
Rectal biopsy	Ganglion cells	No ganglion cells

Modified from Wyllie R: Motility disorders and Hirschsprung disease. *In* Nelson Textbook of Pediatrics, 15th ed. Philadelphia, W.B. Saunders, 1996, p. 1071.

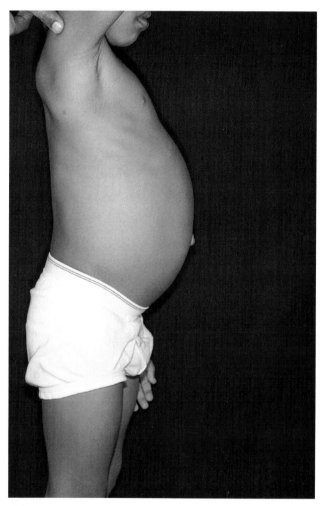

FIGURE 9–22. Distended abdomen in a 4-year-old child who had a chronic history of constipation since early infancy. He was treated on numerus occasions with rectal suppositories.

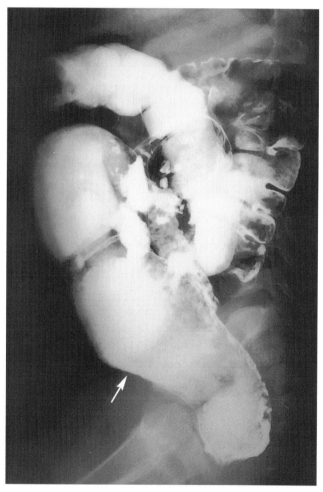

FIGURE 9–23. Lateral view of the bowel using barium contrast shows a transition zone (a funnel-shaped area; *arrow*) between the distended normal (ganglionic) proximal sigmoid colon and the normal-caliber (non-distended) aganglionic distal rectosigmoid segment.

Preauricular Sinus

DEFINITION
A minor developmental defect of the pinna

ANATOMY/PATHOGENESIS
1. Pinna of the external ear develops from a fusion of six hillocks derived from the upper ends of the 1st and 2nd pharyngeal (brachial) arches.
2. Imperfect fusion of the tubercles of the pharyngeal arches results in various anomalies; preauricular sinuses are the most common among these minor anomalies.
3. Sinus tract is lined with keratinized squamous epithelium (epidermis) and can become filled with debris followed by suppuration.

EPIDEMIOLOGY
1. More common in African-Americans than in whites
2. Female-male ratio: 2:1
3. Unilateral involvement: 75%
4. Bilateral involvement: 25%
5. Usually an isolated anomaly; at times may be associated with other anomalies of the face or ears or may be part of anomalies such as Treacher-Collins syndrome or brachio-otorenal dysplasia.

INHERITANCE
Autosomal dominant with incomplete penetrance

CLINICAL FEATURES
1. Appears as a pinhole-sized pit or cutaneous depression
2. Most common location
   a. A pit located anteriorly on the ascending rim of the helix
   b. A sinus tract about 1.0 to 2.0 cm long is present deep to this opening, and this sinus tract is firmly attached to the underlying perichondrium.
3. Less common variant
   a. A pit located in the helical crus just above the external auditory meatus
   b. A deeper sinus tract may be present that penetrates the cartilage of the pinna and passes posteriorly just above the external canal.
   c. When infected, this sinus tract may present as a cyst or inflammatory mass in the postauricular sulcus.
4. Middle ear examination and hearing are usually normal.

5. Most patients are asymptomatic; the presence of such a sinus is often unnoticed for months or years.
6. With chronic infection of the sinus tract, a retention cyst may form and may drain intermittently.

LABORATORY
This is a clinical diagnosis.

COMPLICATIONS
1. Sinus tracts are vulnerable to infection and abscess formation.
2. Damage to the auricular cartilage during infection requires incision and drainage. This can lead to chondritis, which can result in significant deformity.

TREATMENT
1. Surgical removal is usually not required unless infections recur, requiring repeated courses of antibiotics. Since complete surgical excision is much easier if the sinus has never been infected, some surgeons recommend removal even in the absence of infection.
2. Infected preauricular sinus
   a. Antibiotic therapy that provides antistaphylococcal coverage (e.g., dicloxacillin or cephalosporins [cefuroxime] or amoxicillin-clavulanate)
   b. Incision and drainage of an abscess
   c. Once inflammation has subsided, surgical excision of the complete sinus tract (about 6 weeks later)
   d. Because the sinus tract frequently arborizes under the skin surface, complete surgical excision can be difficult.

PROGNOSIS
1. Once infected, recurrence is common.
2. If surgical excision of the complete sinus tract is not done, resuppuration of any remnant of the sinus tract will occur.

KEY POINTS

Preauricular Sinus

- A brachial cleft remnant secondary to incomplete fusion
- Most common location is the ascending rim of the helix.
- Usually an isolated anomaly

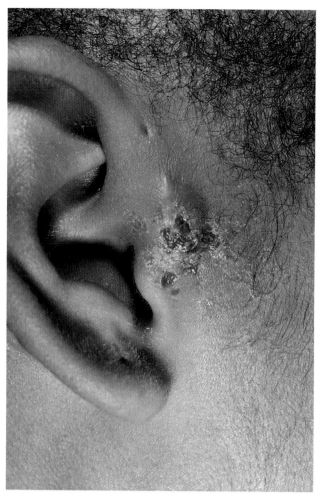

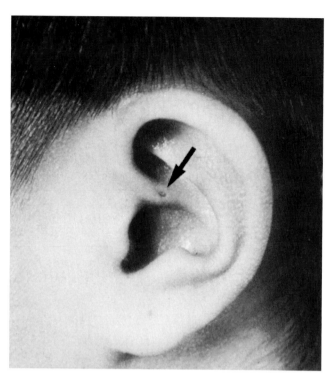

FIGURE 9–25. This auricular pit is less common than the classic preauricular sinus, but it may penetrate the cartilage and extend posteriorly. When the pit is infected, suppuration occurs postauricularly and is easily confused with an infected sebaceous cyst. (From Friedberg JF: Pharyngeal clefts, sinuses and cysts, and other benign neck lesions. Pediatr Clin North Am 36(6):1451, 1989.)

FIGURE 9–24. Preauricular sinus. A pit-like cutaneous dimple is visible in front of the helix and above the tragus, and there are signs of infection (erythema, swelling, and drainage of pus).

Pilonidal Sinus and Abscess

DEFINITION/ANATOMY

Pilonidal sinus presents as a dimple located in the midline at or just superior to the gluteal fold in the sacrococcygeal area. The term pilonidal comes from *pilus* (hair) and *nidus* (nest) and literally means "nest of hair."

ETIOLOGY

1. Usually mixed pathogens
   a. *Staphylococcus aureus*
   b. *Streptococcus pyogenes*
2. Anaerobes
3. Gram-negative organisms

EPIDEMIOLOGY

1. Pilonidal sinus is seen relatively frequently in normal infants.

2. Most common age at presentation
   a. Adolescence
   b. Not seen in younger children
3. Male-female ratio is 3:1

PATHOGENESIS

1. Sinus tract is blocked by keratin or hair, creating a closed space that does not allow drainage.
2. It is thought to be an acquired condition; hairs present in a pilonidal sinus have their roots nearest the opening. The pilonidal sinus results from penetration of shed hair shafts through the skin, which ultimately leads to an acute or chronically infected site.

LABORATORY

A clinical diagnosis

DIFFERENTIAL DIAGNOSIS

Abscess from other causes

1. Hidradenitis suppurativa
2. Anal fistula
3. Inflammatory bowel disease

TREATMENT

1. Incision and drainage of a fluctuant abscess
2. Antistaphylococcal antibiotic coverage (dicloxacillin or cephalosporin)

3. Surgical consultation for recurrent pilonidal sinus infections for definitive treatment (en bloc resection to remove the entire epithelial tract)

PROGNOSIS

1. Recurs in about 20% of patients after simple incision and drainage.
2. Recurrence rate drops to about 6% after surgical excision and marsupialization.
3. Malignant degeneration of pilonidal sinus cyst is reported in patients with chronic infections.

KEY POINTS

Pilonidal Sinus and Abscess

- Almost always occurs in the midline at or just superior to the gluteal fold in the sacrococcygeal area.
- Pilonidal sinus is a benign condition, and patients are asymptomatic.
- Pilonidal abscess occurs in adolescents.

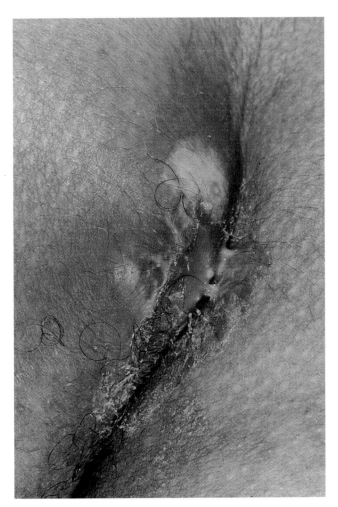

FIGURE 9–26. An infected pilonidal sinus is seen just superior to the gluteal fold in the sacrococcygeal area in this 13-year-old adolescent girl.

TABLE 9–18
Clinical Features of Pilonidal Abscess

Typical Location

At or just superior to gluteal fold in the sacrococcygeal area

Atypical Locations (due to an expanding pilonidal abscess)

May present as a draining abscess laterally
May extend inferiorly, mimicking a posterior perianal abscess

Clinical Features

Swelling
Pain (depending on size or extent)
    Localized in gluteal area
    Pain while sitting
    Low back pain
Purulent drainage
Onset of symptoms either acute or chronic
Usually absence of systemic symptoms
History of recurrence (±)

Thyroglossal Duct Cyst

DEFINITION

A neck mass of embryonic origin arising from the remnants of the thyroglossal duct

EMBRYOLOGY/PATHOGENESIS

1. Thyroid diverticulum arises from the foramen cecum at the base of the tongue, descends in the neck close to the hyoid bone as a thyroglossal duct, and gives rise to the thyroid gland on reaching the final position in the anterior neck.
2. Thyroglossal duct normally disappears by the time the thyroid reaches its final position.
3. Failure of the thyroglossal duct to atrophy can result in cyst formation anywhere along the course of descent. The cyst is usually connected to the foramen cecum by single or multiple tracts, which pass through the hyoid bone.
4. The duct lining contains mucus-secreting glands, and the cyst usually is filled with thick mucus.

EPIDEMIOLOGY

1. Most common age at presentation
   a. Preschool age (2 to 3 years old)
   b. Mid adolescence
2. Rarely presents in the newborn period even though it is embryonic in origin.
3. Location
   a. Most common: anterior midline at or just below the hyoid bone
   b. Uncommon: suprahyoid or suprasternal

CLINICAL FEATURES (see also Box 9–14)

1. Occasionally the cyst or another part of the duct creates a sinus tract to the skin at or just lateral to the midline, and clear or cloudy mucus may escape from the sinus.
2. Rare presentations during infancy
   a. Difficulty in swallowing
   b. Respiratory difficulty
   c. Improvement of above difficulties in the prone position

LABORATORY

1. Diagnosis is clinical by characteristic findings.
2. Thyroid function tests
3. Radionuclide scans prior to surgery to rule out ectopic thyroid gland, especially in the absence of a readily palpable thyroid gland in the normal position

COMPLICATIONS

Infection (by oral flora from the cyst's communication with oropharynx via the foramen cecum)

> **BOX 9–14**   *Clinical Features of Thyroglossal Duct Cyst*
>
> Most common presentation
>   Asymptomatic mass (which may be present intermittently)
> Best visualized as a mass when neck is hyperextended
>   Soft
>   Nontender
>   Round
>   Well-defined margin
>   Usually measures 1–2 cm in diameter (rarely larger)
> Cyst often becomes apparent during an upper respiratory tract infection
> Signs of infected cyst
>   Tenderness
>   Erythema
>   Rapidly increasing swelling with or without drainage

TREATMENT

1. Surgery (Sistrunk procedure): complete excision of the cyst and its tract upward to the base of the tongue, and resection of the central portion of the hyoid bone
2. A course of systemic antibiotics prior to surgery if the cyst is infected
3. Careful follow-up after surgery to check for possible development of hypothyroidism

PROGNOSIS

1. Multiple smaller tracts connecting through the hyoid bone to the floor of the mouth may be present; if these are not completely resected, the cyst may recur.
2. Risk of recurrence is higher with prior infection of the cyst, which makes surgical dissection more difficult.

KEY POINTS

Thyroglossal Duct Cyst

- Most common anterior midline neck mass of embryonic origin during childhood
- Vertical movement of the cyst with tongue protrusion and swallowing is pathognomonic; however, *absence* of this finding *does not* exclude the diagnosis.
- Ectopic thyroid glands have frequently been removed surgically with the mistaken diagnosis of thyroglossal duct cyst, leading to hypothyroidism postoperatively.

TABLE 9–19
Differential Diagnosis of Anterior Neck Masses

Thyroglossal duct cyst
Dermoid cyst (more superficial, attached to the skin and
    moves with it)
Lipoma (more lobulated, softer than thyroglossal duct cyst)
Submental lymph nodes
Cystic hygroma (usually transilluminates)
Ectopic thyroid glands
    Incompletely descended thyroid gland
    Incidence 10% to 45%
    May be present at any point in the normal pathway of
      descent
    These glands are prone to functional insufficiency, and with
      compensatory enlargement may be mistaken for
      thyroglossal duct cyst
    If removed mistakenly as thyroglossal duct cyst, growth
      velocity curve may offer a clue to hypothyroidism

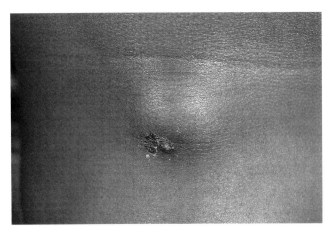

IGURE 9–27. Thyroglossal duct cyst in the anterior midline of the neck. Protrusion of the tongue may cause the cyst to move upward because the tract originates at the base of the tongue.

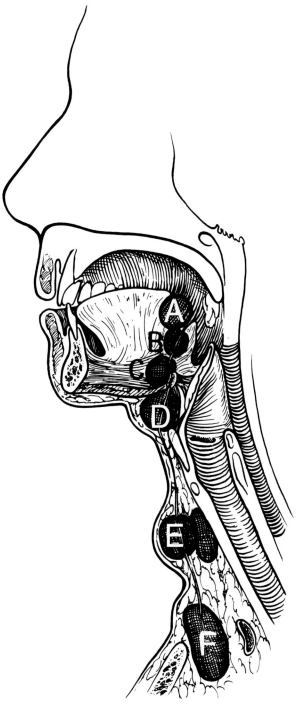

FIGURE 9–28. Thyroglossal duct cysts. These cysts can be located anywhere from the base of the tongue to behind the sternum. *A* and *B,* Lingual (rare). *C* and *D,* Adjacent to the hyoid bone (common), *E* and *F:* Suprasternal fossa (rare). (From Welch K, et al: Pediatric Surgery. Chicago, Year Book Medical Publishers, 1986, p. 549.)

10

Bone Disorders and Orthopedics

Binita R. Shah, M.D.

Acute Hematogenous Osteomyelitis

DEFINITION

Osteomyelitis is an infection that primarily involves the bone. Acute osteomyelitis presents within 2 weeks of onset of disease.

ETIOLOGY (see also Table 10–1)

1. The incidence of osteomyelitis caused by *Haemophilus influenzae* type b is likely to decrease now that the use of routine immunization is common.
2. Osteomyelitis in neonates is caused by *Staphylococcus aureus*, group B streptococci, and coliforms.
3. Uncommon pathogens causing osteomyelitis are *Kingella kingae, Candida* species, and anaerobic bacteria.

EPIDEMIOLOGY

1. Annual incidence: 1 in 5000 children less than 13 years of age in the United States
2. An increased incidence is seen in patients with sickle cell disease.
3. Male-female ratio is 2.5 to 3.7:1.
4. Common age at presentation
   a. About 33% of patients are under 2 years of age.
   b. About 50% of patients are under 5 years of age.

PATHOGENESIS (see Figs. 10–1 and 10–2)

1. Infection of the bone is caused by
   a. Hematogenous seeding (most common in children ≤10 years of age)
   b. Spread from contiguous infected structures (e.g., neonatal heel puncture)
   c. Direct inoculation (open fractures, nail puncture wounds [penetrating injuries to the foot predispose children to *Pseudomonas aeruginosa* osteomyelitis])
2. Acute hematogenous osteomyelitis (see Fig. 10–1).
   a. Infection usually begins in the metaphysis (region of stagnant network of arterioles and capillaries that lacks phagocytic cells) with production of an inflammatory exudate.
   b. Infection rarely spreads down the medullary cavity because the inflammatory response

blocks spread within the bone. Instead, infection spreads to the subperiosteal space, the path of least resistance because the cortex in this area is porous.
   c. As the infection spreads, loosely attached periosteum is stripped off the bone along with the blood supply for the underlying cortex. This results in formation of a sequestrum (a loosely adherent piece of infected dead bone).
   d. Involucrum (periosteal new bone formation enveloping the sequestrum) develops from the periosteum and maintains its blood supply from the overlying muscle.
3. The inflammatory process can also extend into the epiphysis (and into the joint) in infants through the transphyseal vessels (see Fig. 10–2).
4. Septic arthritis may coexist if the infection breaks through the metaphysis, especially in anatomic locations in which the metaphysis lies within the joint capsule (see Box 10–1 and Fig. 10–1).

| BOX 10–1 | *Coexistence of Septic Arthritis with Osteomyelitis* |

Septic arthritis may coexist with osteomyelitis at the following anatomic locations where the metaphysis *lies within* the joint capsule
   Proximal femur–hip joint
   Proximal humerus–shoulder joint
   Distal lateral tibia–ankle joint
   Proximal radius–elbow joint

CLINICAL FEATURES

1. Antecedent infection (with bacteremia) or presence of other foci of infection
2. Infants and young children
   a. Fever, irritability, anorexia, lethargy (infant may appear septic)
   b. Refusal to walk or bear weight (with lower extremity involvement)
   c. Pseudoparalysis (failure to use a limb despite normal neuromuscular structures)

3. Older children
   a. May be able to describe and localize pain
   b. Limping (with lower extremity involvement)
   c. Muscle spasm leading to limitation of active range of motion
4. Physical examination
   a. Soft tissue swelling
   b. Point tenderness
   c. Increased local warmth
   d. Erythema of the skin overlying the infection

LABORATORY

1. Complete blood count
   a. Usually leukocytosis with a left shift
   b. May be normal (in up to 60% of patients) with early disease
   c. Also helps in following response to treatment
2. Erythrocyte sedimentation rate
   a. Elevated
   b. May be normal (in up to 25% of patients) with early disease
   c. Also helps in following response to treatment
3. C-reactive protein
   a. Increased
   b. Also helps in following response to treatment
4. Blood culture: positive (in 36% to 76% of patients)
5. Recovery of bacteria from bone (e.g., drilling to drain the pus) or from subperiosteal needle aspiration (in the area of point tenderness) or joint fluid: positive (in 66% to 76% of patients)

BOX 10-2   *Differential Diagnosis of Acute Hematogenous Osteomyelitis*

Septic arthritis
Fracture
Cellulitis
Toxic synovitis
Pyomyositis
Hemoglobinopathies (bone infarction)
Bone tumors (e.g., osteogenic or Ewing sarcoma)
Malignancies (e.g., leukemia, lymphoma, neuroblastoma)
Acute rheumatic fever
Juvenile rheumatoid arthritis

---

6. Standard radiographs (anteroposterior and lateral views of the suspected area)
   a. To detect soft tissue swelling and/or fluid in the joint
   b. To exclude other conditions (e.g., fracture, bone tumors)
   c. Radiographic evidence includes periosteal elevation and/or subperiosteal new bone formation (changes of periosteal reaction) or rarefaction and/or lysis (changes of bone destruction)

d. Detection of bone destruction and repair is not possible until 10 to 14 days after onset.
7. Bone scan (should be considered when diagnosis is unclear)
   a. Detects evidence of new bone formation and multiple sites of involvement (whole body survey) *earlier* in the course of disease than plain radiographs.
   b. A three-phase bone scan is done with ^{99m}Tc-labeled diphosphonate. The initial phase (blood pool) and the second phase (soft tissue pool) are obtained immediately after injection, while the third phase (bone phase) is a delayed scan that is performed 2 hours after injection.
   c. Increased uptake during the initial phase with subsequent decline in the third phase means increased blood flow and cellulitis (without osteomyelitis). In osteomyelitis and septic arthritis, localized uptake is seen in all three phases.
8. Hemoglobin electrophoresis should be performed in any patient presenting with gram-negative osteomyelitis, especially salmonella osteomyelitis.

TREATMENT

1. Hospitalization and orthopedic consultation
2. Management principles include antibiotic therapy, surgery, and immobilization.
3. Parenteral antibiotic therapy (pending culture results)
   a. In infants and children (coverage for *H. influenzae* in children less than 5 years of age, particularly those who have not been immunized adequately)
      (1) Penicillinase-resistant penicillin (e.g., oxacillin [for *S. aureus* and other gram-positive bacteria]) *and* a cephalosporin (e.g., cefotaxime)
      (2) Cefuroxime alone is another alternative. It covers gram-positive bacteria including *S. aureus* and *H. influenzae.*
   b. Children over 5 years of age: coverage for *S. aureus* and other gram-positive bacteria
   c. Duration of therapy: minimum 4 to 6 weeks
   d. Routes of antibiotics:
      (1) Parenteral antibiotic therapy is usually continued until the patient shows clinical signs of improvement (e.g., afebrile, declining ESR, normal leukocyte count).
      (2) Oral antibiotic therapy can be started if the patient is able to tolerate oral therapy, the etiologic agent and sensitivity have been identified, and the ability to monitor antibiotic level and compliance is ensured.
      (3) Dose of oral antibiotic therapy is *two to three times* the usual dose recommended for common infections.
4. Surgical drainage is indicated for
   a. Soft tissue abscess, subperiosteal abscess, or intramedullary abscess
   b. Presence of sequestra
5. Immobilization of the affected limb in a functional position (usually for 3 weeks or more)

a. To assist the healing process
b. To protect against pathologic fracture (weakening of bone secondary to bony destruction)

COMPLICATIONS/PROGNOSIS

1. Pathologic fracture
2. Chronic osteomyelitis
3. Leg length discrepancy secondary to growth disturbance
4. Destruction of the adjacent joint
5. Limb dysfunction secondary to massive bone defects

KEY POINTS

Acute Hematogenous Osteomyelitis

- Most common site is the rapidly growing end (metaphysis) of long bones
- *S. aureus* is the most common pathogen among patients of all ages
- Clinical symptoms precede the radiographic findings by 7 to 14 days
- Although *Salmonella* osteomyelitis occurs more often in patients with hemoglobinopathies, *S. aureus* remains the predominant pathogen even in this group.

TABLE 10–1
Microbiology of Acute Hematogenous Osteomyelitis

Staphylococcus aureus (most common; [67% to 89%])	*Streptococcus pneumoniae* (2%–6%)
Group A streptococci (second most common [12% to 16%])	*Pseudomonas aeruginosa* (3%)
Haemophilus influenzae type B (5% to 8%)	*Salmonella* (<2%)
	Escherichia coli (<1%)
	Klebsiella

Modified from Krogstad P, Smith AL: Osteomyelitis and septic arthritis. *In* Feigin RD, Cherry JD (eds): Textbook of Pediatric Infectious Diseases. Philadelphia, W.B. Saunders, 1997, p. 684.

TABLE 10–2
Most Common Sites of Bone Involvement: Acute Hematogenous Osteomyelitis

Femur	36%	Radius	3%
Tibia	33%	Ulna	2%
Humerus	10%	Clavicle	1%
Fibula	7%		

Modified from Krogstad P, Smith AL: Osteomyelitis and septic arthritis. *In* Feigin RD, Cherry JD (eds): Textbook of Pediatric Infectious Diseases. Philadelphia, W.B. Saunders, 1997, p. 685.

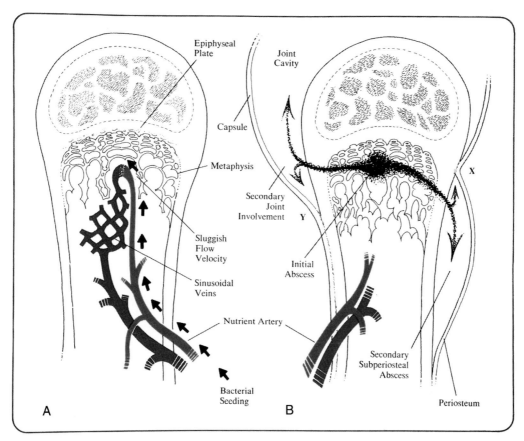

FIGURE 10-1. *A,* Route of bacterial growth. Diagram of the course of blood vessels in the marrow of a young rabbit shows the source of bacteria and how it travels through the nutrient artery to the dilated capillary loops of the metaphysis, where bacterial growth and eventual abscess take place. *B,* Spread of infection. Diagram illustrates the usual course of spread of infection in acute hematogenous osteomyelitis. X represents the point of firm attachment of the capsule and periosteum in the region of the epiphyseal disk when the metaphysis is extracapsular. Y is the fixation point of the capsule and periosteum when the metaphysis is intracapsular. (From Hart VL: Acute hematogenous osteomyelitis in children. JAMA 108:524, 1937.)

FIGURE 10-2. *A,* In the immature infant before the epiphysis has formed, the end of the bone is all cartilage. This cartilage is in the joint, is the precursor of the future bone that will form one side of the joint, and is penetrated by the transphyseal blood vessels. Infection can easily begin and flourish at the end of these vessels because there are no phagocytic cells. Such an infection will rapidly destroy the joint. *B,* After formation of the epiphysis, these transphyseal vessels stop beneath the epiphyseal plate (after 15 to 18 months of age); the physis acts as a physical barrier to the spread of infection from the metaphysis into the joint. (From Morrissy RT, Shore SL: Bone and joint sepsis. Pediatr Clin North Am 33: 1555, 1986.)

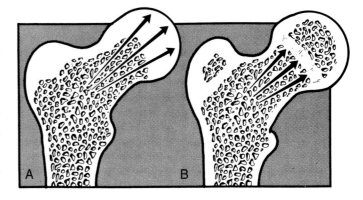

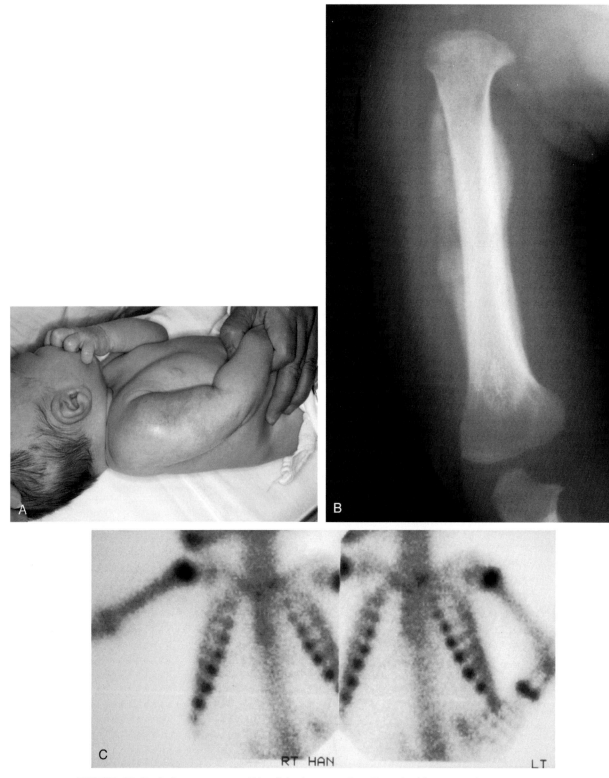

FIGURE 10-3. *A,* Acute osteomyelitis of the humerus in a 3-week old neonate. In acute osteomyelitis soft tissue swelling and local warmth and tenderness are seen in direct proportion to the dissection of pus through the periosteum and soft tissues. Blood culture was positive for *Staphylococcus aureus.* (Courtesy of Nathan Rudolph, M.D., State University of New York, Brooklyn, NY.) *B,* Frontal view of the right humerus demonstrates cortical thickening with diffuse periosteal reaction 10 days after the initial presentation. *C,* Nuclear bone scan (99mTC-labeled diphosphonate) confirmed an increased uptake of radionuclide throughout the right humerus, particularly along the diaphysis, during the delayed phase of the bone scan.

Chronic Osteomyelitis

DEFINITION

Osteomyelitis is an infection that primarily involves the bone. Acute osteomyelitis presents within 2 weeks of onset of disease. Chronic osteomyelitis is an infection of the bone of one to several months' duration.

PREDISPOSING CONDITIONS

1. Inadequately treated acute hematogenous osteomyelitis (see Acute Hematogenous Osteomyelitis)
2. Major trauma
3. Infection secondary to a surgical procedure

PATHOGENESIS (see Pathogenesis, under Acute Hematogenous Osteomyelitis)

Sequestrum of necrotic bone harboring bacteria is the characteristic feature of chronic osteomyelitis.

CLINICAL FEATURES

1. Localized signs of inflammation
   a. Pain
   b. Nonfunctional extremity
   c. A chronically draining sinus
2. Absence of systemic signs and symptoms (e.g., fever)

LABORATORY

1. Complete blood count: usually normal
2. Erythrocyte sedimentation rate: usually normal
3. Blood culture: usually negative
4. Culture of purulent exudate from the surface wound
   a. Often contaminated or colonized with skin flora
   b. Secondary infection of the wound can occur independent of the osteomyelitis, thus not necessarily reflecting the same pathogen
5. Needle biopsy of the bone or culture of the necrotic bone: more often identifies the pathogen
6. Radiographs of the involved extremity
7. Computed tomography: for demonstration of sequestrum
8. Magnetic resonance imaging (MRI): for detailed, precise evidence of inflammation in the soft tissue or bone; delineates anatomy in a localized area (helpful prior to operative intervention)

TREATMENT

1. Orthopedic and infectious disease consultations
2. Principles of management
   a. Antimicrobial therapy has no well-defined time limit in chronic osteomyelitis, although long-term (usually several weeks to months) administration of appropriate antibiotic therapy (depending on culture and sensitivity results) is prescribed.
   b. Antibiotic therapy is given parenterally initially, then orally.
   c. Length of therapy is dictated by clinical and radiographic responses.
   d. Surgical modalities
      (1) Resection of any necrotic bone and avascular tissue
      (2) Close open wounds and improve blood flow after débridement with mobilized tissue flaps.
3. Various adjunctive measures used in management (with variable success) include
   a. Hyperbaric oxygen therapy
   b. Local irrigation with antibiotic solutions
   c. Surgically implanted polymethylmethacrylate beads impregnated with an antibiotic (e.g., gentamicin)
   d. Laser Doppler flowmetry

COMPLICATIONS/PROGNOSIS

1. Local sarcomatosis or carcinomatous changes (squamous cell carcinoma) at the site of chronic draining sinus
2. Secondary amyloidosis

KEY POINTS

Chronic Osteomyelitis

- Common presenting signs are a painful, nonfunctional extremity with a chronically draining sinus.
- Perpetuation of chronic infection is due to the presence of avascular bone and tissue; thus, removal of any necrotic debris is essential.

TABLE 10–3
Microbiology of Chronic Osteomyelitis

Staphylococcus aureus	Anaerobes
Coagulase-negative staphylococci	Fungi
Gram-negative bacteria	
Pseudomonas aeruginosa	
Haemophilus influenzae	

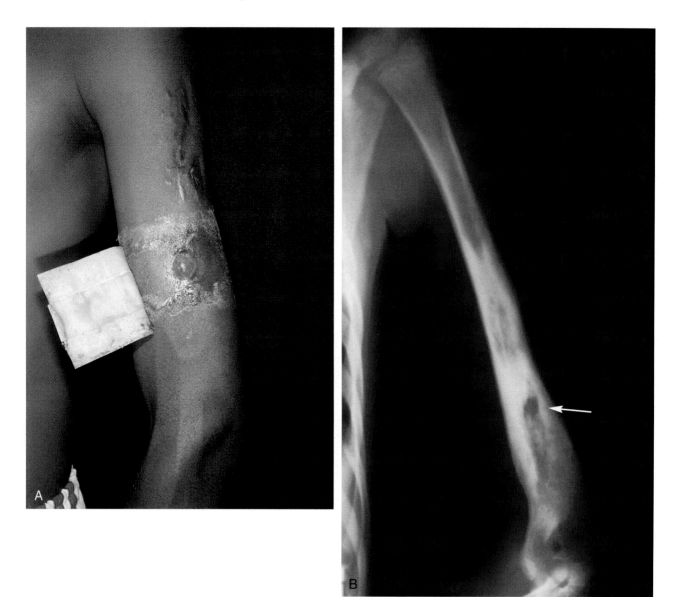

FIGURE 10–4. *A,* Chronic osteomyelitis in a 14-year-old adolescent boy, who presented with yellowish drainage from a sinus tract in his arm. He received a course of antibiotic therapy for 21 days for acute osteomyelitis that he had developed 6 months prior, following an injury. Culture of the purulent drainage was positive for *Pseudomonas aeruginosa.* However, the culture sample obtained in the operating room during irrigation and removal of the necrotic bone grew *Staphylococcus aureus. B,* There is significant widening of the distal humerus with dense sclerosis and a lucent area distally representing a draining sinus *(arrow).*

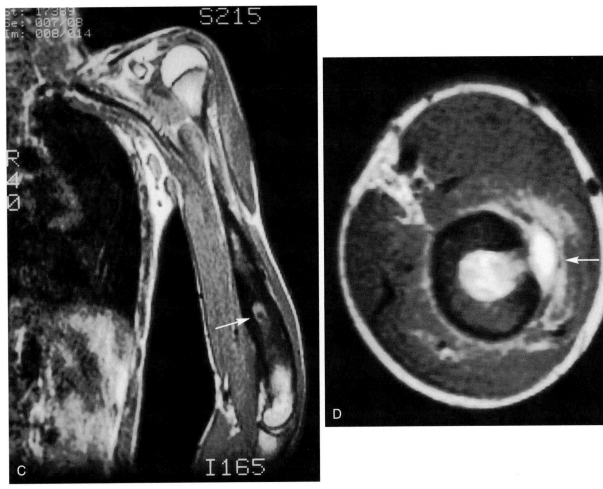

FIGURE 10–4. *Continued C,* Coronal T1-weighted MRI scan demonstrates low signal intensity involving the mid and distal humerus. There is a focal central area of high signal intensity representing the draining sinus (*arrow*). *D,* Corresponding axial T2-weighted MRI shows high signal intensity within the medullary cavity. The draining sinus is visualized (*arrow*) extending into the adjacent soft tissues.

Septic Arthritis

SYNONYMS Acute Suppurative Pyarthrosis
Infected Joint

DEFINITION

A microbial invasion of the joint space

ETIOLOGY (see also Table 10–4)

1. Acute septic arthritis is bacterial regardless of the age of the patient.
2. *Haemophilus influenzae* is an important pathogen in young children (<5 years of age), but with routine vaccination, septic arthritis secondary to *H. influenzae* may be waning.
3. *Streptococcus pneumoniae* septic arthritis is seen mostly in young children.
4. Adolescent intravenous drug abusers are at risk for gram-negative septic arthritis (e.g., *Pseudomonas ae-*

ruginosa septic arthritis of the sternoclavicular joint).

EPIDEMIOLOGY

1. Septic arthritis occurs most commonly in children.
2. Incidence: 5.5 to 12 cases in 100,000 population
3. Salmonella septic arthritis occurs with increased frequency in patients with hemoglobinopathies (mainly sickle cell disease)

PATHOGENESIS

1. Invasion of the joint (synovial) space
   a. Hematogenous seeding
   b. Contiguous spread from an adjacent osteomyelitis (intra-articular metaphysis of the involved bone (see Box 10–1 and Figs. 10–1 and 10–2)
   c. Direct inoculation (penetrating trauma or aspiration of the joint through cellulitis)

2. Hematogenous seeding of bacteria to a highly vascular synovium ⇒ triggers a marked inflammatory response ⇒ release of leukocyte-initiated cytokine mediators and bacterial toxins ⇒ synovial inflammation ⇒ increased vascular permeability ⇒ increased fluid production ⇒ collection of fluid under increased pressure ⇒ compression and/or thrombosis of intra-articular vessels (e.g., avascular necrosis of the femoral head)

CLINICAL FEATURES

1. Constitutional signs and symptoms: fever, arthralgia
2. Clinical signs of arthritis (inflammation) of the involved joint
   a. Erythema, swelling, increased localized warmth, and decreased range of motion
   b. Excruciating pain with passive joint motion (which stresses the joint capsule)
   c. Refusal to walk when the lower limb is involved
   d. Infants with hip joint involvement
      (1) Above signs of inflammation may be absent
      (2) Typical posture: involved leg flexed, abducted, and externally rotated
3. Prior history or presence of skin or soft tissue infection adjacent to the joint (more commonly seen with *Staphylococcus aureus* septic arthritis)
4. Newborns with septic arthritis
   a. Nonspecific signs and symptoms (fever, irritability, poor feeding)
   b. Multiple joint involvement and contiguous osteomyelitis is common
   c. Pseudoparalysis of the involved extremity and pain during diaper changes
   d. Usual joints involved are knees, ankles, and metatarsals
5. Adolescents with gonococcal arthritis (disseminated gonococcemia; see pp. 102–104)
   a. Sepsis with fever and chills
   b. Skin rash
   c. Multiple joint involvement; often tenosynovitis

LABORATORY

1. Complete blood count with differential; helps in following response to treatment
2. Erythrocyte sedimentation rate: elevated; helps in following response to treatment
3. C-reactive protein: increased; also helps in following response to treatment
4. Blood culture: positive (30%)
5. Joint aspiration for synovial fluid examination (the "gold standard" test; see Table 10–6):
   a. Gram stain
      (1) Gram stain of the joint aspirate *must* be done. It is positive in 50%.
      (2) It may show bacteria, which may not grow in the culture because of the bacteriostatic property of synovial fluid.
   b. Cultures: bacterial (aerobic, anaerobic)
      (1) Positive in 70% to 80% of patients (20% to 30% of aspirates are sterile even in the

---

| BOX 10–3 | *Differential Diagnosis of Pediatric Septic Arthritis* |

Acute rheumatic fever
Serum sickness
Inflammatory bowel disease
Juvenile rheumatoid arthritis
Henoch-Schönlein purpura
Kawasaki disease
Lyme disease
Osteomyelitis
Deep cellulitis
Prepatellar bursitis
Reactive arthritis
Toxic synovitis
Leukemia
Hemarthrosis (trauma or spontaneous [hemophilia])
Infectious arthritis from other causes
    Viral (rubella, varicella-zoster, parvovirus B19)
    Mycobacterial (chronic septic arthritis)
    Fungal (chronic septic arthritis)

---

presence of other evidence of septic arthritis)
      (2) If no fluid is obtained on diagnostic aspiration, irrigate the joint space with preservative-free saline and send the irrigated fluid for culture.
   c. Cell count with a leukocyte differential count
   d. Glucose (glucose and electrolyte concentrations in synovial fluid are similar to those in plasma)
   e. Mucin clot test:
      (1) Add 4 mL of water to 1 mL of synovial fluid supernatant. Mix in 2 drops of glacial acetic acid.
      (2) Normal: a tight rope of mucin forms
      (3) With infection or inflammation: clot will flake and shred
6. Plain radiographs of the involved joint (anteroposterior and lateral views)
   a. Increased joint space
   b. Local soft tissue swelling (obliteration of fat pads)
   c. Helps to exclude other pathology (e.g., neoplasm, fracture)

TREATMENT

1. Hospitalization and orthopedic consultation
2. Management principles include:
   a. Antibiotic therapy (given immediately after joint aspiration)
   b. Irrigation and drainage of the joint
   c. Immobilization of the joint in a functional position (until improvement in signs of synovial inflammation occurs) to reduce pain and prevent dislocation
3. Parenteral antibiotic therapy (pending culture results)

a. In infants and children (coverage for *H. influenzae* in children <5 years of age; particularly those who have not been immunized adequately)
   (1) Penicillinase-resistant penicillin (e.g., oxacillin [for *S. aureus* and other gram-positive bacteria]) *and* cephalosporin (e.g., cefotaxime)
   (2) Cefuroxime alone is another alternative. It covers gram-positive bacteria including *S. aureus* and *H. influenzae*).
b. Neonates or adolescents: Gonococcus coverage
c. Duration of antimicrobial therapy
   (1) *S. aureus* septic arthritis: usually 4 to 6 weeks
   (2) Uncomplicated group A streptococci or *S. pneumoniae* or *H. influenzae* septic arthritis: usually 14 to 21 days
   (3) Gonococcal arthritis: usually 7 to 10 days
   (4) Important: longer duration of antibiotic therapy is needed if there is concomitant osteomyelitis
4. Open surgical drainage and irrigation is indicated for:
   a. Septic arthritis of hip or shoulder joint *(as soon as diagnosis is apparent)*
   b. Joints from which frank pus is obtained on initial diagnostic aspiration
   c. Presence of large amount of fibrin or tissue debris or loculated fluid prevents adequate drainage by needle aspiration
5. Joint drainage by repeated needle aspiration or arthroscopy or arthrotomy may be considered for other joints (e.g., knee joint).
6. Radiographs *should* be repeated during therapy to look for changes suggestive of osteomyelitis (periosteal reaction, which usually appears in 7 to 10 days)

COMPLICATIONS/PROGNOSIS

Permanent disability due to destruction of the articular cartilage or epiphysis (especially when diagnosis and treatment are delayed)

1. Osteonecrosis of femoral head with septic arthritis of the hip joint.
2. Severe joint contracture with scarring of the capsule
3. Secondary degenerative arthritis
4. Limb length shortening
5. Angular deformity
6. Impairment of ambulation

KEY POINTS

Septic Arthritis

- Septic arthritis is a surgical emergency.
- About 80% of all cases in children occur in weight-bearing joints.
- Septic arthritis in children is monarticular in 93% of cases.
- *S. aureus* is the most common bacterial pathogen, followed by *Streptococcus pyogenes* and *S. pneumoniae*.
- *N. gonorrhoeae* is the most common cause of polyarticular septic arthritis in children.
- Aspiration of the synovial fluid is the diagnostic examination of choice.
- Gram stain of joint aspirate *must* be done; it may show the presence of bacteria, which may not grow in culture (secondary to the bacteriostatic properties of the synovial fluid).

TABLE 10–4
Microbiology of Pediatric Septic Arthritis

Staphylococcus aureus (most common [48%])
Group A streptococcus (25%)
Streptococcus pneumoniae (4%)
Haemophilus influenzae type b (16%)
Gram-negative bacteria (Enterobacteriaceae [7%])
Salmonella (1%)
Group B beta-hemolytic streptococci (neonates)
Neisseria gonorrhoeae (sexually active adolescents or neonates; <10%)

Modified from Krogstad P, Smith AL: Osteomyelitis and septic arthritis. *In* Feigin RD, Cherry JD (eds): Textbook of Pediatric Infectious Diseases. Philadelphia, W.B. Saunders, 1997, p. 699.

TABLE 10–5
Joint Involvement in Pediatric Septic Arthritis

Knee	38%
Hip	32%
Ankle	11%
Elbow	8%
Shoulder	5%
Wrist	4%
Small synovial joints	2%

Modified from Krogstad P, Smith AL: Osteomyelitis and septic arthritis. *In* Feigin RD, Cherry JD (eds): Textbook of Pediatric Infectious Diseases. Philadelphia, W.B. Saunders, 1997, p. 699.

TABLE 10–6
Synovial Fluid Characteristics

	Appearance	Leukocytes (cells/mm³)	% Neutrophils	% Glucose Synovial/Blood	Mucin Clot
Normal	Clear	<200	25	>50	Good
Septic Arthritis	Purulent, turbid	>50,000	>90	<50	Poor
Inflammatory	Clear or turbid	500–75,000	50–80	>50	Fair to poor
Traumatic	Bloody or clear or straw color	<5000	<50	>50	Good

Modified from Fink PC, Dufort JE, Smith-Wright DL: Orthopedic disorders. *In* Barkin RM (ed): Pediatric Emergency Medicine, 2nd ed. St. Louis, Mosby-Year Book, 1992; p. 1040.

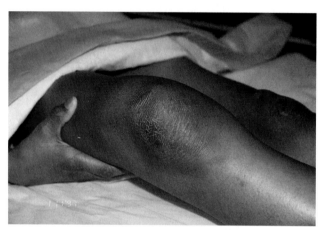

FIGURE 10–5. Septic arthritis of the knee. Swelling (note also the suprapatellar fullness), decreased movements, and tenderness were present in this 8-year-old child. The limb in such cases is typically held in a position that allows the greatest comfort of the joint; as seen here, the knee joint is held in flexion. Joint aspirate was positive for *Staphylococcus aureus*.

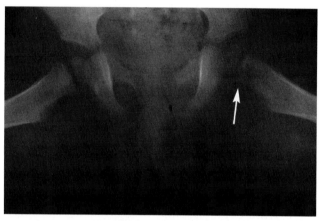

FIGURE 10–6. Frog-leg lateral view in a 5-year-old boy who presented with a left leg limp. Note lytic lesion on the medial femoral metaphysis (*arrow*), osteopenia of the femoral head, widening of the joint space, and soft tissue swelling. Aspiration of joint fluid was positive for *Staphylococcus aureus*.

Nutritional Vitamin D Deficiency Rickets (NR)

SYNONYM   Nutritional Rickets

DEFINITION

1. Rickets
   a. Rickets is undermineralization of the cartilaginous epiphyseal growth plate resulting in excessive accumulation of unmineralized matrix (osteoid).
   b. Rickets is seen only in childhood because the growth plate exists only when the skeleton is growing.
2. Osteomalacia is undermineralization after growth is completed and is seen in adults.

ETIOLOGY/EPIDEMIOLOGY (see Box 10–4)

1. Deficiency of metabolites of vitamin D
   a. "Sunshine deficiency"
      (1) Inadequate exposure to sunlight
      (2) Factors preventing ultraviolet (UV) light

penetration (industrial pollution, darkly pigmented skin, abundant clothing)
   b. Dietary vitamin D deficiency
      (1) Exclusive breastfeeding without vitamin D supplements
      (2) Food faddism (e.g., strict vegan diet; usually combined deficiencies of vitamin D and calcium [Ca] are seen)
   c. Fat malabsorption (usually causes deficiencies of both vitamin D and Ca)
      (1) Celiac disease
      (2) Extrahepatic biliary atresia
      (3) Short bowel syndrome

PATHOPHYSIOLOGY (see Box 10–5)

1. The main function of the vitamin D–parathormone (PTH)–endocrine axis is to maintain the extracellular fluid concentration of Ca and phosphorus (PO_4) at appropriate levels to permit mineralization.
2. The normal critical product of serum $Ca \times PO_4$ concentration, each measured in milligrams per

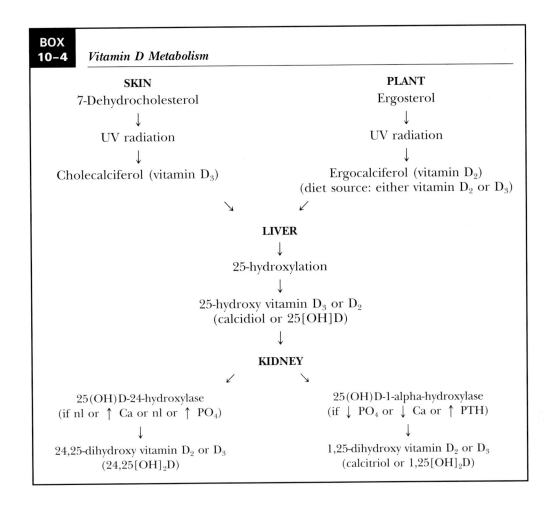

BOX 10–4 *Vitamin D Metabolism*

SKIN	**PLANT**
7-Dehydrocholesterol	Ergosterol
↓	↓
UV radiation	UV radiation
↓	↓
Cholecalciferol (vitamin D₃)	Ergocalciferol (vitamin D₂)
	(diet source: either vitamin D₂ or D₃)

LIVER
↓
25-hydroxylation
↓
25-hydroxy vitamin D₃ or D₂
(calcidiol or 25[OH]D)
↓
KIDNEY

25(OH)D-24-hydroxylase	25(OH)D-1-alpha-hydroxylase
(if nl or ↑ Ca or nl or ↑ PO₄)	(if ↓ PO₄ or ↓ Ca or ↑ PTH)
↓	↓
24,25-dihydroxy vitamin D₂ or D₃	1,25-dihydroxy vitamin D₂ or D₃
(24,25[OH]₂D)	(calcitriol or 1,25[OH]₂D)

deciliter, is 40; rickets occurs when the product of $Ca \times PO_4$ is less than 30.

TREATMENT

1. "Stosstherapy" (a single-day large dose of vitamin D)
   a. A total of 600,000 IU of ergocalciferol (or cholecalciferol) is given by mouth in six divided doses (100,000 IU/dose every 2 hours)
   b. Safe, effective, and obviates problems of poor compliance seen with the daily therapy
   c. Vitamin D is efficiently stored in adipose and muscle tissue. A continued conversion to its active metabolite (calcitriol) occurs for many weeks and sustains healing of rickets.
   d. Stosstherapy helps to distinguish NR from familial hypophosphatemic rickets (FHR)
      (1) Patients with NR show a rise in serum PO_4 in 4 to 7 days and radiographic evidence of healing of rickets in 7 to 10 days.
      (2) Patients with FHR *remain hypophosphatemic* and do not show a rise in serum PO_4 value.
   e. *Do not use the following preparations for stosstherapy:*
      (1) Ergocalciferol in propylene glycol preparation (amount of propylene glycol given with this large dose would cause alcohol intoxication)

   (2) Calcitriol or calcidiol or dihydrotachysterol (each has a short half-life)
2. Calcium supplement (500 to 1000 mg of elemental Ca) given orally until serum Ca normalizes and dietary counseling and modification (including dairy products in the diet) has been accomplished.
3. Maintenance daily vitamin D (400 IU) is started about 12 weeks after stosstherapy.

PREVENTION

1. Exposure to ultraviolet light
2. Daily oral intake of 400 IU of vitamin D
3. Dairy products; dietary intake of Ca 800 to 1200 mg/day

KEY POINTS

Nutritional Vitamin D Deficiency Rickets

- Human milk provides little vitamin D (22 IU/L); exclusively breastfed infants with deeply pigmented skin or infants from the inner city should be given supplements of vitamin D
- Stosstherapy is the preferred method of treating NR
- Serum calcidiol concentration accurately reflects vitamin D status of the body; calcidiol values are low in vitamin D deficiency rickets

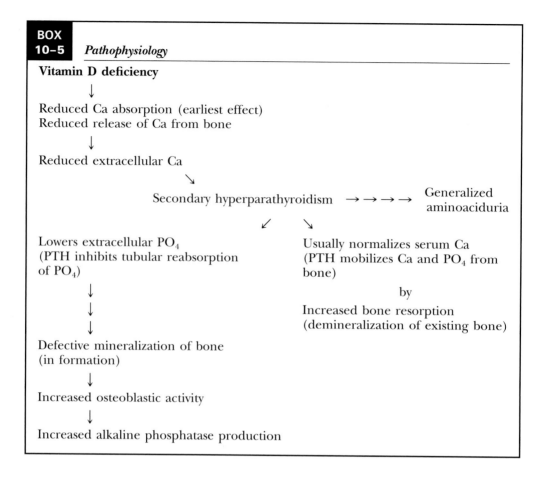

BOX 10–5 *Pathophysiology*

Vitamin D deficiency
↓
Reduced Ca absorption (earliest effect)
Reduced release of Ca from bone
↓
Reduced extracellular Ca
↘
Secondary hyperparathyroidism → → → → Generalized aminoaciduria
↙   ↘
Lowers extracellular PO_4 Usually normalizes serum Ca
(PTH inhibits tubular reabsorption   (PTH mobilizes Ca and PO_4 from
of PO_4)   bone)
↓   by
↓   Increased bone resorption
↓   (demineralization of existing bone)
Defective mineralization of bone
(in formation)
↓
Increased osteoblastic activity
↓
Increased alkaline phosphatase production

TABLE 10–7
Clinical Features of Nutritional Vitamin D Deficiency Rickets

Rachitic deformities
    Bowlegs (genu varum—most common)
    Prominent wrists (excessive accumulation of osteoid)
    Prominent ankles with Marfan sign (impression of double malleolus)
    Rachitic rosary (enlargement of costochondral junction)
    Harrison groove (weakened ribs pulled by muscles producing flaring over the diaphragm) and pigeon breast deformity
    Craniotabes (a Ping-Pong–ball sensation)
    Frontal bossing
    Craniosomatic disproportion
    Knock-knee (genu valgus)
    Windswept deformities (a combination of genu varus and genu valgus deformities)
    Kyphoscoliosis (secondary to vertebral softening)
Generalized hypotonia
Failure to thrive
Hypocalcemia
    Asymptomatic
    Seizures (with or without fever)
    Tetany (latent or manifest)

TABLE 10–8
Laboratory Diagnosis of Nutritional Vitamin D Deficiency Rickets

Serum

Ca: low or normal
PO_4: low for age (*reminder:* PO_4 values vary with age)
Alkaline phosphatase: elevated
PTH: elevated
Calcidiol: decreased
Calcitriol: decreased, normal, or elevated

Urine

Generalized aminoaciduria (secondary to hyperparathyroidism)

Radiograph

AP view of knee (metaphyses/epiphyses of femur and tibia; most rapidly growing bones in infants)

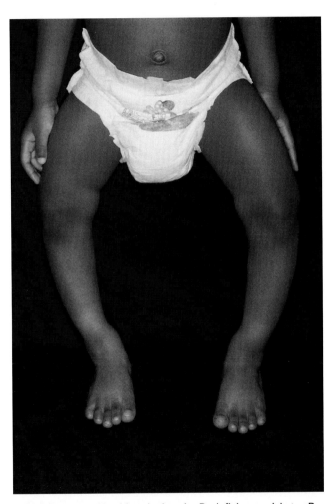

FIGURE 10–7. Nutritional vitamin D deficiency rickets. Rachitic deformities are shown in Figures 10–7 through 10–11. Here, bowlegs (genu varum) and prominent ankles with "double" malleolus are seen in a toddler who refused to eat dairy products and received no vitamin D supplement.

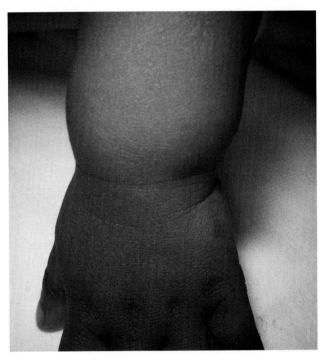

FIGURE 10–8. Prominent wrists (excessive accumulation of osteoid) occured in an infant fed exclusively on breast milk with no vitamin D supplement.

TABLE 10–9
Differential Diagnosis of Nutritional Vitamin D Deficiency Rickets

Rickets	Bowing
Familial hypophosphatemic rickets (FHR)	Physiologic bowing
Vitamin D-dependent rickets, type I	Blount disease
Vitamin D-dependent rickets, type II	
Rickets from other causes (e.g., liver disease)	
Metaphyseal dysplasia, Schmid type	

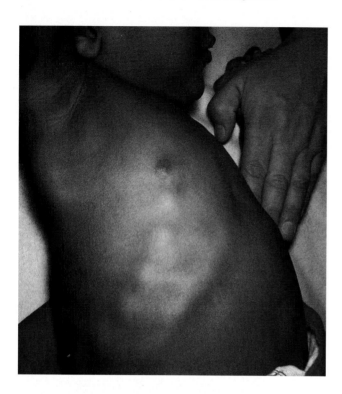

FIGURE 10-9. Rachitic rosary (enlargment of costochondral junctions) in a toddler who was thought to be "allergic to milk" and was not receiving any dairy products or vitamin D supplement.

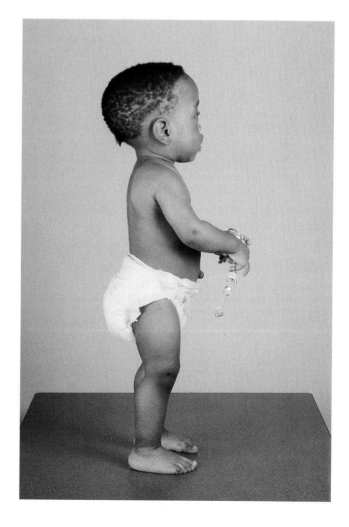

FIGURE 10-10. Frontal bossing with craniosomatic disproportion in a 14-month-old infant (exclusively breastfed with no vitamin D supplement) who presented with delayed milestones (inability to stand or walk without support). He was thought to have "achondroplasia" and was referred to a geneticist. This picture was taken 4 weeks after he received stosstherapy.

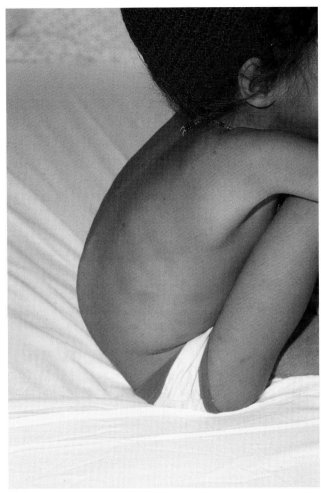

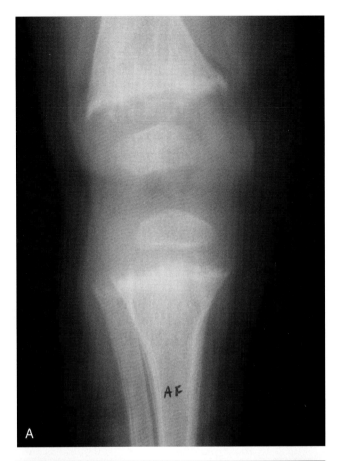

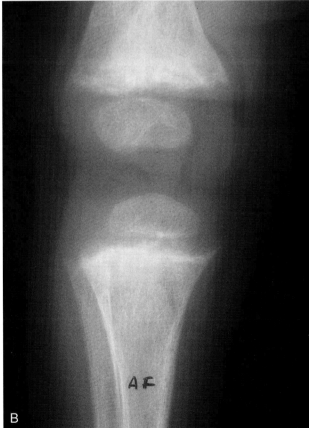

FIGURE 10–11. Kyphosis (secondary to vertebral softening) in an 8-year-old malnourished child who was fed a strict vegan diet (boiled vegetables and rice) with no dairy products.

FIGURE 10–12. *A,* Frontal view of the knee showing evidence of florid rickets. Note metaphyseal widening, cupping, and fraying of the distal femur and proximal tibia and fibula. Normally, the epiphyses should be "hugging" the metaphyses. The increased distance seen here between the metaphyses and the epiphyses is due to the presence of radiolucent osteoid. Generalized osteopenia is also visualized. *B,* Note significant improvement in healing consisting of decreased cupping, straightening of the metaphyses, and position of the epiphyses closer to the metaphyses 7 days after stosstherapy (see also Fig. 2–39, p. 48).

Familial Hypophosphatemic Rickets (FHR)

SYNONYMS   Familial Hypophosphatemia
Vitamin D-Resistant Rickets
X-linked Hypophosphatemic
Rickets

DEFINITION

A genetically determined inability to reabsorb phosphate (PO_4) from the proximal renal tubule, resulting in phosphaturia and hypophosphatemia with or without rickets

EPIDEMIOLOGY

1. Most common type of rickets encountered in North America
2. Prevalence: 1 in 20,000 births

PATHOPHYSIOLOGY (see Box 10–4)

1. The kidney plays a major role in PO_4 homeostasis by regulating tubular reabsorption of phosphate (TRP).
2. FHR is a selective disorder of TRP leading to a massive PO_4 leak ("diabetes of phosphorus"). TRP is reduced to 42% to 72% of normal (normal TRP ranges from 80% to 95%).
3. Impaired conversion of calcidiol (25-[OH]-D) to calcitriol (1,25[OH]$_2$D) occurs in the renal tubules. In these patients, the calcitriol value is normal or low, and the calcidiol value is normal.
4. Since hypophosphatemia is a strong stimulus for mitochondrial 1-hydroxylase activity, a higher than normal value of calcitriol would be expected. Thus, a "normal" value of calcitriol is actually inappropriately low for the degree of hypophosphatemia.
5. Defective transport of PO_4 across the intestinal mucosa
6. The term vitamin D–resistant rickets is a misnomer. The "high doses" of vitamin D required to treat this kind of rickets (as originally described by Albright in 1937) do not "overcome the resistance."

INHERITANCE

1. Most common inheritance: X-linked dominant; males more severely affected than females
2. Uncommon: autosomal recessive or autosomal dominant inheritance or sporadic cases
3. Gene mapped to chromosome Xp22.31-p21.3

BOX 10–6   *Familial Hypophosphatemic Rickets*

Examine all family members for any of the following:
   Short stature and/or
   Rachitic deformities (e.g., bowlegs) and/or
   Fasting hypophosphatemia only

CLINICAL FEATURES

1. An affected infant
   a. Is normal at birth (serum PO_4 normal, skeleton normally mineralized)
   b. Continues to grow normally during the first few months (phosphaturia is minimal because of the physiologically low glomerular filtration rate [GFR] of early infancy)
   c. Serum PO_4 usually decreases in the second half of the first year, coincident with diminished growth velocity.
   d. A rise in serum alkaline phosphatase level is often the first biochemical abnormality noted.
2. Rachitic deformities (seen during second year)
   a. Genu varum (most common), prominent wrists and ankles, genu valgum
   b. Short stature (secondary to rachitic deformities and growth failure)
3. Craniosynostosis
4. Spontaneous tooth abscess; dental eruption occurs normally, and teeth are normal.
5. Absent: generalized muscular hypotonia (characteristic of vitamin D deficiency)

DIFFERENTIAL DIAGNOSIS

1. Nutritional vitamin D deficiency rickets (see Table 10–11)
2. Oncogenous rickets
3. Nutritional phosphate deficiency (e.g., very-low-birth-weight infants)
4. Hereditary hypophosphatemic rickets with hypercalciuria

COMPLICATIONS

1. Vitamin D toxicity
   a. Hypercalciuria
   b. Hypercalcemia
   c. Nephrocalcinosis
   d. Renal failure
2. Secondary hyperparathyroidism related to high doses of PO_4 therapy

TREATMENT

1. Promotion of linear growth (standard therapy)
   a. PO_4 supplements: 1 to 3 g daily, divided in four to six doses to maintain extracellular PO_4 concentration around the clock
   b. Calcitriol therapy: 20 to 60 ng/kg/day (0.5 to 1.5 μg/day as necessary)
2. Monitoring for complications of therapy
   a. Close monitoring of urinary calcium/creatinine (mg/mg) ratio (normal ratio <0.20)
   b. Close monitoring of serum Ca, PO_4, and PTH
   c. Annual renal ultrasound to detect nephrocalcinosis
3. Diuretics (hydrochlorothiazide in combination with amiloride) have been shown (in a small group of patients) to result in elevation of the renal tubular threshhold for PO_4, leading to an elevation of the serum PO_4 concentration. Both

these diuretics, with their hypocalciuric properties, also help to maintain Ca excretion in the normal range, thus allowing continued use of calcitriol. However, long-term studies with a larger number of patients are desirable before such regimens can be used as standard therapy.

4. Currently, the addition of growth hormone therapy to the above regimen is undergoing clinical trials to see if it produces increased linear growth in patients with FHR.
5. Orthopedic consultation for corrective osteotomies for severe deformities
   a. The preferred time depends on severity of disease (and disability) as well as on response to medical therapy
   b. Early surgical intervention without adequate medical therapy may result in reappearance of deformities.
   c. If surgery is warranted, calcitriol therapy should be discontinued several days prior to the operation to avoid immobilization hypercalcemia (and hypercalciuria) and should not be resumed until after complete mobilization has occurred.
6. Medical therapy must be continued at least until skeletal maturation has occurred (completion of puberty).
7. Genetic counseling

PROGNOSIS

1. If medical therapy is initiated early and is optimal, most patients will not develop severe rachitic deformities requiring surgical intervention
2. Some patients may remain symptomatic with bone or joint pain and may need therapy into adulthood to prevent osteomalacia.
3. Despite optimal medical therapy, most patients with FHR exhibit short stature. The adult height of untreated patients is about 130 to 165 cm.

KEY POINTS

Familial Hypophosphatemic Rickets

- Affected infants maintain normal serum PO_4 values during the first several months of life because they have a physiologically low GFR with minimal phosphaturia.
- Hypercalciuria signals vitamin D toxicity, and occurs before hypercalcemia.

TABLE 10–10
Laboratory Diagnosis of Familial Hypophosphatemic Rickets

Serum	Urine
Ca: normal	Selective massive phosphaturia
PO_4: decreased	PO_4 excretion >20 mg/kg/day
Alkaline phosphatase: elevated	Amino acid excretion: normal
Calcidiol: normal	Glucose, protein, or bicarbonate wasting: absent
Calcitriol: "normal" or low	Calcium excretion: reduced
PTH: normal	

TABLE 10–11
Differential Diagnosis: Nutritional Rickets Versus Familial Hypophosphatemic Rickets (FHR)

	Nutritional Rickets	FHR
Serum Values (Prior to Therapy)		
Ca	Low or normal	Normal
PO_4	Low	Low
Alkaline phosphatase	Elevated	Elevated
PTH	Elevated	Normal
Calcidiol	Low	Normal
Calcitriol	Low, normal, or elevated	"Normal" or low
Urine		
Generalized hyperaminoaciduria	Present	Absent
Clinical		
Muscular hypotonia	Present	Absent
Tetany or convulsions	May be present	Absent

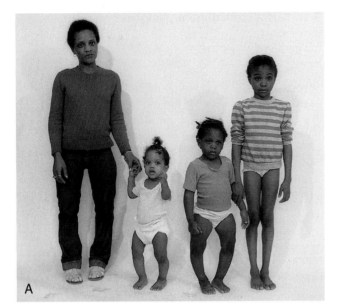

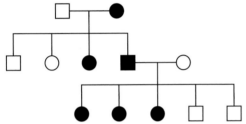

● Female with hypophosphatemia and rickets

○ Normal female

■ Male with hypophosphatemia and rickets

□ Normal male

B

FIGURE 10–13. *A,* Familial hypophosphatemia presenting as bowlegs (genu varum) in mother and her two daughters; one daughter was unaffected. Subsequently, this mother gave birth to one more girl affected with FHR. *B,* Pedigree from another family showing X-linked dominant inheritance of familial hypophosphatemia. Note dominant inheritance with absence of male-to-male transmission, typical of an X-linked trait.

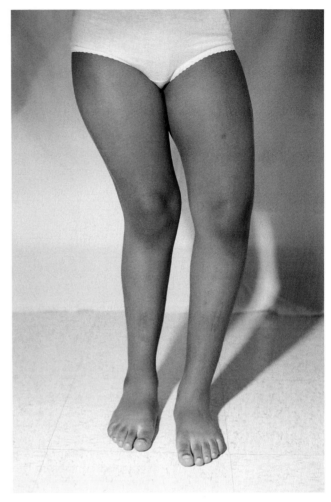

FIGURE 10–14. Windswept deformities (a combination of genu valgum [right extremity] and genu varum [left extremity]) in an 8-year-old girl with FHR.

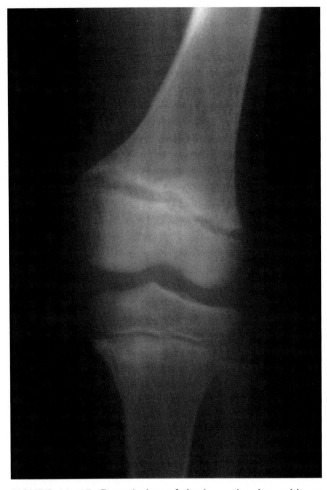

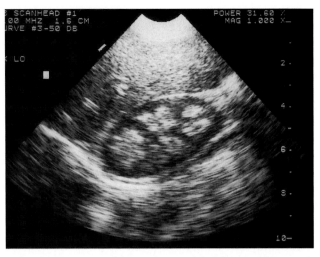

FIGURE 10–16. Medullary nephrocalcinosis secondary to vitamin D toxicity in a 6-year-old girl with FHR. Besides the prescribed dose of calcitriol, this girl was given additional amounts of calcium and vitamin D supplements by her family, leading to hypercalciuria and hypercalcemia. Longitudinal ultrasound examination of the right kidney demonstrates hyperechoic pyramids with some acoustic shadowing.

FIGURE 10–15. Frontal view of the knee showing evidence of rickets. Cupping, sclerosis, and a wedge-shaped metaphyseal defect of the medial aspect of the distal femur and proximal tibia are seen.

Vitamin D-Dependent Rickets, Type I (VDDR, type I)

SYNONYMS   Pseudovitamin D Deficiency Rickets
Hereditary Pseudodeficiency Rickets
Hypocalcemic Vitamin D-Resistant Rickets

DEFINITION/ETIOLOGY

1. Rickets is inadequate mineralization of the organic matrix of the bone in a growing child.
2. Vitamin D-dependent rickets type I refers to rickets secondary to a congenital deficiency or absence of 1-alpha-hydroxylase.

PATHOPHYSIOLOGY (see Boxes 10–4 and 10–5)

1. The enzyme, 1-alpha-hydroxylase activates hydroxylation of 25-hydroxy vitamin D (25[OH]D or cal-

cidiol) to 1,25 dihydroxy vitamin D (1,25[OH]$_2$D or calcitriol) in the renal tubule.
2. Profound hypocalcemia in this disorder illustrates the refractoriness to parathormone (PTH) of vitamin D-depleted individuals.
3. High PO$_4$ despite secondary hyperparathyroidism may be present (secondary to a state of tubular unresponsiveness to PTH as a possible consequence of long-standing severe hypocalcemia).
4. Even though the calcitriol value may be "normal," the value is inappropriate in the presence of enough substrate (25[OH]D) and factors that normally stimulate its production (hypophosphatemia, secondary hyperparathyroidism, and hypocalcemia; see Box 10–4).

INHERITANCE

1. Autosomal recessive
2. Disease caused by a mutation of the gene for 25-OH vitamin D 1-hydroxylase; mutation has been mapped to chromosome 12q 14.

3. Carrier detection in families at risk is available.

CLINICAL FEATURES

1. Age at presentation: 3 to 6 months
2. Common presenting signs/symptoms: tetany or convulsions
3. Nutritional history: adequate intake of vitamin D (which ordinarily would prevent rickets)
4. Failure to thrive
5. Apathy and inactivity because of severe muscle weakness and bone pain
6. Skeletal deformities same as vitamin D deficiency rickets (see Table 10–7)

DIFFERENTIAL DIAGNOSIS

1. Vitamin D deficiency rickets
2. Vitamin D-dependent rickets type II (end-organ receptor defect resulting in variable degree of unresponsiveness to calcitriol)

COMPLICATIONS

Vitamin D toxicity related to therapy

1. Hypercalciuria
2. Hypercalcemia
3. Nephrocalcinosis
4. Renal failure

TREATMENT

1. Vitamin D therapy
   a. Preferred preparation: calcitriol (the missing metabolite)
      (1) Dosage varies among patients
      (2) Usual replacement dose: 10 to 15 ng/kg/ day or 0.50 to 1.0 μg/day
   b. Monitoring for vitamin D toxicity
      (1) Close monitoring of serum Ca, PO$_4$, and alkaline phosphatase
      (2) Close monitoring of urine Ca/Cr ratio (mg/mg); normal ratio is less than 0.2 (random urine sample)
      (3) Annual renal ultrasound examination to detect nephrocalcinosis
   c. Vitamin D$_2$ or D$_3$: supraphysiologic doses (5000 to 10,000 U/day) may also be effective unless the enzyme is completely absent
2. Calcium supplements
   a. Parenteral: Ca gluconate 10% given slowly to patients with hypocalcemic convulsions or tetany
   b. Oral: 500 to 1000 mg elemental Ca/day until healing of rickets has occurred
3. Therapy must be continued for lifetime.

PROGNOSIS

1. Delayed diagnosis or treatment may cause death from profound hypocalcemia.
2. Delayed diagnosis or treatment leads to severe deformities of the long bones and spine.

KEY POINTS

Vitamin D-Dependent Rickets, Type I

- Patients typically present during infancy with tetany or convulsions.
- Profound hypocalcemia, hypophosphatemia, and elevated alkaline phosphatase values despite adequate intake of vitamin D (that ordinarily would prevent rickets)
- Close resemblance to vitamin D deficiency rickets; however, calcidiol value is low in vitamin D deficiency tickets, whereas it is normal or elevated in VDDR, type I

TABLE 10–12

Laboratory Diagnosis of Vitamin D-Dependent Rickets, Type I

Serum	Urine
Ca: low	Generalized hyperaminoaciduria
PO$_4$: low, normal, or high	(secondary hyperparathyroidism)
Alkaline phosphatase: elevated	
PTH: elevated (secondary hyperparathyroidism)	
Calcidiol: normal or increased	
Calcitriol: invariably low or "low normal"	

TABLE 10–13
Differential Diagnosis: Nutritional Rickets Versus Vitamin D-Dependent Rickets, Type I (VDDR, Type I)

	Nutritional Rickets	VDDR, Type I
Serum Values (Prior to Therapy)		
Ca	Low or normal	Low or very low
PO$_4$	Low	Low, normal or high
Alkaline phosphatase	Increased	Increased
PTH	Increased	Increased
Calcidiol	*Low*	*Normal or elevated*
Calcitriol	Low, normal, or increased	Low or "normal"
Urine		
Generalized hyperaminoaciduria	Present	Present
Clinical		
Daily 400 IU of vitamin D	Rickets prevented	Rickets *not* prevented

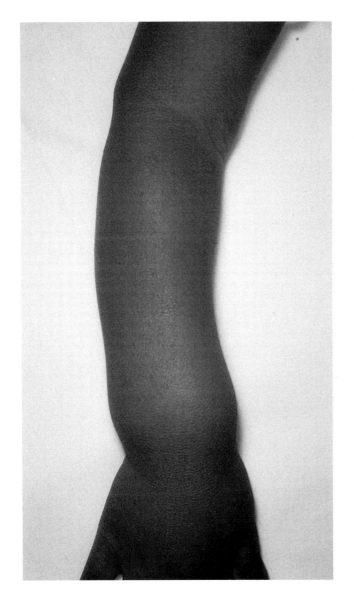

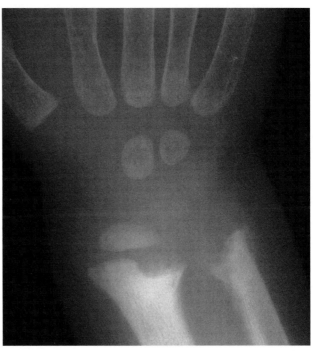

FIGURE 10–18. Frontal view of wrist showing metaphyseal widening, cupping, and fraying of the distal humerus and radius.

FIGURE 10–17. Rachitic deformity showing bowing of the forearm with prominent wrist in an 8-month-old infant who presented with convulsions secondary to hypocalcemia (serum Ca 5.2 mg/dL). This infant was fed human milk supplemented with commercial vitamin D fortified formula, and had received 400 U/day of vitamin D since birth. His serum calcidiol value was 45 ng/mL (normal, 15–50), while the calcitriol value was 20 pg/mL (normal for infants, 70–100).

Metaphyseal Dysplasia, Schmid Type

SYNONYMS   Metaphyseal Chondrodysplasia
Metaphyseal Dysostosis
Primary Chondrodystrophy

DEFINITION

1. Metaphyseal dysplasias are a heterogeneous group of disorders that predominantly involve the metaphyses (with a relatively normal epiphysis and spine).
2. Schmid type is one type of metaphyseal dysplasia that was first described by Schmid in 1949.

ETIOLOGY

1. Mutation in the gene for type X collagen
2. Type X collagen expression is restricted to hypertrophic chondrocytes in areas undergoing endochondral ossification, such as growth plates

EPIDEMIOLOGY

Uncommon

INHERITANCE

Autosomal dominant with variable expression

DIFFERENTIAL DIAGNOSIS

1. Rickets (especially familial hypophosphatemic rickets)
2. Other types of metaphyseal dysplasias (Jansen and McKusick types)

TREATMENT

1. No medical treatment available

TABLE 10–14
Clinical Features of Metaphyseal Dysplasia

Bowlegs (tibial bowing especially at ankle; femoral bowing)
Waddling gait (with coxa vara and genu varum)
Flare to lower rib cage
Enlarged wrists
Short-limbed, short stature; height usually <5th percentile
Increasing shortness with age
Face: usually normal

---

2. Corrective osteotomies for deformities: if indicated, should be done after growth has been completed

PROGNOSIS

1. Short stature; adult height about 130 to 160 cm
2. Intelligence: not affected
3. Life expectancy: not affected

KEY POINTS

Metaphyseal Dysplasia, Schmid Type

- Bowlegs with waddling gait and short stature presenting in the second year in a child who has normal serum values of Ca, PO_4, and alkaline phosphatase.
- Metaphyseal changes visible on radiographs cannot be distinguished from changes seen in rickets.
- Proximal femoral metaphyseal changes are more striking than similar changes seen in rickets (of comparable severity)

TABLE 10–15
Laboratory Diagnosis of Metaphyseal Dysplasia

Serum

Ca: normal
PO_4: normal
Alkaline phosphatase: normal
PTH: normal
Calcidiol: normal
Calcitriol: normal

Radiographic Features

Diffuse metaphyseal flaring
Irregularity and growth plate widening at distal and proximal femur, proximal tibia, proximal fibula, distal ulna and radius
Ribs: anterior cupping, splaying, and sclerosis (100%)
Enlarged capital femoral epiphysis (75%)
Coxa vara (70%)
Femoral bowing (70%)
Mild irregularity of acetabular roof
Hand (metacarpals, phalanges): normal
Spine: usually normal

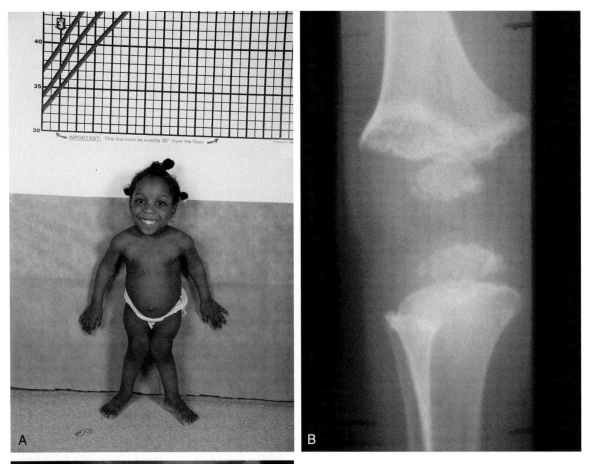

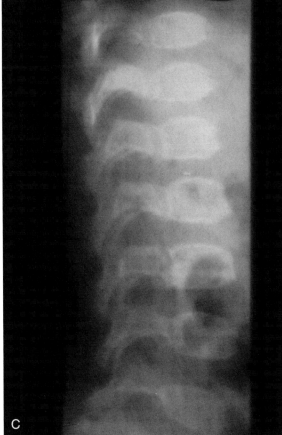

FIGURE 10–19. *A,* Metaphyseal dysplasia presenting in a child with extreme growth failure and rachitic deformities. She was born at 7 months gestation with a birth weight of 2 lb, 6 oz (one of a pair of twins; no other complications). At age 4 years, her weight was 22 lb and height was 28 inches. Serum values of calcium, phosphorus, and alkaline phosphatase were normal. The other twin grew normally. *B,* Frontal view of the knee shows metaphyseal flaring and irregularity of the metaphyses. In contrast to rickets, the zone of provisional calcification is normal. *C,* Lateral view of the spine shows vertebral bodies are ovoid in appearance.

Blount Disease

SYNONYMS   Idiopathic Tibia Vara
             Pathologic Tibia Vara

DEFINITION

Abnormal growth of the medial part of the proximal tibial epiphysis resulting in progressive varus angulation below the knee

ETIOLOGY/PATHOGENESIS

1. The cause is unknown.
2. Abnormal growth at the medial aspect of the proximal tibia involving the epiphysis, physis, and metaphysis.

EPIDEMIOLOGY

Uncommon

CLINICAL FEATURES

1. Tibia vara can occur in any age group in a growing child.
2. Based on three distinct periods of onset, tibia vara is classified as:
   a. Infantile (1 to 3 years)
   b. Juvenile (4 to 10 years)
   c. Adolescent (≥11 years)
   d. The juvenile and adolescent forms are also referred as late-onset tibia vara.
3. Infantile Blount disease (see Box 10–7)
4. Juvenile and adolescent Blount disease
   a. More common in males
   b. More common in African-Americans
   c. Common complaints: pain or stiffness after activity, cosmetic appearance

---

BOX 10–7   *Infantile Blount Disease*

Most common type
Presenting complaint: bowlegs; otherwise patients are asymptomatic
More common in girls
Obesity common
Common in children who walked earlier than 1 year of age
More common in African-Americans
Bowing
  Usually noticed when walking begins and persists without improvement
  Bilateral involvement (about 80%); bowing may resolve on one side and persist on the other
  When a standing child is viewed from behind, bowing is seen to be *below the knee* and does not involve the femur
A prominent medial metaphyseal "beak"
Marked internal tibial torsion
Leg length discrepancy

---

d. Obesity is common
e. Bilateral involvement (about 50% of patients)
f. Absence of palpable proximal medial metaphyseal "beak"
g. Minimal internal tibial torsion
h. Bowing of legs
i. Mild lower extremity length discrepancy

LABORATORY

1. Serum values of calcium, phosphorus, and alkaline phosphatase are normal.
2. Radiographs obtained
   a. Anteroposterior standing views of both lower extremities
   b. Lateral view of the involved extremity
3. Radiographic features
   a. Infantile Blount disease progresses in severity with age.
   b. A staging classification (stages I through VI, reported by Langenskiold) to describe radiologic changes is commonly used.
   c. Radiographic findings that may be seen (few examples):
      (1) Irregular medial tibial metaphysis
      (2) "Beaking" of proximal medial tibial metaphysis
      (3) Fragmentation of medial tibial metaphysis
      (4) Wedging of medial portion of epiphysis
      (5) Deepening depression of medial beak, skip-off
   d. Metaphyseal-diaphyseal angle (tibial metaphyseal angle of Drennan)
      (1) Found by drawing a line parallel to the top of the proximal tibial metaphysis and a line perpendicular to the long axis of the tibial shaft
      (2) Blount disease confirmed: if the angle is more than 20 degrees on a standing radiograph
      (3) Blount disease highly likely: if the angle is more than 15 degrees on a standing radiograph
      (4) Physiologic bowing: if angle is less than 11 degrees

DIFFERENTIAL DIAGNOSIS (see Table 10–16 and Table 10–17)

1. Physiologic bowing
2. Rickets
3. Varus deformity related to trauma (e.g., fracture involving growth plate near the knee with subsequent growth disturbance)
4. Congenital varus deformity

TREATMENT

1. Orthopedic consultation
2. Nonoperative management
   a. For infantile Blount disease in children less than 3 years of age with early stages of disease
   b. Braces usually needed for patients under 4 years of age with tibiofemoral angulation of less than 30 degrees

3. Operative indications and type of surgery
   a. Infantile Blount disease
      (1) Failure of orthotic management
      (2) Severe progressive deformities
      (3) Usual procedures: proximal tibial valgus osteotomy with fibular diaphyseal osteotomy
   b. Juvenile and adolescent-onset Blount disease
      (1) Proximal tibial valgus osteotomy and diaphyseal fibular osteotomy
      (2) Epiphysiodesis for completion of growth arrest
      (3) Contralateral epiphysiodesis may be required in patients with significant leg-length discrepancy.

PROGNOSIS

Premature osteoarthritis secondary to long-standing incongruence of the knee joint

KEY POINTS

Blount Disease

- Bowlegs (bilateral or unilateral) is the most frequent complaint.
- Physiologic bowing is bilateral and usually symmetrical; unilateral or asymmetrical bowing should raise concern about pathologic varus including Blount disease.
- Infantile Blount disease, if not diagnosed and treated early, progresses in severity with age and has the potential for the greatest deformity.

TABLE 10–16
Differential Diagnosis: Physiologic Bowing Versus Infantile Blount Disease

	Physiologic Bowing	Infantile Blount Disease
Etiology	Intrauterine positioning	Growth disorder of proximal tibia
Bowlegs	Bilateral	Bilateral or unilateral
	Usually symmetrical	Asymmetrical
	Spontaneous resolution by $2\frac{1}{2}$ years	Progresses in severity with age
Radiographs	Medial bowing of both proximal tibia and distal femur	Beaking of tibial metaphysis
Metaphyseal-diaphyseal angle	<11 degrees	>11 degrees
Treatment	None	Required

TABLE 10–17
Classification of Genu Varum (Bowlegs)

Physiologic
Asymmetric growth
    Tibia vara (Blount disease: infantile, juvenile, adolescent)
    Focal fibrocartilaginous
Physeal injury
    Trauma
    Tumor
    Infection
    Metabolic disorders
Rickets
    Nutritional
    Familial hypophosphatemia
    Vitamin D-dependent, type I or type II
    Hypophosphatasia
Skeletal dysplasia
    Metaphyseal dysplasia
    Achondroplasia
    Enchondromatosis

Modified from Thompson GH: Angular deformities of the lower extremities. *In:* Chapman MW (ed): Operative Orthopedics, 2nd ed. Philadelphia, JB Lippincott, 1993.

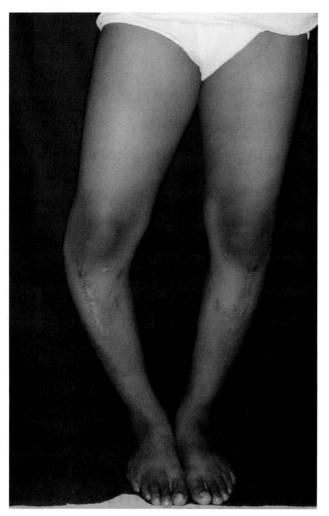

FIGURE 10–20. Asymmetric bowing of the right leg in a 7-year-old African-American male child with infantile Blount disease (onset at 18 months of age). In Blount disease, bowing involves the leg *below the knee* and does not involve the femur. Note the scars from previous osteotomies, which were performed at 4 years of age for severe progressive deformities of both extremities.

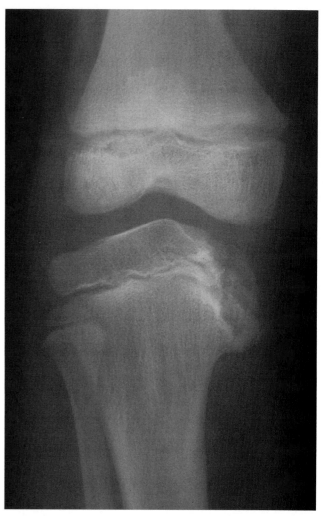

FIGURE 10–21. Frontal view of the knee shows the classic abrupt downsloping of the medial tibial metaphysis with signs of genu varus. In addition, the medial epiphysis is smaller and bends sharply caudad relative to the lateral segment.

Legg-Calvé-Perthes Disease (LCPD)

SYNONYMS   Avascular Necrosis of Femoral
                         Head
                         Aseptic Necrosis of Femoral Head
                         Idiopathic Osteonecrosis of
                         Femoral Head
                         Legg Disease
                         Perthes Disease
                         Legg-Calvé-Waldenstrom Disease

DEFINITION

Legg-Calvé-Perthes disease is an ischemic necrosis of the capital femoral epiphysis (CFE) that occurs in growing children.

ETIOLOGY

1. Uncertain; genetic, hormonal, traumatic or infectious factors may play a role.
2. LCPD is more common among
   a. Boys born with low birth weight
   b. Children with a younger skeletal age than chronological age
   c. Japanese and individuals from central Europe

EPIDEMIOLOGY

1. Incidence: 1 in 1200 to 1 in 12,000
2. Higher incidence in urban areas than rural areas
3. Uncommon in African-Americans
4. Most common age: 4 to 8 years

> ### BOX 10–8   *Differential Diagnosis of Legg-Calvé-Perthes Disease*
>
> | | |
> |---|---|
> | Acute infections (e.g., septic arthritis) | Steroid arthropathy |
> | Chronic infections (e.g., tuberculous arthritis) | Hypothyroidism |
> | Slipped capital femoral epiphysis | Osteoid osteoma |
> | Osteomyelitis of proximal femur | Eosinophilic granuloma |
> | Sickle cell anemia | Lymphoma |
> | Hemophilia | Spondyloepiphyseal dysplasia |
> | Juvenile rheumatoid arthritis | Multiple epiphyseal dysplasia |
> | Gaucher disease | Chondrolysis |
> | Transient synovitis | Traumatic aseptic necrosis |

5. Male-female ratio is 4 or 5:1
6. Unilateral involvement: 90% of patients
7. Bilateral involvement: 10% to 12% of patients; typically seen in young patients

PATHOGENESIS

1. Bulk of the femoral head is composed of the CFE.
2. Blood supply to the CFE comes from retinacular vessels that lie on the surface of the femoral neck (but intracapsularly) and enter the epiphysis from the periphery. Blood supply to CFE can be affected by septic arthritis, trauma, or other insults.
3. Initiating insult ⇒⇒ interference of blood flow to CFE leading to ischemic insult ⇒⇒ avascular necrosis of varying severity (from a small segment to the entire femoral head) ⇒⇒ temporary cessation of growth to the ossific nucleus and loss of structural integrity ⇒⇒ collapse of the articular surface of the femoral head ⇒⇒ residual femoral head deformity ⇒⇒ risk of degenerative arthritis
4. Healing process (takes many months) ⇒⇒ revascularization of the femoral head from the periphery to the center ⇒⇒ removal of necrotic bone ⇒⇒ repair with new and relatively weak bone (woven bone as opposed to strong lamellar bone), which is susceptible to subchondral fracture ⇒⇒ further resorption with subsequent replacement with fibrous bone ⇒⇒ may lead to permanent changes in normal architecture of the femoral head
5. No interventions are available currently that accelerate the healing process after the initial insult.

LABORATORY

1. Plain radiographs
   a. Anteroposterior (AP) and frog-leg lateral views of hip
      (1) Early sign: Increased density of femoral head and widening of joint space
      (2) Crescent sign: indicates a stress fracture in the subchondral bone
   b. With bilateral involvement of the femoral heads AP views of knee and hand are obtained to exclude epiphyseal dysplasia or hypothyroidism
2. Magnetic resonance imaging

3. Bone scan (now rarely done) if radiographs are negative

TREATMENT

1. Orthopedic consultation
2. Majority of patients (about 60%) do not need treatment.
3. Observation and follow-up if
   a. Absence of subluxation at the hip
   b. Abduction of at least 40 to 50 degrees
4. Nonoperative treatment
   a. Bed rest
   b. Traction (to reduce synovitis)
   c. Abduction bracing
      (1) To contain the femoral head within the acetabulum
      (2) Brace is generally worn all day and is discontinued when the lateral portion of the femoral head has regenerated (usually 12 to 18 months)
5. Surgery
   a. Osteotomy
   b. Used for older children with more advanced disease

PROGNOSIS

1. Persistent limp and/or pain may necessitate a change in activities beginning at an early age
2. Although it is a self-limiting disease, 50% of untreated patients develop disabling osteoarthrosis in adulthood.
3. Prognosis is worst for a child in whom onset of disease occurs at an older age or one who has a greater percentage of involvement of the femoral head.

KEY POINTS

Legg-Calvé-Perthes Disease

- A disease of the femoral head characterized by ischemic necrosis, collapse, and subsequent repair
- Typically a male child presenting with pain in the region of the groin, thigh, or knee
- Any child presenting with knee pain requires a thorough hip examination

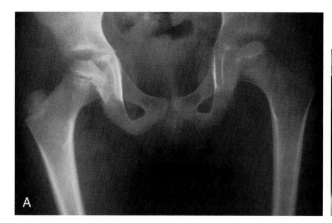
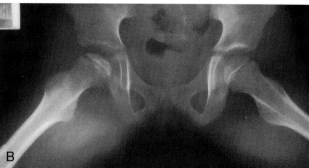

FIGURE 10–22. Legg-Calvé-Perthes disease diagnosed in an 8-year-old girl who presented with persistent bilateral hip pain. In (*A*) standard projection and (*B*), frog-leg lateral projection, flattening, sclerosis, and irregular mineralization of the epiphyseal ossification centers are visible. The right leg is more severely affected than the left. In addition, the right femur shows marked widening of the physis and a medial metaphyseal lucency. (Courtesy of Michael Stracher, M.D., State University of New York, Brooklyn, NY.)

TABLE 10–18
Clinical Features of Legg-Calvé-Perthes Disease

Most common age at onset: 4–8 years (80% of patients)
Average age at presentation: 6 years
Girls or patients with bilateral disease present at younger age
Limp
  Most common complaint
  Painless limp, usually present for several weeks
  Limp becomes worse with activity; is most noticeable
    toward the end of the day
Pain
  Intermittent pain, usually following weight-bearing activities
  Pain referred to the groin, thigh, or knee
Examination of hip: decreased abduction, internal rotation and
  extension
Gait abnormality: secondary to any of the following
  Pain
  Abnormal range of motion
  Limb length discrepancy
    Real discrepancy (secondary to deformity of proximal
      femur)
    Apparent discrepancy (due to flexion and adduction
      contractures)

Osgood-Schlatter Disease

SYNONYMS   Osteochondritis of Inferior Patella
               Osteochondritis of Tibial
                 Tuberosity
               Tibial Tubercle Traction
               Apophysitis

DEFINITION

An inflammatory disorder of the apophyses of the anterior tibial tubercle at the point of insertion of the patellar tendon (quadriceps tendon)

ETIOLOGY/PATHOGENESIS

1. The quadriceps muscle group extends the knee by way of the patella and the patellar tendon (ligament).
2. Apophyses are secondary ossification centers on the tibial tuberosity of the proximal tibia and are sites of insertion of the patellar tendon.
3. Repetitive microtrauma at the bone-tendon junction in the apophyses leads to small avulsion injuries (microscopic stress fractures) and subsequent inflammation, which is referred as apophysitis.

4. The onset of "overuse syndrome" during early adolescence (rapid growth spurt, athletic activity, and skeletal immaturity with unfused apophyses) coincides with the development of secondary ossification centers, which are weak links to repetitive quadriceps contractions.
5. Failure to break the cycle of recurrent microtrauma, inflammation, and calcification of damaged tissue leads to progressive enlargement of the tibial tubercle.

EPIDEMIOLOGY

1. Affects all races
2. A fivefold increased incidence in adolescents who actively participate in sports
3. Most common age at presentation (early adolescence):
   a. Boys: 13 to 14 years
   b. Girls: 10 to 11 years
4. Male-female ratio is 2 to 3:1 (related to gender differences in physical activities)

LABORATORY

1. Plain radiographs (anteroposterior and particularly lateral views of the involved knee)
   a. Radiographs should be used sparingly in evaluating this condition.
   b. Radiographs are indicated in patients with unilateral involvement (to exclude malignancy).
   c. Patients with bilateral signs and symptoms classic for Osgood-Schlatter disease may not need radiographs.
   d. Radiographs may be normal or may show evidence of soft tissue swelling and fragmentation of the growth center of the tibial tubercle where the patellar tendon is inserted.
   e. Repeated radiographs during follow-up visits are rarely of clinical use.

DIFFERENTIAL DIAGNOSIS

1. Sinding-Larsen-Johansson disease or "jumper's knee"
   a. Similar to Osgood-Schlatter disease
   b. Injuries are at the junction of the patellar tendon and inferior pole of the patella
2. Infection
3. Malignancy
   a. Osteogenic sarcoma
   b. Ewing sarcoma

COMPLICATIONS

Uncommon

1. Tibial tubercle fractures are more common in teenagers with a history of Osgood-Schlatter disease.

2. Premature closure of tibial tubercle apophysis, resulting in recurvatum deformity

TREATMENT

1. Reassurance and education for the patient (and family) about the natural course of this disorder
2. Supportive therapy
   a. Use of ice packs after sports
   b. Nonsteroidal anti-inflammatory medications as indicated (e.g., aspirin)
   c. Protective knee pads
   d. Rest and avoidance of activities that normally require usage of quadriceps contractions (to permit healing of avulsion fractures)
   e. Competitive athletes may have to restrict and/or stop full training for several months.
3. Rarely, a knee immobilizer or casts may be required for severe symptoms. A prefabricated knee immobilizer that is worn all day except during bathing and exercise (quadriceps and hamstring stretching exercises) may be used.
4. Surgery is usually not indicated.
5. Rarely, a patient may have persistent symptoms even after reaching skeletal maturity because of the presence of ossicles (calcified fragments within the patellar tendon). Simple surgical excision may be required in such patients.

PROGNOSIS

1. A self-limited disorder that resolves with skeletal maturity (complete ossification of the tibial tuberosity, which usually occurs around 15 years of age)
2. Long-term prognosis is excellent.
3. Disability or chronic pain is uncommon (occasionally pain over the tibial tubercle during kneeling may continue in adults).
4. Residual prominence of the tibial tubercle may persist (especially in patients with fragmentation of the epiphysis and heterotopic ossification during the active phase of the disease).

KEY POINTS

Osgood-Schlatter Disease

- Most common form of traction apophysitis in young adolescents
- Most common cause of chronic knee pain in young adolescents
- Pain (often bilateral) over the tibial tubercle that is exacerbated by kneeling, jumping, or running is a typical presentation.
- Pain (especially unilateral) at rest or pain not directly over the tibial tubercle should raise concern about another cause.

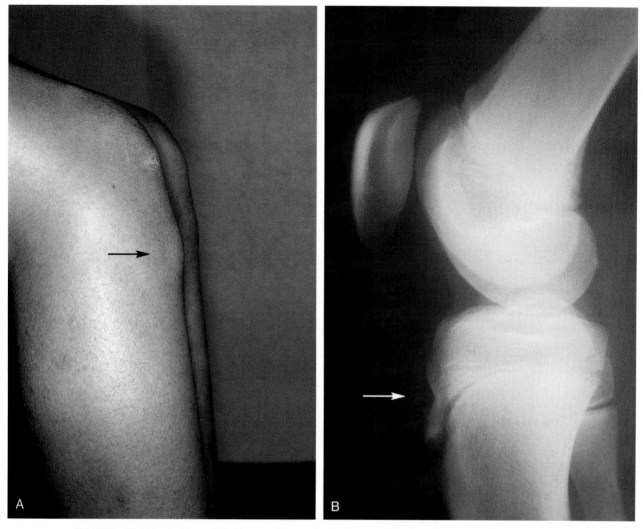

FIGURE 10–23. *A,* Osgood-Schlatter disease in a 13-year-old adolescent male who had complained of knee pain for several weeks. He had localized swelling and tenderness of the tibial tuberosity on the right side *(arrow). B,* Lateral view of the tibia showing fragmentation of the tibial tuberosity; an avulsed fragment is seen superiorly *(arrow).* There is marked soft tissue swelling anteriorly.

TABLE 10–19
Clinical Features of Osgood-Schlatter Disease

Bilateral involvement: 30% to 50% of cases
One side may be more involved than the other
Most common complaint: knee pain
  Usually gradual onset of pain
  Pain localized to tibial tubercle
  Pain accentuated by activities that normally require repeated
    extension of knee (e.g., playing basketball, bicycle riding,
    running, kneeling, or jumping)
  Pain may occur after prolonged sitting with knees flexed
  Pain is relieved by rest
  During examination, pain is exacerbated with resisted knee
    extension
Tibial tubercle
  Swelling may be present
  Point tenderness usually present
Range of motion at knee joint normal; painful kneeling during
  acute phase
Gait normal on a level surface; may have difficulty going up
  or down stairs

Osteogenesis Imperfecta Syndrome (OI)

DEFINITION

An inherited disorder of connective tissue that primarily affects the musculoskeletal system

CLASSIFICATION

1. Clinical classification
   a. OI congenita: extreme bone fragility and fractures, with some patients dying in newborn period
   b. OI tarda: bone fragility manifested later in life, normal lifespan
2. Genetic classification
   a. Four genetic syndromes with variable manifestations
   b. Inheritance
      (1) Type I: autosomal dominant
      (2) Type II: autosomal dominant or recessive
      (3) Type III: autosomal dominant or recessive
      (4) Type IV: autosomal dominant

ETIOLOGY/PATHOGENESIS

1. Osteopenia means insufficiency of bone. It results from either reduced production or increased breakdown of bone or both.
2. Osteoporosis is a clinical syndrome resulting from osteopenia and can lead to
   a. Increased bone fragility
   b. Susceptibility to fractures
   c. Skeletal deformities
3. Osteogenesis imperfecta is the most common type of osteoporosis syndrome in childhood.
4. Osteogenesis imperfecta type 1 results from mutations that cause a quantitative defect in the production of type I collagen; the mutation causes decreased synthesis of the pro-alpha-1 chain of type I procollagen.

EPIDEMIOLOGY

1. Most common type: type I, with an incidence of 1 in 20,000 to 30,000 live births
2. Male-female ratio is 1:1.

PRENATAL DIAGNOSIS

1. Reliable prenatal diagnosis is not available for all types of OI.
2. Ultrasonography demonstrates short, fractured bones that are often curved, and decreased bone density.
3. In utero radiographs at 16 weeks
4. Severely affected fetuses with OI type II may be recognized with the help of ultrasound, radiographs, and biochemical studies.

LABORATORY

1. Radiographs show osteopenia, thin cortices, bowing, angulation of healed fractures, and normal callus formation at the site of recent fractures
2. Biochemical analysis of skin fibroblast collagen

BOX 10-9	*Differential Diagnosis of Osteogenesis Imperfecta*

Child abuse
Achondroplasia
Congenital hypophosphatasia
Idiopathic juvenile osteoporosis
Steroid therapy
Cystinosis
Blue sclera
   Premature infants (normal secondary to underdeveloped sclera)
   Ehlers-Danlos syndrome
   Marfan syndrome
   Trisomy 18 syndrome
   XO syndrome

TREATMENT

1. Multidisciplinary approach with consultations with orthopedist, dentist, geneticist, and social worker for family support
2. Education of family about prevention of fractures (e.g., nursing the newborn on a firm mattress)
3. For OI type II: no therapeutic intervention is effective
4. For other forms of OI, goals of therapy include:
   a. Maximize comfort and function
   b. Aggressive orthopedic regimen aimed at
      (1) Prompt splinting of fractures
      (2) In children with moderate involvement with OI, management of fractures is no different from management of fractures in general population
      (3) Children with increased bone fragility frequently benefit from orthotics (which are used to protect their bones as they are mobilized)
      (4) Correction of deformities arising from fractures and from progressive bowing or bending of skeleton (e.g., osteotomies to straighten bone and intramedullary rods to maintain alignment)
5. Therapeutic regimens have included supplements with sodium fluoride, calcium, vitamin C, or magnesium oxide; none have shown any clear benefit.
6. Calcitonin therapy
   a. Decreases bone resorption
   b. Significant improvement in the fracture rate and in bone density during treatment with salmon calcitonin has been observed in a small number of patients.
   c. Administration of calcitonin by intranasal spray may make the drug an acceptable form of therapy.

PROGNOSIS

Variable among different types of OI

1. Death in perinatal period (type II)
2. Increased mortality in 3rd to 4th decade of life due to cardiopulmonary failure (type III)
3. Limb deformities and disability after fractures
4. Potential normal lifespan with limited morbidity
5. Intelligence normal; every effort should be made to maximize the child's ability to attend school and interact with peers.

KEY POINTS

Osteogenesis Imperfecta Syndrome

- Most common type of osteoporosis syndromes in childhood
- Increased bone fragility, multiple fractures, and skeletal deformities are characteristic findings.
- OI (especially in its milder forms) is often misdiagnosed as child abuse.
- Fractures in patients with OI heal as fast as those in normal individuals.

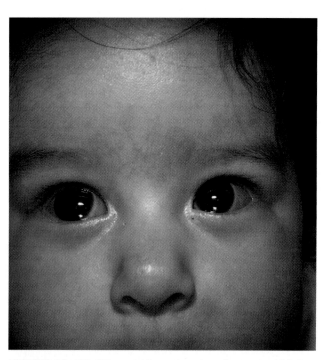

FIGURE 10–24. Bilateral blue sclera in a 3-month-old infant who presented with a femoral fracture.

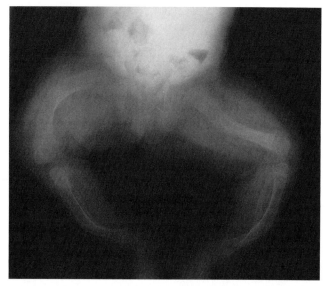

FIGURE 10–26. Frontal view showing severe bowing and deformities of the lower extremities. Diffuse osteopenia and marked hip dysplasia are evident. Periosteal reaction secondary to fracturing is seen along the left femur and right fibula.

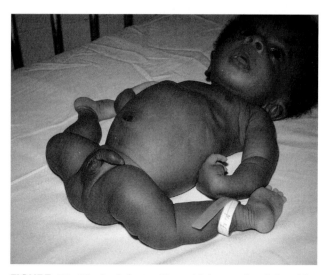

FIGURE 10–25. An infant with multiple angular deformities due to OI, type I.

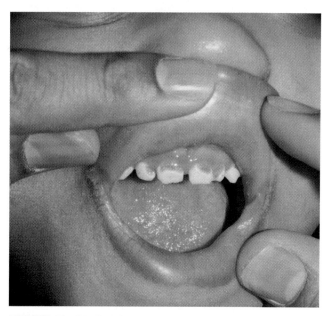

FIGURE 10–27. Dentinogenesis imperfecta showing transparent, prematurely eroded teeth in a patient with OI, type I.

TABLE 10–20
Clinical Features of Osteogenesis Imperfecta Type I

Most common type of OI
Blue sclera (secondary to inadequately developed scleral
    collagen)
Fractures
    Fractures present at birth (10% of cases)
    Frequency of fractures reduced during puberty
    Multiple angular deformities of bones related to fractures
Bowing of long bones
Metatarsus varus
Spine: scoliosis, kyphosis, codfish vertebrae
Wormian bones in cranial sutures
Growth retardation
Defective dentinogenesis
    Transparent teeth, which are distinctly yellow or gray-blue
    Teeth prematurely eroded or broken
Presenile conductive hearing loss caused by otosclerosis (seen
    in adolescents, adults)
Excessive hyperlaxity of ligaments (small joints of hands, feet,
    knees)

TABLE 10–21
Clinical Features of Osteogenesis Imperfecta Type II (Lethal Type)

Stillbirths (50%)	Crumpled long bones
Multiple fractures in utero	Beaded ribs
Death soon after birth (50%)	Abducted thighs, limbs short, bent, deformed
Respiratory failure (thoracic cage deformities)	Multiple palpable bone islands on a soft skull
Skin fragile, thin	

TABLE 10–22
Clinical Features of Osteogenesis Imperfecta Type III

Manifests in neonatal period or infancy	Severe bone fragility
Multiple fractures at birth and during early childhood	Progressive skeletal deformities
Sclera may be blue at birth, become less blue with age	Progressive kyphoscoliosis
Very few patients reach adulthood	No hearing impairment
Macrocephaly with triangular facial appearance	

TABLE 10–23
Clinical Features of Osteogenesis Imperfecta Type IV

Variable age of onset of fractures (birth to adulthood)	Short stature
Significant bowing at birth may be only sign	Normal sclera
Multiple fractures at birth or throughout life	Spontaneous improvement with puberty
Variable deformity of long bones or spine	Dentinogenesis imperfecta

Slipped Capital Femoral Epiphysis (SCFC)

SYNONYM   Slipped Epiphysis

DEFINITION

1. Slipped capital femoral epiphysis is characterized by displacement of the proximal femoral epiphysis (head of the femur) from the neck of the femur through the physeal plate.
2. This name is a misnomer in that it implies that the upper femoral epiphysis is displaced from its usual alignment on top of the metaphysis. In fact, however, the epiphysis remains in its normal position within the acetabulum while the remainder of the femur displaces from the epiphysis because of a loss of mechanical integrity at the proximal femoral physis.

ETIOLOGY/PATHOGENESIS (see also Box 10–10)

1. Etiology of SCFE is believed to be multifactorial.
2. Slippage occurs through the physis (growth plate), which is weaker as it begins to close.
3. Local trauma to the proximal femur is frequently thought to be a contributing factor.
4. Inflammatory factors weaken the physeal plate. Whether synovitis of hip (universal finding) precedes or results from physeal slippage is undermined.
5. Most common path of displacement of the proximal femoral metaphysis is anterolateral and superior, causing the epiphysis to appear to be displaced posteriorly and inferiorly.
6. Paradoxical distribution of pain (to the knee) is secondary to referral within the femoral nerve distribution, which involves both the hip and the knee joint.

EPIDEMIOLOGY

1. Incidence: 2 in 100,000 general population
2. More common in African-Americans than in whites
3. Most common age at presentation:
   a. Peak incidence: at the start of the adolescent growth spurt (about 78% of cases)
   b. Male: average 13.5 years (range 10 to 16 years)
   c. Female: average 11.5 years (range 10 to 14 years; *pre-menarche age*)
4. Male-female ratio is 2.4:1
5. Left hip is affected more often than right hip by a ratio of 2:1
6. Bilateral involvement
   a. Bilateral symptomatic involvement during adolescence: 25% (range 21% to 37%)
      (1) About 50% of these patients have bilateral involvement at presentation
      (2) Remaining 50% show sequential onset
   b. Bilateral involvement is seen more often in males, African-Americans, and obese patients (with younger age at presentation)
   c. Long-term follow-up shows bilateral involvement in 60% to 80% of patients with known unilateral SCFE
7. Endocrine disorders (see Box 10–10) leading to SCFE are typically seen in preadolescent children.

INHERITANCE

1. Definite hereditary pattern has not been established.
2. An autosomal inheritance pattern with incomplete penetrance is suggested, with a 7.1% risk of SCFE in a second family member.
3. Family history is positive in 5% of cases.

CLINICAL FEATURES

1. Onset may be acute or chronic or "acute on chronic"
   a. Acute slip (symptoms < 3 weeks in duration)
      (1) Seen in about 10% to 14% of patients
      (2) Sudden onset of severe pain and inability to walk in a previously asymptomatic patient
   b. Chronic or gradual slip (symptoms of > 3 weeks' duration)
      (1) Secondary to a large sheer force exerted over an extended period of time
      (2) Majority of patients (about 86%) present with chronic, gradual displacement
   c. "Acute on chronic": A child with a chronic slip now experiences acute additional slippage
2. Most common presenting symptoms
   a. Pain: typically referred to groin, anterior or medial thigh, or knee
   b. Altered gait: limp (if unilateral) or waddling gait (if bilateral)

BOX 10–10   *Conditions Frequently Associated with Slipped Capital Femoral Epiphysis*

Obesity (80% of cases)
Delayed skeletal maturation
Tall, thin stature with a recent growth spurt
Growth hormone administration (rapid growth)
Renal osteodystrophy

Endocrine disorders that weaken the physis
  Hypothyroidism (most common)
  Hyperthyroidism
  Hypogonadism
  Hypopituitarism
  Acromegaly, gigantism

3. Limited range of hip movement on the involved side
   a. Loss of internal rotation
   b. Involved leg may be externally rotated and adducted
   c. Exacerbation of pain during internal rotation and abduction
4. Shortening of affected limb (1 to 3 cm shorter than normal limb)
5. Thigh atrophy on the involved side (with long-standing symptoms)

LABORATORY

1. Radiographs (anteroposterior [AP] view of pelvis; frog-leg lateral and true lateral views of both hips)
   a. Lateral view: look for posterior displacement of femoral head
   b. AP view: look for medial displacement of femoral head
   c. Widening of physeal plate may be the only finding in patients without obvious displacement
   d. Severity of slippage is classified radiographically by the degree of displacement of the epiphysis on the femoral neck.
2. Computed tomography
   a. Confirms epiphyseal displacement and accurately measures amount of displacement
   b. Helpful in patients with symptoms that suggest SCFE but are not documented on plain radiographs
3. Tests for endocrine disorders (as clinically indicated) in preadolescent children

DIFFERENTIAL DIAGNOSIS

1. Legg-Calvé-Perthes disease
2. Femoral cutaneous nerve entrapment
3. Endocrine disorders
   a. Hypothyroidism
   b. Hyperthyroidism
   c. Growth hormone deficiency
   d. Multiple endocrine neoplasia
   e. Panhypopituitarism

COMPLICATIONS

1. Avascular necrosis of capital femoral epiphysis
   a. Seen in 10% to 25% of patients with SCFE
   b. Usually seen with manipulative reduction of the slippage

2. Chondrolysis (cartilage necrosis/atrophy of articular cartilage)
   a. Seen in 5% to 55% of patients with SCFE
   b. Results in joint stiffness with joint destruction

TREATMENT

1. Orthopedic consultation
2. Untreated, a slipped epiphysis is likely to progress, leading to greater deformity of the proximal femur.
3. Goals of treatment
   a. To prevent further displacement of the epiphysis
   b. To stabilize the joint until the physis closes
   c. To minimize complications
4. Nonsurgical approach
   a. Bed rest (immediate cessation of weight bearing to protect hip and diminish pain)
   b. Traction
   c. Spica cast immobilization
5. Surgical approach
   a. In situ internal fixation
      (1) With a single or multiple cannulated screw and immobilization
      (2) Most accepted form ("gold standard") of treatment
   b. Bone peg epiphyseodesis
6. Monitor contralateral side for SCFE.

PROGNOSIS

Slipped capital femoral epiphysis during adolescence is associated with development of degenerative joint disease of the hip during middle life.

KEY POINTS

Slipped Capital Femoral Epiphysis

- Most common hip disorder among adolescents
- Patients typically present with pain in the groin or anterior thigh area, but pain may be referred to knee.
- Diagnosis of SCFE is frequently missed when presenting symptom is thigh or knee pain.
- Suspect an endocrine or a systemic disorder when SCFE occurs before puberty in a child.

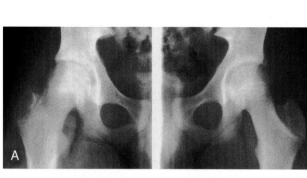

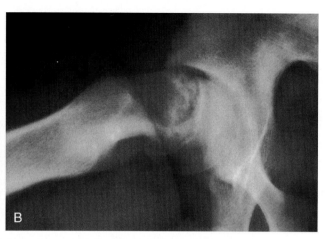

FIGURE 10–28. *A,* Slipped capital femoral epiphysis in a 10-year-old boy with right hip pain. Frontal view of the pelvis demonstrates subtle asymmetry of the femoral heads. The epiphyseal height of the right femur is reduced. A straight line drawn along the lateral femoral neck does not intersect the epiphysis as it does on the normal left side. *B,* The frog-leg lateral view of the right hip shows medial, posterior, and inferior displacement of the epiphysis. SCFE is best seen in the frog-leg lateral view of the pelvis.

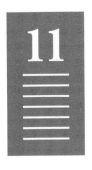

Emergency Pediatrics

Binita R. Shah, M.D.

Anaphylaxis

DEFINITION

Type I IgE-mediated hypersensitive reaction involving several systems (e.g., cutaneous, respiratory, cardiovascular, gastrointestinal, or central nervous system). Two or more systems must be involved to make a diagnosis of anaphylaxis.

EPIDEMIOLOGY

1. An estimated rate of fatal anaphylaxis from any cause is 0.4 incident per million population (about 500 incidents per year in the United States).
2. An estimated rate of fatal anaphylaxis from penicillin is 1 per 7.5 million injections.

PATHOGENESIS

1. Exposure to a sensitizing agent ⟹ formation of IgE antibody, which binds to mast cells and basophils. On reexposure to sensitizing antigen, antigen binds with IgE–mast cell complex ⟹ degranulation of mast cells ⟹ release of preformed and rapidly generated mediators (e.g., histamine, leukotrienes, prostaglandins) ⟹ effects on blood vessels, bronchi, and mucus glands
2. Any route of exposure can cause anaphylaxis: oral, parenteral, inhalation.

BOX 11–1 *Definitions*

ANAPHYLAXIS

IgE-mediated hypersensitivity reaction
Requires previous exposure to an allergen

ANAPHYLACTOID REACTION

Non-IgE-mediated reaction
Clinically indistinguishable from true anaphylaxis
Requires *no* immunologic memory (thus, degranulation of mast cells may occur on first exposure to an allergen)

---

3. Time between exposure to the inciting antigen and onset of symptoms:
   a. Minutes to hours (majority of symptoms occur within 30 minutes)
   b. Interval depends on the route, quantity, and rate of administration of antigen and the sensitivity of the host.
4. Signs and symptoms vary in both severity (ranging from mild urticaria to shock and death) and spectrum of organ involvement.

CLINICAL FEATURES (see also Table 11–2)

1. Clinical manifestations usually occur within seconds to minutes.
2. Clinical course
   a. Uniphasic course
      (1) Seen in about 80% of patients
      (2) Signs and symptoms occur early.
      (3) Good response to therapy, and patients remain symptom-free thereafter.
   b. Biphasic course
      (1) Seen in about 20% of patients
      (2) A second episode of anaphylaxis occurs up to 8 hours following "apparent recovery" from the initial event.
   c. Protracted course (persistence of symptoms for about 3 weeks)

LABORATORY

Anaphylaxis is diagnosed clinically; no laboratory tests are helpful in making a diagnosis.

DIFFERENTIAL DIAGNOSIS

1. Vasovagal syncope (pallor, bradycardia, absence of cutaneous or respiratory findings)
2. Shock from other causes (e.g., septic, cardiogenic, toxic shock syndrome)
3. Other causes of airway obstruction (e.g., croup, epiglottitis, foreign body aspiration)
4. Hereditary angioedema (absence of pruritus, flushing, or respiratory findings)

TREATMENT

1. Anaphylaxis with life-threatening presentation requires *simultaneous evaluation and management* of

ABCs based on a rapid examination and often a minimal history.

2. Secure airway, 100% oxygen, continuous monitoring (pulse oximetry, cardiac, blood pressure), two large-bore intravenous lines, arterial blood gases
   a. Indications for endotracheal intubation: stridor, drooling, labored breathing, altered mental status
   b. Signs of potential airway compromise: voice change, perioral/lingual edema, shortness of breath

3. Epinephrine: first-line therapy for anaphylaxis regardless of cause.
   a. For mild reactions/good perfusion (e.g., urticaria, bronchospasm)
      (1) Subcutaneous
      (2) Dose: 0.01 mL/kg or 0.01 mg/kg (maximum, 0.3 mL); 1:1000 concentration
   b. For moderate to severe reactions (e.g., angioedema, hypotension, laryngeal edema)
      (1) Intravenous (IV) or intraosseous: dose of 0.1 mL/kg (maximum, 5 mL); 1:10,000 concentration *or*
      (2) Endotracheal: dose of 0.1 mL/kg (maximum, 5 mL); 1:1000 concentration

4. Circulatory collapse/hypotension
   a. Intravenous fluid bolus (20 mL/kg) of crystalloid (lactated Ringer's or normal saline)
   b. Trendelenburg position
   c. Epinephrine infusion

5. Remove the antigen if possible; for example
   a. Stop infusion
   b. Remove the insect stinger (*important:* use of tweezers or forceps may release more venom; flick it out with a credit card)

6. To delay absorption from local site (e.g., injection or sting)
   a. Infiltrate epinephrine subcutaneously.
   b. Apply a tourniquet above the site.

7. Antihistamines for cutaneous or systemic reaction
   a. Effect: inhibits vasodilatory effects of histamine
   b. H_1-receptor blocker (e.g., diphenhydramine given IV, intramuscularly (IM), or orally)

8. Corticosteroids
   a. Effects: anti-inflammatory, prevent late-phase response
   b. Parenteral hydrocortisone or methylprednisolone or oral prednisone

9. Inhaled beta-2-agonist (e.g., albuterol) and IV aminophylline for bronchospasm

10. Racemic epinephrine (2.25% diluted in 2.5 mL of normal saline) may be used in patients with signs or symptoms of airway compromise.

11. Hospitalize all patients with moderate-severe reactions requiring resuscitation.

12. All patients must be observed for at least 6 to 8 hours, even if they have responded promptly to therapy. Some patients may experience biphasic reactions with recurrence of signs or symptoms (after initial resolution) within this period of time.

PREVENTION

1. Be prepared. Previous episodes of mild anaphylaxis do not guarantee that future episodes will not be life-threatening.
2. Avoidance of precipitating allergens (e.g., nuts, fish)
3. Children with severe reactions should wear a Medic-Alert bracelet.
4. Parents and older children should be educated about self-administration of epinephrine (e.g., EpiPen Jr, Ana-Kit).

KEY POINTS

Anaphylaxis

■ A potentially life-threatening manifestation of IgE-mediated immediate hypersensitivity reaction involving two or more systems

■ Life-threatening features are upper airway obstruction (laryngeal, pharyngeal, or lingual edema), and hypotensive shock (profound vasodilation and increased vascular permeability)

■ Epinephrine is the mainstay of therapy for anaphylaxis regardless of cause.

TABLE 11–1
Common Causes of Anaphylaxis

Insect venom:	Hymenoptera venom (honeybees, bumblebees, hornets, wasps, fire ants)
Drugs:	Penicillin (leading cause), sulfonamides, cephalosporins, local/topical anesthetics
Foods:	Nuts, peanuts, seafood (fish, shellfish), eggs, milk, monosodium glutamate
Other:	Latex (major cause), blood products, iodinated radiocontrast media

TABLE 11–2
Clinical Features of Anaphylaxis

Organ System	Symptoms/Signs
Skin	Pruritus, warmth, flushing, erythema, urticaria, angioedema
Head, eyes, ears, nose, throat	Conjunctival itching, lacrimation, injection, or chemosis Sneezing, rhinorrhea, stridor, hoarseness Edema of lips, tongue, pharynx, larynx, or nasal turbinates impairing ventilation and swallowing, tingling in lips, mouth or throat itching
Respiratory	Chest pain, tightness, dyspnea, cough, wheezing, intercostal and subcostal retractions
Circulatory	Faintness, palpitations, tachycardia, hypotension, arrythmias, "sense of impending doom," cardiopulmonary arrest
Gastrointestinal	Nausea, vomiting, abdominal cramps, diarrhea, tenesmus
Central nervous system	Dizziness, syncope, seizures, altered level of consciousness
Genitourinary	Genital edema, uterine cramps, urinary urgency

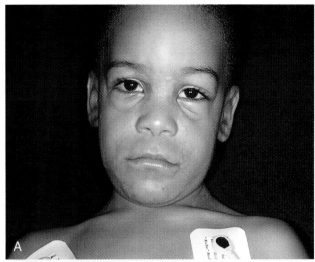

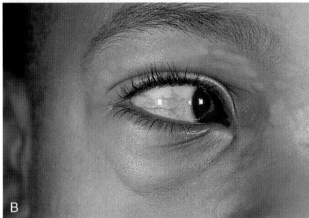

FIGURE 11–2. *A* and *B,* Anaphylaxis presenting with bilateral periorbital swelling, wheezing, hoarseness of voice, and acute urticaria (erythematous, pruritic, well-demarcated flat papules that blanch under pressure). These findings were seen in this child (known to be "allergic" to eggs) 30 minutes after receiving MMR vaccine in a pediatrician's office. Mumps and measles components of MMR vaccine are developed in chick embryo and contain trace amounts of ovalbumin.

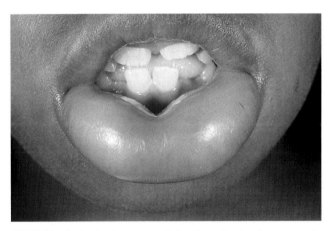

FIGURE 11–1. Angioedema of the lips. Angioedema usually involves the loose connective tissues of the ear or the periorbital or perioral areas but may involve the oropharynx or extremities. The edema is nonpitting, well circumscribed, and usually nonpruritic (unless overlaid by urticaria).

Esophageal Foreign Body

DEFINITION

Impaction of a foreign object into the esophagus

ANATOMY (see also Table 11–3)

1. Most children with impacted foreign bodies (FBs) have a structurally and functionally normal esophagus (unlike adults who may have intrinsic strictures or neuromuscular conditions).
2. Entrapment of FBs occurs at the sites of *normal* anatomic narrowing of the esophagus.
3. If an FB is lodged at any other site, underlying esophageal disease should be suspected.
4. Children who have had prior surgery (e.g., repair of a tracheoesophageal fistula) or strictures (e.g., secondary to caustic ingestion) are at increased risk for recurrent impactions.

EPIDEMIOLOGY

1. Most recent annual report (1996) of the American Association of Poison Control Centers reported a total of 60,579 FB ingestions; 3590 of these FBs were coins.

2. The esophagus is a common site for entrapment of FBs.
3. Most impacted esophageal FBs in children are blunt or smooth.
4. Most common esophageal FBs are coins (50% to 75%).
5. Most ingested coins pass into the esophagus rather than into the airway.
6. Pennies are the most frequently swallowed coins (probably reflecting the frequency with which pennies are accessible to children) followed by quarters, dimes, and nickels.
7. Other swallowed FBs include toys, crayons, marbles, beads, batteries, and chicken or fish bones. Less commonly, sharp objects (e.g., screws, pins) are involved.
8. Most common age
   a. Children under 6 years of age
   b. Peak age: 6 months to 3 years
9. Children's vulnerability to FB ingestion reflects their common practice of placing foreign objects in the mouth as part of play, experimentation, exploration of the environment, and lack of fully developed dentition.

CLINICAL FEATURES

1. A sudden history of choking, gagging, or coughing provoked by swallowing an FB or a complaint of a swallowed FB may be present. However, in the majority of cases, such episodes are usually not witnessed by a caretaker, and the absence of such a history *does not* exclude the diagnosis.
2. Most common presentations
   a. Drooling or excessive salivation
   b. Dysphagia (young infants refuse solid food but may take liquids)
   c. Pain or discomfort on swallowing
   d. Vomiting
   e. Localization or sensation of an FB
   f. Respiratory signs/symptoms: cough, stridor, wheezing, respiratory distress (from external compression of the trachea or larynx), or aspiration (saliva, food)
3. Asymptomatic (7% to 35% of patients with proven esophageal FB are asymptomatic)
4. Uncommon presentations
   a. Symptom-free period followed by edema and inflammation, producing symptoms of esophageal obstruction
   b. Fever, pain (worsening chest pain, pain radiating to neck), crepitus (neck, upper chest), and shock secondary to perforation

LABORATORY

1. Plain radiographs: anteroposterior and lateral views of neck and chest to confirm and localize the FB. Radiopaque FBs are readily seen.
2. Use of a hand-held metal detector (HHMD) for the initial screening:
   a. An alternative approach to initial screening radiographs in *asymptomatic* patients
   b. Used to detect and localize an ingested coin; no side effects, no radiation
   c. If HHMD is positive—confirmation by radiographs
   d. If HHMD is negative—no radiographs
3. Barium swallow may be needed to outline radiolucent FBs (e.g., plastic objects, food boluses) in asymptomatic patients.

TREATMENT

1. Emergent removal of FB by operative endoscopy:
   a. Sharp objects (e.g., open safety pins, straight pins; risk of perforation)
   b. Disc batteries (risk of corrosive injury; see p. 396)
2. Asymptomatic patients with esophageal coins (especially coins at the gastroesophageal junction) may be observed for up to 24 hours after ingestion in the expectation that they will pass spontaneously to the stomach.
3. In symptomatic patients, coins should be removed immediately.
4. Repeat the radiograph just prior to removal to make sure that coin has not passed spontaneously into the stomach.
5. The method of choice for coin retrieval depends on the location, duration of impaction, clinical condition of the patient, prior history of esophageal disease, and availability of a consultant (skilled radiologist, surgeon, gastroenterologist) Several options include:
   a. Rigid endoscopy with forceps extraction under general anesthesia is the standard method of choice. Indications include:
      (1) Patients with any airway compromise
      (2) Patients with prolonged impaction of coin
      (3) Patients with prior history of esophageal disease or surgery
      (4) Allows controlled removal of coin and visualization of the esophagus
   b. Flexible fiberoptic nonoperative endoscopy:
      (1) Patients without respiratory distress (airway control is not guaranteed with this procedure)
      (2) For coin ingestion of less than 1 to 2 weeks' duration
      (3) No risk of general anesthesia; patient may need sedation
   c. Extraction by Foley catheter (by a radiologist under fluoroscopic guidance):
      (1) Patients without airway compromise (clinically or radiographically)
      (2) Patients without underlying esophageal pathology
      (3) Duration of impaction less than 72 hours
      (4) Foley catheter is passed beyond the coin, the balloon is inflated with contrast media, and both the coin and the catheter are removed at the same time.
      (5) No risk of general anesthesia, no hospitalization

d. Indications for thoracotomy for removal of FB:
   (1) Poor endoscopic visualization of FB because of inflammatory tissue
   (2) Herald bleeding during endoscopy
e. Advancement using bougie dilator (with or without fluoroscopy):
   (1) Coin is pushed into the stomach in a patient in an upright or prone position.
   (2) Location in the stomach is confirmed by radiograph.
   (3) May be considered for patients *without* respiratory distress or esophageal pathology, or for coin impacted in the distal esophagus for less than 24 hours
6. Medications (glucagon, diazepam) have been used to relax the lower esophageal sphincter and to enhance esophageal motility. These agents have not been adequately studied in children, and currently their use cannot be recommended.

KEY POINTS

Esophageal Foreign Body

- Coins are the most common esophageal FBs in children.

TABLE 11–3
Esophageal Foreign Bodies

Entrapment occurs at sites of *normal* anatomic narrowing of esophagus
Three most common sites:
  Upper esophageal sphincter at thoracic inlet: 63% to 84%
  Level of aortic arch (crossover of aortic arch in the midesophagus): 10% to 17%
  Lower esophageal sphincter (gastroesophageal junction): 5% to 20%

TABLE 11–4
Complications of Esophageal Foreign Bodies

Impaction of FB for a prolonged period (weeks, months, years)
Mucosal scratch/abrasion, ulceration, and granulation at the point of impaction
Esophageal necrosis (button batteries; see p. 396)
Airway obstruction (wheezing, stridor from external tracheal obstruction)
Lobar atelectasis
Regurgitation and lodging of FB in the trachea
Esophageal diverticulum
Esophageal perforation leading to:
  Paraesophageal abscess
  Mediastinitis
  Pericarditis
  Pericardial tamponade
  Pneumothorax
  Pneumomediastinum
  Tracheoesophageal fistula
  Esophageal-aortic fistula
  Death (related to any of the above)

Modified from Munter DW: Disorders of the esophagus. *In* Howell JM: Emergency Medicine. Philadelphia, W.B. Saunders, 1998.

- Most common site of coin entrapment is thoracic inlet.
- Most common symptoms with an esophageal coin are drooling and dysphagia.
- Presence of symptoms at the time of evaluation often predicts the presence of an esophageal coin; however, absence of symptoms does *not* rule it out.
- Impacted esophageal coin can lead to serious complications and must be removed.

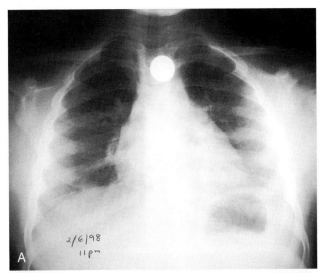

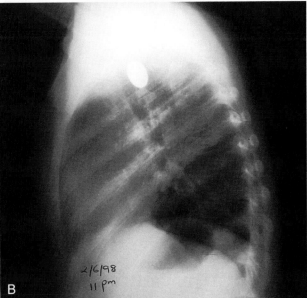

FIGURE 11–3. *A,* Frontal view of chest in a 22-month-old infant showing a coin impacted in the esophagus at the level of the thoracic inlet. Coin is seen in a frontal or transverse orientation (coronal alignment) on this view. *B,* Note the sagittal orientation of the coin (in the plane of the esophagus) on a lateral film. The opposite situation is seen when a coin is lodged in the trachea. Owing to the configuration of the tracheal rings and the incomplete cartilage posteriorly, a coin in the trachea appears in a sagittal orientation in the AP view and in a frontal orientation on a lateral film.

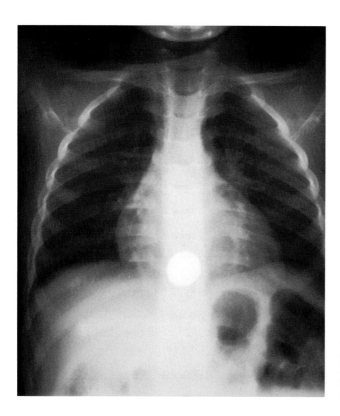

FIGURE 11–4. Coin impacted at the lower esophageal junction in a 3-year-old asymptomatic child who had a history of coin ingestion of less than 24 hours' duration. Patient was observed, and the coin dislodged spontaneously, appearing in the duodenum in a subsequent follow-up radiograph.

Foreign Bodies in Stomach and Lower Gastrointestinal Tract

DEFINITION

An ingestion (either accidental or intentional) of a foreign object in the gastrointestinal tract

EPIDEMIOLOGY

1. Eighty percent of all foreign body ingestions occur in children under 5 years of age with a peak incidence between 6 months and 3 years.
2. Most common foreign objects ingested:
   a. Young children: coins, toys, marbles, buttons, batteries (see p. 395)
   b. Older children, teenagers, and adults: fish or chicken bones, toothpicks, sharp objects
3. Risk of ingestion increases after consumption of alcohol or cold liquids (decrease in oral sensory acuity)
4. Where in the gastrointestinal (GI) tract an FB is retained depends on:
   a. Shape and size of the FB
   b. Diameter of GI tract including normal anatomic narrowings or angulations at the following locations:
      (1) Esophagus (see Table 11–3)
      (2) Pylorus
      (3) Duodenum
      (4) Ligament of Treitz
      (5) Ileocecal valve
      (6) Appendix
      (7) Hepatic and splenic flexures of the colon
      (8) Rectum
   c. Any other location of congenital (e.g., webs, diaphragms, diverticula) or acquired narrowing
   d. Patient with a prior surgical history (e.g., pyloromyotomy) are prone to impaction
   e. GI motility
5. Most likely locations of FBs
   a. Below the diaphragm (55% to 62% of cases)
   b. In the esophagus (20% to 30% of cases)
   c. FB cannot be found in 10% to 20% of reported ingestions.
6. The lower esophageal sphincter (LES) is the narrowest passage in the entire GI tract that a FB must pass. Once in the stomach, 95% of FBs pass through the remainder of the GI tract in an average time of 5 days.

CLINICAL FEATURES

1. Symptoms are uncommon when a swallowed FB has already passed through the gastroesophageal sphincter.
2. Patients may present with a sudden history of choking, coughing, or gagging provoked by ingestion of FB or history of a swallowed FB.
3. These symptoms usually resolve, and most patients have unremarkable findings on physical examination.

LABORATORY

1. Radiographs of neck, chest, and abdomen (antero-posterior and lateral views) to determine the type, location, and number of ingested objects
2. About 90% of ingested foreign bodies are radio-paque.
3. Chicken or fish bones are often poorly visualized because of their varying degree of calcification; only 29% to 50% of endoscopically proven bones are seen on plain radiographs.
4. Computed tomography allows visualization of low-density objects and also delineates adjacent soft tissue inflammation or abscess formation.
5. Esophagogram with contrast may be indicated for patients in whom FBs are not visualized on radiographs and who are thought to have swallowed a radiolucent object (e.g., plastic toy, aluminum tab).

COMPLICATIONS

1. Bowel perforation
   a. Frequency estimated to be less than 1%
   b. Frequency increases with sharp objects (about 15% to 35%)
   c. Sites of perforation
      (1) Areas of previous surgery
      (2) Areas of acute angulation or sites of anatomic narrowing (e.g., pylorus, duodenum, ileocecal valve, appendix)
   d. Complications related to perforation include:
      (1) Peritonitis
      (2) Hemorrhage
      (3) Abscess formation, inflammatory tumors
      (4) Death
2. Bowel obstruction

TREATMENT

1. Conservative management is recommended for most FBs that have already passed the esophagus and entered the stomach.

2. Most FBs pass through the intestine in 4 to 6 days; however, some may take as long as 3 to 4 weeks.
3. Instruct parents to observe the stools for the appearance of the ingested FB. Although this is an unpleasant task, in our experience most parents are willing to accept it.
4. Educate parents about the warning signals (vomiting, abdominal pain, melena, or hematemesis) and advise them to report to a physician immediately if these occur.
5. Stool softeners or cathartics or "special diets" have no proven benefit in the management of FBs.
6. Objects that usually require removal by endoscopy:
   a. Sewing needles or open safety pins (increased risk of perforation)
   b. Infants: FBs longer than 3 cm or larger than 2 cm in diameter usually will not pass through the pylorus.
   c. Older children (and adults): oval-shaped FBs greater than 5 cm in diameter or 2 cm in thickness tend to lodge in the stomach.
   d. Foreign objects more than 10 cm long may have difficulty passing through the duodenal sweep.
7. Once an FB has passed the ligament of Treitz, it cannot be removed endoscopically.
8. Serial abdominal examination and radiographs are needed for a patient with a sharp or long object that has already passed out of the stomach.
9. Immediate surgical consultation is needed for patients with symptoms (perforation or bleeding).

KEY POINT

Foreign Bodies in Stomach and Lower GI Tract

- Once in the stomach, 95% of FBs usually pass through the remainder of the GI tract in an average time of 5 days.

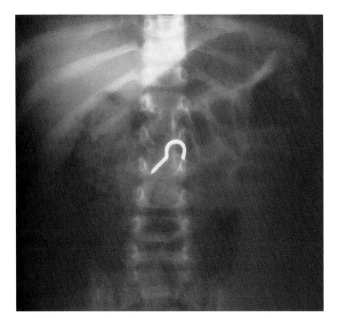

FIGURE 11–5. Swallowed radiopaque hook lodged in the transverse colon. This hook passed spontaneously in 24 hours.

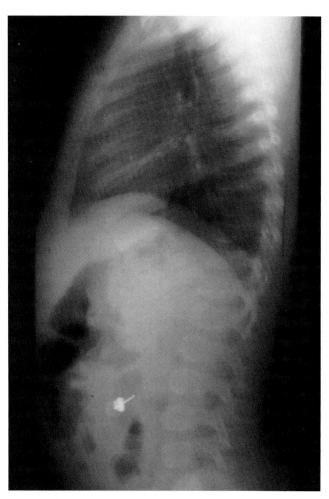

FIGURE 11–7. Abdominal radiograph of a 2-year-old girl showing an earring with a stud situated in the large bowel. She passed this spontaneously in 24 hours. Ear piercing in very young infants (including neonates) is quite common but poses a risk of aspiration or ingestion of the earring by a toddler.

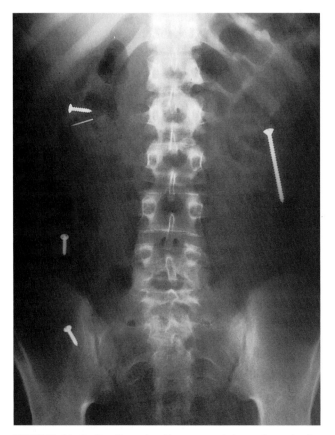

FIGURE 11–6. Swallowed nails scattered throughout the intestines of a teenage psychiatric patient. She spontaneously passed all the nails over a period of 72 hours.

Ingestion of Cylindrical and Button (Disc) Batteries

INTRODUCTION/EPIDEMIOLOGY

1. Both cylindrical and button batteries are found in almost every household.
2. Cylindrical batteries are used for toys and cameras, and button batteries are used for hearing aids, watches, calculators, cameras, and a variety of other small electronic instruments.
3. Important epidemiologic data about battery exposures reported in 1996 by the American Association of Poison Control Centers National Data System, are as follows:
   a. Most ingestions are accidental.
   b. Most ingestions occur in children under 5 years of age; peak incidence is between 1 and 2 years of age.
   c. Hearing aid batteries are the most frequently ingested batteries.
   d. Batteries are often removed by children from their own hearing aids and subsequently ingested.
4. Both size and chemical composition are important in determining the possible consequences and management of ingested batteries.
   a. Most button batteries are 7.9 mm or 11.6 mm in diameter.
   b. Most batteries that lodge in the esophagus and cause tissue injury are large-diameter batteries (20 to 23 mm [size of a quarter]).
   c. Direction of the battery cathode, which produces alkali, is important in determining the severity of complications.
5. Chemical composition of common batteries:
   a. Salts of metals (e.g., mercury, lithium, nickel, zinc, cadmium, silver, manganese) *and* concentrated alkali media (e.g., sodium or potassium hydroxide)
   b. Lithium cells (both larger diameter and greater voltage) are associated more often with adverse effects.
   c. Mercuric oxide cells are more likely to split in the gastrointestinal (GI) tract.

CLINICAL FEATURES

1. Most cases of battery ingestion follow a benign course if the battery has not lodged in the esophagus.
2. Signs and symptoms suggestive of foreign body ingestion and/or esophageal impaction:
   a. Sudden history of choking, coughing, or gagging
   b. Drooling
   c. Refusing food or dysphagia (young infants take liquids but refuse solid food)
   d. Respiratory signs (tracheal compression), including stridor, wheezing, and respiratory distress
   e. Burn in the oral mucosa and pharynx if a battery was chewed

f. Irritability
   g. Retrosternal pain or discomfort
3. Signs and symptoms suggestive of GI tract injury:
   a. Abdominal pain, tenderness
   b. Hematochezia
   c. Vomiting, diarrhea
   d. Bloody or dark stool
4. Nickel hypersensitivity produces skin rashes (if ingested button batteries are nickel-plated)

LABORATORY

1. Radiographs: Posteroanterior (PA) and lateral views of neck and chest and, if required, PA view of abdomen to determine the location of the battery
2. Identification of battery diameter and chemical composition using any of the following:
   a. Imprint code of a duplicate battery
   b. Call for assistance: National Button Battery Ingestion Hotline (202-625-3333)
3. Blood and urine mercury levels (in patients who have ingested mercury oxide batteries and show evidence of radiopaque droplets in the gut or a battery that has split open in the gut)

TREATMENT

(Based on current recommendations of the National Capital Poison Center, Washington, D.C.)

1. Report all battery ingestions to the National Button Battery Ingestion Hotline (202-625-3333).
2. Do not induce vomiting with syrup of ipecac
   a. Risk of perforation of esophagus or stomach in the presence of mucosal burns
   b. Risk of aspiration in the tracheobronchial tree during retrograde movement of the battery during ipecac-induced emesis
3. Batteries impacted in the esophagus
   a. Remove *emergently*
   b. Endoscopy under direct visualization (visualization of esophageal mucosa)
   c. Removal by Foley catheter technique does not allow direct visualization.
   d. Indications for thoracotomy for removal
      (1) Poor endoscopic visualization of a battery because of inflammatory tissue
      (2) Herald bleeding occurring during endoscopy
4. Batteries that have passed beyond the esophagus
   a. Battery retrieval indicated
      (1) In symptomatic patients with significant signs of injury to GI tract (e.g., hematochezia, abdominal pain and tenderness)
      (2) In patients with failure of a large battery to pass through the pylorus; if a battery does not pass within 48 hours, it is unlikely to pass at all.
   b. Battery retrieval in asymptomatic patients
      (1) Follow-up clinically (physical examination, inspection of stools)
      (2) Follow-up by radiographs (to see the passage of the battery)
   c. Most batteries pass through GI tract with no complications (see Table 11–7).

KEY POINTS

Ingestion of Cylindrical and Button Batteries

- Hearing aid batteries are the batteries most frequently ingested by children.
- Location of the ingested battery must be determined promptly by radiographs.

- Batteries impacted in the esophagus should be removed *emergently* by endoscopy under direct visualization.
- It is unsafe to induce vomiting with syrup of ipecac in a child with a battery ingestion.
- Mercuric oxide batteries have a tendency to split open in the GI tract.

TABLE 11–5

Complications Related to Batteries Impacted in the Esophagus*

Pressure necrosis
Leakage of contents producing caustic injury (liquefaction necrosis)
Esophageal burns (seen as early as 4 hours after ingestion)
Electrical injury by conduction to surrounding tissues (from a battery that is not exhausted)
Esophageal perforation (seen as early as 6 hours after ingestion)
Tracheoesophageal fistula
Mediastinitis
Esophageal-aortic fistula
Death (complications related to esophageal perforation)
Aspiration of battery to tracheobronchial tree from esophagus

---

* See also Table 11–4, page 391.

TABLE 11–6

Complications Related to Batteries Impacted in the GI Tract Beyond Esophagus

Leakage and/or split of the cell
Tissue injury *without* leakage as a result of direct current flow from intact button cell
Ulceration ⇒ perforation
Impaction ⇒ obstruction ⇒ perforation in certain locations (e.g., Meckel diverticulum)
Heavy metal absorption (e.g., from a split mercuric oxide cell [usually 15.6-mm diameter cell])

TABLE 11–7

Gastrointestinal Transit Time of 1366 Ingested Batteries*

Passage within 24 hours:	22.6% of cases
Passage within 48 hours:	61.3% of cases
Passage within 72 hours:	78.0% of cases
Passage within 94 hours:	86.4% of cases
Passage >1 week:	4.5% of cases
Passage >2 weeks:	1.1% of cases

---

* Of a total of 2382 cases of battery ingestion, GI transit time was known for 1366 cases. From American Association of Poison Control Centers, National Data System, Washington, D.C., 1992.

From Litovitz TL, Schmitz BF: Ingestion of cylindrical and button batteries: An analysis of 2382 cases. Pediatrics 89:747, 1992.

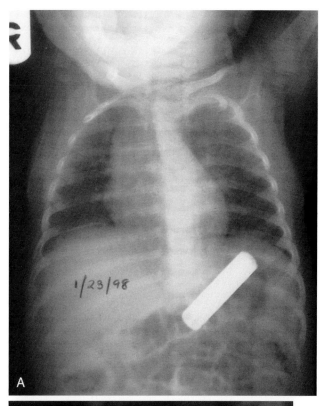

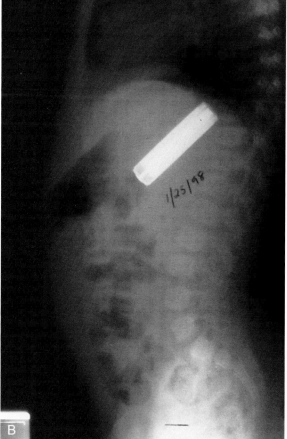

FIGURE 11-8. *A,* Frontal view of the abdomen showing a cylindrical battery lodged in the stomach. The battery was found accidentally in this 5-month-old infant when a chest radiograph was obtained for suspected pneumonia. *B,* Lateral view showing failure of the battery to progress beyond the stomach ("arrested transit") for more than 48 hours. Because of the failure of progression and an unknown exact time of ingestion, the battery was retrieved endoscopically. A severely corroded AAA battery was found.

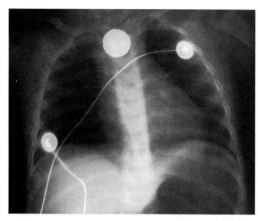

FIGURE 11–9. Button battery "mimicking a coin" that was impacted in the esophagus at the thoracic inlet in this 18-month-old infant who presented with persistent cough and "noisy breathing" of several hours duration. (Courtesy of Richard Scriven, M.D., State University of New York, Brooklyn, NY.)

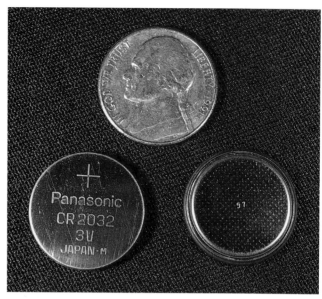

FIGURE 11–11. Compare the size and borders of a button battery (front and back view) with a nickel.

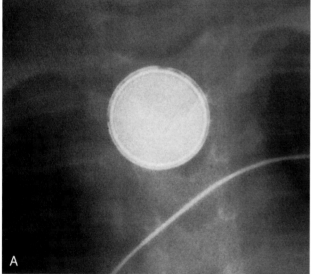

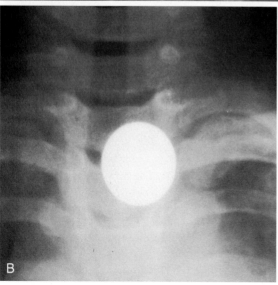

FIGURE 11–10. Compare the magnified views of a battery *(A)* with a coin *(B)* from a different patient. These images clearly demonstrate the radiologic differences between a battery, which has a lucent center and a serrated, "double density" appearance of the borders, and a coin, which has a homogeneous density and smooth borders.

Nursemaid's Elbow

SYNONYMS   Radial Head Subluxation
"Pulled Elbow"
"Temper Tantrum Elbow"

DEFINITION

Subluxation of the radial head caused by a sudden pull on the arm by a caretaker

ETIOLOGY/MECHANISM OF INJURY (see Fig. 11–12)

1. The radial head is not as bulbous in young children as it is in older children. The annular ligament that passes around the neck of the proximal radius just below the radial head provides stability between the radius and the ulna.
2. Sudden longitudinal traction applied by a caretaker on the extended and pronated arm in a young child to prevent a fall or in swinging a child by the arms causes the annular ligament to slide over the radial head in the radiohumeral joint (see Fig. 11–12A).
3. The slipped ligament is entrapped between the articular surfaces of the radial head and capitellum, limiting the arm's motion. Tearing of the ligament does not always occur (see Fig. 11–12B).
4. In infants, a similar injury can occur when an extended arm is trapped beneath the trunk while the infant is rolling over.
5. As a child grows older, the strength of the annular ligament increases, and the radial head also develops sufficiently; thus, this injury is uncommon after 5 years of age.

EPIDEMIOLOGY

1. Very common injury, accounting for 22% of all upper extremity injuries in children
2. Most common age at presentation:
   a. Between 1 and 3 years
   b. Range 6 months to 5 years
3. Most commonly involved side: left elbow (most adults prefer to hold the child's left hand while using their dominant right hand)

CLINICAL FEATURES (see also Box 11–2)

1. Typical complaint: decreased use of the arm in an otherwise happy or playful child
2. A history may be obtained of the child being forcibly lifted by the hand or pulled by the arm during a fall while the hand is held by a parent. However, such a history may be lacking in as many as 50% of cases.

LABORATORY

1. Diagnosis is clinical based on the history (if present) and classic clinical findings.
2. Radiographs are *not* necessary and are not helpful because the radial head and lateral humeral condyle may not be ossified in a young child. When radiographs are obtained, the child often returns

---

BOX 11–2	*Nursemaid's Elbow: Typical Findings*

Child appears playful yet refuses to reach for objects with the affected arm
Forearm is held in pronation with elbow in slight flexion
Child resists all attempts at passive supination
Attempts to supinate, pronate, or flex the elbow elicit pain
Lack of swelling or tenderness over the affected arm
Mild tenderness over the radial head may be present

---

with a normal arm movement following reduction of subluxation that occurs when the forearm is placed in supination for the anteroposterior view by a radiology technician.
3. Indications for radiography (any of the following)
   a. Unsuccessful attempts at reduction
   b. Presence of swelling
   c. Significant tenderness suggesting another diagnosis (e.g., fracture)

DIFFERENTIAL DIAGNOSIS

1. Fracture
2. Bone infections (septic arthritis, osteomyelitis)
3. Soft tissue injury

TREATMENT

1. Most commonly used closed reduction technique: supination and flexion
   a. Grasp the palm of the involved hand as if to shake it, encircle the elbow with the other hand with the thumb placed over the radial head and gently supinate the palm and forearm and in a continuous motion flex the elbow to the shoulder.
   b. Successful reduction on first attempt occurs in 70% to 80% of cases.
   c. A palpable "pop or click" is usually felt by the thumb that lies over the radial head as the annular ligament is freed from the joint. This signals successful reduction in over 90% of patients.
   d. With successful reduction, the child starts using the arm usually within 5 to 15 minutes; however, it may take longer for normal arm movements to return if subluxation has been present for several hours.
2. Absence of a click with an unsuccessful reduction: another attempt is made after 15 minutes
3. Unsuccessful reduction after two to three attempts: consider an alternative diagnosis.
4. In a child with recurrent subluxations: immobilization for a few weeks in a posterior splint with the elbow placed at 90 degrees and the forearm in supination

5. Even when attempts at closed reduction fail, spontaneous reduction almost invariably occurs, and the need for open reduction is exceedingly rare.
6. Educate caretaker about the mechanism of injury to prevent recurrences.

PROGNOSIS

Recurrence rate of subsequent subluxation: 26% to 39%

KEY POINTS

Nursemaid's Elbow

- Most common elbow injury in children between 6 months and 5 years of age
- Caretakers should be counseled to lift a child from the axilla or upper arm and not from the hand or wrist to prevent nursemaid's elbow.

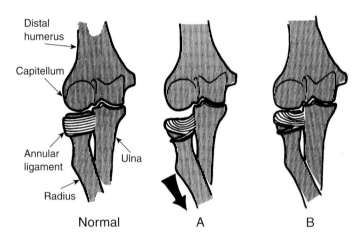

Distal humerus
Capitellum
Annular ligament
Ulna
Radius
Normal　　A　　B

FIGURE 11–12. The pathology of nursemaid's, or pulled, elbow. *A,* Sudden traction on the outstretched arm pulls the radius distally, causing it to slip partially through the annular ligament, and tearing it in the process. *B,* With discontinuation of traction, as the radial head recoils, it traps the proximal portion of the ligament (between it and the capitellum) and carries it into the joint. (Modified from Rang M: *Children's Fractures,* 2nd ed. Philadelphia, J.B. Lippincott, 1983, p. 193.)

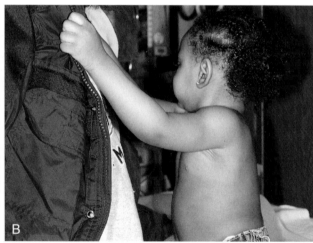

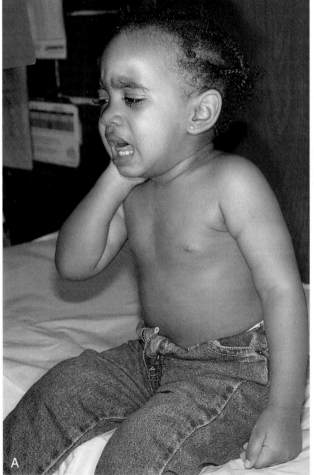

FIGURE 11–13. *A,* A 2-year-old otherwise playful child with left nursemaid's elbow. She was reaching for the object using her right arm, but her left arm was partially flexed, pronated, and close to the body. *B,* Within 5 minutes after reduction, the child started using both arms.

Rheumatology

Teresita A. Laude, M.D. and Binita R. Shah, M.D.

Systemic Lupus Erythematosus (SLE)

DEFINITION

A connective tissue disease that is more acute and more severe in children

ETIOLOGY

It is considered an autoimmune disorder.

EPIDEMIOLOGY

1. Female-male ratio is 3:1 in children under 10 years of age and 9:1 in those over 10 years.
2. More common in African-Americans
3. Most childhood cases present after 8 years of age.

PATHOGENESIS

Factors known to play a role in the pathogenesis

1. Genetics
   a. HLA associations: HLA-DR2 and HLA-DR3
   b. Complement deficiencies
2. Environmental factors
   a. Hormonal
   b. Climate
   c. Infectious agents
   d. Drugs (hydralazine, procainamide)

CLINICAL FEATURES

1. Diagnosis of SLE is established by meeting 4 of the 11 criteria established by the American College of Rheumatology.
   a. Malar rash (see Table 12–1)
   b. Discoid rash (see Table 12–1)
   c. Photosensitivity
   d. Oral ulcers
      (1) They are painless.
      (2) They are often accidental findings.
   e. Arthritis of large joints
   f. Serositis (pleurisy, pericarditis)
   g. Renal involvement
      (1) Persistent proteinuria of more than 0.5 g/day
      (2) RBCs and cellular casts
   h. Neurologic disorder
      (1) Psychosis
      (2) Seizure without a cause

   i. Hematologic disorder
      (1) Anemia
      (2) Leukopenia
      (3) Thrombocytopenia
   j. Immunologic disorder
      (1) Positive LE prep test
      (2) False-positive Venereal Disease Research Laboratory (VDRL) test
      (3) Circulating autoantibodies
   k. Positive antinuclear antibody (ANA) findings
2. Other asssociated findings:
   a. Alopecia
   b. Periungual telangiectasia
   c. Raynaud phenomenon
   d. Embolic episodes
      (1) Deep vein thrombosis
      (2) Cerebrovascular accidents
      (3) Digital ulceration
      (4) Seen in antiphospholipid syndrome
3. Vesicobullous SLE (see Table 12–1)
4. Nonspecific symptoms such as fever, myalgia, arthritis/arthralgia, poor weight gain, depression

LABORATORY

1. Complete blood count
2. Urinalysis
3. Serum complement level
4. Serum electrolytes, blood urea nitrogen (BUN), and creatinine
5. Chest radiograph
6. Assay of autoantibodies in SLE (see Box 12–1)

BOX 12–1	*Assay of Autoantibodies in Systemic Lupus Erythematosus*

Antinuclear antibodies (ANA): screening for connective tissue disease
Anti-nDNA: specific for SLE, correlates with renal disease
Anti-Sm: specific for SLE
Anti-Ro, anti-La: seen in 60% of SLE patients
Antihistone: positive in drug-induced LE
Antiphospholipid antibodies

7. Lupus band test consists of direct immunofluorescence on lesional and normal skin.
   a. Positive in both lesional and normal skin in patients with SLE.
   b. Positive in lesional skin but negative in normal skin in those with discoid cutaneous LE (without systemic involvement)

BOX 12–2	*Differential Diagnosis of Systemic Lupus Erythematosus*

Polymorphous light eruption
Phototoxic and photoallergic drug eruption
Dermatomyositis
Juvenile rheumatoid arthritis

COMPLICATION

Renal disease is the major cause of morbidity and mortality.

TREATMENT

1. Refer patient to a pediatric rheumatologist.

2. Sunscreen, protective clothing
3. Topical corticosteroid for the rash
4. Therapeutic options
   a. Dapsone for vesicobullous LE
   b. Nonsteroidal anti-inflammatory drugs for musculoskeletal manifestations, serositis, and constitutional signs (e.g., fever)
   c. Antimalarial drug (e.g., hydroxycloroquine)
   d. Immunosuppressive agents including systemic corticosteroids
5. Enroll the patient in the

   Lupus Foundation of America. Inc.
   4 Research Place, Suite 180
   Rockville, MD 20850
   Tel. (800) 558-0121

PROGNOSIS

Guarded in the presence of renal involvement

KEY POINTS

Systemic Lupus Erythematosus

- SLE is a more acute and more severe disease in children.
- Renal disease is the major cause of morbidity.

TABLE 12–1
Systemic Lupus Erythematosus— Skin Manifestations

Malar rash
  Butterfly distribution on the face
  Spares the nasolabial fold
  Lesions consist of macular erythema or erythematous papules
Discoid rash
  Characterized by atrophy, adherent scales, hyper and hypopigmentation, and erythema
  Results in scarring
  Most common areas involved: face and head
Vesicobullous SLE
  Variant that has high correlation with kidney involvement
  Lesions consist of vesicles and bullae
  Common areas involved: photosensitive distribution (e.g., face, neck, backs of hands)

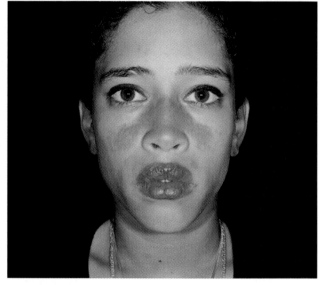

FIGURE 12–1. Butterfly rash.

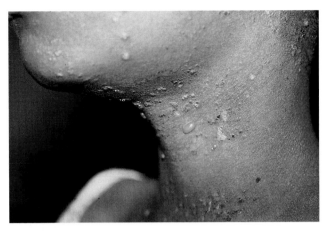

FIGURE 12-2. Vesicobullous eruption of SLE.

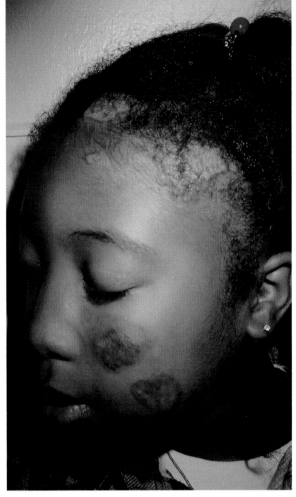

FIGURE 12-3. Discoid LE. Lesions are well circumscribed, atrophic, hyper- and hypopigmented, and have adherent scales.

Neonatal Lupus Erythematosus (NLE)

DEFINITION

A syndrome consisting of skin lesions and/or congenital heart block in the newborn infant.

ETIOLOGY

The syndrome is caused by passively acquired maternal antibodies.

EPIDEMIOLOGY

1. The mother may have overt or latent systemic lupus erythematosus or other connective tissue disease.
2. An infant born to a mother positive for Ro antibodies has a 1:20 chance of developing NLE.
3. Female-male ratio is 3:1 in NLE without cardiac involvement.
4. Female-male ratio is 1.5:1 in NLE with congenital heart block.

PATHOGENESIS

1. The Ro-IgG antibody is responsible for the cardiac muscle damage that leads to conduction defects.
2. Uridine-rich ribonucleoprotein (U^1RNP) antibody does not bind to cardiac muscle and does not produce damage.

LABORATORY

1. Complete blood count
2. Electrocardiography
3. Sjögren syndrome A (SS-A) antibodies (also called Ro) are seen in 95% of patients with NLE. They disappear by 12 months of age.
4. Sjögren syndrome B (SS-B) antibodies (also called La) is seen in 70% of NLE patients.

5. U¹RNP antibodies are seen in 5% of cases.

6. Antinuclear antibody (ANA) may be positive.

DIFFERENTIAL DIAGNOSIS

Atopic dermatitis, seborrheic dermatitis, congenital heart disease

COMPLICATIONS

1. One third of infants with congenital heart block may develop congestive heart failure.

> **BOX 12–3**   *Neonatal Lupus Erythematosus*
>
> Cutaneous findings alone are seen in 45% of all NLE patients.
> Congenital heart block (CHB) alone is seen in 45% of all NLE patients.
> Cutaneous and CHB together are seen in 10% of NLE patients.

---

2. Scarring may result from the discoid lupus erythematosus (DLE)-like skin lesions.

3. SLE may develop later in life.

TREATMENT

1. Sunscreen and protective clothing

2. Mild topical corticosteroid may be used for the rash

3. Cardiology consultation for cardiac evaluation and pacemaker

4. Work-up on the mother is needed for SLE or other connective tissue disease.

KEY POINTS

Neonatal Lupus Erythematosus

- In infants without congenital heart block, neonatal lupus erythematosus is a benign, self-limiting disorder.
- The mother, whether symptomatic or not, must be investigated for SLE or other connective tissue disease.

TABLE 12–2
Neonatal Lupus Erythematosus—Skin Rash

Eruption may be precipitated by sun exposure
Appears within 2 weeks of birth
Appears either as atrophic scaly plaques (like discoid LE) or erythematous macules or annular plaques (like subacute LE)
Most common distribution
    Head
    Face
    Periorbital area
    Upper part of the body
    Occasionally generalized
Natural course
    Disappears in 6–12 months

TABLE 12–3
Noncutaneous Clinical Features of Neonatal Lupus Erythematosus

Congenital heart block (CHB)
    May be diagnosed before or at birth
    Causes morbidity in first few weeks of life
    May require a pacemaker
    Is permanent
Other self-limiting findings
    Hepatomegaly
    Anemia
    Leukopenia
    Thrombocytopenia

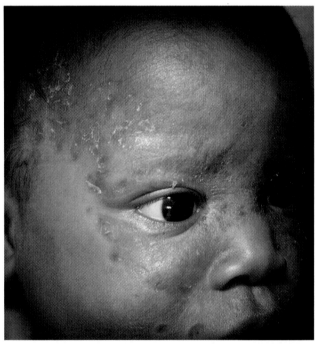

FIGURE 12–4. Skin lesions of NLE in a characteristic periorbital distribution. Lesions are atrophic, scaly, and discoid.

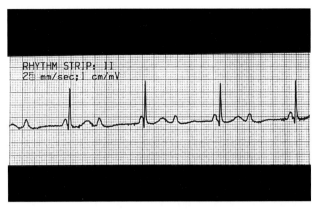

FIGURE 12-6. Neonatal lupus erythematosus. Electrocardiogram showing congenital heart block. (Courtesy of Sudha Rao, M.D., State University of New York, Brooklyn, NY.)

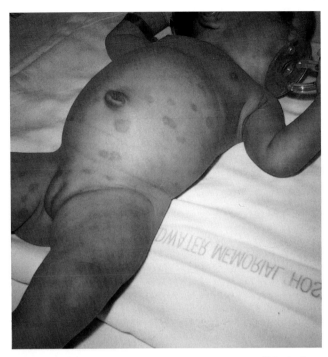

FIGURE 12-5. Neonatal lupus erythematosus. Skin lesions are annular erythematous plaques similar to those of subacute LE.

Juvenile Rheumatoid Arthritis (JRA)

DEFINITION

A chronic disease characterized by inflammation of the joints in a child. It is classified according to mode of onset as systemic, pauciarticular, or polyarticular.

ETIOLOGY

1. The exact cause is unknown.
2. One theory is that the disease results from an abnormal response to a viral infection such as Epstein-Barr (EB) virus or rubella virus.

EPIDEMIOLOGY

1. The incidence is 1:10,000.
2. More common in whites than in African-Americans.

PATHOGENESIS

Genetic and environmental factors including infections probably play a role in the pathogenesis.

CLINICAL FEATURES

There are three clinical types:

1. Systemic JRA (see Table 12–4)
2. Pauciarticular JRA (see Table 12–5)
3. Polyarticular JRA (see Table 12–6)

BOX 12-4	*Differential Diagnosis of Juvenile Rheumatoid Arthritis*

Septic arthritis
Toxic synovitis
Trauma
Serum sickness
Sickle cell disease
Leukemia
Systemic lupus erythematosus
Mixed connective tissue disease
Kawasaki disease

LABORATORY

1. Complete blood count: eosinophilia may be seen in systemic JRA because of vasculitis.
2. ANA is positive in 30% of polyarticular JRA.
3. Rheumatoid factor may be positive in girls with polyarticular JRA.
4. Chest radiograph

COMPLICATIONS

1. Chronic iridocyclitis in pauciarticular JRA (20%)
2. Joint deformities in polyarticular JRA

TREATMENT

1. Refer patient to a pediatric rheumatologist.
2. Therapeutic options
   a. ASA or other nonsteroidal anti-inflammatory agents
   b. IV gamma globulin
   c. Immunosuppressive agents
3. Physical therapy

TABLE 12-4
Clinical Features of Systemic Juvenile Rheumatoid Arthritis

More common in young children
Equal sex incidence
Acute onset
Spiking fever with a quotidian or diquotidian pattern
Lymphadenopathy
Hepatomegaly
Serositis (pericardial and pleural effusion)
Joint involvement
  Pain or swelling of large joints
  May precede, occur, or follow other acute signs or
    symptoms
Skin eruption
  Evanescent
  Morbilliform or salmon-colored macules
  Appears during height of fever
Systemic JRA may be a cause of fever of unknown origin

TABLE 12-5
Clinical Features of Pauciarticular Rheumatoid Arthritis

Only four or fewer large joints are involved
Usually no systemic symptoms
Spondyloarthropathy may be seen in older boys (associated
  with HLA-B27)
Ocular disease (20% of patients)
  Iritis
  Iridocyclitis
  Uveitis

TABLE 12-6
Clinical Features of Polyarticular Rheumatoid Arthritis

More than five joints are involved
Mild systemic complaints such as fever and malaise
Subcutaneous nodules over bony prominences may be seen
One subset characterized by positive rheumatoid factor
  Seen in girls
  10–14 years of age
  Erosive arthritis
  Symmetrical hand involvement
  Rheumatoid nodules
  Rarely uveitis
Second subset characterized by negative rheumatoid factor
  Mild systemic symptoms
  Polyarthritis may involve neck and jaw
  Uveitis (5% of patients)

KEY POINTS

Juvenile Rheumatoid Arthritis

- JRA may mimic any systemic disease.
- Diagnosis is arrived at after exclusion of the other causes of joint disease in children.

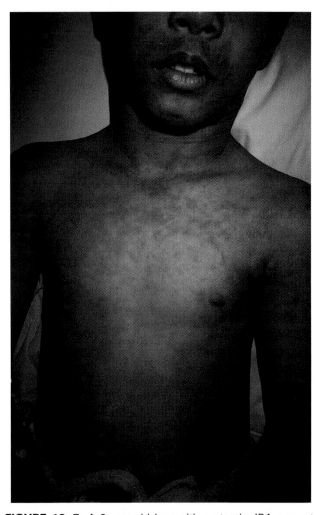

FIGURE 12-7. A 3-year-old boy with systemic JRA presenting with spiking fever and an exanthematous rash, eosinophilia, hepatomegaly, and adenopathy.

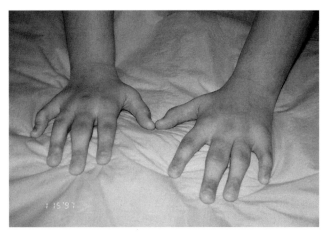

FIGURE 12-8. Pauciarticular JRA.

Juvenile Dermatomyositis (JDM)

DEFINITION

An inflammatory disorder affecting the striated muscles and the skin.

ETIOLOGY

1. The exact cause is unknown.
2. It may be triggered by a viral infection, specifically coxsackie virus B.

EPIDEMIOLOGY

1. JDM comprises 8% to 22% of all dermatomyositides.

BOX 12–5 *Diagnostic Criteria for Juvenile Dermatomyositis*

Characteristic skin rash (see Table 12–7) plus the following:
1. Proximal symmetrical muscle weakness of limbs and shoulder girdle that is progressive over months and years
2. Elevated serum levels of muscle enzymes (creatine phosphokinase, aldolase, lactate dehydrogenase, transaminases)
3. Abnormal electromyographic findings
4. Abnormal muscle biopsy findings

BOX 12–6 *Differential Diagnosis of Juvenile Dermatomyositis*

Systemic lupus erythematosus
Photocontact dermatitis
Myopathies
Knuckle pads
Serum sickness
Mixed connective tissue disease

---

2. There is an association with HLA-B8 and HLA-DR3.
3. More common in African-Americans than in whites
4. Peak age at onset: 5 to 15 years

PATHOGENESIS

Unknown, but genetic and environmental factors including infection play a role

LABORATORY

1. Muscle enzyme elevation is a diagnostic feature of the disease.
2. Triceps muscle biopsy preceded by muscle magnetic resonance imaging (MRI) may be done in doubtful cases.
3. Antinuclear antibody (ANA) may be positive.
4. Mi-2 antibody, which is specific for DM, is positive in 10% of cases.
5. Jo-1 antibody is seen in 25% of adults with DM but not in JDM.
6. The following are useful tools for following the activity of the disease:
   a. MRI of muscle groups
   b. Von Willebrand factor–related antigen (measures endothelial cell damage)
   c. Neopterin levels (released by activated macrophages)
   d. B-lymphocyte activity
   e. Nailfold capillaroscopy

COMPLICATIONS

1. Dystrophic calcification (calcinosis cutis)
   a. Seen in more than 40% of cases
   b. Especially common in those with severe disease and those in whom diagnosis and treatment have been delayed
2. Muscles of gastrointestinal, cardiac, and respiratory systems may also be involved, resulting in dysphagia, cardiac decompensation, or gastric perforation.
3. JDM is not associated with the development of malignancy, unlike adult DM.

TREATMENT

1. Refer the patient to a pediatric rheumatologist.
2. Therapeutic pharmacologic options include
   a. Systemic corticosteroids, oral or pulse dosing
   b. IV gamma globulin
   c. Immunosuppressants (methotrexate)
3. Sunscreen and protective clothing
4. Physical therapy

PROGNOSIS

1. Mortality rate is 7%.
2. Cause of death: overwhelming sepsis, aspiration
3. Natural course
   a. In 30% of patients the disease follows a monophasic or uniphasic course; the patient generally does well and is weaned from steroids.
   b. In the remaining 63% the disease follows a more chronic course that is continuous or marked by inactive relapses complicated by contractures and/or calcification.

KEY POINTS

Juvenile Dermatomyositis

- Juvenile dermatomyositis is characterized by a combination of proximal muscle weakness and characteristic skin rash.
- Calcinosis is more common in juvenile dermatomyositis than adult DM.

TABLE 12–7
Skin Findings in Juvenile Dermatomyositis

Characteristic Rash

Heliotrope (reddish purple) hue with edema of periorbital area
Rash is photosensitive

Gottron Papules

Red telangiectatic and later atrophic papules
Location: over metacarpophalangeal and interphalangeal
  joints, knees and elbows

Other Findings

Abnormal capillary loops in nailfold and cuticle
Poikiloderma on shoulder and upper chest (shawl sign)
Hypertrichosis
Scalp involvement: alopecia, scaliness, pruritus
Partial lipoatrophy

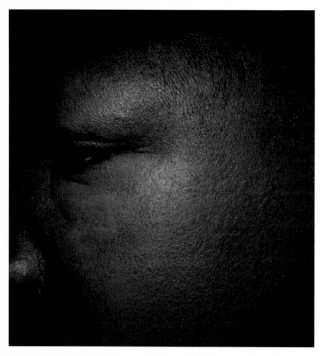

FIGURE 12–9. A 10-year-old boy with dermatomyositis. Heliotrope and facial edema.

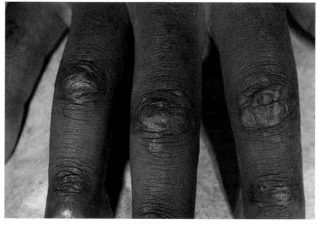

FIGURE 12–10. Gottron's papules in same patient.

Lyme Disease

SYNONYM   Borreliosis

DEFINITION

A multisystem disease caused by a spirochete

ETIOLOGY

The spirochete *Borrelia burgdorferi*, which causes Lyme disease, is transmitted by a deer tick, *Ixodes dammini*.

EPIDEMIOLOGY

1. Endemic areas include the following states:
   a. Massachusetts to Maryland
   b. Wisconsin to Minnesota
   c. California to Oregon
2. The peak season is May to July.
3. Children are affected more often than adults.

CLINICAL FEATURES

1. Stage I: Localized disease

Differential Diagnosis of Lyme Disease

Rheumatic fever
Systemic lupus erythematosus
Rheumatoid arthritis
Septic arthritis
Tinea corporis
Cellulitis
Erysipelas

*Characteristic Rash of Lyme Disease:
Erythema Chronicum Migrans*

Annular erythema
Size: 5 cm or more
Location: initial rash at site of tick bite (in 80%
of patients)
Appears 8 or 9 days after the tick bite
Solitary or multiple lesions (secondary to hema-
togenous spread of spirochetes)
May be asymptomatic, burning, or painful

   a. Characteristic rash (erythema chronicum migrans, see Box 12-8).
   b. There may be minor constitutional symptoms
such as fever and regional adenopathy.
2. Stage II: Disseminated disease
   a. Malaise, fever
   b. Neurologic signs (Bell's palsy, aseptic meningitis, radiculitis)
   c. Arthritis affecting the large joints
   d. Cardiac signs (arrhythmias)
3. Stage III
   a. Prolonged neurologic problems
   b. Recurrent joint symptoms
   c. Chronic fatigue

LABORATORY

1. Lyme titer
   a. Enzyme-linked immunosorbent assay (ELISA):
IgM antibodies
     (1) Develop 3 to 4 weeks after infection begins
     (2) Levels peak at 6 to 8 weeks
     (3) Subsequently decline
     (4) Positive titer: 1:160 or more
   b. IgG levels
     (1) Positive titer: 1:320 or more
     (2) Peak at 3 to 6 months
   c. ELISA may be negative if erythema chronicum
migrans is treated early.
   d. Western blot test: confirms a positive ELISA result
2. Polymerase chain reaction (PCR) on skin tissue
3. Culture of skin tissue on modified Kelly medium
4. Skin biopsy: positive direct immunofluorescence
provides a rapid test.

COMPLICATION

Chronic arthritis (10% of patients)

TREATMENT

1. For patients less than 9 years of age:
   a. Amoxicillin 250 mg three times a day for 10 to
30 days
   b. For patients allergic to penicillin, erythromycin
30 mg/kg/day for 10 to 30 days
2. For patients over 9 years of age:
   a. Doxycycline 100 mg twice a day for 10 to 30
days
   b. Amoxicillin 500 mg four times a day for 10 to
30 days

PROGNOSIS

Guarded in the presence of neurologic and cardiac
involvement

KEY POINTS

Lyme Disease

- Majority of cases of Lyme disease start with the
distinct rash of erythema chronicum migrans.
- The disease is endemic in certain areas of the
United States.

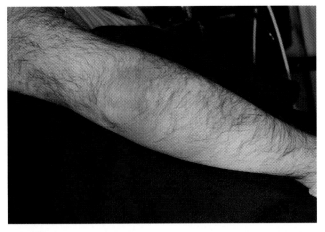

FIGURE 12-11. Erythema chronicum migrans in a patient
presenting with radiculitis.

Kawasaki Disease

SYNONYMS   Kawasaki Syndrome
            Mucocutaneous Lymph Node
            Syndrome

DEFINITION

A disease of unknown etiology and pathogenesis that affects young children

ETIOLOGY

1. The exact cause is unknown.
2. It is most probably an immune-mediated disorder in a genetically predisposed child.

EPIDEMIOLOGY

1. A disease of young children
2. Majority of patients are less than 5 years of age; peak incidence: 2 to 3 years of age
3. It is more common in Asians than in whites and is least common in African-Americans.

PATHOGENESIS

An unknown superantigen results in heavy cytokine release, which is responsible for the multiple clinical findings.

CLINICAL FEATURES (see Table 12–8)

1. Atypical Kawasaki disease (see Box 12–10)
2. Later findings in the skin
   a. Perineal desquamation (seen within the first week of illness)
   b. Desquamation of the fingertips
   c. Beau's line (transverse grooves) in the nails
3. Other, less common associated findings
   a. Hydrops of the gallbladder

BOX 12–9   *Differential Diagnosis of Kawasaki Disease*

Measles
Scarlet fever
Toxic shock syndrome (staphylococcal or streptococcal)
Viral infections (e.g., Epstein-Barr virus, enterovirus, adenovirus)
Rocky Mountain spotted fever
Stevens-Johnson syndrome
Hypersensitivity reactions
Juvenile rheumatoid arthritis

BOX 12–10   *Kawasaki Disease in Young Infants*

Presentation often atypical
Two or three criteria are not fulfilled

---

   b. Aseptic meningitis
   c. Uveitis
   d. Pneumonitis
   e. Erythema and induration at the site of bacille Calmette-Guérin (BCG) inoculation
   f. Urethritis giving rise to sterile pyuria

LABORATORY

1. There is *no* specific test for Kawasaki disease (see Table 12–8).
2. Acute phase reactants (e.g., erythrocyte sedimentation rate [ESR]) are elevated.
3. Significant thrombocytosis (up to 1 million platelet count) occurs in the second week.
4. Chest radiograph (for cardiomegaly)
5. Electrocardiogram may show evidence of myocarditis, pericarditis, or arrhythmias (e.g., prolonged PR interval, decreased QRS voltage, flat T waves, and ST changes).
6. Echocardiography, baseline and follow-up, must be done to detect coronary aneurysm.

COMPLICATIONS

1. Coronary artery disease and coronary aneurysm
   a. Incidence: 20%
   b. At risk for this complication are:
      (1) Young male infants
      (2) Those with delayed treatment
   c. Most complications are reversible.
2. Aneurysm of the peripheral arteries

TREATMENT

1. Hospitalization and cardiology consultation
2. Cardiac monitoring
3. Intravenous gamma globulin
   a. Dose: 2 g/kg single dose to run in 10 to 12 hours
   b. This results in rapid resolution of clinical symptoms and findings.
4. Aspirin
   a. Dose: 80 to 100 mg/kg/day until fever subsides, followed by
   b. 3-4 mg/kg/day until platelet count, ESR, and echocardiogram are normal.

PROGNOSIS

Since high-dose IV gamma globulin therapy was instituted for this disease, mortality has decreased to 0.5%.

KEY POINTS

Kawasaki Disease

- Not all clinical criteria for a diagnosis of Kawasaki disease may be present in a young infant.
- Perineal desquamation seen within the first week of illness is an important diagnostic clue.
- High-dose IV gamma globulin, when used early, results in dramatic clinical improvement.
- Coronary aneurysm is a major complication in untreated patients.

TABLE 12-8
Clinical Features of Kawasaki Disease

Diagnosis is established clinically by fulfilling five of six
 criteria:
   1. Fever
      High, unremitting
      Lasting 5 days or more
      Unresponsive to antipyretics and antibiotics
   2. Skin rash
      Polymorphic
      Nonvesicular
      Erythematous papular lesions
      Scarlatiniform (15% of cases)
      Commonly seen on trunk and extremities
   3. Mucous membrane changes
      Erythematous dry cracked lips
      Erythema of buccal mucosa
      Strawberry tongue
   4. Conjunctivitis
      Bulbar involvement
      Nonexudative
      Bilateral
   5. Changes in distal extremities
      Erythema
      Indurative edema of hands and feet
   6. Cervical lymphadenitis
      Unilateral
      Nonpurulent
      Least constant finding

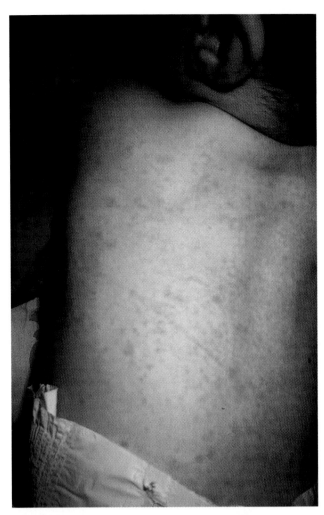

FIGURE 12-13. Erythematous papular eruption.

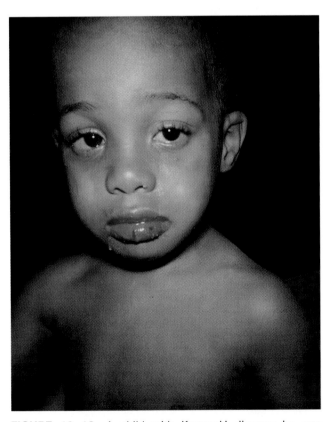

FIGURE 12-12. A child with Kawasaki disease; he was highly febrile and acutely ill.

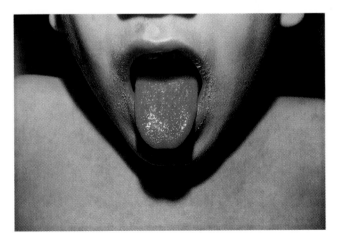

FIGURE 12-14. Strawberry tongue.

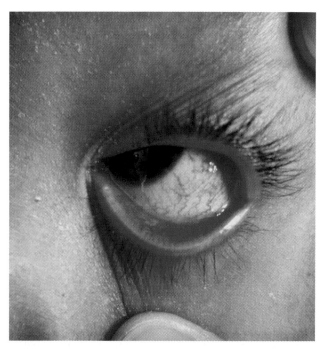

FIGURE 12-15. Kawasaki disease. Nonexudative conjunctivitis.

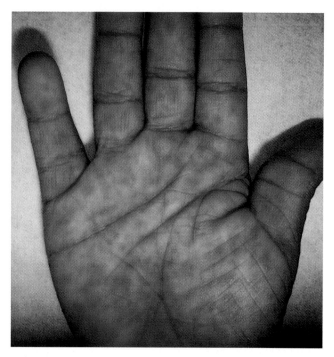

FIGURE 12-17. Hand of a child with measles showing the rash on the palm. In Kawasaki disease, the rash is a diffuse erythema of the hand.

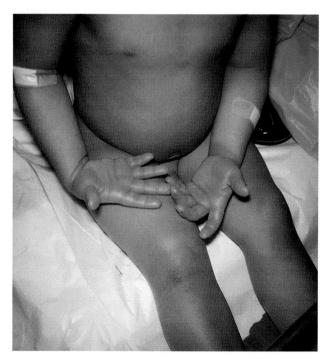

FIGURE 12-16. Kawasaki disease. Erythema and swelling of the hands.

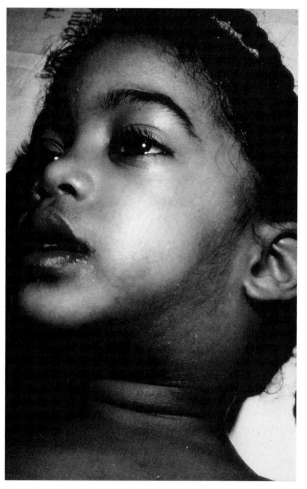

FIGURE 12-18. Kawasaki disease. Nonpurulent unilateral cervical lymphadenitis.

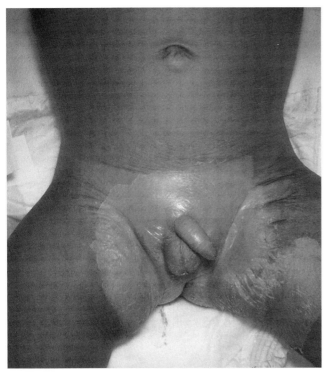

FIGURE 12–19. Kawasaki disease. Perineal desquamation.

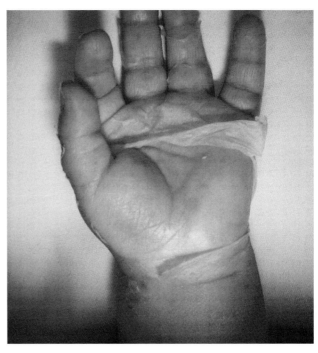

FIGURE 12–21. Desquamation of the palm in a 5-month-old infant with atypical Kawasaki disease.

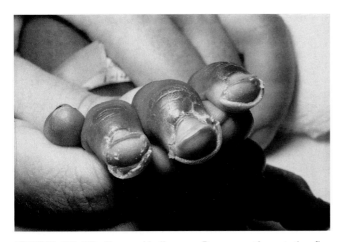

FIGURE 12–20. Kawasaki disease. Desquamation at the fingertips.

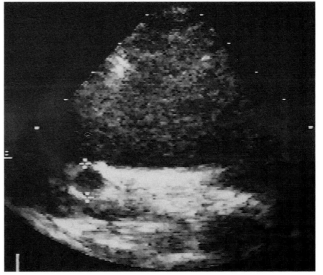

FIGURE 12–22. Kawasaki disease. Two-dimensional echocardiogram showing a giant aneurysm of the right main coronary artery (parasternal short axis view). (Courtesy of Sudha Rao, M.D., State University of New York, Brooklyn, NY.)

Serum Sickness

DEFINITION

A delayed hypersensitivity reaction, type IV immune response, characterized by involvement of the joint, skin, and reticuloendothelial systems.

ETIOLOGY/EPIDEMIOLOGY

1. Animal serum
   a. A prominent cause in the past
   b. Less commonly used now except as antitoxins for clostridial infections, diphtheria, tetanus, and spider and snake envenomations

2. Medications
    a. Antibiotics (penicillin, cephalosporins, strepto-mycin)
    b. Others (hydantoins, thiouracil)
    c. Serum sickness response occurs 2 to 3 weeks after exposure to the medication.

> ### BOX 12–11   *Differential Diagnosis of Serum Sickness*
>
> Acute hypersensitivity drug reaction
> Rheumatic fever
> Systemic lupus erythematosus
> Infectious mononucleosis

PATHOGENESIS

1. Serum sickness is a type IV reaction (Gell and Coombs classification).
2. The molecule of the medication acts as a hapten (incomplete antigen), combines with the patient's protein, and incites antibody production.
3. The antigen-antibody complexes are deposited in the basement membrane of the blood vessels and activate the complement system.
4. Clearance of the immune complexes depends on their size and the effectiveness of the reticuloen-dothelial system.

LABORATORY

1. Complete blood count; leukocyte count and eosin-ophil counts are variable; thrombocytopenia may be seen.

2. Erythrocyte sedimentation rate (ESR) is often in-creased.
3. Decreased serum complement values (C3 and C4)
4. Proteinuria, microscopic hematuria, and hemoglo-binuria may be present.

COMPLICATION

1. Anaphylaxis
2. Carditis (rare)
3. Glomerulonephritis (rare)

TREATMENT

1. The patient recovers in 7 to 10 days if exposure to the offending antigen is discontinued.
2. Antihistamines and nonsteroidal anti-inflammatory agents may be used.
3. In severe cases, systemic corticosteroids may be used.
    a. Prednisone (dose: 1 to 1.5 mg/kg/day)
    b. Duration: 1 to 2 weeks

PROGNOSIS

Self-limiting

KEY POINTS

Serum Sickness

- Antibiotics are now the most common cause of serum sickness.
- The prominent symptoms are rash, joint involve-ment, and lymphadenopathy.

TABLE 12–9
Clinical Features of Serum Sickness

Skin Lesions

Pruritic
Urticaria
Angioedema (face, neck)
Faint erythema with serpiginous border at margins of palmar or plantar skin of the hands, feet, and toes
Onset within 7–14 days after primary exposure

Other Features

Lymphadenopathy (10% to 20%)
Fever and malaise
Myalgia, arthralgia
GI (diarrhea, nausea, abdominal cramps)
Arthritis (10% to 50%)
Multiple joint involvement (knee, wrist, ankle, fingers, toes)

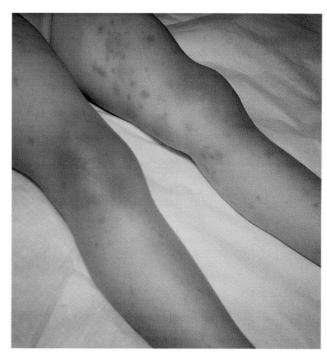

FIGURE 12–23. Serum sickness. Swelling of both knees and urticarial skin eruption.

Sarcoidosis

DEFINITION

A systemic granulomatous disorder of unknown etiology with multisystem involvement, prominently involving the skin, eyes, lungs, and reticuloendothelial system

ETIOLOGY/PATHOGENESIS

1. The exact cause is unknown.
2. T cell-mediated disease resulting in noncaseating granuloma in affected organs

EPIDEMIOLOGY

1. It occurs worldwide but is reported largely in the United States, England, Scandinavian countries, and Japan.
2. In the United States it is seen mostly in the rural communities of the southeastern states.
3. It is 20 times more common in African-Americans than in whites.
4. In children, 75% of cases occur between 9 and 15 years of age.
5. There is equal sex distribution.

BOX 12–12

Clinical Features of Sarcoidosis

Age 4 years and under
  Triad of rash, arthritis, and uveitis
Age 8–15 years
  A multisystem disease that involves primarily the lungs, lymph nodes, and eyes

---

LABORATORY

1. Biopsy of the skin lesion, lymph node, or other tissue demonstrates noncaseating granulomas.
2. Hypergammaglobulinemia
3. Eosinophilia
4. Elevated erythrocyte sedimentation rate (ESR)

TABLE 12–10
Skin Manifestations of Sarcoidosis

Skin Lesions

Papules
Plaques
Nodules
Distribution
  Face
  Extremities
  Buttocks
  Shoulders
  Scars

Other Skin Presentations

Lupus pernio
Erythroderma
Erythema nodosum

---

5. Elevated angiotensin-converting enzyme levels
   a. Correlates with disease activity
   b. Can be used to follow response to treatment
6. Hypercalcemia, hypercalciuria
7. Chest radiograph: bilateral hilar adenopathy, pulmonary infiltrate
8. Abnormal pulmonary function test

BOX 12–13

Differential Diagnosis of Sarcoidosis

Tuberculosis
Rheumatoid arthritis
Systemic lupus erythematosus
Deep fungal infections (e.g., pulmonary mycosis)
Lymphoma
Inflammatory ocular lesions

COMPLICATIONS

1. Pulmonary insufficiency
2. Blindness
3. Renal impairment (secondary to hypercalciuria)

TREATMENT

1. Sarcoidosis in children is usually a self-limiting disease that requires no treatment and resolves in 2 to 3 years.
2. In severely symptomatic cases, systemic corticosteroid may be used (prednisone 1 to 2 mg/kg/day for several weeks, tapering to alternate-day regimen)

PROGNOSIS

Self-limiting in many cases

KEY POINTS

Sarcoidosis

- Sarcoidosis is a multisystem disease that is more common in some population groups.
- Skin, eyes, joints, and lungs are the most commonly affected organ systems.

TABLE 12–11
Clinical Features of Sarcoidosis

Arthritis
  Involves large joints
  Nondestructive in nature
Ocular findings
  Uveitis
  Conjunctival nodules
  Secondary glaucoma
Pulmonary findings
  Bilateral hilar adenopathy
  Pulmonary infiltrates
  Abnormal pulmonary function test results (restrictive lung disease)

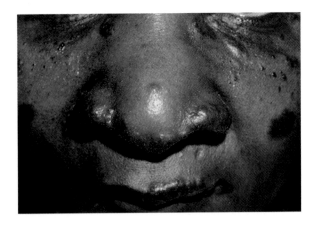

FIGURE 12–24. Sarcoidosis, Nodules on the face.

Acute Rheumatic Fever (ARF)

DEFINITION

An inflammatory illness following group A beta-hemolytic streptococcal (GAS) pharyngeal infection that affects the heart, joints, central nervous system, skin, and subcutaneous tissues.

ETIOLOGY/PATHOGENESIS (see Fig. 12–28)

1. The period of latency between GAS infection and onset of ARF:
   a. For manifestations of arthritis or carditis: about 3 to 4 weeks
   b. For manifestations of Sydenham chorea: about 3 months or longer
2. Acute glomerulonephritis occurs after either GAS skin or pharyngeal infection; ARF occurs *only* after GAS pharyngeal infection.

EPIDEMIOLOGY

1. ARF is the most common cause of acquired heart disease in children and young adults.
2. Affects both sexes equally
3. Age at presentation
   a. Peak incidence: 5 to 15 years of age
   b. Infrequent in early infancy and after age 30
4. An increased number of ARF cases are seen in fall, winter, and early spring.
5. Attack rate of ARF: about 3% following untreated or inadequately treated GAS infection.

CLINICAL FEATURES (see also Table 12–12 and Boxes 12–14 to 12–18)

1. Diagnosis of ARF is suspected when patient presents with any of the major criteria with or without minor criteria.
2. None of the symptoms by themselves, except for chorea, are sufficiently characteristic or pathognomonic of ARF.

LABORATORY

1. Supporting evidence of antecedent GAS infection:

| BOX 12–14 | *Subcutaneous Nodules and ARF* |

Seen in 3% to 5% of patients
Characteristics of nodules: firm, nontender, freely movable, pea-sized
Locations: extensor surfaces of wrists, elbows, knees; scalp, over bony prominences of spinal column
Their presence heralds severe carditis
Usually last for a shorter period of time; rarely may persist up to 4 weeks

---

| BOX 12–15 | *Carditis and ARF* |

Seen in 35% to 40% of patients
Pancarditis (involves pericardium, epicardium, myocardium, and endocardium)
Most frequent murmurs: mitral insufficiency followed by aortic insufficiency (20%)
Pulmonic and tricuspid valves rarely involved
Can potentially cause death of the patient during active phase of illness
Other features:
 Tachycardia (disproportionate to degree of fever, and persistent during sleep)
 Congestive heart failure
 Hyperactive precordium
 Friction rub (pericarditis)

---

   a. Positive throat culture or rapid streptococcal antigen test
   b. Elevated or rising streptococcal antibody titer (antistreptolysin O [ASO] and antideoxyribonuclease B [anti-DNase B])
2. Complete blood count (leukocytosis, normocytic anemia)
3. Erythrocyte sedimentation rate (ESR)

| BOX 12–16 | *Erythema Marginatum and ARF* |

Seen in 5% to 15% of patients
Skin rash
  Begins as pink macule or papules
  Expands to form annular plaques
  Annular plaques with fairly distinct and serpiginous borders
  Lesions vary in size and number
  Evanescent
  Nonpruritic
  Accentuated by warm bath or hot towels
  Confined to trunk and proximal extremities
  Spares face, hands, and feet
  Typically observed at peak activity of carditis and arthritis
  Unaffected by treatment of ARF with anti-inflammatory drugs or other agents

| BOX 12–17 | *Migratory Polyarthritis and ARF* |

Seen in 85% to 95% of patients
Joint involvement
  Polyarticular
  Asymmetrical
  Migratory arthritis of large joints (ankles, knees, wrists, elbows)
  Small joints rarely involved
Develops acutely (hours to overnight)
Joints red, hot, swollen, and *exquisitely tender* (patient will not tolerate even a bed sheet on an affected joint)
Dramatic response to salicylates
Validity of ARF diagnosis should be questioned with lack of resolution of arthritis 48–72 hours after initiation of therapy
Lasts 2–4 weeks with or without treatment
Does not result in chronic joint disease
Described by Lasegue in 1884: *"Rheumatic fever is a disease that licks the joints but bites the heart."*

4. C-reactive protein (CRP)
5. Urine analysis (absence of proteinuria, hematuria)
6. Chest radiograph (cardiomegaly, pulmonary edema)
7. Electrocardiogram
8. Doppler echocardiography (pericardial effusion, valvulitis, myocarditis)
9. To exclude collagen diseases (as indicated): serum antinuclear antibody (ANA), anti-DNA, complement

DIFFERENTIAL DIAGNOSIS

1. Collagen vascular diseases (e.g., juvenile rheuma-

| BOX 12–18 | *Sydenham Chorea (St. Vitus Dance) and ARF* |

Seen in 5% to 10% of patients
Seen predominantly in teenage girls
Presents as
  Sudden, purposeless, jerking, involuntary movements of extremities
  Movements subside during sleep, and are exaggerated by emotions
  Facial grimacing
  Inability to write
  Inability to hold the tongue still when protruded
  Emotional lability
  "Pronator sign": a gradual pronation of hands when arms are raised above the head
Benign manifestation reflecting involvement of basal ganglia and caudate nuclei
Complete resolution of symptoms occurs with no neurologic sequelae

toid arthritis, systemic lupus erythematosus, Lyme disease)
2. Poststreptococcal arthritis
3. Septic arthritis (e.g., gonococcal)
4. Postinfectious reactive arthritides
5. Myocarditis or pericarditis from other causes (e.g., coxsackie virus)
6. Leukemia
7. Huntington chorea

TREATMENT

1. Hospitalization and cardiology consultation
2. Bed rest (for the period of acute carditis)
3. Penicillin or erythromycin (if patient is allergic to penicillin), even if culture for GAS is negative
4. Arthritis or carditis (mild/moderate):
   a. Anti-inflammatory dose of aspirin (usually 90 to 120 mg/kg/day in four divided doses)
   b. Aim for a serum salicylate level of between 20 and 25 mg/dL.
   c. Duration depends on patient's clinical course and response.
5. Severe carditis (pancarditis and/or cardiac failure)
   a. A short course of steroids (e.g., prednisone 2 mg/kg/day given in two divided doses for 2 to 3 weeks)
   b. Digitalis (if indicated)
6. Chorea with severe symptoms: haloperidol, phenobarbital, or valproic acid

PREVENTION

1. Primary prophylaxis: antibiotic treatment of GAS infection to prevent an initial attack of ARF
2. Secondary prophylaxis: continuous antibiotic prophylaxis (as per guidelines of American Heart Association) to prevent colonization or infection by GAS in people in whom ARF has already been diagnosed

PROGNOSIS

1. ARF subsides in 6 weeks in 80% of patients and by 12 weeks in over 90%.
2. Of the five major clinical manifestations of ARF, all eventually disappear with or without treatment leaving no sequelae, with the important exception of carditis.
3. Up to 70% of patients with ARF who develop carditis during the initial episode recover with no residual valvular disease.
4. Between 50% and 100% of patients with two or more recurrences of ARF with carditis experience permanent valvular damage.
5. Patients with chorea (without carditis) may present years later with mitral stenosis.

KEY POINTS

Acute Rheumatic Fever

- No specific laboratory test exists for the diagnosis of ARF.
- Modified Jones criteria form the basis for making the diagnosis of an initial attack of ARF.
- Prevention and treatment of GAS upper respiratory tract infection can prevent ARF.
- Presence of chorea, even without evidence of an antecedent streptococcal infection, indicates ARF until proved otherwise.

TABLE 12–12
Modified Jones Criteria, 1992

Major Criteria	Minor Criteria
Carditis	Arthralgia
Migratory polyarthritis	Fever
Chorea	Elevated acute phase reactants: ESR, C-reactive protein
Erythema marginatum	Prolonged PR interval
Subcutaneous nodules	

An illness characterized by two major criteria or one major and two minor criteria *and* evidence of antecedent GAS infection indicates a high probability of ARF.

Pure chorea and late-onset carditis are exempted from fulfilling the Jones criteria because of their long latent period.

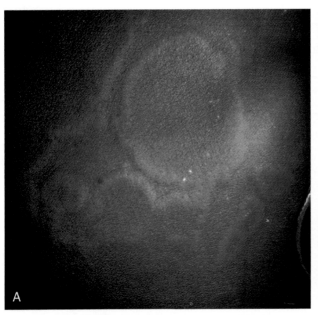
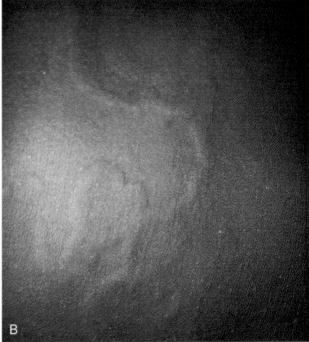

FIGURE 12–25. *A,* Erythema marginatum. Annular plaques (complete rings) of varying sizes with flat, pale centers and fairly distinct, raised erythematous margins. *B,* Note the serpiginous borders formed by a coalescence of several partial rings.

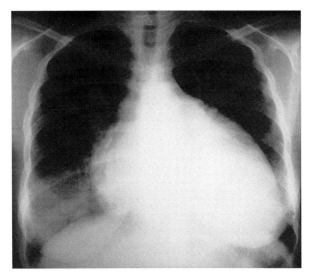

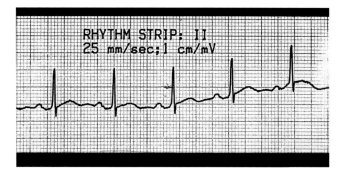

FIGURE 12–27. Electrocardiogram demonstrating prolonged PR interval (0.2 seconds) in a patient with ARF. (Courtesy of Sudha Rao, M.D., State University of New York, Brooklyn, NY.)

FIGURE 12–26. Rheumatic carditis presenting as mitral and aortic insufficiency in a 14-year-old girl with an initial attack of ARF. Frontal view of the chest demonstrating severe cardiomegaly, particularly of the left atrium and left ventricle. There is mild prominence of the central pulmonary vasculature.

FIGURE 12–28. Outline of the various factors involved in the pathogenesis of rheumatic fever. (From Ayoub EM: Acute rheumatic fever. *In* Moss and Adams: Heart Disease in Infants, Children, and Adolescents Including the Fetus and Young Adult, 5th ed. Baltimore, Williams & Wilkins, 1995.)

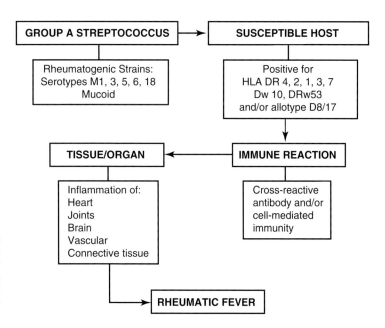

Neurology

Binita R. Shah, M.D. and Teresita A. Laude, M.D.

Neurofibromatosis (NF)

SYNONYMS Von Recklinghausen Disease (NF1)
Acoustic Neurofibromatosis (NF2)

DEFINITION

A hereditary neurocutaneous disorder

ETIOLOGY

1. NF is transmitted as an autosomal dominant trait, with 50% incidence of spontaneous mutation.
2. The gene locus for NF1 is in chromosome 17q; that for NF2 is in chromosome 22q.

EPIDEMIOLOGY

1. The incidence of NF1 is 1 in 3000. It comprises 85% of all cases of NF.
2. The incidence of NF2 is 1 in 35,000. It comprises 15% of all cases of NF.
3. There is equal sex distribution.

PATHOGENESIS

Neurofibromin, a tumor suppressor, is defective. This results in tumor progression.

CLINICAL FEATURES

1. The clinical types of NF are

   NF1: classic or peripheral (see Box 13–1)
   NF2: central or acoustic (see Box 13–2)
   NF3: mixed
   NF4: variant
   NF5: segmental
   NF6: café-au-lait macules only
   NF7: late-onset NF
   NF8: not otherwise specified
2. Associated central nervous system (CNS) findings
   a. Seizures
   b. Learning disability
   c. Hydrocephalus
   d. Headaches
3. Other system findings
   a. Hypertension
   b. Precocious puberty
   c. Hemihypertrophy

BOX 13–1 *Diagnosis of Neurofibromatosis 1 (NF1)*

NIH consensus criteria for diagnosis: two or more of the following:
1. Five or more café-au-lait macules >5 mm in greatest diameter in prepubertal children and >15 mm in postpubertal individuals
2. Two or more neurofibromas (dermal, subcutaneous) or one plexiform neurofibroma
3. Freckling in axillae (Crowe sign) or inguinal regions
4. Optic glioma
5. Two or more Lisch nodules (iris hamartomas); these are seen in >90% of patients >6 years of age
6. Bone lesions (sphenoid dysplasia, scoliosis)
7. A first-degree relative with NF1 by the above criteria

BOX 13–2 *Diagnosis of Neruofibromatosis 2 (NF2)*

Diagnosis is made in the presence of:
1. Bilateral 8th nerve masses (visualized with CT or MRI) *or*
2. First-degree relative with NF2 *and either*
   a. Unilateral 8th nerve deafness *or*
   b. Any two of the following: neurofibroma, meningioma, spinal glioma, schwannoma, juvenile posterior subcapsular lenticular opacity

---

LABORATORY

1. Prenatal diagnosis is possible by DNA analysis.
2. Magnetic resonance imaging (MRI) of the brain and spinal cord
3. Ophthalmologic examination

TREATMENT

1. Genetic counseling
2. Neurologic evaluation and treatment
3. Referral to subspecialists
4. Enroll the patient in the

> National Neurofibromatosis Foundation
> 141 Fifth Avenue, Suite 7-S
> New York, NY 10010
> Tel. (800) 323-7938
>   (212) 460-4980
>
> NF2 Sharing Network
> 10074 Cabachon Court
> Ellicott City, MD 21042
> Tel. (410) 461-5213

PROGNOSIS

In the absence of complications, many patients with neurofibromatosis lead normal long lives.

KEY POINTS

Neurofibromatosis

- Diagnosis is made by fulfilling the criteria set up by the National Institutes of Health.
- A young infant with multiple café-au-lait spots (>5) must be followed carefully for other signs of neurofibromatosis, whether the family history is positive for NF or not.

TABLE 13–1
Complications of Neurofibromatosis

Severe scoliosis
Pheochromocytoma
Neurofibrosarcoma
Chronic myeloid leukemia (may be seen in children with NF and juvenile xanthogranulomas)
Severe hearing loss (NF2)
Blindness (NF2)
Severe cosmetic disability (innumerable neurofibromas)

TABLE 13–2
Differential Diagnosis of Neurofibromatosis

McCune-Albright syndrome
Proteus syndrome
LEOPARD syndrome

LEOPARD stands for: (*l*entigines, *e*lectrocardiographic abnormalities, *o*cular hypertelorism, *p*ulmonic stenosis, *a*bnormal genitalia, *r*etardation of growth, *d*eafness)

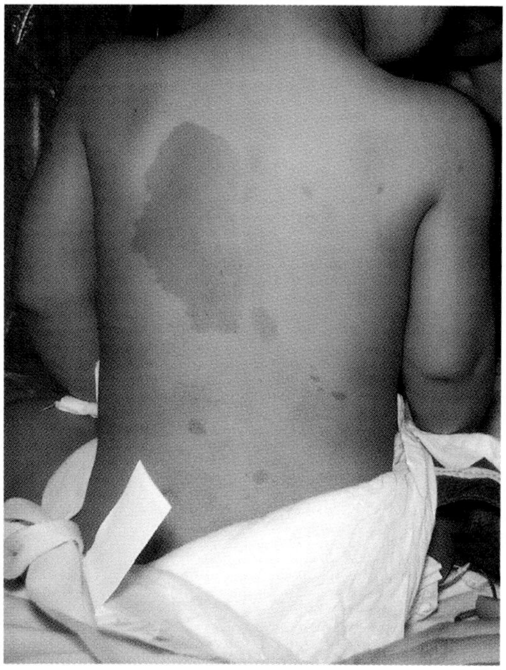

FIGURE 13–1. An 11-month-old with multiple café-au-lait spots who presented with status epilepticus. His mother was known to have neurofibromatosis.

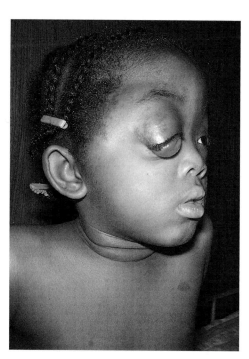

FIGURE 13–2. Optic glioma.

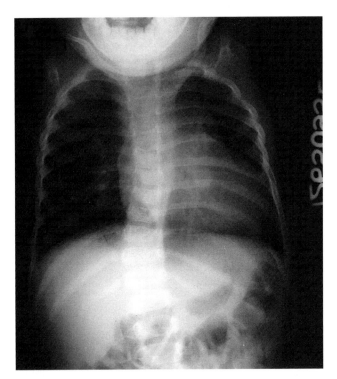

FIGURE 13-3. Severe scoliosis in a 4-year-old girl with neurofibromatosis.

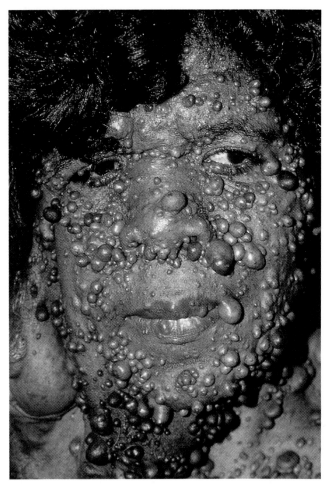

FIGURE 13-4. An adult with neurofibromas covering 98% of the body surface area. She had twin children who both had neurofibromatosis.

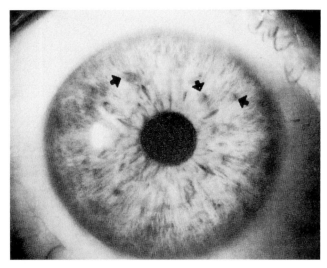

FIGURE 13-5. Lisch nodules.

Tuberous Sclerosis

SYNONYMS   Epiloia
               Bourneville Disease

DEFINITION

Tuberous sclerosis is a hereditary neurocutaneous disorder.

ETIOLOGY/INHERITANCE

1. It is inherited as an autosomal dominant trait with a 50% incidence of spontaneous mutation.
2. The gene loci are in chromosomes 9q and 16p.

EPIDEMIOLOGY

1. It is seen in all races at an incidence of 1 in 10,000.
2. Sex distribution is equal.

PATHOGENESIS

Tuberin, a tumor suppressor, is defective. This results in tumor progression.

LABORATORY

1. Prenatal diagnosis is made by DNA analysis.
2. Computed tomography (CT) scan or magnetic resonance imaging (MRI)

BOX 13–3   *Differential Diagnosis of Tuberous Sclerosis*

Nevus depigmentosus
Idiopathic epilepsy
Periungual wart
Acne vulgaris
Congenital heart disease

---

3. Electroencephalography (EEG)
4. Funduscopic examination
5. Echocardiogram
6. Renal ultrasound
7. Wood lamp examination to detect hypopigmented macule in a white infant

COMPLICATIONS

1. Status epilepticus
2. Malignant brain tumor

TREATMENT

1. A child presenting initially with the characteristic skin lesions must be closely followed.
2. Neurologic evaluation and management
3. Laser removal of the adenoma sebaceum (angiofibromas)
4. Genetic counseling
5. Enroll the patient in the

> National Tuberous Sclerosis Association (NTSA)
> 8000 Corporate Drive, Suite 120
> Landover, MD 20785
> Tel. (800) HURTFUL

PROGNOSIS

Seizures and mental retardation are the major causes of morbidity.

KEY POINTS

Tuberous Sclerosis

- Tuberous sclerosis is characterized by a triad of mental retardation, seizure disorder, and characteristic skin findings.
- The skin findings are hypopigmented macule, adenoma sebaceum, shagreen patch, and periungual fibroma.

TABLE 13–3
Clinical Features of Tuberous Sclerosis

Central Nervous System

Mental retardation (60%)
Seizures, infantile spasms (hypsarrhythmia)
Periventricular calcification

Skin

Hypopigmented (ash leaf) macule
Adenoma sebaceum (angiofibroma)
Shagreen patch (connective tissue nevus)
Periungual fibromas (Koenen tumors)
Facial plaques

Other Findings

Retinal phakomas
Cardiac rhabdomyoma (may be diagnosed intrauterinely from maternal sonogram)
Enamel pits
Gingival fibromas
Renal cysts
Pulmonary cysts

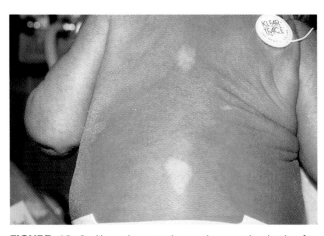

FIGURE 13–6. Hypopigmented macules on the back of a newborn in whom cardiac rhabdomyoma was diagnosed during maternal ultrasound. There was no family history of tuberous sclerosis.

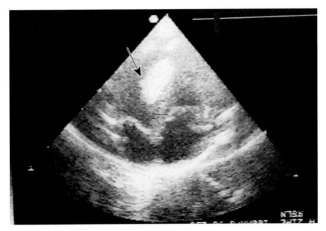

FIGURE 13–7. Cardiac sonogram of the patient in Figure 13–6 shows the intracardiac tumor (*arrow*).

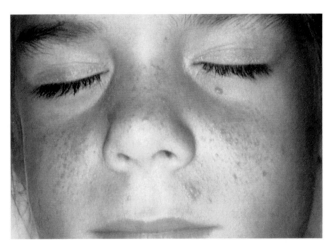

FIGURE 13–9. Adenoma sebaceum. (From Hurwitz S: Clinical Pediatric Dermatology, 2nd ed. Philadelphia, W.B. Saunders, 1993.)

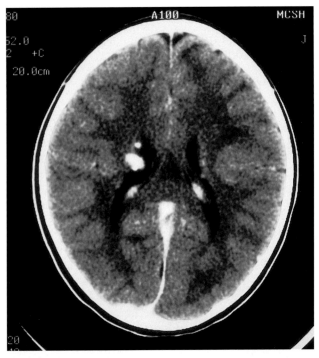

FIGURE 13–8. CT scan in a 2-year-old with tuberous sclerosis demonstrating multiple calcified subependymal nodules extending into the right ventricle.

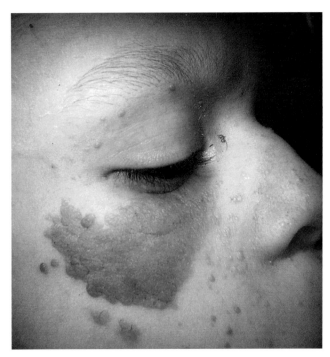

FIGURE 13–10. Facial fibrous plaque in a severely retarded child with tuberous sclerosis.

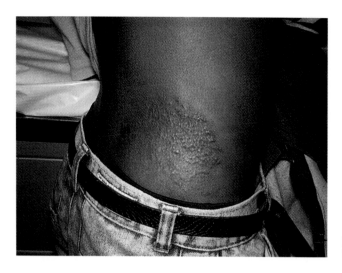

FIGURE 13–11. Tuberous sclerosis. Shagreen patch on the lower back.

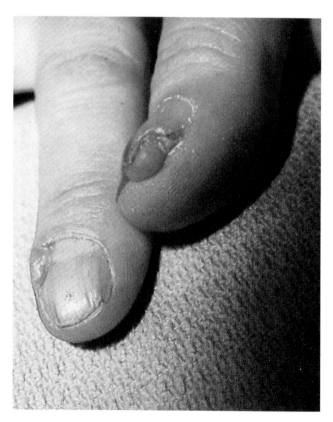

FIGURE 13–12. Tuberous sclerosis. Periungual fibroma.

Sturge-Weber Syndrome

DEFINITION

A nonhereditary or sporadic neurocutaneous disorder

ETIOLOGY

The exact cause is unknown.

EPIDEMIOLOGY

1. It is rare.
2. It has equal sex distribution.

BOX 13–4	*Differential Diagnosis of Sturge-Weber Syndrome*
	Hemangioma PHACE syndrome (*p*osterior fossa brain defects, *h*emangiomas, *a*rterial abnormalities, *c*oarctation of the aorta/cardiac defects, *e*ye abnormalities) Idiopathic epilepsy

LABORATORY

1. Magnetic resonance imaging (MRI)
2. Ophthalmologic examination

COMPLICATION

Progressive soft tissue hypertrophy underlying the port wine stain.

TREATMENT

1. Refer the patient to an ophthalmologist and a neurologist.
2. Laser surgical removal of the port wine stain as early as possible to encourage cosmetic improvement.
3. Enroll the patient in the

    The Sturge-Weber Foundation
    P.O. Box 418
    Mt. Freedom, NJ 07970
    Tel. (800) 627-5482
        (201) 895-4445

PROGNOSIS

The major causes of morbidity are central nervous system and ocular involvement.

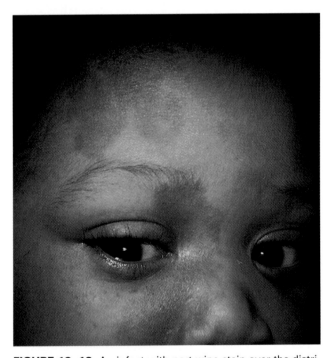

FIGURE 13–13. An infant with port wine stain over the distribution of the trigeminal nerve (V1). He presented with seizures involving the left side of the body.

KEY POINTS

Sturge-Weber Syndrome

- An infant with a port wine stain over the distribution of the ophthalmic division of the trigeminal nerve (V1) must have a screening MRI. Repeat in 2 years if initially negative.
- If the port wine stain is over the maxillary division of the trigeminal nerve (V2), an ophthalmologic examination is necessary to rule out glaucoma.

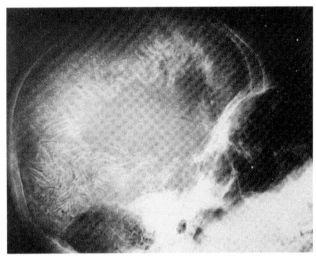

FIGURE 13–14. Sturge-Weber syndrome. Tram-track calcification in the brain cortex (From Spitz JL: Genodermatosis. Baltimore, Williams & Wilkins, 1996.)

TABLE 13–4
Clinical Features of Sturge-Weber Syndrome

Central Nervous System

Seizures (70%)
Mental retardation (50%)
Contralateral hemiparesis
Ipsilateral tram-track intracranial calcification (leptomeningeal angiomatosis)
Cerebral atrophy

Skin

Port wine stain
Over distribution of trigeminal nerve (V1 with or without involvement of V2 and V3)

Eyes

Ipsilateral glaucoma (with V2 involvement)

Spinal Dysraphism

DEFINITION

Incomplete fusion of the midline structures of the embryo's dorsal median region that results in spinal abnormalities that may cause irreversible neurologic damage.

ETIOLOGY

The exact cause is unknown.

EPIDEMIOLOGY

Fifty percent of children with paraspinal skin lesions have underlying spinal dysraphism.

LABORATORY

Magnetic resonance imaging (MRI) of the spine

TREATMENT

Neurosurgical intervention

PROGNOSIS

In diastematomyelia, the neurologic symptoms become progressive.

KEY POINTS

Spinal Dysraphism

- In a child with a paraspinal skin lesion present from birth, an MRI is indicated to detect spinal defects.
- Early recognition and treatment of spinal dysraphism can prevent neurologic damage.

BOX 13–5   *Clinical Features of Spinal Dysraphism*

Paraspinal (lumbosacral) skin birthmarks, except Mongolian spot, may be a marker for spinal dysraphism
Cutaneous lesions (in order of reported frequency)
  Lipomas
  Hypertrichosis
  Dimples
  Hyperpigmentation
  Dermal sinuses
  Atrophic or denuded skin
  Undefined nevus
  Teratoma
Spinal defects include
  Spina bifida
  Tethered cord (diastematomyelia)

TABLE 13–5
Complications of Spinal Dysraphism

Neurologic Symptoms

Urinary or fecal incontinence
Recurrent urinary tract infections
Muscle atrophy
Foot deformities
Weakness and pain
Diminished sensation

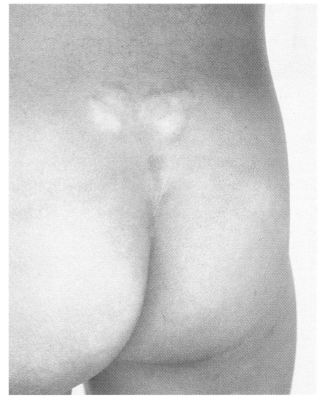

FIGURE 13–16. Midline lipoma.

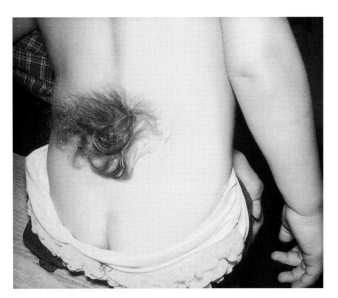

FIGURE 13–15. Sacral hypertrichosis in a child who had a tethered spinal cord.

Bell's Palsy

DEFINITION

1. Bell's palsy is an acute, idiopathic, and unilateral peripheral facial nerve dysfunction.
2. A complete loss of facial movement is defined as paralysis. Paresis refers to an incomplete paralysis. Palsy refers to either a complete or an incomplete paralysis.

ANATOMY (see Fig. 13–17)

1. Bell's palsy is a lower motor neuron facial palsy.
2. It results from a lesion of the 7th nerve nucleus or emergent facial nerve.
3. The most commonly affected portion of the facial nerve lies within the temporal bone; as the facial nerve traverses this bone, three branches arise at different levels:
   a. Greater superficial petrosal nerve, which exits at the geniculate ganglia and innervates the lacrimal and salivary glands
   b. Chorda tympani nerve, which exits near the stylomastoid foramen and supplies taste sensation to anterior two thirds of tongue
   c. Nerve to stapedius muscle, which exits at the posterosuperior portion of the middle ear

---

BOX 13–6   *Differential Diagnosis of Bell's Palsy*

CENTRAL FACIAL PALSY (Upper Motor Neuron Palsy)

Caused by a lesion above the level of the facial nerve nucleus (e.g., brain stem tumors)

Weakness of lower half or two thirds of the face on contralateral side (of the lesion)

Sparing of upper part of the face on contralateral side (of the lesion)

Ability to wrinkle forehead preserved

Ability to close eyes on both sides preserved

Flattening of nasolabial fold on contralateral side (of the lesion)

Inability to retract (drooping) corner of mouth on contralateral side (of the lesion)

Usually results in permanent deficit

Associated neurologic signs and cranial neuropathies

---

4. The facial nerve has motor, sensory, and autonomic functions. It supplies the muscles of the face.

EPIDEMIOLOGY

1. Bell's palsy is the most common type of facial palsy and accounts for 80% of all facial palsies.
2. Annual incidence
   a. About 3 per 100,000 in first decade
   b. About 10 per 100,000 in second decade
   c. About 25 per 100,000 in adults

3. There is no predilection for age, sex, or race.

PATHOGENESIS

1. There is no readily identifiable cause for Bell's palsy.
2. Pathogenesis is still poorly understood. Several postulated theories include:
   a. An immune-mediated demyelination
   b. Entrapment theory:
      (1) Edema and compression of the facial nerve within the bony facial canal leads to ischemia.
      (2) Narrowest part of the facial canal is at the meatal foramen at the distal end of the internal auditory canal, and is the site of ischemia.

CLINICAL FEATURES

1. Onset is heralded by:
   a. Preceding upper respiratory tract infection (in >50% of patients)
   b. First sign: usually pain or tingling in the ear ipsilateral to the site of subsequent facial palsy
   c. Rapid progression occurs over the next 48 hours.
2. Typical and uncommon features (see Table 13–6)
3. Otoscopic examination and remainder of neurologic examination are normal.

LABORATORY (as indicated)

1. Other causes of facial palsy must be excluded by a thorough history and physical examination including a neurologic examination.
2. Complete blood count
3. Lyme titers
4. Electromyography of the facial nerve to determine the degree of neural degeneration and to predict recovery
5. Topognostic tests (to determine the site of the lesion—e.g., Schirmer tear test, stapedial reflex test, evaluation of salivation and taste) generally are not necessary.

BOX 13–7   *Bell's Palsy*

Recovery from palsy confirms the diagnosis of Bell's palsy

TREATMENT/PROGNOSIS

1. Complete recovery occurs in 60% to 80% of children beginning in the 2nd to 3rd week of illness.
2. In a large series of 1011 patients:
   a. In 85% of patients the first sign of recovery became evident within 3 weeks after onset.
   b. For the remaining 15%, recovery occurred 3 to 6 months later.
3. Most patients recover completely without treatment.

4. Corticosteroid therapy
   a. Despite a lack of proven efficacy, steroids within 5 days of onset of palsy are commonly used.
   b. Prednisone 60 mg/day orally for 3 days followed by a tapering dose over the next 7 days is one suggested regimen.
5. Corneal protection to prevent exposure keratopathy is the most important treatment.
   a. Application of artificial tears during daytime
   b. Eyeglasses while outdoors
   c. Ointment at bedtime
   d. A moisture chamber at night is preferred.
   e. Eye patch has a potential risk of scratching the cornea and should be avoided.

KEY POINTS

Bell's Palsy

- Most common type of facial palsy
- Causes unilateral weakness of the entire face
- Diagnosis is made largely by excluding infectious or noninfectious diseases, trauma, and central nervous system tumors causing facial palsy.
- In an upper motor neuron facial palsy, the ability to close the eye and to wrinkle the forehead is preserved because the upper face is innervated bilaterally from the motor cortex.

TABLE 13–6
Clinical Features of Bell's Palsy

Typical Features

All muscles on affected side of face are involved
Flattening of nasolabial fold
Drooping of corner of mouth
Inability to close eye ipsilaterally
Inability to wrinkle forehead ipsilaterally
Facial weakness when asked to puff out cheeks against resistance

Other Features (May Be Present)

Impairment of ipsilateral lacrimation
Hyperacusis (painful sensitivity to loud sounds) in affected ear (if stapedial nerve is affected)
Heaviness or numbness in the face (sensory loss is rarely demonstrable)
Loss of taste on anterior two thirds of tongue
Difficulty in eating and drinking with dribbling of liquids from the weak corner of the mouth

---

TABLE 13–7
Differential Diagnosis of Bell's Palsy

Central facial palsy (see Box 13–6)
Facial palsy from other causes; examples:
  Infections
    Lyme disease
    Acquired immune deficiency syndrome (AIDS)
    Otitis media (see p. 158)
    Mastoiditis
    Temporal lobe abscess
    Chickenpox
    Infectious mononucleosis
    Ramsay-Hunt syndrome
      Herpes zoster infection of geniculate ganglia
      Presents with facial palsy, vesicles on pinna or in external auditory canal
  Noninfectious diseases
    Guillain-Barré syndrome
    Diabetes
    Sarcoidosis
    Blunt or penetrating temporal bone or facial trauma
    Parotid gland tumors

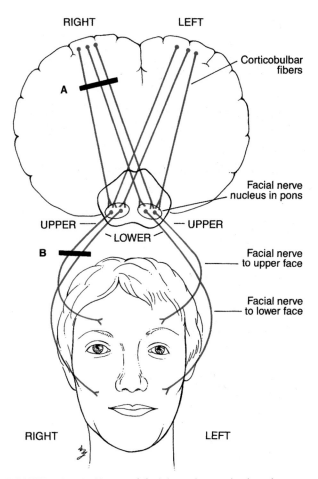

FIGURE 13–17. Types of facial weakness. Lesion *A* causes an upper motor nerve palsy that produces contralateral weakness of the lower face but spares the contralateral forehead. Lesion *B* causes a lower motor nerve palsy that produces total paralysis of the ipsilateral face. (From Swartz MH: Textbook of Physical Diagnosis, 2nd ed. Philadelphia, W.B. Saunders, 1994.)

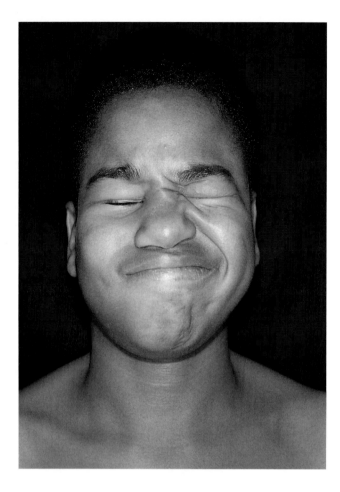

FIGURE 13–18. Bell's palsy in a 12-year-old adolescent (onset 12 hours prior to this picture). When the patient was asked to smile, close the eyes, raise the eyebrows, whistle, or puff out the cheeks, flattening of the nasolabial fold and incomplete closure of the eye were seen on the right side. The remainder of the neurologic examination was completely normal. He completely recovered from Bell's palsy in 4 weeks with no therapy.

Craniosynostosis

DEFINITION

Craniosynostosis is premature closure of one or more of the cranial sutures.

ANATOMY/PATHOGENESIS

1. Principal sutures of the infant's skull:
   a. Sagittal
   b. Coronal
   c. Lambdoid
   d. Metopic
2. Normally, skull growth occurs perpendicular to suture lines.
3. If fusion of a suture takes place before or soon after birth, it inhibits the growth of adjacent bone perpendicular to the course of the fused suture.
4. Rapid brain growth during early infancy requires expansion of the skull, which is forced to grow parallel to the fused suture (e.g., premature closure of the sagittal suture prevents growth in the coronal dimension, causing skull growth parallel to the sagittal suture, resulting in an elongated, narrow head).

5. Deformity of skull results from
   a. Reduced skull diameter in the perpendicular direction
   b. Compensatory and abnormal skull growth in directions permitted by open sutures and fontanels
6. Types of craniosynostosis
   a. Simple craniosynostosis: a single suture is involved
   b. Compound craniosynostosis: multiple sutures are involved

ETIOLOGY

1. Craniosynostosis can occur as an isolated defect or as part of a syndrome with other malformations.
2. Primary craniosynostosis
   a. Etiology is unknown.
   b. One or more sutures are closed owing to abnormality of skull development.
   c. Deformity is present at birth, and synostosis can lead to restriction of brain growth.
3. Secondary craniosynostosis
   a. Sutures close and skull fails to grow *secondary to* failure of brain growth (e.g., brain atrophy or agenesis, microcephaly).

b. Secondary to a known disorder
   (1) Hyperthyroidism
   (2) Mucopolysaccharidosis
   (3) Rickets (familial hypophosphatemic rickets)
   (4) Thalassemia
4. Syndromic
   a. With scaphocephaly: Marfan, trisomy 18, or Russell-Silver syndrome
   b. With brachycephaly: Crouzon, Down, Carpenter, Apert, or Pfeiffer syndrome
   c. With trigonocephaly: 9p-, 13q-, or fetal valproate syndrome

EPIDEMIOLOGY

1. Estimated incidence of single or multiple sutures: about 1 in 2000 live births
2. No racial predilection
3. Most common types of simple craniosynostosis (in decreasing order of frequency):
   a. Sagittal synostosis (about 55% of cases)
   b. Unilateral or bilateral coronal synostosis (about 20% to 25% of cases)
   c. Lambdoid synostosis
   d. Metopic synostosis
4. Compound craniosynostosis (affecting two or more sutures): about 15% of cases

INHERITANCE

1. Majority of cases of simple craniosynostosis are sporadic.
2. Familial (autosomal dominant more common than autosomal recessive)
   a. Coronal synostosis (about 10% of cases; especially when coronal synostosis occurs in association with Apert, Crouzon, or Carpenter syndrome)
   b. Sagittal synostosis (about 2% of cases)

CLINICAL FEATURES (see also Table 13–8)

1. Scaphocephaly or dolichocephaly (sagittal synostosis)
   a. Secondary to early fusion of sagittal suture
   b. Male-female ratio is 4:1
   c. As the brain expands, the coronal and lambdoidal sutures are widened and fronto-occipital elongation takes place while the parietal protuberances are absent.
2. Brachycephaly (bilateral coronal synostosis)
   a. Short, broad head
   b. Slight predilection for females

LABORATORY

1. Diagnosis is usually made clinically by the configuration of the head.
2. Affected suture can usually be palpated as a prominent, elevated bony ridge in majority of patients.
3. Funduscopy (to look for papilledema and/or optic atrophy)

4. Radiographs of skull (show fusion of the suture(s) and configuration of the skull)
5. Computed tomography scan of head
6. Cytogenetic studies—in a child with craniosynostosis and multiple malformations that do not fit one of the known disorders

COMPLICATIONS

1. Increased intracranial pressure (ICP)
2. Papilledema
3. Optic atrophy
4. Severe unilateral coronal synostosis can cause exophthalmos, strabismus, nystagmus, blindness.

TREATMENT

1. Neurosurgical consultation
2. Principles of management
   a. Correction of the cranial deformity
   b. Prevention or relief of the effects of cranial or orbital compression
   c. Patients with stenosis of multiple cranial sutures should be operated on as soon as possible after birth to prevent the effects of cerebral compression during the period of most rapid growth.
   d. Patients with stenosis of one cranial suture can be operated on electively in early infancy (at 6 weeks of life).
3. Indications for surgery
   a. Evidence of increased ICP
   b. Presence of optic atrophy or papilledema
   c. Presence of severe exophthalmos with exposure keratitis
   d. Cosmetic reasons
4. For a single suture synostosis, the usual approach is a linear craniectomy (parallel to the prematurely fused suture).
5. For a patient with multiple suture synostosis, a staged operation with or without orbital decompression may be required.

KEY POINTS

Craniosynostosis

- Patients with craniosynostosis have a hard, nonmovable bony ridge over the involved suture and an *abnormally shaped* skull.
- A *normally shaped* small head with closed sutures is secondary to failure of the brain to grow (e.g., microcephaly).
- Most common type of primary craniosynostosis results from premature fusion of the sagittal suture.
- With premature closure of one suture, the consequences are usually cosmetic.
- With closure of two or more sutures, the consequences include restricted brain growth, increased ICP, and visual complications.

TABLE 13–8
Craniosynostosis

Sutures Involved	Cranial Shape

Sagittal	Scaphocephaly or dolichocephaly
	    Boat-shaped, long, narrow head; absent parietal protuberances
	    Prominent occiput, broad forehead, a small or absent anterior fontanel

Coronal	Brachycephaly Broad, short, square head; limited growth in occipitofrontal diameter
Lambdoid	Brachycephaly Small, flattened occiput with a broad and increased height of calvaria
Metopic	Trigonocephaly Bullet-shaped head (keel-shaped forehead), hypotelorism

Unilateral coronal	Frontal plagiocephaly
	    Unilateral flattening of forehead, elevation of ipsilateral orbit and eyebrow, accentuation of frontal
	        bone on opposite side

Unilateral lambdoid	Occipital plagiocephaly Unilateral occipital flattening, accentuation of ipsilateral frontal bone
Coronal and sagittal	Oxycephaly or acrocephaly or turricephaly Growth excessive toward vertex; pointed, narrow, tower-shaped head

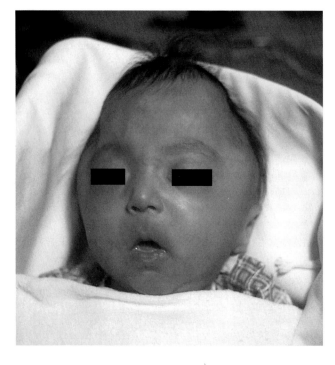

FIGURE 13–19. Trigonocephaly in a neonate due to closure of metopic sutures.

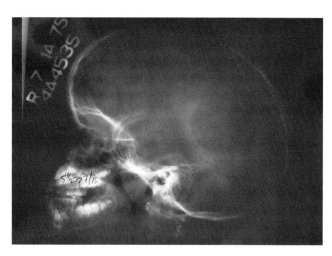

FIGURE 13–20. Sagittal craniosynostosis. Lateral view of the skull demonstrates a long, narrow skull (scaphocephaly) secondary to premature closure of the sagittal suture.

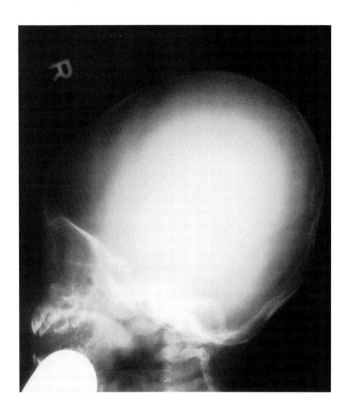

FIGURE 13-21. Coronal craniosynostosis (brachycephaly). Lateral view of the infant skull demonstrates an abnormally short cranium due to prematurely fused coronal sutures.

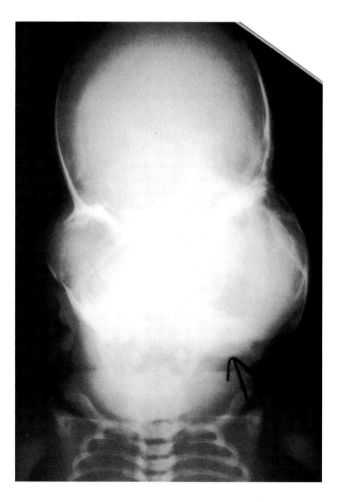

FIGURE 13-22. Cloverleaf skull in thanatophoric dysplasia resulting from intrauterine sutural synostosis and hydrocephalus. AP view of the skull demonstrates its characteristic trilobed appearance (*arrow*).

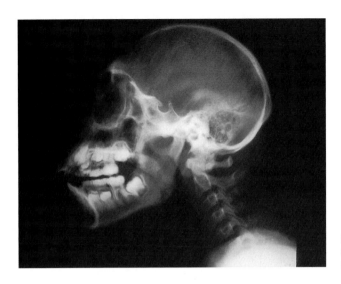

FIGURE 13–23. Microcephaly. Lateral skull view in a 6-year-old girl clearly demonstrates a markedly small but "normally shaped" cranium. Note the ape-like slope of the forehead.

Neural Tube Defects

DEFINITION

A group of clinically apparent or occult congenital malformations resulting from failure of neural tube closure. *Patterns of neural tube defects include:*

1. Anencephaly (see p. 437)
2. Meningomyelocele (see p. 438)
3. Meningocele (see p. 440)
4. Encephalocele (see p. 441)
5. Spina bifida occulta
6. Dermal sinus
7. Tethered cord
8. Syringomyelia
9. Diastematomyelia
10. Lipoma involving conus medullaris

ETIOLOGY/INHERITANCE

1. The precise cause of neural tube defects remains unknown.
2. Factors that have been implicated in producing neural tube defects include:
   a. Maternal nutritional or vitamin (folic acid) deficiencies
   b. Gestational diabetes
   c. Maternal hyperthermia during days 20 to 28 of gestation
   d. Chemicals
   e. Environmental factors (exposure to radiation)
   f. Low socioeconomic status
   g. Genetic susceptibility
   h. Drugs used during pregnancy (1st trimester)
      (1) Valproic acid (neural tube defects seen in 1% to 2% of pregnancies)
      (2) Carbamazepine
      (3) Alcohol
3. Recurrence risk of neural tube defects in subsequent pregnancies after the birth of an anencephalic infant is about 4% to 5%; this risk in-

creases to 10% if the couple has had two previously affected pregnancies.

EPIDEMIOLOGY

1. Neural tube defects account for most congenital anomalies of the central nervous system (CNS).
2. Incidence in the United States is 1 in 1000 live births (not including occult defects).
3. A continuous decline in the incidence of all forms of neural tube defects has been seen for the following reasons:
   a. Prophylactic periconceptional use of folic acid in women who have had an infant with a neural tube defect
   b. Prenatal diagnosis and termination of the affected pregnancy

PATHOGENESIS (see Fig. 13–24)

1. Neural tube defects result from failure of the neural tube to close spontaneously between the 3rd and 4th weeks of gestation.

> **BOX 13–8**   *Prevention of Neural Tube Defects*
>
> United States Public Health Service recommendations for prevention of neural tube defects:
> All women of childbearing age
>   Folic acid 0.4 mg/day (minimum daily requirement of folic acid is 0.4 mg) in order to reduce risk of conceiving a child with a neural tube defect
> Women who previously have given birth to an affected infant with a neural tube defect:
>   Folic acid: 4.0 mg/day beginning 1 month prior to conception through 3 months of pregnancy

2. Normally, the rostral end of the neural tube closes on the 23rd day, and the caudal neuropore closes by the 27th day.

ANTENATAL DIAGNOSIS

1. Amniotic fluid alpha-fetoprotein (AFP) measurement
   a. Elevated values at the beginning of the 2nd trimester
   b. Detected in early pregnancy so that termination of pregnancy is possible
   c. Extremely high levels indicate a large open defect.
   d. False-negative results are unusual except when the lesion is completely covered by skin.
2. Maternal serum AFP measurement
   a. Less reliable than amniotic fluid AFP levels
   b. Detects 50% to 90% of open defects
   c. False-negative rate may be as high as 20%
3. Fetal real-time ultrasonography
   a. Between 14th and 16th weeks of gestation

b. Sensitivity approaches almost 100% in diagnosis of myelomeningocele and anencephaly (absence of fetal skull).

PREVENTION

1. Folic acid supplements (see Box 13–8)
2. Close monitoring of successive pregnancies in couples who have had an infant with a neural tube defect; monitoring includes amniocentesis, determination of AFP, and sonogram.

KEY POINTS

Neural Tube Defects

■ Neural tube defects account for most congenital anomalies of the CNS.
■ Failure of the neural tube to close allows excretion of fetal substances such as AFP into the amniotic fluid.
■ Amniotic fluid or maternal serum AFP values serve as biochemical markers for a neural tube defect.

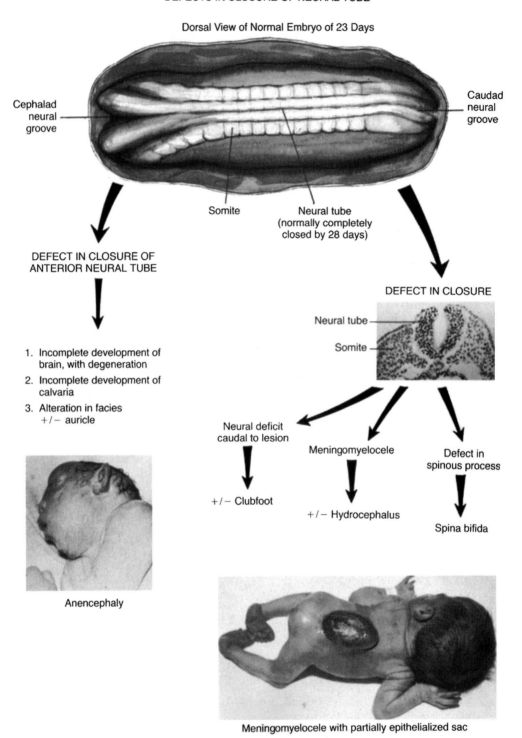

DEFECTS IN CLOSURE OF NEURAL TUBE

Dorsal View of Normal Embryo of 23 Days

Cephalad neural groove

Caudad neural groove

Somite

Neural tube (normally completely closed by 28 days)

DEFECT IN CLOSURE OF ANTERIOR NEURAL TUBE

1. Incomplete development of brain, with degeneration
2. Incomplete development of calvaria
3. Alteration in facies +/− auricle

DEFECT IN CLOSURE

Neural tube

Somite

Neural deficit caudal to lesion

Meningomyelocele

Defect in spinous process

+/− Clubfoot

+/− Hydrocephalus

Spina bifida

Anencephaly

Meningomyelocele with partially epithelialized sac

FIGURE 13–24. Developmental pathogenesis of anencephaly and meningomyelocele. (From Jones KL: Smith's Recognizable Patterns of Human Malformations, 5th ed. Philadelphia, W.B. Saunders, 1997.)

Anencephaly

SYNONYM   Aprosencephaly with Open
                    Cranium

DEFINITION

A severe defect in closure at the anterior portions of the neural tube

ETIOLOGY (see p. 434)

EPIDEMIOLOGY

1. Incidence: about 1 to 5 per 1000 live births
2. Greatest frequency of anencephaly is seen in Ireland and Wales.
3. It occurs more frequently in girls than in boys.
4. It occurs more frequently in whites than in African-Americans.
5. About 50% of anencephalic pregnancies are associated with polyhydramnios.

PATHOGENESIS/CLINICAL FEATURES (see Fig. 13–24)

1. Normally the neural tube is completely fused by 28 days.
2. A defect in closure of the neural groove to form an intact neural tube is the initiating event, which is subsequently followed by secondary consequences.
3. Anencephaly ⇒ secondary consequences
   a. Major portions of the central nervous system are either absent or malformed.
      (1) Forebrain: unfused, incompletely developed; usually degenerates in utero, producing a hemorrhagic, fibrotic, nonfunctioning mass
      (2) Cerebral hemispheres and cerebellum: usually absent
      (3) Hypothalamus, pituitary glands: usually absent
      (4) Brain stem, spinal cord, optic nerve: usually malformed
      (5) Cervical vertebral abnormalities
   b. Calvarium: incompletely developed; frontal, parietal, and portions of occipital bones are usually absent

   c. Facial features, auricular development: variable degree of deformities
   d. Cleft palate
   e. Malformations of other organs: gastrointestinal tract, kidneys, heart, lungs, skeleton, and adrenal glands (hypoplasia)

ANTENATAL DIAGNOSIS (see p. 435)

1. Amniotic fluid alpha-fetoprotein (AFP) measurement
2. Maternal AFP measurement
3. Ultrasonography (between 14th and 16th weeks of gestation) reveals absence of the fetal skull, confirming the diagnosis.

LABORATORY

Clinical diagnosis based on a distinct appearance

TREATMENT

1. No specific treatment is available for a newborn with anencephaly.
2. Because anencephaly is incompatible with life, such a newborn may be considered a potential organ donor for transplantation.
3. Counseling and moral support are needed for the family.

PREVENTION (see Box 13–8)

1. Close monitoring of successive pregnancies in couples who have had an anencephalic infant is needed, including amniocentesis, determination of AFP, and sonogram.
2. Antenatal detection of anencephaly is usually followed by elective termination of the pregnancy.

KEY POINTS

Anencephaly

- A defect in closure at the anterior portion of the neural tube
- Incompatible with survival
- Fetuses that are not aborted are stillborn, or newborns die within several days.

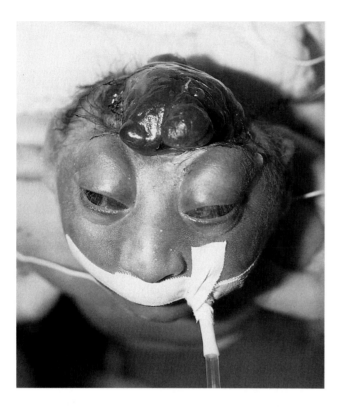

FIGURE 13–25. Anencephaly. A newborn with a distinct appearance with a large defect of calvarium, meninges, and scalp associated with a rudimentary brain. (Courtesy of Nathan Rudolph, M.D., State University of New York, Brooklyn, NY.)

Meningomyelocele

SYNONYM   Myelomeningocele

DEFINITION

Meningomyelocele results from failure of the posterior neural tube to close. Both meningeal and neural components protrude through a defect in the vertebral column.

ETIOLOGY/INHERITANCE (see Fig. 13–24)

1. Etiology of meningomyelocele is poorly understood.
2. Genetic susceptibility
   a. Risk of recurrence after one affected child: about 3% to 4%
   b. Risk of recurrence after two affected children: about 10%
   c. Multifactorial inheritance; occasionally mendelian or chromosomal

EPIDEMIOLOGY

1. Incidence: 1 in 500 to 1000 live births
2. Lesion may arise at any point on the vertebral column from C1 to the coccyx.
3. Most common site:
   a. Lumbosacral region: 75% of cases
   b. Lumbar or sacral segments

ANTENATAL DIAGNOSIS (see p. 435)

CLINICAL FEATURES

1. A cystic sac covered by a thin layer of partially epithelialized tissue in the lumbosacral region (most common site). Neural tissue may be visible beneath the membrane.
2. Leakage of cerebrospinal fluid (CSF) may be present.
3. Neurologic deficits in motor and sensory functions (below the level of the lesion and depending on

---

BOX 13–9   *Meningomyelocele*

Lesion is similar to meningocele but has associated abnormalities in structure and position of spinal cord or cauda equina
It contains
  Meninges
  Nerve roots of cauda equina
  Neural tissue including dysplastic spinal cord
It produces dysfunction of
  Peripheral and central nervous system
  Genitourinary tract
  Skeleton
  Skin

extent of neural involvement) involving the lower extremities and bladder and bowel functions
   a. Lesions at L1–L2 or above: complete paraplegia with no functional ability
   b. Lesions at L3–S1: able to ambulate with or without leg braces
   c. Lesions in the lower sacral region: No impairment of motor function; bowel and bladder incontinence with lack of sensation in the perineal area
4. Associated congenital anomalies are present in all patients except a few (see Table 13–9).

LABORATORY

1. Diagnosis is usually apparent at birth.
2. Computed tomography or magnetic resonance imaging of the head can detect Arnold-Chiari malformation and/or hydrocephalus.
3. Electromyography assesses motor function in the lower extremity.
4. Baseline assessment of serum electrolytes, urea nitrogen, and creatinine.

COMPLICATIONS

1. Meningitis
2. Ventriculitis
3. Urinary tract infection
4. Pyelonephritis
5. Reflux leading to hydronephrosis

TREATMENT

1. Counseling about the neurologic disabilities, treatment plan, and emotional support for the family
2. Multidisciplinary team approach that includes pediatrician, neurosurgeon, neurologist, orthopedist, urologist, gastroenterologist, social worker, and physical therapist
3. Surgery for repair of meningomyelocele:
   a. Controversial whether urgent repair is required to preserve existing neurologic function and prevent further deterioration. Delays in surgery for several days have shown similar long-term results.

TABLE 13–9
Meningomyelocele and Associated Congenital Anomalies

Arnold-Chiari malformation type II
  Present in 100% of cases
  Complex anomaly with skull, dura, brain, spine, and cord manifestations
  Hind brain abnormality consisting of a small posterior fossa and impaction of posterior cerebellar vermis through the foramen magnum
Noncommunicating hydrocephalus
  About 80% of cases
  Secondary to aqueductal forking
Other anomalies include syringomyelia, double spinal cord (50% to 90% of cases)
Congenital heart disease
Intestinal anomalies (duodenal atresia or pyloric stenosis)
Klippel-Feil anomaly

---

b. Immediate repair is indicated in the presence of a CSF leak (to prevent meningitis).
4. Surgery for a shunting procedure for patients with hydrocephalus
5. Functional ambulation is assisted with the use of braces or canes.
6. For a neurogenic bladder:
   a. Parents are taught about regular intermittent catheterization of bladder to reduce residual volume and prevent recurrent urinary tract infections.
   b. Urine cultures, renal function tests, renal ultrasound examinations, and renal scans are monitored as required.
7. For patients with bowel incontinence, enemas or suppositories, that allow bowel evacuation at a predetermined time, are used as required (e.g., once or twice a day).

PROGNOSIS

1. Mortality rate (in children who are treated aggressively): approximately 10% to 15%
2. Increased incidence of seizures and learning disabilities compared with general population
3. Intelligence is normal in about 70% of survivors.

KEY POINTS

Meningomyelocele

- Most severe form of dysraphism involving the vertebral column
- Most common location is in the lumbosacral region
- The more rostral the meningomyelocele, the more likely hydrocephalus will be present.

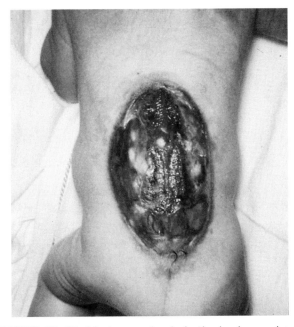

FIGURE 13–26. Meningomyelocele in the lumbosacral area (Courtesy of Sanjivan Patel, M.D., Long Island College Hospital, Brooklyn, NY.)

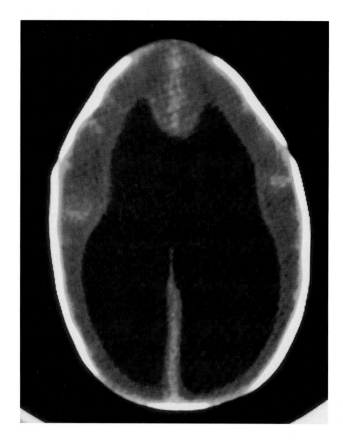

FIGURE 13-27. Severe hydrocephalus. CT scan of an infant with Arnold-Chiari malformation, type II and meningomyelocele. There is marked ballooning of both ventricles, causing the septum to be thinned to the point of nonvisualization.

Meningocele

DEFINITION

A herniation of the meninges through a defect in the posterior vertebral arches

CLINICAL FEATURES (see also Table 13-10)

Anterior meningocele

1. Projects into pelvis through a defect in the sacrum
2. Common presenting signs and symptoms secondary to compression by the increasing size of the meningocele:
   a. Constipation
   b. Bladder dysfunction
3. Associated anomalies include rectovaginal fistula and vaginal septa in female patients.

LABORATORY

1. Plain radiographs of the underlying spine
2. To exclude the presence of neural tissue or associated anomalies (e.g., tethered spinal cord)
   a. Computed tomogram (CT) with metrizamide, *or*
   b. Magnetic resonance imaging
3. CT scan of head to exclude hydrocephalus

TREATMENT

1. Most meningoceles are well covered with full-thickness skin and usually pose no immediate threat to the patient.
2. Surgery
   a. Indicated immediately: if cerebrospinal fluid (CSF) is leaking or skin covering the sac is thin
   b. Elective: Asymptomatic patients with a normal neurologic examination

PROGNOSIS

Excellent

KEY POINTS

Meningocele

- Fluctuant midline cystic mass most frequently seen along the vertebral column in the low back
- Meningocele may transilluminate.

BOX 13-10	*Meningocele*
Does not contain neural tissue Patients have no neurologic deficits	

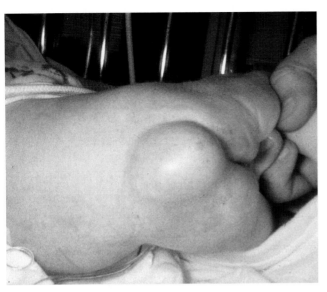

FIGURE 13–28. Meningocele covered with full-thickness skin in the lumbosacral area. (Courtesy of Sanjivan Patel, M.D., Long Island College Hospital, Brooklyn, NY.)

TABLE 13–10
Clinical Features of Meningocele

Most common location: low back
Uncommon location: cranium (see p. 10)
A cystic dilatation of the meninges associated with spina bifida and a defect in the overlying skin
Fluctuant midline mass along the vertebral column
Usually well covered with full-thickness skin
Rarely, cerebrospinal fluid may be leaking and skin may be thin
Transillumination may be positive
Spinal cord and nerve roots assume a normal position in the spinal canal
Spinal cord is usually normal in structure
Tethering, syringomyelia, or diastematomyelia may be present

Encephalocele

SYNONYM   Exencephaly

DEFINITION

A herniation of the neural tissue (meningeal sac and brain) through a congenital midline cranial defect (cranium bifidum).

EPIDEMIOLOGY

1. Estimated incidence: 1 to 3 per 10,000 live births
2. One tenth as common as neural tube closure defects involving the spine
3. Europe and North America: occipital encephaloceles are most common
4. Southeast Asia (especially Thailand): frontal encephaloceles are more common
5. Encephalocele may occur as an isolated anomaly or may be associated with meningomyelocele or amniotic band syndrome or with some genetic syndromes (e.g., Meckel-Gruber syndrome).

> **BOX 13–11**   *Locations of Encephalocele*
>
> Occipital (posterior) encephalocele: about 75% of cases
> Anterior encephalocele: about 20% of cases; includes any of the following
> Frontal
> Nasofrontal
> Nasopharyngeal
> Orbital region
> Parietal region: unusual

ETIOLOGY (see p. 434)

PATHOLOGY

1. Neural tissue may include cerebral cortex, cerebellum, and portions of the brain stem, ventricular system, or choroid plexuses.
2. Meninges and neural tissue within the encephalocele may be completely dysplastic or may retain a relatively well organized architecture.
3. Calcifications are common, and lesion may also contain ectopic ossified fragments.
4. Intracranial brain may be malformed but not as severely as neural tissue within the encephalocele.

ANTENATAL DIAGNOSIS (see p. 435)

1. Ultrasound diagnosis: protrusion of brain tissue within a meningeal sac *with* a bony calvarial defect
2. Maternal serum alpha-fetoprotein level

CLINICAL FEATURES (see also Tables 13–11 to 13–14 and Box 13–11)

1. Nearly always a midline mass
2. Size varies
   a. May be a very small sac that may be covered by hair and thus go unnoticed
   b. May be a very large cyst-like mass that may be larger than the cranium
   c. Although some encephaloceles may reach gigantic proportions, the size of the external lesion gives little information about its contents.
3. Sac
   a. May be pedunculated or sessile
   b. May be completely covered by skin (with or without some denuded area) or by just a thin, parchmentlike membrane

4. Other associated findings:
   a. Obstructive hydrocephalus due to aqueduct stenosis, Arnold-Chiari malformation
   b. Agenesis of a portion of the corpus callosum
   c. Vascular abnormalities of the scalp adjacent to the overlying mass

LABORATORY

1. Transillumination of the sac (indicates presence of solid neural tissue)
2. Chromosomal studies
3. Plain radiograph of skull and cervical spine (for anatomy of the vertebrae)
4. Ultrasonography (for determining the contents of the sac)
5. Computed tomography (CT) or magnetic resonance imaging (MRI) of the brain (for detection of hydrocephalus or intracranial malformations)
6. Electroencephalogram

DIFFERENTIAL DIAGNOSIS

Cranial meningocele (herniation of cerebrospinal fluid [CSF] filled meningeal sac only)

TREATMENT

1. Surgical removal of the sac and closure of the defect in a patient who is not severely affected
2. Prevention of infection (meningitis/sepsis) by surgical closure for
   a. Encephalocele not covered by skin
   b. Those leaking CSF
3. Early resection of nasal encephalocele to decrease the risk of meningitis and prevent marked nasal

deformity related to progressive growth of encephalocele
4. Supportive therapy
   a. Hydrocephalus: a shunting procedure
   b. Epilepsy: anticonvulsant therapy

PROGNOSIS (long-term disabilities)

1. Profound mental retardation
2. Microcephaly
3. Spasticity
4. Blindness
5. Epilepsy (secondary to dysplasia of the cerebral cortex remaining in the cranium)

KEY POINTS

Encephalocele

- A pulsating, fluctuant cyst that increases with crying or coughing or can be reduced partly by digital pressure suggests an orbital encephalocele.
- Frontal or nasopharyngeal encephalocele usually indicates a severe malformation of the brain.
- Any infant with an intranasal mass should be evaluated, using MRI to assess for skull base involvement and intracranial extension before any intervention is planned. Biopsy of an unsuspected nasal encephalocele may lead to CFS leak, meningitis, and death.
- Slowly progressive proptosis that pulsates with the vascular pulse or is accentuated by coughing is diagnostic of orbital encephalocele.

TABLE 13–11
Clinical Features of Occipital Encephalocele

Associated with hypoplasia of occipital bones
Severity of intracranial cerebral malformations usually not predictable from size alone (except when extremely large, which is a marker of severe malformations)
Cortical blindness (if occipital lobes are contained within encephalocele)

TABLE 13–13
Clinical Features of Nasal Encephalocele

Herniated brain tissue, dura, and CSF constitute this mass
Originates through defective ethmoid bones into nasopharynx
Usually not diagnosed in neonatal period
May be confused with a nasal polyp
May present with signs/symptoms of nasal obstruction
May present with watery nasal secretions (if perforated)

TABLE 13–12
Clinical Features of Orbital Encephalocele

Unilateral proptosis or orbital cyst
Either present at birth or appears in later years
Originates through a defective wall between the cranial cavity and the orbit at suture lines
Herniation of brain or meninges or both into orbit (at inner angle of orbit at root of nose), with an increase in cranial pressure

---

TABLE 13–14
Clinical Features of Frontal Encephalocele

Frequently seen in midline just above nasion
Produces wide lateral displacement of orbit (seen as hypertelorism)

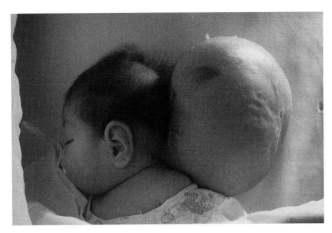

FIGURE 13–29. Occipital encephalocele. Patient was delivered by cesarean section.

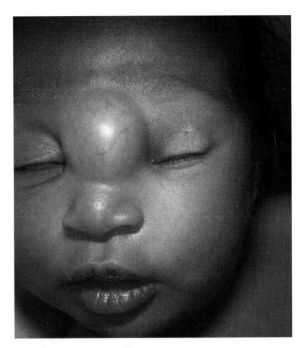

FIGURE 13–31. Nasofrontal encephalocele.

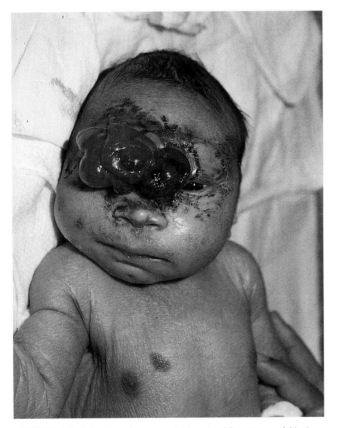

FIGURE 13–30. Anterior encephalocele. (Courtesy of Nathan Rudolph, M.D., State University of New York, Brooklyn, NY.)

Genetics

Binita R. Shah, M.D. and Teresita A. Laude, M.D.

Trisomy 21 Syndrome

SYNONYM   Down Syndrome

DEFINITION

1. A chromosomal syndrome consisting of multiple abnormalities including hypotonia, flat facies, slanted palpebral fissures, and small ears
2. After first description by John Langdon Down in 1866, the condition was labeled "mongolism" because of the facial resemblance between patients with Down syndrome and Asiatic people.

ETIOLOGY/PATHOGENESIS

1. Abnormality of chromosome number; thus, patients carry three representatives (trisomy) of chromosome 21 instead of the usual two (a total of 47 chromosomes).
2. Nondisjunction (failure of a chromosome pair to segregate) at chromosome 21 during meiosis (about 95% of cases)
3. Translocation Down syndrome (seen in about 4% to 5% of cases)
   a. Transfer of chromosomal material from one chromosome to another
   b. Translocations occur between chromosomes 21 and 14 or 13 or 15
   c. Fifty percent of translocations are inherited from a translocation carrier parent.
   d. Fifty percent of translocations occur as sporadic de novo events.
4. Mosaic with some normal cells (about 1% to 2%)

EPIDEMIOLOGY

1. Incidence: 1 in 600 to 800 live births
2. Male-female ratio is 1 : 1
3. More than 50% of trisomic 21 conceptions abort spontaneously in early pregnancy.
4. Translocations account for 9% of children with Down syndrome born to mothers under 30 years of age.
5. Incidence of Down syndrome increases with advancing maternal age (see Box 14–1).

BOX 14–1	*Maternal Age and Down Syndrome*	
MATERNAL AGE (YEARS)		**INCIDENCE OF DOWN SYNDROME**
15–29		1 in 1500
30–34		1 in 800
35–39		1 in 270
40–44		1 in 100
Over 45		1 in 50

BOX 14–2	*Down Syndrome Patients at Increased Risk for*

Atlantoaxial instability (12% to 20%)
Serous otitis media (50% to 70%)
Sinus, nasolacrimal duct, and pulmonary infections
Autoimmune hypothyroidism (more common) or hyperthyroidism
Leukemia
  1 in 95 (~1%)
  Risk is 10-fold to 30-fold greater than that in general population
  Most common type: acute lymphoblastic leukemia, acute myeloid leukemia
Cataracts (young child [60%], adolescents [100%])
Myopia (70%)
Diabetes
Obstructive sleep apnea (33%)

LABORATORY

1. A presumptive diagnosis is often made after birth based on the phenotypic features. However, because of lifelong implications, cytogenetic studies must be done.
2. Chromosomal karyotype is performed on cultured lymphocytes from peripheral blood.
3. Bone marrow-derived chromosomes or cord blood

444

lymphocyte chromosomes (for making a therapeutic decision in emergencies, if indicated)
4. Cardiac evaluation (before 6 months of life):
   a. Performed in all children even in the absence of heart murmur or symptoms
   b. Chest radiograph, electrocardiogram, and echocardiogram
5. Thyroid function tests
   a. Newborn screening
   b. Periodic thyroid-stimulating hormone and T_4 levels throughout childhood
6. Auditory brain stem evoked response within first 6 to 8 months of life
7. Ophthalmologic examination at 4 years of age
8. Lateral cervical spine radiographs for screening for atlantoaxial instability (see p. 446)

TREATMENT

1. Supportive, including social and educational support
2. Referral to specialists (symptom-specific, e.g., cardiologist, endocrinologist)
3. Genetic counseling. Chromosomal analysis for both parents to exclude translocation carrier (if patient has translocation)
4. Periodic evaluation by physical examination for atlantoaxial dislocation
5. Periodic thyroid function tests

PRENATAL DIAGNOSIS/PREVENTION

1. Presence of Down syndrome in fetus in women under 35 years of age may be suggested by:
   a. Lower maternal serum alpha-fetoprotein values
   b. Decreased maternal serum unconjugated estradiol values
   c. Increased maternal serum human chorionic gonadotropin values

2. Amniocentesis or chorionic villus sampling for chromosomal analysis is indicated:
   a. Routinely for maternal age 35 or over at the time of conception
   b. For women with previous child with chromosomal abnormality
3. Ultrasonographic findings may show any of the following:
   a. Duodenal atresia
   b. Tracheoesophageal fistula
   c. Atrioventricular canal, ventricular septal defect, atrial septal defect
   d. Hypoplasia of middle quadrant of the 5th finger
   e. Thickened nuchal folds
4. Risk of having another child with Down syndrome is about 1%.
5. Down syndrome secondary to inherited translocation occurs in approximately 2% of cases.

PROGNOSIS

1. Major cause of mortality in infancy: congenital heart defects
2. Primary gonadal deficiency: no male has reproduced; rarely females have reproduced
3. Average life expectancy: 35 years, although many live up to the 6th decade

KEY POINTS

Trisomy 21 Syndrome

- Most common chromosomal abnormality in humans
- Congenital heart defects are present in 30% to 50% of patients and are the most common cause of early death.

TABLE 14-1
Clinical Features of Down Syndrome

Brachycephaly, microcephaly, flat occiput, loose folds in posterior neck during infancy
Flat face, flat nasal bridge with small nose, short and broad neck, protruding tongue
Hypotonia; hypotonia tends to improve with age
Mental retardation (IQ range 25–50; mean: 24), seizures
Upslanting palpebral fissures, epicanthal folds, speckling of iris (Brushfield spots), strabismus
Small, prominent, and low-set ears; hearing loss (sensorineural and conductive [in 75% of patients])
Endocardial cushion defect, ventricular septal defect, atrial septal defect, tetralogy of Fallot, patent ductus arteriosus
Simian crease, small, broad hands with short metacarpals and phalanges, clinodactyly and hypoplasia of mid-phalanx of 5th finger
Wide gap between 1st and 2nd toes
Pelvis hypoplastic with wide, flat iliac wings and narrow acetabular angle
Short stature
Hair sparse, fine, and soft; alopecia areata; straight pubic hair at adolescence
Small penis with decreased testicular volume
Gastrointestinal malformation, duodenal atresia (most common)

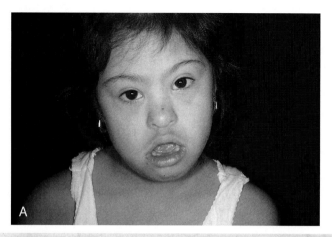

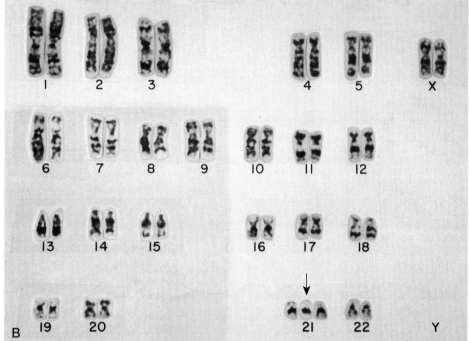

FIGURE 14–1. *A*, A young girl with some of the typical features of Down syndrome (up-slanting palpebral fissures, flat nasal bridge with small nose, short and broad neck, and protruding tongue). She also had simian crease. *B*, Her karyotype indicates trisomy 21 (*arrow*). (Courtesy of Qutubuddin Qazi, M.D., State University of New York, Brooklyn, NY.)

Trisomy 21 and Atlantoaxial Instability

DEFINITION

1. Trisomy 21 (Down Syndrome) patients are susceptible to atlantoaxial instability (or atlantoaxial subluxation).
2. Atlantoaxial instability (AAI) denotes increased mobility at the articulation of the first (C1 or atlas) and second (C2 or axis) cervical vertebra.
3. AAI is defined as excessive mobility of C2 in relation to C1, resulting in an abnormally large distance (>5 mm) between the anterior arch of the atlas and the odontoid process of the axis.

ETIOLOGY/CONTRIBUTORY FACTORS

1. Laxity of the transverse ligaments that maintain the integrity of the C1 and C2 articulation

2. Bony abnormality of C1 or C2 or both (e.g., hypoplasia or dysplasia of the odontoid process)
3. Periods of rapid growth

EPIDEMIOLOGY

AAI is seen in approximately 15% (range 12% to 20%) of pediatric patients with Down syndrome (age <21 years old)

CLINICAL FEATURES

1. AAI is usually seen in patients less than 10 years of age, when ligamentous laxity is most severe.
2. AAI can be either symptomatic or asymptomatic.
3. Asymptomatic AAI
   a. Most common; includes almost all patients with AAI (98% to 99%)
   b. Diagnosed by radiographs

4. Symptomatic AAI
   a. Rare; may be seen in 1% to 2% of patients
   b. Signs and symptoms of spinal cord compression (see Box 14–3)

BOX 14–3	*Signs and Symptoms of Spinal Cord Compression*

Neck posturing or head tilt or limited neck mobility
Neck pain
Sleep apnea
Loss of ambulatory skills
Abnormal gait
Difficulties in walking
Ataxia
Incoordination and clumsiness
Hyperreflexia, extensor-plantar reflex, clonus
Paresthesias of upper extremities
Upper motor neuron and posterior column signs or symptoms
Distal muscle weakness
Spasticity
Paraplegia
Hemiplegia
Quadriplegia
Urinary or fecal incontinence
Death

---

   c. Such signs and symptoms often remain relatively stable for months or years; occasionally they progress.
   d. Almost all patients who experience catastrophic injury to the spinal cord have had a prior history of less severe neurologic signs and symptoms for weeks to years.
   e. Trauma may cause the initial appearance or progression of these symptoms.

LABORATORY/RADIOGRAPHS

1. Lateral radiographs of the neck in the neutral, flexion, and extension positions
   a. During periods of rapid growth
      (1) At 5 to 8 years old
      (2) At 10 to 12 years old
      (3) At 18 years old
      (4) Every decade
   b. Prior to participation in sports
   c. Prior to any therapeutic programs or any operative procedures that involve active neck manipulation
2. Some patients with initially normal radiographs may have abnormal radiographic signs at a follow-up visit. Others with initially abnormal radiographs have normal follow-up radiographs.
3. Patients with symptoms or signs of spinal cord compression
   a. Computed tomography (CT): delineates bone abnormalities
   b. Magnetic resonance imaging (MRI): delineates cord involvement

CURRENT RECOMMENDATIONS

1. Thorough history, physical, and neurologic examination before participation in sports, preferably by the same physician who is familiar with the baseline examination
2. The Special Olympics recommend that all athletes with Down syndrome undergo radiographs of the cervical spine.
3. Children with asymptomatic AAI are not allowed to participate in sports such as football, soccer, diving, gymnastics, high jump, butterfly stroke, and diving starts in swimming or tumbling (all the "risky" sports thought to have a high risk for spinal cord injury).
4. Hospitalization and emergent neurosurgical consultation for patients with signs or symptoms of spinal cord compression for possible operative intervention

KEY POINTS

Trisomy 21 and Atlantoaxial Instability

- Although asymptomatic AAI occurs in 12% to 20% of patients with Down syndrome, compression of the spinal cord leading to symptoms is rare.
- Many patients with symptomatic AAI have signs or symptoms of spinal cord compression for weeks or years before neurologic symptoms are recognized.
- Parents should be educated about the signs and symptoms of spinal cord compression and instructed to seek medical care immediately if any symptoms develop.

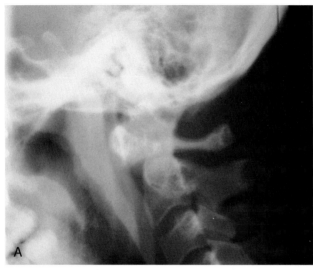

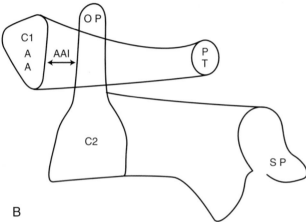

FIGURE 14–2. Atlantoaxial instability in a child with Down syndrome. *A,* Cross-table lateral radiograph of the cervical spine. Anterior arch of C1 is sublaxed anteriorly. It is 9 mm in front of the anterior cortex of the odontoid process (dens). The posterior tubercle of C1 is also anteriorly displaced from its usual position, producing a decrease in the anteroposterior diameter of the spinal canal (i.e., a decreased space for the cord). (Courtesy of Drs. Siegel and Hotson, State University of New York, Brooklyn, NY.) *B,* Schematic drawing of findings seen in *A.* First cervical vertebrae (C1 or atlas) is a bony arch with lateral masses. It supports the skull above and articulates with C2 below. (AA = anterior arch, PT = posterior turbercle.) The second cervical vertebra (C2 or axis) is a large vertebral body from which extends superiorly the dens or odontoid process (OP) (SP = spinous process). The pre-dens space is the space (a synovial joint) formed by the posterior surface of the AA of C1 with the anterior surface of OP. The pre-dens space or atlantoaxial interval (AAI) measures less than 5 mm in children and less than 3 mm in adults when viewed on the cross-table lateral radiograph.

Turner Syndrome

SYNONYMS   Gonadal Dysgenesis
XO Syndrome
Ullrich-Turner Syndrome

DEFINITION

A syndrome characterized by a female phenotype, sexual infantilism, short stature, streak gonads, absence of a second sex chromosome, and a diverse array of other somatic anomalies

EPIDEMIOLOGY

1. Seen in about 1 in 2500 to 3000 live-born females
2. The frequency of 45,X karyotype at conception is about 3%.
3. About 98% of pregnancies involving Turner syndrome abort spontaneously.
4. About 10% of fetuses from pregnancies that have spontaneously aborted have Turner syndrome.

PATHOGENESIS

1. About 50% of affected patients have the 45,X karyotype; about 15% of patients are mosaic for 45,X

and a normal cell line (45,X/46,XX; 45,X/46,XY). Other mosaics are seen less frequently.
2. The cause of chromosome loss is unknown; the maternal chromosome is missing in two thirds of patients.

CLINICAL FEATURES

1. Newborn
   a. Small for gestational age
   b. Redundant skinfolds at nape of neck
   c. Lymphedema of dorsa of hands and feet
2. Phenotype:
   a. Webbing of neck
   b. Small mandible
   c. A low posterior hairline
   d. Prominent ears
   e. Appearance of widely spaced nipples on a broad chest
   f. Hyperconvex nails and cubitus valgus
3. Gonadal dysgenesis and sexual maturation (see Box 14–4)
4. Short stature (see Box 14–5)
5. Cardiac anomalies

<table>
<tr><td>

BOX 14-4 *Turner Syndrome: Gonadal Dysgenesis and Sexual Maturation*

</td></tr>
</table>

Lack of sexual maturation with primary amenorrhea in a teenager

At puberty, sexual maturation normally caused by estrogen secretion is lacking in the majority; thus:

Breast development lacking

Menses lacking

Development of pubic and axillary hair progresses *normally*

Residual ovarian function may lead to:

Spontaneous pubertal development in 20% to 25% of girls

Spontaneous menses in 2% to 5% of girls

Females with mosaicism

May develop some sexual maturation because of functioning ovarian tissue

May present with primary or secondary amenorrhea, early menopause, infertility or recurrent miscarriage in adulthood

<table>
<tr><td>

BOX 14-5 *Turner Syndrome and Short Stature*

</td></tr>
</table>

A cardinal feature

Untreated patients show a progressive deviation of height away from normal growth curve during infancy and childhood; pronounced lack of pubertal growth results in a mean adult height of 143 cm (range 130–155 cm)

a. Bicuspid aortic valves (50%)
b. Coarctation of the aorta (20%)
c. Aortic root dilatation (10%)
d. Aortic stenosis, or anomalous pulmonary venous drainage

6. Renal anomalies (seen in one third to one half of patients)
   a. Double collecting systems
   b. Horseshoe kidneys
   c. Ureteropelvic junction obstruction or absence of one kidney
7. Skeletal involvement
   a. Shortened 4th and 5th metacarpal and metatarsal bones
   b. Osteopenia
8. Normal intelligence with specific impairment in cognitive functioning (deficits in visual-spatial processing, visual memory)
9. Other associated diseases
   a. Primary hypothyroidism (10% to 30%)
   b. Diabetes mellitus
   c. Frequent ear infections

d. Ulcerative colitis
e. Crohn disease
f. Gastrointestinal telangiectasia presenting as rectal bleeding

LABORATORY

1. Chromosome analysis *must be* performed in all cases.
2. Buccal smear is chromatin negative in most patients. However, the diagnosis cannot be made by the buccal smear alone because it is also positive in approximately 20% of patients with mosaicism or a structurally abnormal X chromosome.
3. Serum gonadotropins (luteinizing hormone, follicle-stimulating hormone)
   a. Markedly elevated from birth to about 4 years of age
   b. During mid childhood gonadotropin levels fall to normal prepubertal levels (normal central nervous system suppression of gonadotropins at this age).
   c. Levels again rise abnormally high at the usual age of puberty (indicating primary ovarian failure).
4. Bone age
5. Pelvic ultrasound
   a. In 50% of patients small ovaries are seen in first 4 years of life.
   b. In 90% of patients ovaries are seen as streaks between 4 and 10 years of age.
6. Renal ultrasound
7. Echocardiogram: monitor progressive dilatation of aortic root in patients with bicuspid aortic valve
8. Baseline and periodic screening for thyroid autoimmunity leading to hypothyroidism

DIFFERENTIAL DIAGNOSIS

1. Noonan syndrome
2. Syndromes associated with short stature
3. Milroy disease

TREATMENT

1. Refer the patient to a pediatric endocrinologist.
2. To maximize the final height:
   a. Growth hormone (GH) therapy is begun as soon as patient starts falling below 5th percentile on the normal female growth curve (usually between 2 and 5 years of age).
   b. Combination therapy with GH and anabolic steroids (e.g., oxandrolone) is begun between 9 and 12 years of age.
   c. Therapy is continued until growth velocity decreases to less than 2.5 cm/year with a bone age of over 15 years.
3. To promote development of secondary sex characteristics:
   a. Estrogen therapy is usually begun at time of puberty (14 to 15 years of age).
   b. Progestin therapy is added (for 12 days each

month) either with first vaginal breakthrough bleeding or in second year of therapy.

4. Refer the patient to a cardiologist (cardiac evaluation, bacterial endocarditis prophylaxis).
5. Audiologic and cognitive evaluation
6. Counseling of patient and family and referral to a support group
7. Because of increased risk of gonadoblastoma, prophylactic gonadectomy is indicated for
   a. Patients with Y-chromosome mosaicism (45,X/46,XY)
   b. Patients with a fragment of Y chromosome (45,X +mar)

KEY POINTS

Turner Syndrome

- All phenotypic characteristics except short stature may be absent in Turner syndrome; thus, any girl with short stature of unknown etiology must have a karyotype analysis.
- Exclude Turner syndrome by karyotype analysis in any girl with primary amenorrhea or coarctation of aorta.
- Most common cause of lack of sexual maturation associated with increased serum gonadotropins.

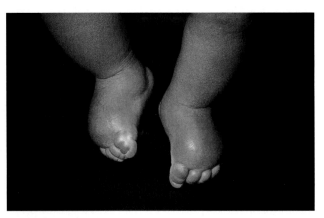

FIGURE 14–3. Lymphedema (manifesting as puffiness) on the dorsa of the feet in a newborn girl with Turner syndrome.

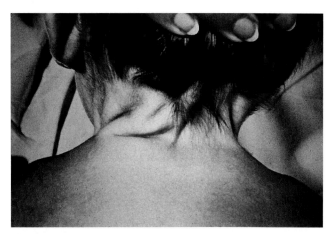

FIGURE 14–4. Webbed neck with low hairline in a girl with Turner syndrome. (Courtesy of Max Salas, M.D., St. Peter's University Hospital, New Brunswick, NJ.)

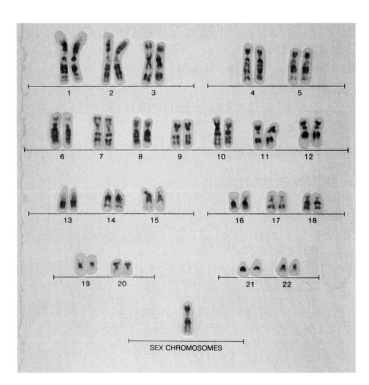

FIGURE 14–5. Karyotype of a patient with TS showing XO pattern. (Courtesy of Qutubuddin Qazi, M.D., State University of New York, Brooklyn, NY.)

Sotos Syndrome

SYNONYM Cerebral Gigantism

DEFINITION

A clinical entity of cerebral gigantism (with no identified endocrine abnormality) and a nonprogressive neurologic disorder. This entity was first described by Sotos in 1964.

ETIOLOGY

The cause is unknown.

EPIDEMIOLOGY

1. Seen in all ethnic groups
2. Prevalence of this syndrome is unknown but is estimated to be 1 in 10,000 to 50,000.

INHERITANCE

1. Most cases are sporadic.
2. Usual mode of inheritance in familial cases: autosomal dominant; occasionally autosomal recessive
3. Prenatal diagnosis: not available

LABORATORY

1. No distinctive laboratory marker
2. Bone age: advanced over chronologic age but compatible with height age
3. Endocrine studies
   a. Insulin-like growth factor (IGF-1 or somatomedin C): normal
   b. Growth hormone (GH) levels: normal
   c. Testicular and ovarian function: normal
   d. No endocrine abnormality present to explain the rapid growth.

DIFFERENTIAL DIAGNOSIS

1. Beckwith-Wiedemann syndrome (neonate with macrosomia, macroglossia, omphalocele, hypoglycemia)
2. Growth hormone-secreting pituitary tumors: (elevated IGF-1 and GH levels)
3. Extrahypothalamic tumors that secrete growth hormone–releasing hormone and stimulate the pituitary to produce excess growth hormone

TREATMENT

1. Management of mental retardation
2. Excessive height
   a. Usually not a problems for males
   b. For girls
      (1) Consult pediatric endocrinologist
      (2) May consider giving high doses of estrogen to curtail linear growth

PROGNOSIS

1. Affected patients have increased risk of malignancy (like patients with overgrowth syndromes)
   a. Hepatic carcinoma
   b. Wilms
   c. Ovarian
   d. Parotid tumors
2. Fertility is normal, and affected individual has a 50% chance of transmitting the disorder to offspring.

KEY POINTS

Sotos Syndrome

- A syndrome characterized by prenatal and postnatal overgrowth
- Large size, large hands, and feet

BOX 14–6 *Growth Characteristics of Cerebral Gigantism*

NEWBORN

Large for gestational age at birth
Mean length: 21.7 inches; 97th percentile
Mean weight: 3.4 kg; between 75th and 95th percentiles

INFANCY

Growth velocity excessive in first 3–4 years of life
Rapid growth continues for first 4–5 years of life and then returns to normal (but in a higher percentile)

PUBERTY/ADULTS

Adult height: usually exceeds 50th percentile of normal
Excessive heights in some adults (e.g., males with height up to 6 ft 8 inches; females with height up to 6 ft 2 inches)

TABLE 14–2
Clinical Features of Cerebral Gigantism

Appearance	Premature eruption of teeth
Coarse-looking facies	Hands and feet: large, acromegalic appearance
Large dolichocephalic head	Gait: awkward, clumsy
Prominent jaw	Kyphoscoliosis
Frontal bossing	Hypotonia during 1st year of life
Eyes with antimongoloid slant	Some degree of mental retardation
Hypertelorism	Perceptual deficiencies, poor coordination
Strabismus	
Large ears	Mild hydrocephalus
High narrow palate	Seizures

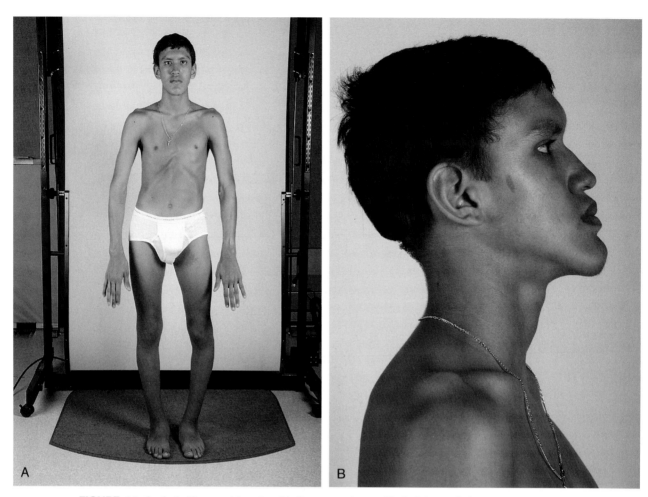

FIGURE 14–6. *A,* A 13-year-old male with Sotos syndrome. He is 6 feet tall, has very large hands and feet, and wears size 14 shoes. He has been slow in learning and attends special classes. (Courtesy of Ernesto Jule, M.D., State University of New York, Brooklyn, NY.) *B,* Prominent jaws with a pointed chin, dolichocephalic head, and prominent forehead. Craniofacial characteristics may improve with age.

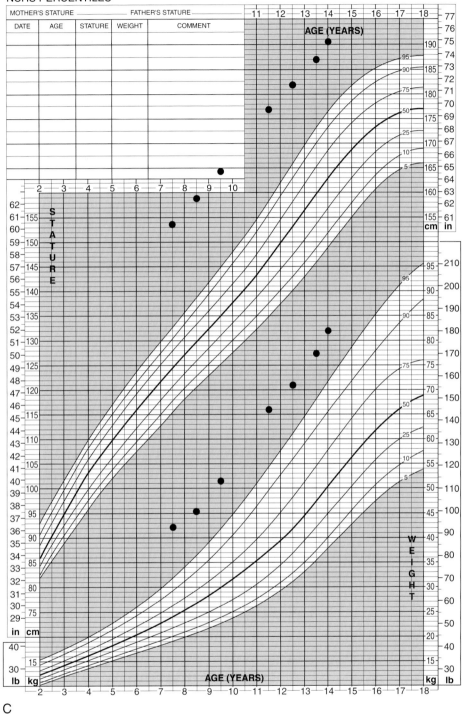

BOYS: 2 TO 18 YEARS
PHYSICAL GROWTH
NCHS PERCENTILES

FIGURE 14–6. *Continued C,* Growth velocity curve of this patient. He was born at term with a birth weight of 10 lb, 12 oz and a length of 61 cm. He continued to grow at over 95% in both height and weight (growth parameters prior to age 7 are not available). Mother's height is 64 inches, and father's height is 68 inches. At present (age 14) the patient's height is 75 inches, and his weight is 180 lb.

C

TAR Syndrome

SYNONYMS   Thrombocytopenia-Absent Radius Syndrome
Thrombocytopenia-Radial Aplasia Syndrome

DEFINITION

Absent radii with thrombocytopenia

ETIOLOGY/INHERITANCE

1. Congenital disorder

2. Autosomal recessive mode of inheritance in the majority of patients
3. Gene(s) responsible for this condition: unknown
4. Etiology of thrombocytopenia
   a. Megakaryocytes absent (66%)
   b. Megakaryocytes decreased (12%)
   c. Megakaryocytes inactive (12%)

EPIDEMIOLOGY

1. Seen in all ethnic groups
2. Rare cause of neonatal thrombocytopenia

ANTENATAL DIAGNOSIS

1. Demonstration of upper limb defects on sonography
2. Platelet count from fetal blood obtained in mid trimester

CLINICAL FEATURES

1. Great variability of expression among patients
2. Hematologic abnormalities
   a. Thrombocytopenia
      (1) Congenital
      (2) May present at birth with severe hemorrhagic manifestations
      (3) Platelet count in neonates with condition: usually less than 50,000/mm^3
   b. Precipitating factors for thrombocytopenia
      (1) Infection
      (2) Nonspecific stress
      (3) Cow's milk (some cases)

BOX 14–7 *Hallmark of TAR Syndrome*

Hypomegakaryocytic thrombocytopenia with bilateral radial aplasia

---

3. Limb abnormalities
   a. Upper extremity involvement ranges from isolated absent radii to true phocomelia
      (1) Bilateral absence of radius (100%)
      (2) Abnormalities of ulna, humerus, and shoulder girdle (hypoplasia or absent; bilateral or unilateral)
      (3) Hands and feet: thumbs present, club hand, syndactyly (abnormal fusion) or clinodactyly (abnormal deflection) of fingers and toes
   b. Lower extremity: dislocated hips, hypoplasia or aplasia of lower limbs
4. Other abnormalities (reported in some cases)
   a. Cardiac: tetralogy of Fallot, ventricular or atrial septal defect
   b. Renal (absent kidney)
   c. Gastrointestinal

LABORATORY

1. Complete blood count
   a. Thrombocytopenia
   b. Anemia (out of proportion to apparent blood loss)
   c. Leukemoid reaction and eosinophilia (especially during bleeding episodes)
2. Bone marrow examination (usually not required to make the diagnosis)

DIFFERENTIAL DIAGNOSIS

1. Congenital leukemia (thrombocytopenia with hematologic picture of leukemia)
2. Fanconi anemia (see Table 14–3)
3. Holt-Oram syndrome (heart-hand syndrome)
   a. Thumb abnormality (absent or triphalangeal)
   b. Atrial septal defect
   c. *Absence* of hematologic involvement

COMPLICATIONS

1. Death in early infancy (usually during first year) from hemorrhage
2. Hemorrhage
   a. Intracranial hemorrhage
   b. Visceral hemorrhage
   c. Pulmonary hemorrhage

TREATMENT

1. Pediatric hematology consultation
2. Platelet transfusions
   a. Mainstay of treatment
   b. Transfused platelets survive normally
   c. Current recommendations
      (1) Provide HLA-matched platelet transfusions; this reduces the chances of platelet antibody development.
      (2) Administer transfusions as necessary to maintain platelet count above 10,000 to 20,000/mm^3 (to prevent potentially fatal hemorrhage until a spontaneous recovery occurs).
3. Antifibrinolytic agent (e.g., epsilon aminocaproic acid) may be used to decrease bleeding (e.g., gingival bleeding), thus reducing requirements for platelet transfusions.
4. Bone marrow transplant for the rare patient who does not improve by early childhood.
5. Therapies that are *not* effective and *not* indicated
   a. Splenectomy
   b. Administration of corticosteroids
   c. Administration of androgens
6. Orthopedic consultation and early intervention for deformities

PROGNOSIS

1. Thrombocytopenia is most severe in early infancy and tends to remit spontaneously in 2nd to 3rd year of life. Periodic episodes of thrombocytopenia (with leukocytosis and eosinophilia) continue until remission occurs.

2. Mental retardation (seen in some) is thought to be secondary to intracranial bleeding (related to severe thrombocytopenia).
3. Majority of mortality occurs in the first few months of life. The survival curve for these patients plateaus above 70% by 4 years of age.
4. Risk of malignancy
   a. Until recently, it was thought that, unlike Fanconi syndrome, patients with TAR syndrome do not develop leukemia or aplastic anemia. However, recently a child with TAR syndrome who developed acute lymphoid leukemia was described in the literature.
   b. Recently an increased cellular radiation sensitivity has been described in a patient with TAR syndrome. A 70-year-old woman with TAR syndrome was reported in the literature who showed an increased risk of neoplasia (three separate primary cancers involving the small bowel, ovary, and bladder).

PREVENTION

1. With antenatal diagnosis, a fetus can be monitored with serial ultrasound examinations for evidence of internal bleeding.

2. A complete blood count can be obtained by cordocentesis, and platelet transfusion into the umbilical vein can be carried out to correct thrombocytopenia prior to delivery.

KEY POINTS

TAR Syndrome

- An infant with purpura and characteristic limb deformities
- Thrombocytopenia is present at birth but tends to remit spontaneously in the 2nd to 3rd year of life.
- Thumbs are present with radial aplasia in patients with TAR syndrome; thumbs are absent or hypoplastic with radial aplasia in those with Fanconi anemia.

TABLE 14–3
Comparison of TAR Syndrome with Fanconi Anemia

	TAR Syndrome	**Fanconi Anemia**
Thrombocytopenia	Present at birth	Rare in neonatal period
Radial anomalies	100%	30%
Thumb	Present with absence of radii	Always absent or hypoplastic with absence of radii
Diagnosis	At birth	8 years (mean age)
Hematology	Thrombocytopenia Other cell lines *normal*	Pancytopenia; may present as isolated thrombocytopenia initially
Chromosomal fragility	Absent	Present
Incidence of malignancy	Increased ?	Increased

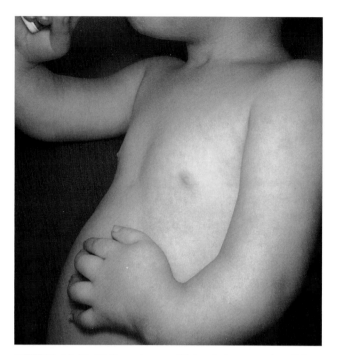

FIGURE 14-7. TAR syndrome. Bilateral absence of radii in a patient with a presence of thumb on both hands.

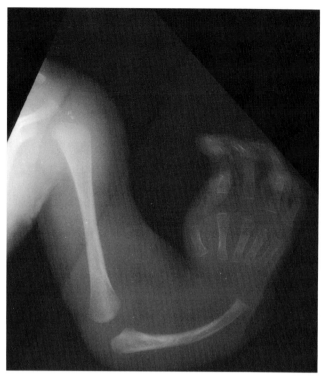

FIGURE 14-8. TAR syndrome. Anteroposterior view of left upper extremity shows absence of radius and curvature of ulna. First phalanx (thumb) is present. (Courtesy of George Kassner, M.D., Maimonides Medical Center, Brooklyn, NY.)

Albinism

DEFINITION

A hereditary disorder of pigmentation characterized by a normal number of melanocytes but absent or defective tyrosinase activity, resulting in diminished or absent melanin production

ETIOLOGY

1. An autosomal recessive trait
2. Gene locus in chromosome 15q for tyrosinase-positive albinism (TPA); in chromosome 11q for tyrosinase-negative albinism (TNA)

EPIDEMIOLOGY

1. TPA: 1 in 5000 African-Americans; 1 in 37,000 whites TNA: 1 in 28,000 African-Americans; 1 in 39,000 whites
2. Male-female ratio is 1 : 1.

LABORATORY

1. Hair bulb incubation test: incubation of a hair bulb in L-tyrosine 1 mg/mL in 0.1 M phosphate buffer at pH 6.8
2. In TPA, melanin production is detected in the hair bulb.
3. In TNA, no melanin production is detected.

> **BOX 14-8** *Differential Diagnosis of Albinism*
>
> Chediak-Higashi syndrome
> Vogt-Koyanagi-Harada syndrome

COMPLICATIONS

1. Severe sun damage
2. Skin cancers at an early age
3. Bleeding in patients with Hermansky-Pudlak syndrome (TPA seen mostly in Puerto Rico and Holland; associated with platelet aggregation, prolonged beeding time and ceroid deposits in bone marrow macrophages, reticuloendothelial system, and other organs.)

TREATMENT

1. Sun avoidance
2. Vigilant use of sunscreen
3. Skin cancer surveillance every 6 months
4. Genetic counseling
5. Enroll the patient in the

National Organization for Albinism and Hypopigmentation
1530 Locust Street #29
Philadelphia, PA 19102-4316
Telephone (800) 473-2310
                (215) 545-2322

PROGNOSIS

Normal life span in the absence of skin cancers

KEY POINTS

Albinism

- There are two types of albinism. Tyrosinase-positive albinism, which is the more common type, is characterized by reddish blonde hair. Tyrosinase-negative albinism is characterized by white hair.
- The major complications are sun damage and early development of skin cancers.

TABLE 14–4
Clinical Features of Albinism

Skin
Generalized pink to cream color

Hair
TPA: cream to yellow brown in color
TNA: snow white in color

Eyes
Blue to yellow brown
Photophobia
Nystagmus
Diminished visual acuity
Strabismus
Foveal hypoplasia

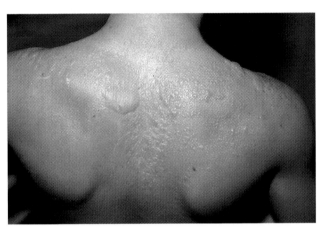
FIGURE 14–10. An albino child with severe sunburn.

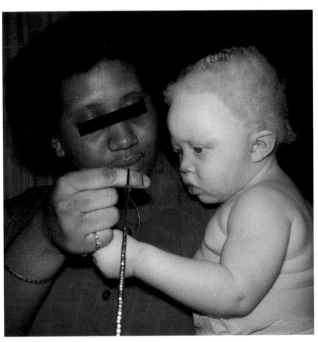
FIGURE 14–9. An African-American albino infant.

Piebaldism

SYNONYMS   Familial White Spotting
            Partial Albinism

DEFINITION

A hereditary disorder characterized by a distinct pattern of localized skin depigmentation present from birth

ETIOLOGY/INHERITANCE

1. Autosomal dominant inheritance
2. Gene locus on chromosome 4q12

EPIDEMIOLOGY

1. Incidence: 1 in 20,000
2. No racial predilection
3. Male-female ratio is 1:1

PATHOGENESIS

Defect in migration and differentiation of melanoblasts from the neural crest

LABORATORY

Skin biopsy of a depigmented patch shows absence of melanocytes

COMPLICATION

The depigmented patches may be severely sunburned.

BOX 14-9   *Differential Diagnosis of Piebaldism*

Vitiligo
Waardenburg syndrome
Nevus depigmentosus

TREATMENT

1. Camouflage make up
2. Sunscreen use
3. Genetic counseling

PROGNOSIS

1. Depigmented patches are stable and permanent.
2. Normal life span

KEY POINTS

Piebaldism

- Piebaldism consists of a white forelock and depigmented patches on the forehead, anterior chest, abdomen, and mid-extremities.
- These areas must be protected against the sun because they are devoid of pigment.

TABLE 14-5
Clinical Features of Piebaldism

White forelock
Depigmented patches at following sites
    Forehead
    Anterior chest
    Abdomen
    Mid-extremities
    Spares hands, feet, shoulders, hips
White patch on forehead is triangular with angle pointing
    downward
There may be islands of normal skin within white patches
Normal intelligence

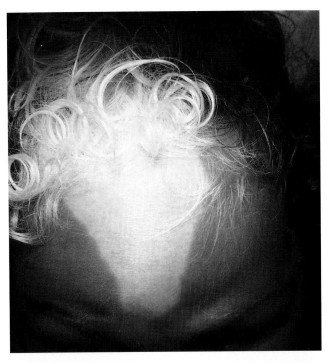

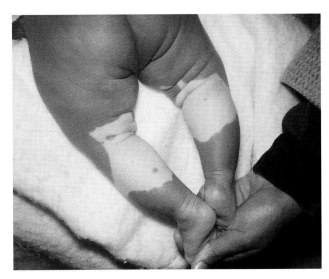

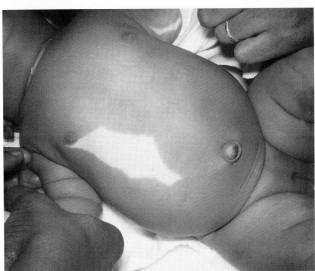

FIGURES 14–11, 14–12, and 14–13. A 7-week-old infant with piebaldism. Her father was similarly affected.

Waardenburg Syndrome

DEFINITION

A hereditary disorder transmitted as an autosomal dominant trait

ETIOLOGY/INHERITANCE

1. Inherited as an autosomal dominant trait
2. Gene locus is in chromosome 2q.

EPIDEMIOLOGY

1. Incidence: 1 in 42,000
2. Male-female ratio is 1:1.

3. One to three percent of all children with congenital sensorineural deafness have Waardenburg syndrome.

BOX 14–10	*Differential Diagnosis of Waardenburg Syndrome*
Piebaldism
Hypertelorism (increased distance between the pupils)	

LABORATORY

Hearing evaluation test

COMPLICATION

Hirschprung disease (5%)

TREATMENT

1. Refer patient to an audiologist and otolaryngologist for early hearing evaluation and use of hearing aid.
2. Genetic counseling

KEY POINT

Waardenburg Syndrome

■ The most prominent features of Waardenburg syndrome are heterochromia irides, white forelock, and sensorineural deafness.

TABLE 14–6
Features of Waardenburg Syndrome

Dystophia canthorum or lateral displacement of medial canthi (99%)
Broad nasal root (80%)
Synophrys (70%)
White forelock (50%)
Heterochromia irides (25%)
Congenital sensorineural deafness (20%)

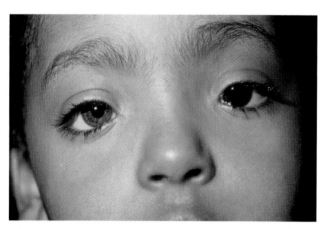

FIGURE 14–14. Child with Waardenburg syndrome. He had heterochromia irides, dystophia canthorum, synophrys, and deafness.

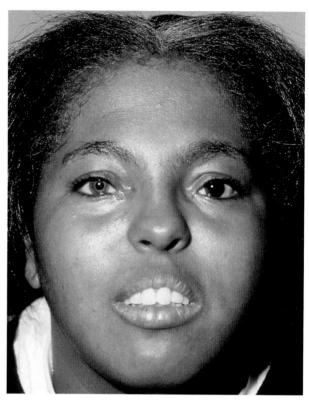

FIGURE 14–15. The mother of child in Figure 14–14 was similarly affected.

Miscellaneous

Binita R. Shah, M.D.

Oral Electrical Burns

DEFINITION

Electrical burns involving the oral tissues

ETIOLOGY/PATHOGENESIS

1. Most oral electrical burns are caused by biting, chewing, or sucking on any of the following:
   a. Female end of a live extension cord (most frequent cause)
   b. Exposed live wire
   c. Junction of an extension cord and a partially plugged-in appliance
   d. A wall socket (least common)
2. Types of electrical burns
   a. Arc burns
      (1) Arc burns are responsible for most burns involving the commissure of the lips.
      (2) When a live extension cord is placed in the mouth, a short circuit between the cord terminals results in an electrical arc; saliva serves to complete the circuit between the electrical elements and the tissues.
      (3) Arc burns can generate intense heat (between 2000 and 3000 degrees Celsius), causing heat necrosis.
   b. Contact burns
      (1) May cause additional damage to oral tissues
      (2) Contact burns are caused by passage of electricity through the body and transformation of electrical energy into heat (resulting from the resistance of body tissue).

PATHOLOGY

1. Usually a full-thickness burn involving the mucosa, submucosa, muscle, nerves, and blood vessels
2. Characterized by fat liquefaction, protein coagulation, and fluid vaporization proportional to the source voltage and the tissue conductance
3. Extensive deep damage may be hidden between the entrance and exit wounds.

EPIDEMIOLOGY

1. Most common age:
   a. Peak: 1 to 2 years; age range: 1 to 4 years
   b. Young children are vulnerable, especially at the age when oral tactile stimulation and curiosity are part of their desire to explore.
2. Male-female ratio is 3:1.
3. Seasonal variation: most frequent in winter

LABORATORY

1. A clinical diagnosis supported by the history
2. Electrocardiogram
3. Hematologic evaluation: complete blood count and coagulation profile (baseline and monitoring for intravascular coagulopathy)

TREATMENT

1. Dental and plastic surgery consultations
2. To control hemorrhage:
   a. Direct pressure
   b. Application of epinephrine-soaked sponges
   c. Suture ligation
3. Wound treatment (controversial; treatment should be individualized according to consultants' advice)
   a. Early excision and closure or nonoperative management
   b. Usually more aggressive early excision is reserved for more extensive lesions.
4. Local wound care
   a. Cleanse the site with mild surgical soap and water and irrigate with hydrogen peroxide and saline solution.
   b. Do not cover the burn site; leave open to air to allow coagulum to form.
   c. Apply topical antibiotic (e.g., bacitracin)
   d. Do not remove the eschar that forms over the wound; it will slough in about 2 weeks, leaving an ulcer to heal secondarily.
   e. Daily wound debridement and evaluation
   f. Tetanus immunization (if required based on child's immunization status)
   g. Prophylactic antibiotics are not given for minor to moderate burns, but may be considered for severe burns.
5. Dietary modification
   a. A clear liquid diet $\Rightarrow$ nutrient liquid diet $\Rightarrow$ soft diet
   b. Soft diet minimizes perioral muscle use (reduces probability of bleeding)
6. With superficial burns, patient can be treated con-

servatively on an outpatient basis (if family is compliant).

7. Hospitalize patients with extensive full-thickness burns.

8. To prevent facial deformity caused by contracture of the oral and perioral tissue:

   a. A removable acrylic prosthesis (fabricated by a dentist) is recommended; it should have extraoral extensions located at the commissures to deflect the burn side.

   b. Should be worn for 1 year (even though the wound heals in 4 to 6 weeks)

BOX 15–1 *Complications of Oral Electrical Burns*

Microstomia from extensive scarring
Abnormal development of dental arches
Devitalization of deciduous and secondary teeth
Lip eversion from scarring
Labial alveolar adhesions
Speech problems
Ankyloglossia

PROGNOSIS

Although oral electrical burns are rarely fatal, they result in long-term morbidity owing to disfiguring scars and dysfunction of oral sphincter.

PREVENTION

1. Use of safety caps on wall outlets
2. Use of well-insulated electric cords
3. Installation of wall switches for open wall sockets

KEY POINTS

Oral Electrical Burns

■ Best defense against oral electrical burns is prevention.

■ Most frequent location of oral electrical burn is commissure of the lips.

■ Parents must be alerted to the fact that profuse bleeding from the labial or lingual artery may occur about 1 to 2 weeks after the burn when sloughing of the eschar occurs.

TABLE 15–1
Clinical Features of Oral Electrical Burns

Localized burn to the mouth
Usually involves upper and lower commissure (which come in contact with the extension cord)
Drooling
Injured tissue is usually:
  Pale (bloodless)
  Painless
  Has a well-demarcated depressed center with surrounding pale gray area with an erythematous border
Delayed bleeding
  Seen in about 6% to 20% of cases
  Severe bleeding from labial or lingual artery as eschar sloughs in 1–2 weeks

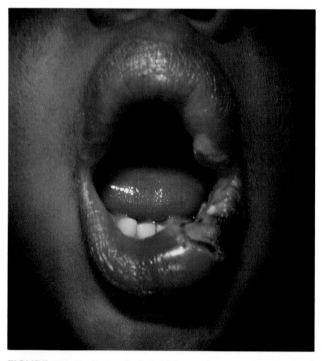

FIGURE 15–1. A classic full-thickness burn at the corner of the mouth in this 18-month-old toddler resulted from chewing on an extension cord.

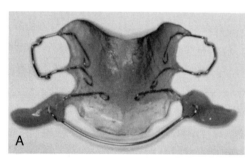
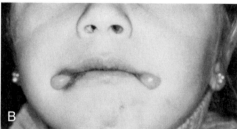

FIGURE 15–2. A, Removable maxillary appliance is used to help healing and limit lip scarring and contractures. B, Appliance being worn by patient. (From Josell SD, Abrams, RG: Managing common dental problems and emergencies. Pediatr Clin North Am 38(5): 1327, 1991.)

Nursing-Bottle Caries

SYNONYMS Milk Bottle Syndrome
Baby Bottle Syndrome
Nursing Caries
Bottle Mouth Syndrome

DEFINITION

The term nursing-bottle caries refers to tooth decay caused by prolonged use of a nursing bottle; however, this pattern of tooth decay is also seen in breastfed infants and infants regularly given pacifiers that have been dipped in honey, sugar, or other sweetened substances.

ETIOLOGY/PATHOGENESIS

1. Interaction of several interdependent variables is required to initiate caries.
   a. Susceptible host: abnormal structure or alignment of teeth; abnormal flow or composition of saliva
   b. Cariogenic diet: sucrose is the principal substrate; other carbohydrates (glucose, lactose, fructose, maltose) are also implicated.
   c. Microorganism with cariogenic potential: *Streptococcus mutans* is an initiating offender; other pathogens include *Lactobacillus* sp. and *Actinomyces* sp.
2. Bacterial fermentation of dietary carbohydrates: formation of organic acids leads to demineralization of the tooth surface.
   a. Time: prolonged contact with carbohydrate-containing fluid retained in the oral cavity
   b. Frequency: frequency of carbohydrate consumption is more important than the actual amount

EPIDEMIOLOGY

1. Prevalence rate: 3% to 6% of pediatric population
2. Common age at start of decay: 1 to 2 years

LABORATORY

Diagnosis is made by the classic pattern of tooth involvement in association with an appropriate feeding history.

PROGNOSIS

Patients with nursing bottle caries are more likely to develop additional cavities.

BOX 15-2 | *Prevention and Treatment of Nursing-Bottle Caries*

Counseling on feeding and nutrition and dental caries:

- Feeding of any fluid other than water to an infant during prolonged sleeping periods may serve as a substrate for bacteria capable of causing dental caries.
- Bottles given at bedtime (if required) should contain only water after the primary teeth have erupted.
- Remove the nursing bottle from the mouth immediately after the infant goes to sleep.
- Nursing bottle should not be propped in the crib for the infant to suck on intermittently through the night.
- Start weaning from the bottle or nursing as soon as infant starts drinking from a cup (usually by 1 year of age).
- If weaning from the bottle is difficult, the contents of the bottle should be increasingly diluted with water.
- Avoid offering pacifiers dipped in honey or sugar.
- Prolonged periods of nursing or breastfeeding on demand during sleep after eruption of primary teeth also promote caries.
- Start brushing the teeth as soon as they erupt.
- Dental consultation is needed for patients with established nursing-bottle caries.

KEY POINTS

Nursing-Bottle Caries

- Nursing-bottle caries is a preventable disease.
- Caries in infants prior to 18 months of age are almost invariably nursing-bottle caries.
- Cariogenic fluids such as sweetened beverages or milk that constantly bathe the teeth while the infant is sleeping with the bottle lead to nursing-bottle caries.
- After eruption of primary teeth, bottles given at bed time should contain only water.

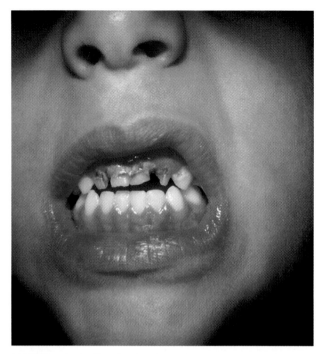

FIGURE 15-3. Nursing-bottle caries showing characteristic involvement of anterior maxillary central and lateral incisors. Lower anterior mandibular teeth are uninvolved. This child slept every night with a juice bottle until he was 2 years old. Severe tooth erosion occurs in advanced cases. These teeth are nonrestorable and must be extracted. Breast-fed infants (especially infants allowed to nurse "at will" during sleep) can develop similar caries. Prolonged nocturnal bathing of anterior teeth in lactose-rich human milk (approximately 7% lactose compared with bovine milk [4.5%]) may be a contributory factor.

TABLE 15-2
Clinical Features of Nursing-Bottle Caries

Dental caries involving primary teeth in sequence
Most commonly involved: maxillary anterior teeth
  Maxillary central and lateral incisors (facial surfaces and proximal ends) are first to be affected
  Followed by maxillary first primary molars (palatal surfaces)
  Primary canines are affected last
Least affected: mandibular teeth
  Tongue, salivary secretions, and lower lip usually protect mandibular teeth during sucking
  Anterior mandibular teeth and second molar involvement indicate advanced caries

Ranula

SYNONYMS   Mucocele
            Mucus Retention Cyst

DEFINITION

A large mucocele that occurs in the floor of the mouth

ETIOLOGY/PATHOGENESIS

1. Mucocele results from traumatic severance (rupture) of the submucosal excretory ducts of the minor salivary glands, with subsequent pooling of saliva in the connective tissue.
2. Ranula is a large mucocele that results from either severance or obstruction of the duct of a major salivary gland, usually the sublingual gland. Salivary gland calcium precipitates, mucin, and cellu-

lar debris may combine to produce a sialolith duct obstruction.
3. Even though a mucocele appears cystic, it is not a true cyst because it is not lined with epithelium.

BOX 15-3   *Clinical Features of Ranula*

A large, soft, mucus-containing cyst
Compressible swelling
Translucent, bluish color
Unilateral
Painless
Located in the floor of the mouth
Presents at any age including infancy
May persist for weeks to months, then rupture
Recurrences are common

TREATMENT

1. Consultation with a dentist
2. Conservative treatment: marsupialization (unroofing the lesion) to evacuate the contents
3. Aggressive treatment: excision of the lesion, adjacent salivary gland tissue, and severed duct (exteriorized)

KEY POINTS

Ranula

■ Most common cystic structures in the oral cavity are mucoceles.
■ Ranula is a large mucocele that occurs in the floor of the mouth (sublingual area).

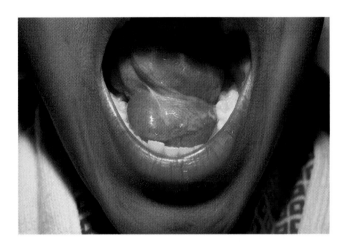

FIGURE 15–4. Ranula. A large translucent ranula with a bluish color is visible on the floor of the mouth in this 6-year-old patient. This was the 3rd recurrence in a period of 8 months. Previously the cyst had been unroofed to evacuate the contents.

Minimal Change Nephrotic Syndrome (MCNS)

SYNONYMS   Lipoid Nephrosis
"Nil Disease"
Minimal Change Disease

DEFINITION

The term nephrosis or nephrotic syndrome (NS) implies heavy proteinuria, hypoproteinemia (hypoalbuminemia), edema, and hyperlipidemia.

ETIOLOGY

1. Primary or idiopathic (90%)
   a. Minimal change nephrotic syndrome: most common type (85%)
   b. Focal segmental glomerulosclerosis (10%)
   c. Mesangial proliferation (5%)
2. Secondary cases (10%)
   a. Associated with systemic disease (e.g., systemic lupus erythematosus, Henoch-Schönlein purpura, IgA nephropathy)
   b. Associated with infections (bacterial [e.g., syphilis], viral [e.g., hepatitis], protozoal [e.g., malaria], helminthic)
   c. Drug-induced (e.g., penicillamine, gold, nonsteroidal anti-inflammatory drugs)
   d. Allergen-induced (e.g., bee stings, snake bites)

EPIDEMIOLOGY

1. Prevalence of NS: 16 in 100,000 population under 16 years old
2. Age at presentation
   a. Preschool-age children between 2 and 6 years old
   b. About 80% of children are less than 6 years of age; median age at diagnosis: 2.5 years
3. Male-female ratio is 3:2.

PATHOGENESIS

1. An increase in glomerular capillary wall permeability ⇒ protein loss, primarily of albumin
2. Hypoalbuminemia ⇒ decrease in plasma oncotic pressure permitting transudation of intravascular fluid into the interstitial space
3. Depleted intravascular volume activates renin-angiotensin-aldosterone system (reabsorption of sodium in distal tubules) and release of antidiuretic hormone (reabsorption of water in collecting duct). Reabsorbed sodium and water are lost into the interstitial space secondary to reduced oncotic pressure; thus edema becomes worse.
4. Hypoalbuminemia stimulates protein synthesis in the liver including synthesis of lipids (cholesterol, triglycerides) and lipoproteins.

LABORATORY (see also Table 15–4)

1. Complete blood count: high hemoglobin and hematocrit (hemoconcentration) and thrombocytosis
2. Serum values of electrolytes are normal; hyponatremia may be seen (pseudohyponatremia because of hyperlipidemia)
3. Serum values of creatinine and complement: normal
4. Hypocalcemia (secondary to hypoalbuminemia)

5. Antinuclear antigen and serologic tests for hepatitis and syphilis: negative
6. Renal biopsy (see Box 15–4)
   a. *Not* indicated to confirm the diagnosis of MCNS
   b. Minimal histologic changes in the glomeruli are seen on light microscopy; negative immunofluorescence and fusion of foot processes are seen on electron microscopy.

BOX 15–4   *Renal Biopsy Indications in Nephrotic Syndrome*

Usually indicated for children whose initial presentation suggests a diagnosis *other than* MCNS
Infants <12 months or children >6 years of age
Presence of renal failure (not secondary to hypovolemia)
Decreased serum complement
Gross hematuria (in absence of infection)
Persistent hypertension
Persistent microscopic hematuria
Failure to respond to initial course of steroids
Steroid-dependent or steroid-resistant patient
Multiple relapses (four episodes or more per year)

COMPLICATIONS

1. Infections
   a. Spontaneous bacterial peritonitis
      (1) *Streptococcus pneumoniae* (most common cause)
      (2) Gram-negative organisms
   b. Other: sepsis, cellulitis (skin breakdown from edema), pneumonia
2. Hypovolemia: despite the edematous appearance with fluid and salt retention, children are actually intravascularly depleted, and injudicious use of diuretics can lead to shock.
3. Respiratory compromise due to ascites, pleural effusion
4. Hypercoagulability may lead to venous thrombosis (e.g., in deep veins in the legs or pelvis or pulmonary or renal veins) and rarely to arterial thrombosis (e.g., pulmonary).

TREATMENT

1. Hospitalize patients with severe nephrosis.
2. With first episode of nephrosis, family needs to be educated about chronic relapsing nature of the disease, home monitoring of urine by Albustix, diet, and complications related to both the disease and therapy.
2. Specific therapy
   a. Prednisone therapy for a period of 8 weeks
      (1) Prednisone 2 mg/kg/day or 60 mg/m²/day (maximum 60 mg/day) given orally every

morning in one dose or in two divided doses (preferably after meals) for the first 4 weeks, followed by 40 mg/m²/day given every other day for the next 4 weeks
      (2) Therapy is then abruptly discontinued without tapering.
   b. Majority of children (80% to 85%) respond with remission of proteinuria and resolution of edema by 4 weeks (average time, about 2 weeks)

BOX 15–5   *Periorbital Edema of Nephrotic Syndrome*

- Often mistaken for an allergic reaction
- Absence of itching and a dipstick check for proteinuria in such cases should alert one to the possibility of NS
- Edema is gravity-dependent; thus, early morning periorbital or facial edema may not be apparent by the time the child is seen later in the day

---

3. For symptomatic edema
   a. Salt and fluid restriction and, if indicated, judicious use of diuretics (e.g., spironolactone, furosemide) during periods of edema
   b. Infusion of concentrated albumin followed by a loop diuretic (e.g., in patients with respiratory symptoms or profound edema). This therapy should be used with extreme caution (owing to risk of fluid overload and hypertension).
4. Lipid lowering agents: usually not indicated since hyperlipidemia disappears with resolution of proteinuria.
5. For child with relapse (presence of proteinuria >1+ on a urinary dipstick on three consecutive days):
   a. Treatment with prednisone 60 mg/m²/day until the urine is protein-free for 3 consecutive days
   b. Followed by prednisone 40 mg/m² every other day for 4 weeks
6. Pediatric nephrology consultation for:
   a. A child requiring frequent courses of steroid therapy and steroid toxicity (e.g., growth retardation, cushingoid features)
   b. Failure to respond to steroid treatment despite good compliance, or occurrence of frequent relapses
   c. A steroid-resistant child (continuous proteinuria [>2+] after 4 weeks of daily prednisone therapy for possible renal biopsy and further management with cytotoxic therapy [e.g., cyclophosphamide, chlorambucil, or macrolide immunosuppressants such as cyclosporine A])
7. Prevention of infection

a. Polyvalent pneumococcal vaccine (current recommendation)
   (1) Children over 2 years old: one dose
   (2) Revaccination once after 3 to 5 years for children under 10 years old
b. Daily penicillin prophylaxis for edematous children with ascites until edema resolves

PROGNOSIS

1. Relapse is the rule, and children with steroid-responsive MCNS usually have repeated relapses until the disease resolves spontaneously toward the end of the second decade of life.
2. Most children with MCNS do not develop progressive renal disease. It is essentially a benign disorder.

3. Overwhelming infection is one of the major causes of death in patients with NS.
4. Mortality rate is less than 1%.

KEY POINTS

Minimal Change Nephrotic Syndrome

- Term NS implies heavy proteinuria, hypoproteinemia (hypoalbuminemia), edema, and hyperlipidemia.
- Most common variety among primary NS is MCNS.
- Presence of fever, abdominal pain, and rebound tenderness in an edematous patient with ascites suggests spontaneous bacterial peritonitis.

TABLE 15-3
Clinical Features of Minimal Change Nephrotic Syndrome

Cardinal Features	Other Features
Edema	Oliguria
Often periorbital	Weight gain (edema, ascites)
Most common sign heralding the diagnosis	Hypertension (10%)
Pedal edema (difficulty putting on regular-sized shoes)	Pleural effusion
Leg (pretibial) edema	Bowel wall edema
Edema of the scrotum, penis or vulva, sacrum	Abdominal pain
Ascites	Diarrhea, vomiting

TABLE 15-4
Laboratory Features of Minimal Change Nephrotic Syndrome

Heavy proteinuria (sine qua non of NS)
  Nephrotic-range proteinuria (any of the following):
    Proteinuria >40 mg/m^2/hour in 24 hours
    (normal <4 mg/m^2/hour in 24 hours)
    Urine protein/creatinine ratio (mg/mg) >3.0
    (normal ratio: [infants <0.5, child <0.2])
Hypoproteinemia and hypoalbuminemia
  (serum albumin <2.5 g/dL)
Hyperlipidemia (increased cholesterol, triglycerides, low-density and very-low-density lipoproteins)
Elevated serum urea nitrogen (seen in 15% to 30% of patients)
Urinalysis
  High specific gravity (intravascular volume depletion)
  Proteinuria 3+ or 4+
  Microscopic hematuria (20% to 25%); gross hematuria (rare)
  Lipid droplets and broad waxy casts

TABLE 15-5
Differential Diagnosis of Minimal Change Nephrotic Syndrome

Edema

Periorbital edema due to infections or allergies
Protein-losing enteropathy
Kwashiorkor (protein-energy malnutrition)
Proteinuria from other causes (proteinuria *rarely* exceeds 1 g/24 hours, and is *not* associated with edema)
  Transient proteinuria (e.g., fever, dehydration, exercise)
  Orthostatic proteinuria
  Tubular proteinuria (e.g., Fanconi syndrome, myoglobin, hemoglobin)

Nephrotic Syndrome (Other Types)

Focal glomerulosclerosis
Membranoproliferative glomerulonephritis
Membranous glomerulonephritis

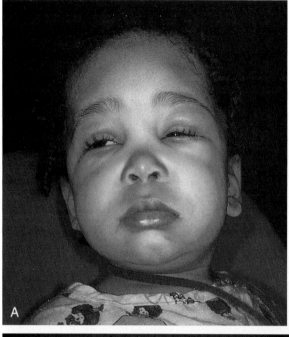

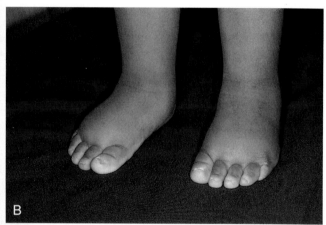

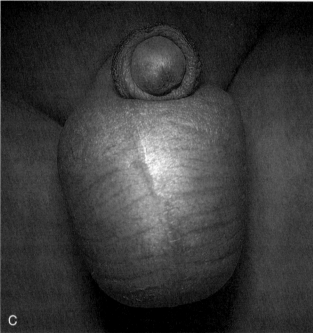

FIGURE 15-5. Minimal change NS in an 18-month-old child presenting with periorbital and facial edema (A), (picture taken right after he awakened in the morning) and edema of the feet (B), and scrotum (C).

Acute Poststreptococcal Glomerulonephritis (APSGN)

DEFINITION

Acute glomerulonephritis (AGN) constitutes varying degrees of hematuria, hypertension, proteinuria, and occasionally impaired renal function. Acute glomerulonephritis following group A beta-hemolytic streptococcus (GABS) infection is referred to as acute poststreptococcal glomerulonephritis.

ETIOLOGY

1. APSGN follows a throat infection (usually in winter) or a skin infection (usually in summer) with nephritogenic strains of GABS (e.g., M-type 49 or 12).
2. Latent period between GABS infection and development of AGN:
   a. Between throat infection and APSGN: usually 7 to 10 days

b. Between skin infection and APSGN: 1 to 3 weeks

EPIDEMIOLOGY

1. Most common infectious agent associated with acute glomerulonephritis is GABS.
2. Most common form of immune-mediated nephritis in children is APSGN.
3. Age at presentation
   a. Most common in school-aged children
   b. Mean age: 7 years; range 5 to 10 years
   c. Rare: less than 3 years of age
4. Male-female ratio is 2:1.

PATHOGENESIS

1. Immune complexes mediate glomerular damage.
2. Immune complex deposits are present on the subepithelial side of the glomerular basement membrane. Immune complexes are predominantly composed of IgG and complement C3.
3. The precise mechanism by which nephritogenic streptococci induce immune complex formation is not clearly defined.

LABORATORY

1. Evidence of preceding GABS infection
   a. Throat culture (positive in 15% to 20% of patients with APSGN)
   b. Rise in antistreptolysin O titers (follows streptococcal pharyngeal infection)
   c. Streptozyme test (detects antibodies to hyaluronidase, streptolysin O, DNase B, and NADase).
2. Serum electrolytes, urea nitrogen, and creatinine
3. Serum complement C3 value
   a. Reduced in 90% of cases
   b. Returns to normal by 8 weeks in 94% of cases
   c. Persistent hypocomplementemia: suspect another cause of glomerulonephritis (see Table 15-7)
4. Urinalysis
   a. Gross hematuria (blood in the urine visible to naked eye) or microscopic hematuria (>5 red blood cells/high power field in a centrifuged urine detected only by microscopic examination)
   b. Red blood cell casts (pathognomonic of glomerulonephritis)

BOX 15-6 *Hematuria*

- Brown color of the urine is produced because hemoglobin is converted to hematin by the acid urine; it indicates blood coming from the upper urinary tract.
- Bleeding from the lower urinary tract is associated with terminal hematuria with passage of blood clots.

---

c. Proteinuria
d. Hyaline and granular casts
5. Chest radiograph (to evaluate cardiac size and pulmonary edema in patients with hypertension, oliguria, and renal insufficiency)

COMPLICATIONS

1. Complications related to acute renal failure
   a. Volume overload (edema, congestive heart failure, pulmonary edema)
   b. Electrolyte imbalance (e.g., hyperkalemia, acidosis, hyperphosphatemia, hypocalcemia)
   c. Uremia
   d. Hypertension
2. Complications related to hypertensive encephalopathy

BOX 15-7 *Renal Biopsy and APSGN*

Not indicated routinely to confirm the diagnosis
May be considered for patients with:
   Acute renal failure
   Nephrotic syndrome
   Persistence of significant hematuria and/or proteinuria
   Persistence of hypocomplementemia
   Renal insufficiency *beyond* 12 weeks after onset of AGN

BOX 15-8 *Renal Involvement in APSGN* (any of the following):

Asymptomatic microscopic hematuria
Acute *nephritic syndrome* presentation
   Sudden onset of hematuria
   Gross (30% to 50% of cases) or microscopic hematuria
   Proteinuria (minimal to moderate)
   Hypertension (50% to 90% of cases)
   Edema (salt/water retention)
   Renal insufficiency
Nephrotic syndrome presentation
   Seen in 10% to 20% of patients
   Heavy proteinuria
   Hypoproteinemia
   Edema
   Hypercholesterolemia

TREATMENT

1. Hospitalization for monitoring of blood pressure and other vital signs (signs of pulmonary edema, congestive heart failure) and urinary output
2. Treatment of hypertension

a. Calcium channel blockers (e.g., nifedipine) for mild to moderate elevation of blood pressure
   b. Intravenous therapy (e.g., diazoxide, nitroprusside) for hypertensive encephalopathy
3. Salt and fluid restrictions to prevent further fluid retention (especially in patients with oliguria).
4. Diuretic therapy may be considered in patients with edema.
5. Penicillin or other antistreptococcal antibiotic therapy
   a. Antibiotic therapy for all patients who either did not receive therapy for preceding GABS infection or have evidence of ongoing GABS infection
   b. Antibiotic therapy does not affect the natural course of APSGN.
   c. Antibiotic therapy is recommended to prevent the spread of nephritogenic strains of GABS.

PREVENTION

1. Early antibiotic therapy for GABS infections does *not* eliminate the risk of APSGN.

2. All family members of a patient should be screened for GABS and treated appropriately, if cultures are positive.

PROGNOSIS

1. About 95% of patients recover spontaneously; 5% develop chronic glomerulonephritis.
2. Recurrences are extremely rare.
3. Gross hematuria usually disappears in a few days; microscopic hematuria may persist for 1 year or longer.

KEY POINTS

Acute Poststreptococcal Glomerulonephritis

■ Most common cause of acute nephritis
■ Acute nephritic syndrome associated with hypocomplementemia and antecedent streptococcal infection strongly suggests the diagnosis.
■ Hallmark of APSGN is hematuria and urinary red blood cell casts, with only minimal to moderate proteinuria.

TABLE 15–6
Clinical Features of Acute Poststreptococcal Glomerulonephritis

Hematuria	Hypertensive encephalopathy
Most common presentation	Headache
Painless hematuria	Convulsions
Tea-colored, cola-colored, or smoky urine	Somnolence, coma
Gross or microscopic hematuria	Aphasia, transient blindness
Hypertension	Pulmonary edema or congestive heart failure
Nonspecific symptoms	Orthopnea, dyspnea
Fever, malaise	Rales, cough
Flank pain	Gallop rhythm

See also Box 15–6.

TABLE 15–7
Differential Diagnosis: Poststreptococcal Glomerulonephritis

Hematuria

IgA nephropathy/Berger disease (hematuria within 1–2 days of acute infection)
Benign hematuria
Sickle cell disease or trait
Hypercalciuria
Urinary tract infection
Hereditary nephritis

Acute Nephritic Syndrome

IgA nephropathy
Membranoproliferative glomerulonephritis
Hereditary nephritis
Vasculitides (e.g., systemic lupus erythematosus, Henoch-Schönlein purpura)

Other Conditions Associated With Hypocomplementemia

Lupus nephritis
Membranoproliferative glomerulonephritis
Shunt nephritis
Subacute bacterial endocarditis

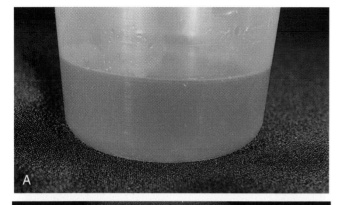

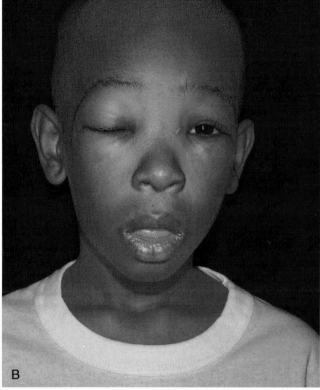

FIGURE 15-6. Acute poststreptococcal glomerulonephritis in an 8-year-old child who presented with tea-colored urine *(A)*, bilateral periorbital edema *(B)*, and hypertension following streptococcal pharyngitis (2 weeks prior to this photo).

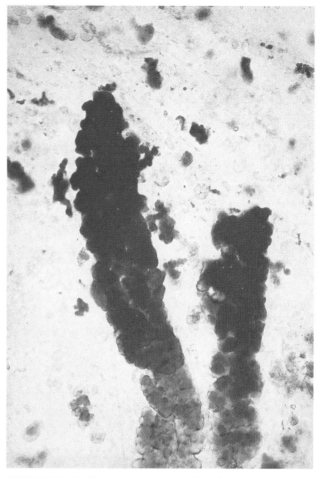

FIGURE 15-7. Microscopic examination of the urine showing red blood cell cast. (From Jao W, Padleckas R, Swerdlow MA: An Atlas of Urinary Sediment. Abbott Laboratories, North Chicago, Illinois, 1980.)

Lymphedema

DEFINITION

1. Lymphedema is the accumulation of interstitial fluid secondary to obstruction of lymphatic flow.
2. Lymphangiectasia is a dilation of the lymphatics.
3. Lymphangioma (or cystic hygroma) is a mass of dilated lymphatics.

ETIOLOGY (see also Tables 15-8 and 15-9)

1. Most cases of lymphedema in children are primary.

2. Primary lymphedema is further divided into
   a. Congenital lymphedema (onset of lymphedema within few months after birth)
   b. Lymphedema praecox or Meige disease (onset of lymphedema at 10 to 25 years of age)
   c. Lymphedema tarda (onset of lymphedema after 35 years of age)

EPIDEMIOLOGY

1. Prevalence of primary lymphedema: about 1 in 10,000 population

2. Of primary lymphedema cases:
   a. Congenital lymphedema: about 10% of cases
   b. Lymphedema praecox: about 71% of cases
   c. Lymphedema tarda: about 19% of cases
3. Lymphedema praecox and tarda: seen predominantly in females (about 64% to 90% of cases)
4. Congenital lymphedema: female-male ratio is 1 : 1.

ANATOMY/PATHOPHYSIOLOGY

1. Hydrostatic and osmotic pressures operating in the capillary beds force fluid out of the blood at the arterial ends of the capillary beds and cause most of it to be reabsorbed at the venous ends.
2. The protein-rich fluid that remains behind in the tissue spaces becomes interstitial fluid. Lymphatic circulation is involved in the absorption of interstitial fluid.
3. About 3 liters of lymph enters the blood stream daily (a volume almost exactly equal to the amount of fluid lost to the tissue space from the blood stream every 24 hours).
4. The lymphatic system is pumpless, and under normal conditions the lymphatic vessels are very low-pressure conduits.
5. Lymphatic vessels form a one-way system in which lymph flows only toward the heart. Lymphatic capillaries begin as blind-ended channels formed by a single layer of endothelial cells; ⇒ ⇒ they merge to form larger vessels (small and medium-sized vessels with smooth muscles), ⇒ ⇒ and empty into progressively larger channels ⇒ ⇒ that empty into the thoracic duct. Movement of lymph depends on contraction of the smooth muscles of the lymphatic trunks and on extrinsic factors (e.g., milking action of skeletal muscles, pressure changes during respiratory movements, arterial pulse).
6. Lymphatic malformations can occur in any lymphatic-bearing anatomic region; however, they are frequent in lymphatic-rich areas (neck, mediastinum, axilla, groin, and retroperitoneum).
7. Lymph capillaries are normally absent in the following anatomic regions:
   a. Entire central nervous system
   b. Bone and bone marrow
   c. Teeth
8. In primary lymphedema the lymphatic vessels are absent or hypoplastic or ectatic.
9. In secondary lymphedema the lymphatic vessels are usually dilated.

INHERITANCE

1. Hereditary or familial lymphedema
   a. Autosomal dominant with variable penetrance
   b. Examples: familial Milroy lymphedema and familial lymphedema praecox
2. Many chromosomal disorders are associated with lymphedema (see also Table 15–9).

CLINICAL FEATURES

1. Most common location of lymphedema: lower extremity
2. Most frequent complaint: a gradual, painless swelling of one leg in an otherwise healthy person
3. Early stages of lymphedema
   a. Edema soft
   b. Pitting present
   c. Usually painless
   d. Chronic, heavy sensation of the extremity
4. Chronic stages of lymphedema
   a. Woody texture of the extremity
   b. Involved tissues are indurated and fibrosed
   c. Pitting absent
   d. Loss of normal contour of the extremity
   e. Loss of hair and skin changes (hyperkeratosis) of the extremity

LABORATORY (as Clinically Indicated)

1. Complete blood count: eosinophilia frequently seen (in up to 25% of cases) in the early inflammatory phase of filariasis.
2. Serum values of total protein and albumin (to exclude hypoproteinemia)
3. Urinalysis (to exclude proteinuria)
4. Assay for circulating filarial antigen.
5. With lower extremity lymphedema:
   a. Ultrasound examination of abdomen and pelvis
   b. Computed tomography of abdomen and pelvis
6. Doppler ultrasound to exclude deep vein thrombosis
7. To differentiate primary from secondary lymphedema, to confirm the diagnosis, or to see the level of obstruction following tests (rarely indicated in clinical practice):
   a. Lymphangiography: requires cannulation of a distal lymphatic vessel followed by injection of contrast material
   b. Lymphoscintigraphy: involves injection of radioactively labeled technetium-containing colloid into the distal subcutaneous tissue of the affected extremity

COMPLICATIONS

1. Infections (seen in 25% to 50% of patients)
   a. Lymphangitis (inflammation of lymphatics seen as tender red streaks extending proximally from the infected site)
   b. Cellulitis
   c. Most common bacteria: group A streptococci and *Staphylococcus aureus*
2. Lymphosarcoma (extremely rare)

DIFFERENTIAL DIAGNOSIS (see also Tables 15–8 and 15–9)

1. Conditions with unilateral leg swelling
   a. Deep vein thrombosis
   b. Chronic venous insufficiency
2. Hypoproteinemia with edema (e.g., nephrotic syndrome, Menetrier disease)

TREATMENT

1. No specific treatment for lymphatic malformations; however, supportive care is very important.
2. Principles of therapy

a. Decrease risk of infections in the swollen extremity
  (1) Meticulous skin care, use of emollients to prevent drying
  (2) Properly fitting shoes
  (3) Education about warning signs of infection (e.g., "red streaks," fever, swollen lymph glands)
  (4) Parenteral antibiotic therapy for cellulitis or lymphangitis
  (5) Prophylactic antibiotic therapy for patients with recurrent cellulitis or lymphangitis
b. Maintain or possibly try to reduce the swelling
  (1) Frequent elevation of the extremity
  (2) Jobst (compression) stockings. Patient can be fitted with graduated stockings to reduce the amount of lymphedema that develops with upright posture.
  (3) Manual massage or intermittent pneumatic machines to reduce edema
  (4) Encourage exercise to enhance lymph return
  (5) Diuretic use is associated with metabolic alterations (e.g., hypokalemia, metabolic alkalosis, hypocalcemia) and risk of depletion of intravascular volume
c. Psychological and "social" support (disability and job limitations related to deformities)
3. Surgery
  a. Removal of excess edematous tissue
  b. Microsurgical lymphovenous anastomotic procedures to restore lymph drainage
4. Benzopyrone (5, 6-benzo-[α]-pyrone)
  a. Results in slow reduction of lymphedema of the extremities
  b. Stimulates proteolysis by tissue macrophages (removes excess protein and its consequent edema)
  c. Given orally; not available in North America for general use at the present time.

PROGNOSIS

1. Lymphedema persists throughout life.
2. Natural progression of lymphedema
  a. Plateaus in severity after early years of progression in 50% of cases
  b. Slow constant progression in 50% of cases
3. Lymphedema of contralateral extremity may develop in up to 10% of cases over a long period of time.

KEY POINTS

Lymphedema

- Most common location of lymphedema is lower extremity.
- Most common cause of secondary lymphedema worldwide is filariasis.

TABLE 15–8
Etiology of Lymphedema

Primary (Congenital Lymphedema)—Absent or Hypoplastic or Ectatic Lymphatic Vessels	Secondary (Acquired Condition)—Previously Normal Lymphatic Vessels
Milroy disease	Filariasis
Lymphedema praecox	Malignancy (e.g., lymphoma)
Lymphedema tarda	Following surgery
Turner syndrome	Postradiation fibrosis
Noonan syndrome	Recurrent lymphangitis (e.g., secondary to erysipelas)
Intestinal lymphangiectasia syndrome	Tuberculosis
Yellow nail syndrome	Pregnancy
Lymphangiomyomatosis	Factitious (application of tourniquets)
	Lymphogranuloma venereum
	Rheumatoid arthritis

TABLE 15–9
Multiple Malformation Syndromes and Associated Lymphatic Malformations

Turner syndrome	Lymphedema, cystic hygroma, webbed neck, intestinal lymphangiectasia, hydrops fetalis
Trisomy 21	Lymphedema, cystic hygroma
Trisomy 18	Lymphedema, cystic hygroma, webbed neck
Trisomy 13	Lymphedema, cystic hygroma
Klinefelter syndrome	Lymphedema, cystic hygroma
Noonan syndrome	Lymphedema, intestinal lymphangiectasia
Klippel-Trenaunay-Weber syndrome	Lymphedema, cystic hygroma
Milroy lymphedema	Lymphedema, intestinal lymphangiectasia
Meige disease	Lymphedema

Modified from Greenlee R, Hoyme H, Witte M, Crowe P, Witte C: Developmental disorders of the lymphatic system. Lymphology 1993; 26:156–168.

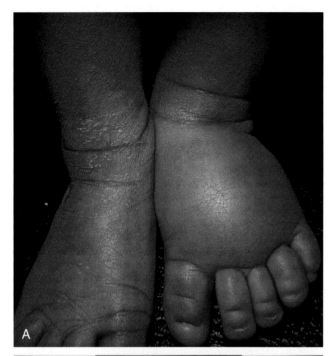

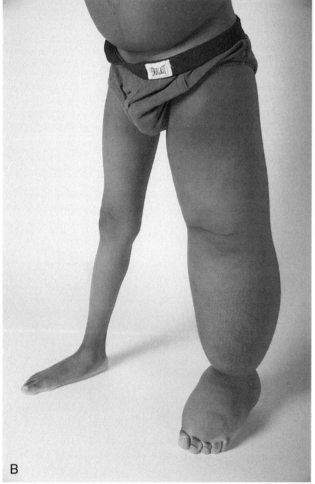

FIGURE 15-8. *A,* Congenital lymphedema presenting at birth. *B,* Extreme swelling of the extremity at 10 years of age. This patient also had pulmonary, mediastinal, neck, groin and retroperitoneal involvement. Since the CNS is devoid of lymph capillaries, this patient has no CNS involvement; he has been an honor student who is currently attending 7th grade.

Suggested Readings

1. American Academy of Pediatrics, Committee on Child Abuse and Neglect: Guidelines for the evaluation of sexual abuse of children. Pediatrics 1991;87:254–260.
2. American Academy of Pediatrics, Committee on Child Abuse and Neglect: Shaken baby syndrome: Inflicted cerebral trauma. Pediatrics 1993;92:872–875.
3. American Academy of Pediatrics, Section on Child Abuse and Neglect: A Guide to References and Resources in Child Abuse and Neglect. Elk Grove Village, IL, American Academy of Pediatrics, 1994.
4. American Academy of Pediatrics, Section on Child Abuse and Neglect: A Guide to References and Resources in Child Abuse and Neglect 2nd ed. Elk Grove Village, IL, American Academy of Pediatrics, 1998.
5. American Academy of Pediatrics, Section on Radiology: Diagnostic imaging of child abuse. Pediatrics 1991;87:262–264.
6. American Academy of Orthopaedic Surgeons, American Academy of Pediatrics: Essentials of Musculoskeletal Care. Snider RK (ed). Elk Grove Village, IL, American Academy of Pediatrics, 1997.
7. American Academy of Pediatrics: Red Book. Elk Grove Village, IL, American Academy of Pediatrics, 1997.
8. American Academy of Pediatrics, Committee on Infectious Diseases: Report. In Red Book, 24th ed. Elk Grove Village, IL, American Academy of Pediatrics, 1997.
9. Aslan Y, Mocan H, Erduran E, Aynaci M, Okten A: Asymmetric crying facies: An index of other malformations. Turk J Pediatr 1996;38:271–276.
10. Ashcraft KW (ed): Pediatric Surgery, 2nd ed. Philadelphia, W.B. Saunders, 1985.
11. Augsburger JJ: Ocular tumors in children. Pediatr Clin North Am 1983;30(6):1071–1086.
12. Ayoub EM: Acute rheumatic fever. In Emmanouilides GC (ed): Moss and Adams' Heart Disease in Infants, Children, and Adolescents Including the Fetus and Young Adult, 5th ed. Baltimore, Williams & Wilkins, 1995, pp. 1400.
13. Barkin RM (ed): Pediatric Emergency Medicine Concepts and Clinical Practice, 2nd ed. St. Louis, Mosby-Year Book, 1997.
14. Barratt TM, Clark G: Minimal change nephrotic syndrome and focal segmental glomerulosclerosis. In Holliday MA, Barratt TM, Avner ED (eds): Pediatric Nephrology, 3rd ed. Baltimore, Williams & Wilkins, 1994, p. 767.
15. Behrman RE, Kliegman RM, Arvin AM (eds): Nelson Textbook of Pediatrics, 15th ed. Philadelphia, W.B. Saunders, 1996.
16. Bloom JN: Traumatic hyphema in children. Pediatr Ann 1990; 19(6):368–375.
17. Botulism in infants. In Katz SL, Gershon AA, Hotez PJ (eds): Krugman's Infectious Diseases of Children, 10th ed. St. Louis, Mosby-Year Book, 1998, pp. 25–28.
18. Braunstein GD: Gynecomastia. N Engl J Med 1993;328(7):490–495.
19. Brodeur GM, Castleberry RP: Neuroblastoma. In Pizzo PA, Poplack DG (eds): Principles and Practice of Pediatric Oncology, 3rd ed. Philadelphia, Lippincott-Raven, 1997, pp. 761.
20. Calhoun JH: Cataracts in children. Pediatr Clin North Am 1983;30(6):1061–1069.
21. Camitta BM, Rock A: Acute lymphoblastic leukemia in a patient with thrombocytopenia/absent radii (TAR) syndrome. Am J Pediatr Hematol Oncol 1993;15(3):335–337.
22. Carraccio C, Sacchetti A, Lichenstein R: A new way to locate swallowed coins. Contemp Pediatr 1996;13(5):49–54.
23. Centers for Disease Control and Prevention: Recommendations for use of folic acid to reduce number of spina bifida cases and other neural tube defects. JAMA 1993;269:1233.
24. Centers for Disease Control and Prevention: 1998 Guidelines for Treatment of Sexually Transmitted Diseases. Atlanta, 1998.
25. Chew E, Morin JD: Glaucoma in children. Pediatr Clin North Am 1983;30(6):1043–1060.
26. Comerci JT Jr, Licciardi F, Bergh PA, Gregori C, Breen JL: Mature cystic teratoma: A clinicopathologic evaluation of 517 cases and review of the literature. Obstet Gynecol 1994;84:22–28.
27. Conners GP, Chamberlain JM, Ochsenschlager DW: Symptoms and spontaneous passage of esophageal coins. Arch Pediatr Adolesc Med 1995;149:36–39.
28. Danon M, Friedman SC: Ambiguous genitalia, micropenis, hypospadia and cryptorchidism. In Lifshitz F (ed): Pediatric Endocrinology, 3rd ed. New York, Marcel Dekker, 1996, pp. 281–303.
29. Dyment PG: Osgood-Schlatter disease and other apophysitides. In Finberg L (ed): Saunders Manual of Pediatric Practice. Philadelphia, W.B. Saunders, 1998, pp. 998–999.
30. Dyson M, Beckerman RC, Brouillette RT: Obstructive sleep apnea syndrome. In Beckerman RC, Brouillette RT, Hunt CE (eds): Respiratory Control Disorders in Infants and Children. Baltimore, Williams & Wilkins, 1992, pp. 212–230.
31. Ein SH, Shandling B, Wesson D, Filler RM: Recurrent pheochromocytomas in children. J Pediatr Surg 1990;25(10):1063–1065.
32. Espinoza LR (ed): Acute rheumatic fever. Rheum Dis Clin North Am 1993;19(2):333–349.
33. Fairbanks DNF, Milmoe GJ: Complications and sequelae: An otolaryngologist's perspective. Pediatr Infect Dis 1985;4(6):S75–S79.
34. Fanaroff A, Martin RJ: Neonatal-Perinatal Medicine. Diseases of the Fetus and Infant, 6th ed. St. Louis, Mosby-Year Book, 1997.
35. Feigin RD, Cherry JD (eds): Textbook of Pediatric Infectious Disease, 4th ed. Philadelphia, W.B. Saunders, 1998.
36. Finberg L: Nutritional rickets. In Finberg L (ed): Saunders Manual of Pediatric Practice. Philadelphia, W.B. Saunders, 1998, pp. 24–26.
37. Finberg L: Metabolic bone disorders. In Finberg L (ed): Saunders Manual of Pediatric Practice. Philadelphia, W.B. Saunders, 1998, pp. 216–218.
38. Finberg L (ed): Saunders Manual of Pediatric Practice. Philadelphia, W.B. Saunders, 1998.
39. Fiordalisi I, Shah BR, Finberg L: Rickets. In Castells S, Finberg L (eds): Metabolic Bone Disease. New York. Marcel Dekker, 1990, pp. 83–98.
40. Fisher MC: Conjunctivitis in children. In Pediatric ophthalmology. Pediatr Clin North Am 1987;34(6):1447–1456.
41. Fleisher GR, Ludwig S (eds): Textbook of Pediatric Emergency Medicine, 3rd ed. Baltimore, Williams & Wilkins, 1993.
42. Friedberg JF: Pharyngeal clefts, sinuses and cysts, and other benign neck lesions. Pediatr Clin North Am 1989;36(6):1451–1455.
43. Giardino AP, Christian CW, Giardino ER: A Practical Guide to the Evaluation of Child Physical Abuse and Neglect. Thousand Oaks, CA, Sage Pub, 1997.
44. Gilchrist BF, Lobe TE: The acute groin in pediatrics. Clin Pediatr 1992;31(8):488–496.

45. Ginsburg CM: Buccal cellulitis. Pediatr Infect Dis 1983;2(5): 381–382.

46. Glass AR: Gynecomastia. Endocrinol Metab Clin North Am 1994;23(4):825–837.

47. Greene JP, Guay AT: New perspectives in pheochromocytoma. Urol Clin North Am 1989;16(3):487–503.

48. Greenlee R, Hoyme H, Witte M, Crowe P, Witte C: Developmental disorders of the lymphatic system. Lymphology 1993; 26:156–168.

49. Fonkalsrud EW: Pheochromocytoma in children. Prog Pediatr Surg 1991;26:103–111.

50. Halperin DS, Doyle JJ: Is bone marrow examination justified in idiopathic thrombocytopenic purpura? Am J Dis Child 1988;142:508–511.

51. Hammerschlag MR: Sexually transmitted diseases in sexually abused children: Medical and legal implications. Sex Transm Inf 1998;74:167–174.

52. Hamre MR, Harmon EP, Kirkpatrick DV, Stern MJ, Humbert JR: Priapism as a complication of sickle cell disease. J Urol 1991;145:1–5.

53. Hedberg VA, Lipton JM: Thrombocytopenia with absent radii. A review of 100 cases. Am J Pediatr Hematol Oncol 1988; 10(1):51–64.

54. Henretig FM, King C (eds): Textbook of Pediatric Emergency Procedures. Baltimore, Williams and Wilkins, 1997.

55. Himelstein BP, Dormans JP: Malignant bone tumors of childhood. Pediatr Clin North Am 1996;43(4):967–984.

56. Hughes GB: Practical management of Bell's palsy. Otolaryngol Head Neck Surg 1990;102(6):658–663.

57. Hurwitz S: Clinical Pediatric Dermatology, 2nd ed. Philadelphia, W.B. Saunders, 1993.

58. Jacobsson M, Nylen O, Tjellstrom A: Acute otitis media and facial palsy in children. Acta Paediatr Scand 1990;79:118–120.

59. Johnson KB, Oski FA (eds): Oski's Essential Pediatrics. Philadelphia, Lippincott-Raven, 1997.

60. Jones KL: Smith's Recognizable Patterns of Human Malformations, 5th ed. Philadelphia, W.B. Saunders, 1997.

61. Katz, SL, Gershon AA, Hotez PJ (eds): Krugman's Infectious Diseases of Children, 10th ed. St. Louis, Mosby-Year Book, 1998.

62. Kehl DK: Slipped capital femoral epiphysis. *In* Morrisey RT, Weinstech SL (eds): Lovell and Winter's Pediatric Orthopedics, 4th ed. Philadelphia, Lippincott-Raven, 1996, pp. 993–1009.

63. Kliegman RM (ed): Practical Strategies in Pediatric Diagnosis and Therapy. Philadelphia, W.B. Saunders, 1996.

64. Krane SM, Schiller AL: Hyperostosis, neoplasms, and other disorders of bone and cartilage. *In* Isselbacher KJ, Braunwald E, Wilson JD, et al (eds): Harrison's Principles of Internal Medicine, 13th ed. New York, McGraw-Hill, 1994, pp. 2197–2199.

65. Krogstad P, Smith AL: Osteomyelitis and septic arthritis. *In* Feigin RD, Cherry JD (eds): Textbook of Pediatric Infectious Diseases, 4th ed. Philadelphia, W.B. Saunders, 1998, pp. 683–704.

66. Lane PA: Sickle cell disease. Pediatr Clin North Am 1996; 43(3):639–662.

67. Litovitz TL, Schmitz BF: Ingestion of cylindrical and button batteries: An analysis of 2382 cases. Pediatrics 1992;89(4):747–757.

68. Litovitz TL: Battery ingestions: Product accessibility and clinical course. Pediatrics 1985;75(3):469–476.

69. Luzzatto L: G6PD deficiency and hemolytic anemia. *In* Nathan DG, Oski FA (eds): Hematology of Infancy and Childhood, 4th ed. Philadelphia, W.B. Saunders, 1993.

70. Lynn M, Snoey E, Bosker G: Allergic disease update—Sneezing, wheezing, and getting the red out: Clinical classification and outcome—Effective pharmacotherapy. Emerg Med Rep 1997;18(25):245–256.

71. Mahoney CP: Adolescent gynecomastia. Differential diagnosis and management. Pediatr Clin North Am 1990;37(6):1389–1404.

72. Mangurten HH: Birth injuries. *In* Fanaroff AA, Martin R (eds): Neonatal-Perinatal Medicine, 6th ed. St. Louis, Mosby-Year Book, 1997, p. 425.

73. Morrissy RT, Shore SL: Bone and joint sepsis. Common orthopedic problems. Pediatr Clin North Am 1986;33(6):1551–1564.

74. Neely EK, Rosenfeld RG: Turner syndrome. *In* Lifshitz F (ed): Pediatric Endocrinology, 3rd ed. New York, Marcel Dekker, 1996, pp 267–280.

75. O'Brien KL, Dowell SF, Schwartz B, et al: Acute sinusitis—Principles of judicious use of antimicrobial agents. Pediatrics (Suppl) 1998;101:174–177.

76. O'Hara MA: Ophthalmia neonatorum. Pediatr Clin North Am 1993;40(4):715–725.

77. Pagon RA: Diagnostic approach to the newborn with ambiguous genitalia. Pediatr Clin North Am 1987;34(4):1019–1031.

78. Palin WE, Sadove AM, Jones JE, Judson WF, Stambaugh HD: Oral electrical burns in a pediatric population. J Oral Med 1987;42(1):17–21.

79. Parks RW, Parks TG: Pathogenesis, clinical features and management of hidradenitis suppurativa. Ann R Coll Surg Engl 1997;79(2):83–89.

80. Peitersen E: The natural history of Bell's palsy. Am J Otol 1982;4(2):107–111.

81. Pizzo PA, Poplack DG (eds): Principles and Practice of Pediatric Oncology, 3rd ed. Philadelphia, Lippincott-Raven, 1997.

82. Potsic WP: Obstructive sleep apnea. Pediatr Clin North Am 1989;36(6):1435–1442.

83. Potter WS: Pediatric cataracts. Pediatr Clin North Am 1993; 40(4):841–853.

84. Pounds LA: Neck masses of congenital origin. Pediatr Clin North Am 1981;28(4):841–844.

85. Rao SP: Glucose 6-Phosphate Dehydrogenase deficiency. *In* Finberg L (ed): Saunders Manual of Pediatric Practice. Philadelphia, W.B. Saunders, 1998, pp 395–397.

86. Rao SP: Iron deficiency Anemia and Other Microcytic Anemias. *In* Finberg L (ed): Saunders Manual of Pediatric Practice. Philadelphia, W.B. Saunders, 1998, pp 384–386.

87. Reece RM: Child abuse: Medical Diagnosis and Management. Philadelphia, Lea & Febiger, 1994.

88. Rosenstein N, Phillips WR, Gerber MA, et al: The common Cold—Principles of Judicious Use of Antimicrobial Agents. Pediatrics. Supplement. 1998;101:181–184.

89. Rudolph AM, Hoffman JIE, Rudolph CD (eds): Rudolph's Pediatrics, 20th ed. Stamford, CT, Appleton and Lange, 1996.

90. Rudoy PC, Nelson JD: Breast abscess during the neonatal period. Am J Dis Child 1975;129:1031–1034.

91. Saenger P: Turner's syndrome. N Engl J Med 1996;335(23): 1749–1754.

92. Schachner LA, Hansen RC (eds): Pediatric Dermatology, 2nd ed. New York, Churchill Livingston, 1995.

93. Schwartz MW (ed): The 5-Minute Pediatric Consult. Baltimore, Williams & Wilkins, 1997.

94. Schul MW, Keating MA: The acute pediatric scrotum. J Emerg Med 1993;11:565–577.

95. Schunk JE, Harrison AM, Corneli HM, Nixon GW: Fluoroscopic Foley catheter removal of esophageal foreign bodies in children: Experience with 415 episodes. Pediatrics 1994;94(5): 709–714.

96. Schweich PJ: Management of coin ingestion: Any change? Pediatr Emerg Care 1995;11(1):37–39.

97. Secord E, Emre U, Shah BR, Tunnessen WW Jr: Erythema marginatum in acute rheumatic fever. Am J Dis Child 1992; 146:637–638.

98. Selesnick SH, Patwardhan A: Acute facial paralysis: Evaluation and early management. Am J Otolaryngol 1994;15(6):387–408.

99. Shah BR, Finberg L: Single-day therapy for nutritional vitamin D-deficiency rickets: A preferred method. J Pediatr 1994;125: 487–490.

100. Shah BR, Fiordalisi I, Finberg L: Familial hypophosphatemia. *In* Castells S, Finberg L (eds): Metabolic Bone Disease in Children. New York. Marcel Dekker, 1990, pp. 151–169.

101. Shah BR, Fiordalisi I, Sheinbaum K, Finberg L: Familial glucocorticoid deficiency in a girl with familial hypophosphatemic rickets. Am J Dis Child 1988;142:900–903.

102. Shah BR, Tunnessen WW Jr: Urethral prolapse. Arch Pediatr Adolesc Med 1995;149:462–463.

103. Shelton PG, Ferretti GA: Maintaining oral health Pediatr Clin North Am 1982;29(3):653–668.

104. Sonnen GM, Henry NK: Pediatric bone and joint infections. Pediatr Clin North Am 1996;43(4):933–947.

105. Sotos JF: Overgrowth. Clin Pediatr 1997;36(2):91–103.

106. Spitz JL: Genodermatoses. Baltimore, Williams & Wilkins, 1996.

107. Stack LB, Munter DW: Foreign bodies in the gastrointestinal tract. Emerg Med Clin North Am 1996;14(3):493–521.

108. Swartz MH: Textbook of Physical Diagnosis. History and Examination, 2nd ed. Philadelphia, W.B. Saunders, 1994.

109. Surrell JA: Pilonidal disease. Surg Clin North Am 1994;74(6): 1309–1315.

110. Thompson JC, Ashwal S. Electrical injuries in children. Am J Dis Child 1983;137:231–235.

111. Wagner RS: Glaucoma in children. Pediatr Clin North Am 1993;40(4):855–867.

112. Wald ER, Pang D, Milmoe GJ, Schramm VL Jr: Sinusitis and its complications in the pediatric patient. Pediatr Clin North Am 1981;28(4):777–796.

113. Wald ER: Sinusitis in children. Pediatr Infect Dis J 1988;7: S150–S153.

114. Walsh M, McIntosh K: Neonatal mastitis. Clin Pediatr 1986; 25(8):395–399.

115. Warren FH: Genu varum and genu valgum. *In* Finberg L (ed): Saunders Manual of Pediatric Practice. Philadelphia, W.B. Saunders, 1998, pp. 994–996.

116. Warren FH: Legg-Calvé-Perthes disease. *In* Finberg L (ed): Saunders Manual of Pediatric Practice. Philadelphia, W.B. Saunders, 1998, pp. 996–997.

117. Warshaw BL: Nephrotic syndrome in children. Pediatr Ann 1994;23(9):495–504.

118. Wartofsky L: Diseases of the thyroid. *In* Isselbacher KJ, Braunwald E, Wilson JD, et al (eds): Harrison's Principles of Internal Medicine, 13th ed. New York, McGraw-Hill, 1994, pp. 1942–1946.

119. Weinblatt M, Petrikovsky B, Bialer M, Kochen J, Harper R: Prenatal evaluation and in utero platelet transfusion for thrombocytopenia absent radii syndrome. Prenatal Diagn. 1994;14(9):892–896.

120. Williams GH, Dluhy RG: Diseases of the adrenal, cortex. *In* Isselbacher KJ, Braunwald E, Wilson JD, et al (eds): Harrison's Principles of Internal Medicine, 13th ed. New York, McGraw-Hill, 1994, pp. 1970–1973.

Index

Note: Page numbers in italics refer to illustrations; page numbers followed by the letter b refer to boxed material, and those by t to tables.

Abscess(es), breast, neonatal, 19–20, 19b, 20, 20t
  pilonidal, 346–347, 347, 347b, 347t
Abuse, child. See *Child abuse.*
  sexual. See *Sexual abuse.*
Acanthosis nigricans, 238–239, 238b, 239, 239t
Acetaminophen, drug eruption from, 179, 180
Acne, 195–197, 195b, 195t, 196–197, 196t
Acoustic neurofibromatosis, 420b, 421–422, 421–422, 421t
Acrodermatitis, papular, of childhood, 68, 68, 68b, 68t
Acropustulosis, infantile, 198, 198, 198b, 198t
Acute glomerulonephritis, 468
Acute lymphoblastic leukemia, 273–275, 273b, 274t, 275–276, 275t
Acute poststreptococcal glomerulonephritis (APSGN), 468–471, 469b, 470t, 471
Acute rheumatic fever, 416–418, 416b, 417b, 418–419, 418t
Addison disease, 301–303, 302b, 303t, 304
Addisonian crisis, 303t
Adenoma sebaceum, 424
Adenoviral conjunctivitis, 131–132, 133, 133t
Adrenal crisis, acute, 303t
Adrenocortical deficiency, primary, 301–303, 302b, 303t, 304
Adrenocorticotropic hormone (ACTH) unresponsiveness, 304–306, 304b, 305t, 306
Aganglionic megacolon, congenital, 342–344, 342b, 343b, 343t, 344, 344t
Albinism, 456–457, 456b, 457, 457t
  partial, 458–459, 458b, 458t, 459
Albright syndrome, 314–316, 314b, 315–316, 315t
Allergic contact dermatitis, 168–170, 168b, 168t, 169–170
Allgrove syndrome, 304–306, 304b, 305t, 306
Alopecia areata, 210–211, 210b, 211, 211t
Alopecia universalis, 211
Amniotic constriction bands, 17–18, 18
Ampicillin, drug eruption from, 179, 180
Anaphylactoid purpura, 186–188, 186b, 187t, 188
Anaphylactoid reaction, 387b
Anaphylaxis, 387–389, 387b, 388t, 389, 389t
Ancylostoma, cutaneous larva migrans from, 125–126, 126
Anemia, acute hemolytic, 248–250, 249t, 250, 250t
  hypochromic microcytic, 247t
  iron deficiency, 245–247, 245b, 246t, 247, 247t
Anencephaly, 437–438, 438
Angioedema, in anaphylaxis, 389
Angio-osteohypertrophy syndrome, 215, 215, 215b, 215t

Anhidrotic ectodermal dysplasia, 236, 236–237, 236b, 236t
Antihemophilic factor deficiency, 268–272, 269b, 270t, 271–272, 271t
Aplasia, of depressor anguli oris muscle, 15–17, 16b, 16t, 17
Aplasia cutis congenita, 5–6, 5b, 6, 6t
Apnea, 159
  obstructive sleep, 159–161, 160b, 161, 161t
Apophysitis, tibial tubercle traction, 378–380, 380, 380t
Appendix testis, torsion of, 330–332, 331–332, 331t
Aprosencephaly with open cranium, 437–438, 438
Arachnidism, 243–244, 243b, 243t, 244
Arthritis, rheumatoid, juvenile, 405–407, 405b, 406, 406t
  septic, 357–360, 358b, 359t, 360, 360t
  with osteomyelitis, 350b
Arthropod bites, 173–175, 174b, 174t, 175
Aseptic necrosis of femoral head, 376–378, 377b, 378, 378t
Aspirin, urticaria from, 173
Asymmetric crying facies, 15–17, 16b, 16t, 17
Athlete's foot, 116–117, 117, 117t
Atlantoaxial instability, in trisomy 21, 446–448, 447b, 448
Atopic dermatitis, 162–166, 163b, 163t, 164–166, 164t
  vs. seborrheic dermatitis, 164t
Auricular pit, 346
Autoimmune disease(s), 297b, 300t
  Addison disease as, 301–303, 302b, 303t, 304
  Graves disease as, juvenile, 296–298, 297b, 297t, 298
  systemic lupus erythematosus as, 401–403, 401b, 402–403, 402b, 402t
  thyroiditis as, 298–301, 300t, 301
Autoimmune thyroiditis, 298–301, 300t, 301
Avascular necrosis, of femoral head, 376–378, 377b, 378, 378t

Baby bottle syndrome, 463–464, 463b, 464, 464t
Bacillary angiomatosis, with HIV infection, 81
Bacteria. See also specific type, e.g., *Streptococcus.*
  "flesh-eating," 91–92, 91t, 92
Balanitis, 334, 335b
Balanoposthitis, 334–336, 335b, 336, 336t
Barium enema, intussusception and, 339b
Batteries, ingestion of, 395–397, 396t, 397–398
Bee stings, 173–175, 174b, 174t, 175
"Bell-clapper" deformity, 326, 328
Bell's palsy, 428–430, 428b, 429–430, 429t
Belt buckle mark, 28
Bite(s), arthropod, 173–175, 174b, 174t, 175

Bite marks, 28
  spider, 243–244, 243b, 243t, 244
Black eyes, 42, 46
Black widow spider, 244
  bite from, 243–244, 243b, 243t
Blennorrhea, inclusion, 129–130, 130, 130b, 130t
  neonatal, 127–129, 127b, 129, 129t
Blistering distal dactylitis, 87, 88
  vs. child abuse, 43
Bloch-Sulzberger syndrome, 232–233, 232b, 233, 233t
Blount disease, 374–376, 374b, 375t, 376
  infantile, 374b
Bockhart impetigo, 92–93
Bone tumors, differential diagnosis of, 282b
  osteosarcomas as, 281–284, 282b, 282t, 283–284, 284t
Bordetella pertussis, pertussis from, 100–101, 100b, 100t, 101
Borrelia burgdorferi, 408
Borreliosis, 408–409, 409, 409b
Bottle mouth syndrome, 463–464, 463b, 464, 464t
Botulism, infant, 109–112, 111–112, 111t
Bourneville disease, 423–425, 423–425, 423b, 423t
Bowing, physiologic, vs. Blount disease, 375t
Bowlegs (genu varum), 375t
Brachial palsy, 8–9, 8b, 9, 9t
Breast abscess, neonatal, 19–20, 19b, 20, 20t
Brown recluse spider, 244
  bite from, 243–244, 243b, 243t, 244
Bruise(s), from child abuse, 24–25, 25b, 26t, 27
  black eye as, 42, 46
  of pinna, 46
Buccal cellulitis, 101–102, 101b, 102, 102t, 176b
Bucket handle fracture, from abuse, 36
Bug bites, 173–175, 174b, 174t, 175
Bullous dermatosis, benign chronic, of childhood, 203–204, 203b, 204, 204t
Bullous impetigo, 92, 93
Bullous pemphigoid, 208–209, 208b, 209, 209t
Burns, accidental, 29
  from child abuse, 25, 28–29
  oral electrical, 461–462, 462, 462b, 462t

Café-au-lait spots, 314b, 315, 421
Candidal diaper dermatitis, 120, 120, 120b, 171
Candidal paronychia, with HIV, 81
Candidiasis, 120–121, 120–121, 120b
Cao gio (coin rubbing), vs. child abuse, 41, 43
Capital femoral epiphysis, ischemic necrosis of, 376–378, 377b, 378, 378t
  slipped, 384–386, 384b, 386
Caput succedaneum, 11–12, 12–13, 12t
Carbunculosis, 92–93, 94

Cardiofacial syndrome, 15–17, 16b, 16t, *17*

Carditis, in acute rheumatic fever, 416b, *419*

Caries, nursing-bottle, 463–464, 463b, *464*, 464t

Cataract, 140–142, 141b, *142*, 142t

Catecholamine, synthesis and metabolism of, 278b

Catecholamine-secreting tumor(s), differential diagnosis of, 311b

  pheochromocytoma as, 311–313, 311b, 312t, *313*, 313t

Cayler syndrome, 15–17, 16b, 16t, *17*

Cellulitis, buccal, 101–102, 101b, *102*, 102t, 176b

  orbital, 149–152, 149b, 150t, *151–152*, 151t

    with proptosis, *152, 155*

  perianal, streptococcal, 87, *88*

  preseptal, 147–148, *148*, 148t

  staphylococcal, 92–93, *94*

Cephalhematoma, 9–11, 9b, *10–11*, 10t

  vs. caput succedaneum, 12t

Cerebral gigantism, 451–453, 451b, 451t, *452–453*

Chalazion, 140, *140*, 140t

Chest syndrome, acute, sickle cell anemia and, 261–263, 262t, *263*

Chickenpox (varicella), 50–55, 51t, *52–55*

  congenital syndrome of, 50b, *53*

  distribution of, *52*

  lesions of, *52–53*

  with HIV, *80*

Child abuse, 24–36

  bite marks in, *28*

  bruises in, 24–25, 25b, 26t, *27*

  burn marks in, *28–29*

  clinical features of, 24–25, 24b

  condition(s) mistaken for, 41–49, 41b

    acute immune thrombocytopenic purpura as, 42, *44*

    black eyes as, 42, *46*

    blistering distal dactylitis as, *43*

    cao gio (coin rubbing) as, 41, *43*

    cupping (ventosa) as, 41, *44*

    hemarthrosis of elbow as, *47*

    hemophilia A as, 42, *47*

    Henoch-Schönlein purpura as, 42, *45*

    lichen sclerosus et atrophicus as, *43*

    Mongolian spots as, 41, *43*

    osteogenesis imperfecta as, 42, *48*

    perianal streptococcal infection as, 43

    petechiae as, *45*

    protein C deficiency as, 41, *44*

    purpura fulminans as, 41, *44*

    "raccoon eyes" as, 42, *46*

    rickets as, 42, *48*

    scurvy as, 42, *47*

    urethral prolapse as, 42–43, *49*

  differential diagnosis of, 26, 34t

  full skeletal survey in, 25–26, 25b

  object marks in, *27–28*

  rib fractures in, 32b, *34*

  sexual. See *Sexual abuse.*

  shaken impact syndrome in, 30–31, 30b, *31–32*, 31t

  skeletal injuries in, 32–35, 32b, 33b, 33t, *34–36*, 34t

    differential diagnosis of, 34t

Chlamydial ophthalmia, 129–130, *130*, 130b, 130t

Chondrodysplasia, metaphyseal, 372–373, 372t, *373*

Chondrodystrophy, primary, 372–373, 372t, *373*

Christ-Siemens-Tourraine syndrome, 236, *236–237*, 236b, 236t

Circle of Willis, *265*

Clostridium botulinum, infant botulism from, 109–112, *111–112*, 111t

Clouston syndrome, 236b

Coin rubbing, vs. child abuse, 41, *43*

Collodion baby, *227*

Condylomata acuminata, *39*, 39t

Condylomata lata, *40*

Congenital adrenal hyperplasia from 21-hydroxylase deficiency, 317t, 318t

Congenital adrenocortical unresponsiveness to ACTH, 304–306, 304b, 305t, *306*

Congenital aganglionic megacolon, 342–344, 342b, 343b, 343t, *344*, 344t

Congenital hypoplasia, of depressor anguli oris muscle, 15–17, 16b, 16t, *17*

Congenital muscular torticollis, 20–21, *21*, 21t

Congenital pigmented nevus, 216–217, 216b, *217*, 217t

Congenital rubella syndrome, 62b, *63–64*

Congenital varicella syndrome, 50b, *53*

Conjunctivitis, acute, 131–133, 131b, 132t, *133*, 133t

  adenoviral, 131–132, *133*, 133t

  allergic, 132, 132t

  bacterial, 131, 132t

  gonococcal, *40*

  herpes, 131, 132t, *133*

  neonatal, 127–129, 127b, *129*, 129t

    inclusion, 129–130, *130*, 130b, 130t

  vernal, 132, 132t, *133*

Constipation, differential diagnosis of, 343t

  vs. Hirschsprung disease, 344t

Contact dermatitis, allergic, 168–170, 168b, 168t, *169–170*

  irritant, 168t

Contusions, from child abuse, 24–25, 25b, 26t

Corynebacterium minutissimum, erythrasma from, 97–98, 97b, *98*, 98t

Coxsackievirus, Gianotti-Crosti syndrome from, 68, *68*, 68b, 68t

  hand-foot-mouth disease from, 72–74, 72b, *73–74*

  herpangina from, 74–75, 74t, *75*

Cradle cap, 189–190, *189–190*, 189b

Craniosynostosis, 430–434, *432–434*, 432t

Creeping eruption, 125–126, *126*

Cupping (ventosa), vs. child abuse, 41, *44*

Cushing disease, 307

Cushing syndrome, 307–310, 308t, *309–310*, 309t, 310t

Cushingoid syndrome, 307

Cutaneous larva migrans, 125–126, *126*

Cyst(s), dermoid, 240–241, 240b, *241*, 241t

  in thyroglossal duct, 348–349, 348b, *349*, 349t

  mucus retention, 464–465, 464b, *465*

Cystic hygroma, *471*

Cystic ovarian teratoma, mature, 285–287, *286–287*, 286t, 287t

Dactylitis, blistering distal, 87, *88*

  vs. child abuse, 43

Dandruff, 189–190, *189–190*, 189b

Darier sign, positive, 223b

Depressor anguli oris muscle, aplasia of, 15–17, 16b, 16t, *17*

Dermal melanocytosis, 217–219, 217b, *218–219*, 218t

Dermatitis, 162–244

  atopic, 162–166, 163b, 163t, *164–166*, 164t

Dermatitis *(Continued)*

  erythroderma from, *166*

  from herpes simplex virus, *166*

  from *Staphylococcus aureus, 166*

  vs. seborrheic, 164t

  contact, allergic, 168–170, 168b, 168t, *169–170*

    irritant, 168t

  dermatitis herpetiformis as, *207–208*, 207b, 207t

  diaper, 170–171, 170b, *171*

    candidal, 120, *120*, 120b, *171*

  exfoliative, 176–177, *177*, 177b, 177t

    with psoriasis, *177*

  from poison ivy, 168–169, 168b, 168t, *169*

  Gianotti-type perioral, 200, *200*, 200b, 200t

  papular acrodermatitis as, 68, *68*, 68b, 68t

  perianal streptococcal, 87, *88*

  perioral granulomatous, 200, *200*, 200b, 200t

  phytophotodermatitis as, 239–240, 239b, 239t, *240*

  seborrheic, 189–190, *189–190*, 189b

    vs. atopic, 164t

Dermatomyositis, juvenile, 407–408, 407b, *408*, 408t

Dermatosis, bullous, benign chronic, of childhood, 203–204, 203b, *204*, 204t

Dermoid cyst, 240–241, 240b, *241*, 241t

Dermoids, 285–287, *286–287*, 286t, 287t

Diaper dermatitis (diaper rash), 170–171, 170b, *171*

  candidal, 120, *120*, 120b, *171*

Down syndrome (trisomy 21), 444–446, 444b, 445t, *446*

  atlantoaxial instability in, 446–448, 447b, *448*

Drug eruption(s), 179–181, 179b, *180–181*

Drug reaction(s), erythema multiforme major as, 181–183, 181b, *182–183*, 182t

  erythema multiforme minor as, 179, *181*

Duhring's disease, *207–208*, 207b, 207t

Dysostosis, metaphyseal, 372–373, 372t, *373*

Dysplasia, metaphyseal, Schmid type, 372–373, 372t, *373*

Dystrophic epidermolysis bullosa, 230–232, *232*

EBV. See *Epstein-Barr virus (EBV).*

Ecchymosis, periorbital, 42, *46*

Echovirus, herpangina from, 74–75, 74t, *75*

Ecthyma, 87, *88*

Ecthyma gangrenosum, 99, *99*, 99b, 99t

Eczema herpeticum, *166*

Elbow, hemarthrosis of, vs. child abuse, *47*

  nursemaid's (pulled), 399–400, 399b, *400*

Electrical burns, oral, 461–462, *462*, 462b, 462t

Encephalocele, 441–443, 441b, 442t, *443*

Enema, barium, intussusception and, 339b

Epidermal nevus, 221, *221–222*, 221b, 221t

Epidermolysis bullosa, 230–231, 230b, *231–232*

Epidermolytic hyperkeratosis, *228*

Epidermophyton, tinea corporis from, 115–116, *116*, 116t

Epididymitis, 332

Epididymo-orchitis, 332–334, 333b, 333t, *334*, 334t

Epiloia, 423–425, *423–425*, 423b, 423t

Epiphysis, slipped capital femoral, 384–386, 384b, *386*

Epstein-Barr virus (EBV), Gianotti-Crosti syndrome from, 68, *68*, 68b, 68t

Epstein-Barr virus (EBV) *(Continued)*
  infectious mononucleosis from, 66–67, 66b, 66t, *67*, 67t
Erb-Duchenne (Erb) palsy, 8–9, 8b, *9*, 9t
Erysipelas, 82–83, 82b, *83*, 83t
Erythema chronicum migrans, in Lyme disease, *409*, 409b
Erythema infectiosum, 70–72, *71–72*, 71b, 71t
Erythema marginatum, in acute rheumatic fever, 417b, *418*
Erythema multiforme major, 181–183, 181b, *182–183*, 182t
Erythema multiforme minor, 179, *181*
Erythema nodosum, 177–178, *178*, 178b, 178t
Erythema toxicum neonatorum, 2–3, *3*, 3t
Erythrasma, 97–98, 97b, *98*, 98t
Erythroderma, from atopic dermatitis, *166*
  generalized, 176–177, *177*, 177b, 177t
Esophageal foreign body, 389–392, *391–392*, 391t
Ewing sarcoma, vs. osteosarcoma, 284t
Exanthem subitum, 69–70, *69–70*, 69b, 70t
Exencephaly, 441–443, 441b, 442t, *443*
Exfoliative dermatitis, 176–177, *177*, 177b, 177t
Eye, normal angle structures in, *138*

FACE (Facial Afro-Caribbean Childhood Eruption), 200, *200*, 200b, 200t
Facial nerve palsy, traumatic neonatal, 13–15, 14b, *15*
Facial palsy, Bell's palsy as, 428–430, 428b, *429–430*, 429t
  peripheral, 158b
  with acute otitis media, 158–159, 158b, *159*
Factor VIII deficiency, 268–272, 269b, 270t, *271–272*, 271t
Familial glucocorticoid deficiency (FGD), 304–306, 304b, 305t, *306*
Familial hypophosphatemic rickets (FHR), 366–369, 366b, 367t, *368–369*
Familial white spotting, 458–459, 458b, 458t, *459*
Fanconi anemia, vs. TAR syndrome, 455t
Fasciitis, necrotizing, 91–92, 91t, *92*
Fat necrosis, subcutaneous, 3–4, 3b, *4*, 4t
Femoral head, avascular (aseptic) necrosis of, 376–378, 377b, *378*, 378t
  idiopathic osteonecrosis of, 376–378, 377b, *378*, 378t
Fibroma, periungual, *425*
Fifth disease (erythema infectiosum), 70–72, *71–72*, 71b, 71t
"Flesh-eating bacteria," 91–92, 91t, *92*
Follicular occlusion triad, 241b
Folliculitis, staphylococcal, 92–93
Foreign body(ies), batteries as, 395–397, 396b, *397–398*
  in esophagus, 389–392, *391–392*, 391t
  in stomach and lower GI tract, 392–394, *394*
Foreskin, anatomy of, 334, *336*, 336–337
Fox metal shield, 137, *138*
Fracture(s), from child abuse, 32–35, 32b, 33b, 33t, *34–36*, 34t
  bucket handle, *36*
  differential diagnosis of, *34t*
  humeral, *35*
  pathognomic or "classic," 33b

Fracture(s) *(Continued)*
  rib, 32t, *34*
  tibial, *36*
Furunculosis, 92–93, *93*

Gangrene, streptococcal (hospital), 91–92, 91t, *92*
Gastrointestinal tract, lower, foreign bodies in, 392–394, *394*
Genitalia, ambiguous, 316–319, 317t, 318t, *319*
Genu varum (bowlegs), 375t
German measles (rubella), 62–64, 62t, *63–64*
  congenital syndrome of, 62b, *63–64*
Gianotti-Crosti syndrome, 68, *68*, 68b, 68t
Gianotti-type perioral dermatitis, 200, *200*, 200b, 200t
Gigantism, cerebral, 451–453, 451b, 451t, *452–453*
Gingivostomatitis, herpetic, *57*, 57t
Glaucoma, 134
  infantile (congenital), 134–136, 134b, 135t, *136*
Glomerulonephritis, acute, 468
  poststreptococcal, 468–471, 469b, 470t, *471*
Glucocorticoid deficiency, familial, 304–306, 304b, 305t, *306*
Glucose-6-phosphate dehydrogenase (G6PD) deficiency, 248–250, 249t, *250*, 250t
Goiter, lymphadenoid, 298–301, 300t, *301*
Gonadal dysgenesis, 316–319, 317t, 318t, *319*
  in Turner syndrome, 448–450, 449b, *450*
Gonococcal infections, 102–104, 103b, 103t, *104*
  conjunctivitis as, *40*, 127–129, 127b, *129*, 129t
Gottron's papules, *408*
Granuloma, Jacquet, *171*
  Kaposi sarcomalike, 201, *201*, 201b, 201t
  pyogenic, 185–186, 185b, 185t, *186*
Granuloma annulare, 199, *199*, 199b
Granuloma gluteale infantum, 201, *201*, 201b, 201t
Granuloma intertriginosum infantum, 201, *201*, 201b, 201t
Graves disease, juvenile, 296–298, 297b, 297t, *298*
Group A beta-hemolytic streptococcus (GABS). See *Streptococcus, group A beta-hemolytic.*
Guttate psoriasis, 192–194, 193b, 193t, *194*
Gynecomastia, 292
  adolescent, 292–294, 292b, 293t, *294*, 294t

Hand-foot-mouth disease, 72–74, 72b, *73–74*
Hashimoto thyroiditis, 298–301, 300t, *301*
Head injuries, traumatic, *13*
Hemangioma, 212–214, 212b, *213–214*, 213t
Hemarthrosis, in hemophilia, 269b, *271–272*
  of elbow, vs. child abuse, *47*
Hematocolpos, 320
Hematometrocolpos, 320
Hematuria, 469b
Hemolytic anemia, acute, 248–250, 249t, *250*, 250t
Hemophilia, 268

Hemophilia A, 268–272, 269b, 270t, *271–272*, 271t
  vs. child abuse, 42
Henoch-Schönlein purpura, 186–188, 186b, 187t, *188*
  vs. child abuse, 42, *45*
Hepatitis B virus, Gianotti-Crosti syndrome from, 68, *68*, 68b, 68t
Hereditary adrenocortical unresponsiveness, to ACTH, 304–306, 304b, 305t, *306*
Hereditary pseudodeficiency rickets, 369–371, 370t, *371*, 371t
Herpangina, 74–75, 74t, *75*
Herpes simplex virus (HSV) infection(s), 56–58, *57–58*, 57t
  atopic dermatitis from, *166*
  gingivostomatitis from, *57*, 57t
  herpes labialis from, *57*
  keratoconjunctivitis from, 132t, *133*
  neonatal, 4–5, 4b, *5*, 5t
  vulvovaginitis from, *58*
  with HIV, *80*
Herpes zoster, 54–55, 54t, *55*
  Ramsay Hunt syndrome from, 54b
Hidradenitis suppurativa, 241–242, 241b, *242*, 242t
Hidrotic ectodermal dysplasia, 236b
Hirschsprung disease, 342–344, 342b, 343b, 343t, *344*, 344t
Histiocytosis X, 224–225, 224b, 224t, *225*
Hives, 171–173, *172–173*, 172t
Hodgkin lymphoma, 288–291, 288b, 289t, *290–291*
Hookworm, cutaneous larva migrans from, 125–126, *126*
Hordeolum, 139, *139*, 139t
Hospital gangrene, 91–92, 91t, *92*
Human herpesvirus (HHV), roseola infantum from, 69–70, *69–70*, 69b, 70t
Human immunodeficiency virus (HIV) infection, 78–81, *79*, 79t
Human papillomavirus, warts from, 76–78, *77–78*, 77t
Human parvovirus B19 infection, erythema infectiosum from, 70–72, *71–72*, 71b, 71t
  with sickle cell anemia, *261*
    transient aplastic crises from, 260–261, *261*, 261t
Humeral fractures, from abuse, *35*
Hutchinson triad, 107b
Hydatid of Morgagni, torsion of, 330–332, *331–332*, 331t
Hydrocolpos, 320
Hydrometrocolpos, 320
  with imperforate hymen, 320–321, 320b, *321*, 321t
Hygroma, cystic, 471
Hymen, imperforate, with hydrometrocolpos, 320–321, 320b, *321*, 321t
Hyperkeratosis, epidermolytic, *228*
Hyperpigmentation, Addison disease and, 302b
  postinflammatory, 167, *167*, 167b
Hypersensitivity reaction(s), allergic contact dermatitis as, 168–170, 168b, 168t, *169–170*
  anaphylaxis as, 387–389, 387b, 388t, *389*, 389t
  Henoch-Schönlein purpura as, 186–188, 186b, 187t, *188*
  serum sickness as, 413–414, *414*, 414b, 414t
Hypertension, 312t
Hypertrichosis, sacral, *427*

Hyphema, 136–138, 136b, *138*, 138t
Hypocalcemic vitamin D–resistant rickets, 369–371, 370t, *371*, 371t
Hypochromic microcytic anemia, 247t
Hypohidrotic ectodermal dysplasia, 236, *236–237*, 236b, 236t
Hypomelanosis of Ito, 233–234, *234*, 234b, 234t
Hypophosphatemia, familial, 366–369, 366b, 367t, *368–369*
Hypopigmentation, postinflammatory, 167, *167*, 167b
Hypopnea, 159

Ichthyosis, 226–227, 226b, 226t, *227–228*
Ichthyosis hystrix, 221, *221–222*, 221b, 221t
Ichthyosis linearis circumflexa, 228–230, *229–230*, 229t
Immune thrombocytopenic purpura, acute, 250–253, 251b, 252b, 252t, *253*, 253t
    vs. child abuse, 42, *44*
Impetigo, Bockhart, 92–93
    bullous, 92, *93*
Impetigo contagiosa, 86–88, *88*
Inclusion blennorrhea, 129–130, *130*, 130b, 130t
Incontinentia pigmenti, 232–233, 232b, *233*, 233t
Incontinentia pigmenti achromians, 233–234, *234*, 234b, 234t
Infantile acropustulosis, *198*, 198, 198b, 198t
Infectious diseases. See specific diseases, e.g., *Varicella.*
Infectious mononucleosis, 66–67, 66b, 66t, *67*, 67t
Inflammatory proptosis, 149b
Insect bites, 173–175, 174b, 174t, *175*
Intraocular pressure, 134b
Intussusception, 338–342, 339b, *340–342*, 340t
Iron deficiency anemia, 245–247, 245b, 246t, *247*, 247t
Irritant contact dermatitis, 168t

Jacquet granuloma, *171*
Jock itch, 117, *118*
Joint, infected, 357–360, 358b, 359t, *360*, 360t
Junctional epidermolysis bullosa, 230, 230b, *231*
Juvenile dermatomyositis, 407–408, 407b, *408*, 408t
Juvenile plantar dermatosis, *118*
Juvenile rheumatoid arthritis, 405–407, 405b, *406*, 406t

Kaposi sarcoma-like granuloma, 201, *201*, 201b, 201t
Kawasaki disease, 410–413, 410b, *411–413*, 411t
Keloids, 237–238, 237b, 237t, *238*
Keratoconjunctivitis, herpes, 132t, *133*
Keratosis pilaris, *165*
Klippel-Trenaunay syndrome, 215, *215*, 215b, 215t
Koplik spots, 59, *61*
Kyphosis, *365*

Labia minor, fusion of, 321–323, 322b, 322t, *323*
Labial adhesions, 321–323, 322b, 322t, *323*

Labial fusion, 321–323, 322b, 322t, *323*
Labial synechiae, 321–323, 322b, 322t, *323*
Langerhans' cell histiocytosis, 224–225, 224b, 224t, *225*
Latrodectus mactans, 244
    bite from, 243–244, 243b, 243t
Legg-Calvé-Perthes disease, 376–378, 377b, *378*, 378t
Legg-Calvé-Waldenstrom disease, 376–378, 377b, *378*, 378t
Letterer-Siwe disease, 224–225, 224b, 224t, *225*
Leukemia, acute lymphoblastic, 273–275, 273b, 274t, *275–276*, 275t
    conditions with, 273, 273b
Lice, in scalp, 124–125, *125*
Lichen sclerosus et atrophicus, 202–203, *202–203*, 202b, 202t
    vs. child abuse, 43
Lichen striatus, 191–192, 191b, *192*, 192t
Linear IgA disease, of childhood, 203–204, 203b, *204*, 204t
Lines of Blaschko, *222*
Lipoid nephrosis, 465–468, 466b, 467t, *468*
Lips, angioedema of, *173*, *389*
Lithium batteries, ingestion of, 395–397, 396t, *397–398*
Looped cord mark, *28*
Loxosceles reclusa, 244
    bite from, 243–244, 243b, 243t, *244*
Lues (acquired syphilis), 106–107, 106t, *107*
Lupus erythematosus, neonatal, 403–405, *404–405*, 404b, 404t
    systemic, 401–403, 401b, *402–403*, 402b, 402t
Lyme disease, 408–409, *409*, 409b
Lymph node syndrome, mucocutaneous, 410–413, 410b, *411–413*, 411t
Lymphadenoid goiter, 298–301, 300t, *301*
Lymphadenopathy, Hodgkin disease and, 288b
Lymphangiectasia, 471
Lymphangioma, 471
Lymphedema, 471–474, 473t, *474*
Lymphoblastic leukemia, acute, 273–275, 273b, 274t, *275–276*, 275t
Lymphocytic thyroiditis, chronic, 298–301, 300t, *301*
Lymphoma, Hodgkin, 288–291, 288b, 289t, *290–291*

Malignant melanoma, from congenital pigmented nevus, 216b
Mast cell disease, 222–223, *223*, 223b, 223t
Mastitis neonatorum, 19–20, 19b, *20*, 20t
Mastocytosis, 222–223, *223*, 223b, 223t
Mastoid osteitis, acute, 156–158, 157b, *158*, 158t
Mastoiditis, 156
    acute, 156–158, 157b, *158*, 158t
Mature cystic ovarian teratoma, 285–287, *286–287*, 286t, 287t
McCune-Albright syndrome, 314–316, 314b, *315–316*, 315t
Measles, 59–61, 59b, *60–61*, 60t
    rash in, *412*
Megacolon, congenital aganglionic, 342–344, 342b, 343b, 343t, *344*, 344t
Melanocytosis, dermal, 217–219, 217b, *218–219*, 218t
Melanoma, malignant, from congenital pigmented nevus, 216b
Melanosis, transient neonatal pustular, 1–2, *1–2*, 1t, 2t

Meningocele, 440–441, 440b, *441*, 441t
Meningococcemia, 104–105, 104b, *105*, 105t
Meningomyelocele, 438–440, 438b, *439–440*, 439t
Metaphyseal chondrodysplasia (dysostosis), 372–373, 372t, *373*
Metaphyseal dysplasia, Schmid type, 372–373, 372t, *373*
Microsporum, tinea capitis from, 112–115, 112b, *113–115*, 113t
    tinea corporis from, 115–116, *116*, 116t
Migratory polyarthritis, in acute rheumatic fever, 417b
Minimal change disease, 465–468, 466b, 467t, *468*
Minimal change nephrotic syndrome, 465–468, 466b, 467t, *468*
Molluscum contagiosum, 75–76, *76*, 76t
    with HIV, 80
Mongolian spot, 7, *7*, 7t
    vs. child abuse, 41, *43*
Mononucleosis, infectious, 66–67, 66b, 66t, *67*, 67t
Mosquito bites, 173–175, 174b, 174t, *175*
Mucocele, 464–465, 464b, *465*
Mucocolpos, 320
Mucocutaneous lymph node syndrome, 410–413, 410b, *411–413*, 411t
Mucus retention cyst, 464–465, 464b, *465*
Multiple malformation syndromes, 473t
Mumps, 64–65, *65*, 65t
Munchausen syndrome by proxy, 25
Myelomeningocele, 438–440, 438b, *439–440*, 439t

Napkin dermatitis, 170–171, 170b, *171*
Napkin psoriasis, *194*
Neck, surface anatomy of, *291*
Neck masses, anterior, 349t
Necrotizing fasciitis, 91–92, 91t, *92*
Neisseria gonorrhoeae, gonococcal infections from, 102–104, 103b, 103t, *104*
Neisseria meningitidis, meningococcemia from, 104–105, 104b, *105*, 105t
Neonatal lupus erythematosus, 403–405, *404–405*, 404b, 404t
Nephrosis, 465
Netherton syndrome, 228–230, *229–230*, 229t
Neural tube defects, 434–436, *436* . See also specific defects, e.g., *Anencephaly.*
Neuroblastomas, 276–281, *280*
    anatomic locations of, 277b
    catecholamine synthesis/metabolism and, 278b
    clinical features of, 279t
    differential diagnosis of, 281t
    epidemiology of, 276
    laboratory studies of, 277, 279t
    paraneoplastic syndromes and, 276b
    pathology of, 277
    prognosis of, 279t
    treatment of, 277
Neurofibromatosis, 420b, 421–422, *421–422*, 421t
    acoustic, 420b, 421–422, *421–422*, 421t
    café-au-lait spots in, 314b
Nevus fuscoceruleus acromiodeltoidalis, 217–219, 217b, *218–219*, 218t
Nevus fuscoceruleus ophthalmomaxillaris, 217–219, 217b, *218–219*, 218t
Nevus of Ito, 217–219, 217b, 218t, *219*
Nevus of Ota, 217–218, 217b, *218*, 218t
Nevus sebaceus of Jadassohn, 219–220, 219b, *220*, 220t

Nevus unius lateris, 221, *221–222*, 221b, 221t
Nevus verrucous, 221, *221–222*, 221b, 221t
Nickel contact dermatitis, 168–169, 168b, 168t, *170*
Nikolsky sign, 95b
"Nil disease," 465–468, 466b, 467t, *468*
Nursemaid's elbow, 399–400, 399b, *400*
Nursing-bottle caries, 463–464, 463b, *464*, 464t
Nutritional vitamin D deficiency rickets (NR), 360–365, 361b, 362b, 362t, *363–365*, 363t. See also *Rickets, nutritional vitamin D deficiency.*

Obesity, exogenous, vs. Cushing syndrome, 310t
Obstructive sleep apnea, 159–161, 160b, *161*, 161t
Onychomycosis, 117, *118*
 with HIV, *81*
Ophthalmia neonatorum, 127–129, 127b, *129*, 129t
Oral electrical burns, 461–462, *462*, 462b, 462t
Orbit, eye, 149, *151*
Orbital cellulitis, 149–152, 149b, 150t, *151–152*, 151t
 with proptosis, *152, 155*
Orchitis, 332
Osgood-Schlatter disease, 378–380, *380*, 380t
Osteitis, acute mastoid, 156–158, 157b, *158*, 158t
Osteochondritis, of inferior patella, 378–380, *380*, 380t
 of tibial tuberosity, 378–380, *380*, 380t
Osteogenesis imperfecta syndrome, 381–383, 381b, *382*, 383t
 vs. child abuse, 42, *48*
Osteomalacia, 360
Osteomyelitis, 350
 acute hematogenous, 350–354, 350b, 351b, 352t, *353–354*
  clinical features of, 350–351, 352t, *354*
  complications/prognosis in, 352
  differential diagnosis of, 351b
  epidemiology of, 350
  etiology of, 350, 352t
  laboratory studies of, 351
  pathogenesis of, 350, *353*
  treatment of, 351–352
 chronic, 355–357, 355t, *356–357*
 with septic arthritis, 350b
Osteoneogenesis imperfecta, 381
Osteopenia, 381
Osteoporosis, 381
Osteosarcoma, 281–284, 282b, 282t, *283–284*
 vs. Ewing sarcoma, 284t
Otitis media, acute, facial palsy with, 158–159, 158b, *159*
Ovarian teratoma, mature cystic, 285–287, *286–287*, 286t, 287t

Palm, hyperlinear, *165*
Palsy, 428
 Bell's, 428–430, 428b, *429–430*, 429t
 brachial, 8–9, 8b, *9*, 9t
 facial nerve, traumatic neonatal, 13–15, 14b, *15*
  with acute otitis media, 158–159, 158b, *159*
Panniculitis, popsicle, 176, *176*, 176b, 176t

Papular acrodermatitis of childhood, 68, *68*, 68b, 68t
Papular urticaria, *175*
Paralysis, 428
Paramyxovirus, measles from, 59–61, 59b, *60–61*, 60t, 412
 mumps from, 64–65, *65*, 65t
Paranasal sinuses, 153, 153b
Paraneoplastic syndromes, 276b
Paraphimosis, 336–338, *338*, 338t
Paresis, 428
Paronychia, candidal, with HIV, *81*
Parotitis, epidemic, 64–65, *65*, 65t
Parvovirus B19 infection, erythema infectiosum from, 70–72, *71–72*, 71b, 71t
 with sickle cell anemia, 261
  transient aplastic crises from, 260–261, *261*, 261t
Patella, inferior, osteochondritis of, 378–380, *380*, 380t
Pediculosis capitis, 124–125, *125*
Pediculus humanus var. *capitis,* 124
Pemphigus, 205–206, *205–206*, 205b, 205t
Penicillin, erythema multiforme minor from, 179, *181*
Penis, anatomy of, *267, 334, 336*
Perianal dermatitis/cellulitis, streptococcal, 87, *88*
Perianal infection, streptococcal, vs. child abuse, 43
Perioral granulomatous dermatitis, 200, *200*, 200b, 200t
Periorbital ecchymosis, 42, *46*
Periungual fibroma, *425*
Perthes disease, 376–378, 377b, *378*, 378t
Pertussis (whooping cough), 100–101, 100b, 100t, *101*
Petechiae, vs. child abuse, *45*
Pheochromocytoma, 311–313, 311b, 312t, *313*, 313t
Phimosis, 336
Phytophotodermatitis, 239–240, 239b, 239t, *240*
Piebaldism, 458–459, 458b, 458t, *459*
Pilonidal sinus and abscess, 346–347, *347*, 347b, 347t
Pinnae, preauricular sinus of, 345–346, *346*
Pityriasis alba, *165*
Pityriasis rosea, 190–191, 190b, *191*
Pityriasis versicolor, 118–119, *119*, 119t
Plantar dermatosis, juvenile, *118*
Poikiloderma congenitale, 235, *235*, 235b, 235t
Poison ivy dermatitis, 168–169, 168b, 168t, *169*
Poisoning, from child abuse, 25
Polyarthritis, migratory, in acute rheumatic fever, 417b
Popsicle panniculitis, 176, *176*, 176b, 176t
Port wine stain, *214, 215*
 in tuberous sclerosis, *426*
Posthitis, 334, 335b, *336*
Postinflammatory hyperpigmentation, 167, *167*, 167b
Postinflammatory hypopigmentation, 167, *167*, 167b
Pox virus, molluscum contagiosum from, 75–76, *76*, 76t
Preauricular sinus, 345–346, *346*
Premature thelarche, 294–296, 295t, *296*, 296t
Preseptal cellulitis, 147–148, *148*, 148t
Priapism, 266, 266b, *267–268*
 sickle cell anemia and, 266–267, 266b, *267–268*, 267t

Proptosis, inflammatory, 149b
 orbital cellulitis with, *152, 155*
Protein C deficiency, vs. child abuse, 41, *44*
Pseudohermaphroditism, 316–319, 317t, 318t, *319*
Pseudomonas aeruginosa, ecthyma gangrenosum from, 99, *99*, 99b, 99t
Pseudomonas septicemia, cutaneous, 99, *99*, 99b, 99t
Pseudovitamin D deficiency rickets, 369–371, 370t, *371*, 371t
Psoriasis, 192–194, *193–194*, 193b, 193t
 exfoliative dermatitis with, *177*
Puberty, precocious, in McCune-Albright syndrome, 314
 incomplete (partial), 294–296, 295t, *296*, 296t
Purpura(s), 252b
 acute immune thrombocytopenic, 250–253, 251b, 252b, 252t, *253*, 253t
  vs. child abuse, 42, *44*
 anaphylactoid, 186–188, 186b, 187t, *188*
 differential diagnosis of, 253t
 fulminans, vs. child abuse, 41, *44*
 Henoch-Schönlein, 186–188, 186b, 187t, *188*
  vs. child abuse, 42, *45*
Pyarthrosis, acute suppurative, 357–360, 358b, 359t, *360*, 360t
Pyogenic granuloma, 185–186, 185b, 185t, *186*

"Raccoon eyes," vs. child abuse, 42, *46*
Radial head subluxation, 399–400, 399b, *400*
Ramsay Hunt syndrome, 54b
Ranula, 464–465, 464b, *465*
Rash, diaper, 170–171, 170b, *171*
"Red eye," 131–133, 131b, 132t, *133*, 133t
Retinal hemorrhage, from shaken impact syndrome, 30b, *32*
Retinoblastoma, 143–146, 143b, 144t, *145–146*, 145t
Rheumatic fever, acute, 416–418, 416b, 417b, *418–419*, 418t
Rheumatoid arthritis, juvenile, 405–407, 405b, *406*, 406t
Rib fractures, from child abuse, 32t, *34*
Rickets, 360
 differential diagnosis of, 367t, 371t
 familial hypophosphatemic, 366–369, 366b, 367t, *368–369*
 nutritional vitamin D deficiency, 360–365, 361b, 362b, 362t, *363–365*, 363t
  clinical features of, 362t
  diagnosis of, 363t
  etiology/epidemiology of, 360, 361b
  pathophysiology of, 360–361, 362b
  prevention of, 361
  treatment of, 361
 vitamin D–dependent, type I, 369–371, 370t, *371*, 371t
 vitamin D–resistant, 366–369, 366b, 367t, *368–369*
 vs. child abuse, 42, *48*
Rickettsia, Rocky Mountain spotted fever from, 81–82, *82*, 82t
Ringworm, of hand, 117, *118*
 of nail, 117, *118*
 of scalp, 112–115, 112b, *113–115*, 113t
 of smooth skin, 115–116, *116*, 116t
Ritter disease, 94–96, *95–96*, 95b, 95t
Rocky Mountain spotted fever, 81–82, *82*, 82t

Rosacea-like eruption of children, 200, *200*, 200b, 200t
Roseola infantum, 69–70, *69–70*, 69b, 70t
Rothmund-Thomson syndrome, 235, *235*, 235b, 235t
Rubella, 62–64, 62t, *63–64*
  congenital syndrome of, 62b, *63–64*
Rubeola (measles), 59–61, 59b, *60–61*, 60t

Sacral hypertrichosis, *427*
Sarcoidosis, 415–416, 415b, 415t, *416*
Sarcoma, osteogenic, 281–284, 282b, 282t, *283–284*, 284t
Sarcoptes scabiei var. *hominus*, 121
Scabies, 121–124, 121b, *122–124*, 122t
  crusted Norwegian, with HIV, 80
Scarlatina, 84–86, 84b, 84t, *85–86*
  staphylococcal, *95, 97*
Scarlet fever, 84–86, 84b, 84t, *85–86*
Scrotum, acute pediatric, causes of, 333
  differential diagnosis of, 326b
Scurvy, vs. child abuse, 42, *47*
Sebaceous follicle, *196*
Seborrheic dermatitis, 189–190, *189–190*, 189b
  vs. atopic, 164t
Septic arthritis, 357–360, 358b, 359t, *360*, 360t
  with osteomyelitis, 350b
Sequestration crisis, acute, sickle cell anemia and, 259–260, *260*, 260t
Serum sickness, 413–414, *414*, 414b, 414t
Sexual abuse, 36–40, 38t, 39t
  clinical findings in, 37, 37b, 38t
  conditions mistaken for, 41, 41b
  urethral prolapse as, 42–43, *49*
  signs and symptoms of, 38t, *39–40*, 39t
Sexual ambiguity, neonatal, 316–319, 317t, 318t, *319*
Sexually transmitted disease(s)
  condylomata acuminata as, *39*, 39t
  condylomata lata as, *40*
  gonococcal conjunctivitis as, *40*
  syphilis as, 39t, *40*
Shagreen patch, *425*
Shaken impact (baby) syndrome, 30–31, 30b, *31–32*, 31t
Shingles (herpes zoster), 54–55, 54t, *55*
Sickle cell anemia, 253–258, 254b, 256t, *257–258*
  acute chest syndrome and, 261–263, 262t, *263*
  acute sequestration crisis and, 259–260, *260*, 260t
  priapism and, 266–267, 266b, *267–268*, 267t
  stroke and, 263–265, *265*, 265t
  transient aplastic crises and, 260–261, *261*, 261t
Sickle cell trait, 254b
Sinusitis, 153
  acute bacterial, 153–156, 153b, 154t, *155–156*
Sixth disease (roseola infantum), 69–70, *69–70*, 69b
Sleep apnea, obstructive, 159–161, 160b, *161*, 161t
Slipped capital femoral epiphysis, 384–386, 384b, *386*
Sotos syndrome, 451–453, 451b, 451t, *452–453*
Spider bites, 243–244, 243b, 243t, *244*
Spinal dysraphism, 426–427, *427*, 427b, 427t

Splenic sequestration, 259–260, *260*, 260t
SSSS of newborn, 94–96, *95–96*, 95b, 95t
St. Anthony's fire, 82–83, 82b, *83*, 83t
St. Vitus dance, in acute rheumatic fever, 417b
Staphylococcal scalded skin syndrome, 94–96, *95–96*, 95b, 95t
Staphylococcus aureus, atopic dermatitis from, *166*
  scalded skin syndrome from, 94–96, *95–96*, 95b, 95t
  skin infections from, localized, 92–94, *93–94*
  toxic shock syndrome from, 96–97, *97*
Steroids, potency ranking of, 164t
Stevens-Johnson syndrome, 181–183, 181b, *182–183*, 182t
Stings, bee, 173–175, 174b, 174t, *175*
Stomach, foreign bodies in, 392–394, *394*
Streptococcus, group A beta-hemolytic, acute glomerulonephritis after, 468–471, 469b, 470t, *471*
  erysipelas from, 82–83, 82b, *83*, 83t
  erythema nodosum from, 177–178, *178*, 178b, 178t
  impetigo contagiosa from, 86–88, *88*
  invasive disease from, 89–90, 89b, *90*, 90t
  rheumatic fever from, acute, 416–418, 416b, 417b, *418–419*, 418t
  scarlet fever from, 84–86, 84b, 84t, *85–86*
  toxic shock syndrome from, 89–90, 89b, *90*, 90t
  necrotizing fasciitis from, 91–92, 91t, *92*
Streptococcus infections, gangrene from, 91–92, 91t, *92*
  perianal, vs. child abuse, 43
  skin, localized, 86–88, *88*
Stroke, sickle cell anemia and, 263–265, *265*, 265t
Sturge-Weber syndrome, 425–426, 425b, *426*, 426t
Stye, 139, *139*, 139t
Subcutaneous fat necrosis, 3–4, 3b, *4*, 4t
Suppurative pyarthrosis, acute, 357–360, 358b, 359t, *360*, 360t
Sydenham chorea, in acute rheumatic fever, 417b
Synovial fluid, 360t
Syphilis, acquired, 106–107, 106t, *107*
  congenital, 107–109, 107b, *108–109*, 108t
Systemic lupus erythematosus, 401–403, 401b, *402–403*, 402b, 402t

TAR syndrome, 453–456, 454b, 455t, *456*
Teeth, natal, 22–23, 22b, *23*, 23t
  neonatal, 22
Temper tantrum elbow, 399–400, 399b, *400*
Teratoma, benign cystic, 285
  mature cystic ovarian, 285–287, *286–287*, 286t, 287t
Testicular appendage, torsion of, 330–332, *331–332*, 331t
Testicular torsion, 325–330, 326b, 327b, 327t, *328–330*
  clinical features of, 326, 327t, *328–330*
  epidemiology of, 326
  etiology/pathogenesis of, 325–326, *328*
  laboratory test for, 326–327
  treatment and prognosis of, 327, 327b, 327t

Testis, anatomy of, *331*
Thelarche, premature, 294–296, 295t, *296*, 296t
Thrombocytopenia, 253t
Thrombocytopenia–absent radius syndrome, 453–456, 454b, 455t, *456*
Thrombocytopenia–radial aplasia (TAR) syndrome, 453–456, 454b, 455t, *456*
Thyroglossal duct cyst, 348–349, 348b, *349*, 349t
Thyroiditis, autoimmune (Hashimoto), 298–301, 300t, *301*
Tibia vara, idiopathic (pathologic), 374–376, 374b, 375t, *376*
Tibial fractures, from abuse, 36
Tibial tubercle traction apophysitis, 378–380, *380*, 380t
Tibial tuberosity, osteochondritis of, 378–380, *380*, 380t
Tin ear syndrome, 24
Tinea capitis, 112–115, 112b, *113–115*, 113t
Tinea circinata, 115–116, *116*, 116t
Tinea corporis, 115–116, *116*, 116t
Tinea cruris, 117, *118*
Tinea faciei, *116*
Tinea manuum, 117, *118*
Tinea pedis, 116–117, *117*, 117t
Tinea unguium, 117, *118*
Tinea versicolor, 118–119, *119*, 119t
Togavirus, rubella from, 62–64, 62b, 62t, *63–64*
Torsion, of hydatid of Morgagni, 330–332, *331–332*, 331t
  testicular. See *Testicular torsion*.
Torticollis, 20
  congenital muscular, 20–21, *21*, 21t
Toxic epidermal necrolysis, 183–185, 183b, *184–185*, 184t
  vs. staphylococcal scalded skin syndrome, 95t
Toxic shock syndrome, staphylococcal, 96–97, *97*
  streptococcal, 89–90, 89b, *90*, 90t
Transient aplastic crises, sickle cell anemia and, 260–261, *261*, 261t
Transient neonatal pustular melanosis, 1–2, *1–2*, 1t, 2t
Treponema pallidum, syphilis from, acquired, 106–107, 106t, *107*
  congenital, 107–109, 107b, *108–109*, 108t
Trichophyton, tinea capitis from, 112–115, 112b, *113–115*, 113t
  tinea corporis from, 115–116, *116*, 116t
Trichorrhexis invaginata, 228, *230*
Triple A syndrome, 304–306, 304b, 305t, *306*
Trisomy 21 (Down syndrome), 444–446, 444b, 445t, *446*
  atlantoaxial instability in, 446–448, 447b, *448*
Tuberous sclerosis, 423–425, *423–425*, 423b, 423t
Tumor(s). See specific type, e.g., *Pheochromocytoma*.
Turner syndrome, 448–450, 449b, *450*
Tzanck test, 50, *58*

Ulrich-Turner syndrome, 448–450, 449b, *450*
Urethral prolapse, 323–325, 324b, 324t, *325*
  vs. child abuse, 42–43, *49*
Urine, red, 250t

Urticaria, 171–173, *172–173,* 172t
  papular, *175*
Urticaria pigmentosa, 222–223, *223,* 223b,
  223t

Vagina, anatomy of, 320
Varicella, 50–55, 51t, *52–55*
  congenital syndrome of, 50b, *53*
  distribution of, *52*
  lesions of, *52–53*
  with HIV, *80*
Varicella-zoster virus, chickenpox from, 50–
  55, 51t, *52–55*
  shingles from, 56–57, 56b, 56t, *57*
Ventosa (cupping), vs. child abuse, 41, *44*

Verruca vulgaris, 77
Verrucae, 76–78, *77–78,* 77t
Virus(es). See specific virus, e.g., *Epstein-Barr
  virus (EBV)*
Vitamin A, for measles, 59b
Vitamin D, metabolism of, 361b
Vitamin D deficiency rickets, nutritional, 360–
  365, 361b, 362b, 362t, *363–365,* 363t
Vitamin D–dependent rickets, type I, 369–
  371, 370t, *371,* 371t
Vitiligo, 209–210, 209b, *210,* 210t
Von Recklinghausen disease, 420b, 421–
  422, *421–422,* 421t
Vulvar agglutination, 321–323, 322b, 322t,
  323
Vulvovaginitis, herpetic, *58*

Waardenburg syndrome, 459–460, 459b,
  460, 460t
Warts, 76–78, *77–78,* 77t
Whiplash shaken baby syndrome, 30–31,
  30b, *31–32,* 31t
White dermographism, *166*
White spotting, familial, 458–459, 458b,
  458t, *459*
Whooping cough (pertussis), 100–101,
  100b, 100t, *101*

X-linked hypophosphatemic rickets, 366–
  369, 366b, 367t, *368–369*
X-linked ichthyosis, 226, 226b, 226t, *227*
XO syndrome, 448–450, 449b, *450*

ISBN 0-7216-7639-1

DATE DUE

APR 0 8 2003			
APR 2 1 2003			
AUG 2 4 2003			
FEB 2 9 2004			
SEP 2 3 2004			